Clinical Biochemistry

Questions and Answers

Clinical Biochemistry

Questions and Answers

Veena Singh Ghalaut MBBS, MD
Sr Professor and Head, Department of Biochemistry
Pt BD Sharma Post Graduate Institute of Medical Sciences, Rohtak, Haryana

Ashuma Sachdeva MBBS, MD
Associate Professor, Department of Biochemistry
Pt BD Sharma Post Graduate Institute of Medical Sciences, Rohtak, Haryana

Piyush Bansal MBBS, MD, DNB
Assistant Professor, ESI Medical College, Mandi, HP

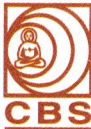

CBS Publishers & Distributors Pvt Ltd

New Delhi • Bengaluru • Chennai • Kochi • Mumbai • Pune
Hyderabad • Kolkata • Nagpur • Patna • Vijayawada

Disclaimer

Science and technology are constantly changing fields. New research and experience broaden the scope of information and knowledge. The authors have tried their best in giving information available to them while preparing the material for this book. Although all efforts have been made to ensure optimum accuracy of the material, yet it is quite possible some errors might have been left uncorrected. The publisher, the printer, and the authors will not be held responsible for any inadvertent errors, omissions or inaccuracies.

Clinical Biochemistry
Questions and Answers

ISBN: 978-81-239-2483-0

Copyright © Publisher

First Edition: 2015

All rights reserved. No part of this book may be reproduced or transmitted in any form or by any means, electronic or mechanical, including photocopying, recording, or any information storage and retrieval system without permission, in writing, from the authors and the publisher.

Published by Satish Kumar Jain and Produced by Varun Jain for

CBS Publishers & Distributors Pvt Ltd
4819/XI Prahlad Street, 24 Ansari Road, Daryaganj, New Delhi 110 002, India.
Ph: 23289259, 23266861, 23266867   Fax: 011-23243014   Website: www.cbspd.com
e-mail: delhi@cbspd.com; cbspubs@airtelmail.in.

Corporate Office: 204 FIE, Industrial Area, Patparganj, Delhi 110 092
Ph: 4934 4934   Fax: 4934 4935   e-mail: publishing@cbspd.com;   publicity@cbspd.com

Branches

- **Bengaluru:** Seema House 2975, 17th Cross, K.R. Road,
  Banasankari 2nd Stage, Bengaluru 560 070, Karnataka
  Ph: +91-80-26771678/79   Fax: +91-80-26771680   e-mail: bangalore@cbspd.com
- **Chennai:** No. 7, Subbaraya Street, Shenoy Nagar, Chennai 600 030, Tamil Nadu
  Ph: +91-44-42032115   Fax: +91-44-42032115   e-mail: chennai@cbspd.com
- **Kochi:** 36/14 Kalluvilakam, Lissie Hospital Road, Kochi 682 018, Kerala
  Ph: +91-484-4059061-65   Fax: +91-484-4059065   e-mail: kochi@cbspd.com
- **Mumbai:** 83-C, Dr E Moses Road, Worli, Mumbai-400018, Maharashtra
  Ph: +91-22-24902340/41   Fax: +91-22-24902342   e-mail: mumbai@cbspd.com
- **Pune:** Bhuruk Prestige, Sr. No. 52/12/2+1+3/2 Narhe, Haveli
  (Near Katraj-Dehu Road Bypass), Pune 411 041, Maharashtra
  Ph: +91-20-64704058/59, 32392317   Fax: +91-20-24300160   e-mail: pune@cbspd.com

Representatives

- **Hyderabad** 0-9885175004
- **Nagpur** 0-9021734563
- **Kolkata** 0-9831437309, 0-9051152362
- **Patna** 0-9334159340
- **Vijayawada** 0-9000660880

Printed at Options Printfast

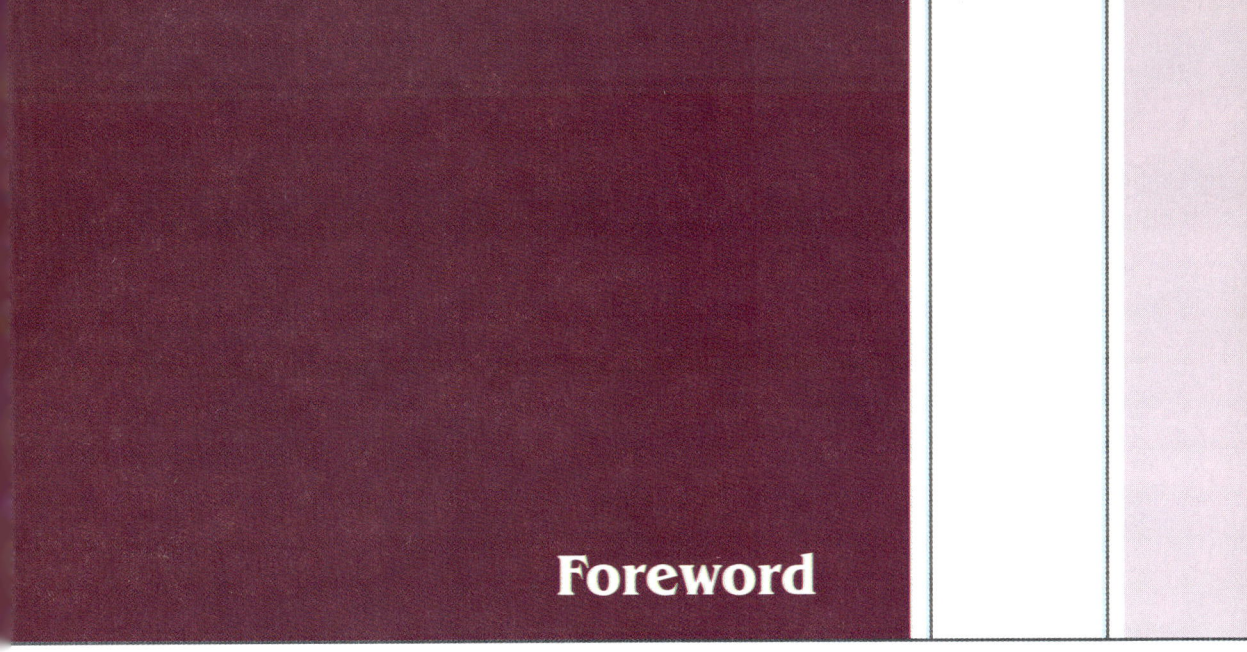

Foreword

Rapid advances in the knowledge about clinical diseases makes it even more difficult for the textbooks to keep up-to-date. More so in the field of clinical biochemistry, as it endeavours to correlate the clinical signs of the diseases with the biochemical changes occurring in the body. To be able to present those changes to the medical student in a lucid language is a herculean task. Precisely for this, I congratulate the authors of this book *Clinical Biochemistry* for coming out with a splendid edition which not only tries to make the students understand the subject but also helps in preparing them for *viva voce* examination. The simple "question and answer" form layout of this textbook will certainly appeal to all the students in medical field as it takes them on a journey of self-learning with in-depth knowledge. It is aptly said that a picture is worth a 100 words. The book has been richly illustrated with diagrams and figures to augment the retentive power of the students.

I am sure that this is just a beginning by the authors and in time to come they will come up with more innovative ideas to make the subject better understandable to the medical students. I wish them all the best for their future projects.

S S Sangwan
Vice Chancellor
Pt BD Sharma Post Graduate Institute of Medical Sciences
Rohtak (Haryana)

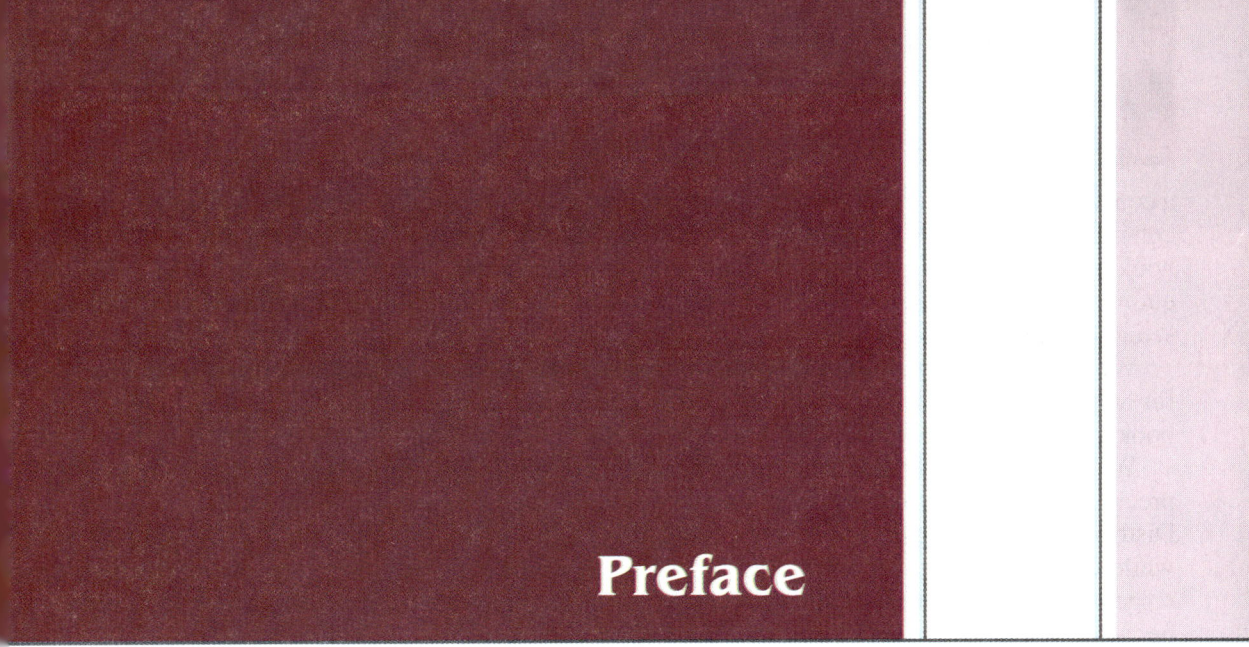

Preface

Understanding the subject of biochemistry is still a difficult proposition for many undergraduate students. Even the postgraduate students find it difficult to correlate the biochemical changes that occur in human body in the state of health and disease. While lot of detailed and up-to-date information is available in textbooks and on internet, our aim is to present the same information on selected crucial concepts of biochemistry in a lucid, mathematical and compact way with suitable illustrations. The aim is to help students digest and assimilate the actual biochemical phenomenon as they occur in human body in health and disease, rather than remembering cycles and facts from books.

Ours is one such effort that has been written keeping in mind the need of a medical student to understand biochemistry at clinical level. A brilliant mind is that which seeks answers to the unknown. Precisely for that matter, the book has been written in a very lucid language and is in a question and answer format, the questions that can arise in the fertile minds of the students who seek to understand this volatile subject.

We have taken all pains to keep it readable and simple so that the person reading it gets a grip of the subject and then is able to understand the subject matter easily when he or she reads the standard textbooks. This book is in no way meant to be a substitute for regular textbooks on the subject but is only meant to be a companion to the students who want to critically understand and revise the matter to be able to apply a similar approach to learning whole biochemistry and answer with confidance and reasoning the difficult questions based on biochemistry asked in various PG entrance examinations. Aim is to stimulate the learner to actively seek relevant information and reasons from multiple sources rather than sticking to one textbook to be able to enjoy learning this dry and boring subject.

This effort would not have been possible without the help and guidance of a number of people. The authors are deeply indebted to Prof SS Sangwan, honourable Vice Chancellor, Pt BD Sharma University of Health Sciences, a giant of a personality in his field, a BC Roy awardee, who has been a constant source of motivation to us for taking up new challenges and seeing them to their fruitful completion. He has also been very kind in accepting our request for writing the Foreword to this book for which we are ever grateful. We are also thankful to our worthy Director, Prof CS Dhull, an eminent ophthalmologist and a philanthropist, for providing us the conducive environment in our setup for taking up this project.

We thank the faculty, students and staff members of Department of Biochemistry, PGIMS, Rohtak, for helping us with their valuable inputs and constructive criticism which enabled us to make this book more crisp and readable.

We thank our family members for their patience and support, as this type of project does steal a precious moment or two from their valuable time too. We are also thankful to CBS Publishers & Distributors for seeing the spark in us, recognizing the need of this book for the medical students while cooperating with us fully even at odd hours and seeing the project through. We take all responsibility for the matter contained herein and any suggestion to improve the book will not only be welcome but highly appreciated.

Last but not the least, we thank the almighty who has kept us under his grace and made us strong and courageous to overcome any obstacles that arose while completing this fine journey.

Jai Hind

Veena Singh Ghalaut
Ashuma Sachdeva
Piyush Bansal

Contents

Foreword v
Preface vii

CHAPTER 1

Water, Amino Acids and Peptides   1

1. Describe the properties of water that make it most fit solvent in biological systems. 1
2. What is pH and pKa? What is their physiological and clinical significance? 4
3. What is viscosity and hyperviscosity syndrome? 9
4. What is selenocysteine? How is it incorporated into proteins? 9
5. Which is the 22nd amino acid? 12
6. What is isoelectric point or isoelectric pH? How to calculate isoelectric pH of amino acids? 13

CHAPTER 2

Protein Chemistry, Structure and Function   16

1. What are the biological functions of proteins? 16
2. Differentiate between configuration and conformation. 19
3. What are unstructured proteins? 20
4. What is salting in and salting out? Why ammonium sulphate is most commonly used for this purpose? 23
5. What are disulfide bonds? How are they formed and what is their significance in protein structure? 27
6. Distinguish between peptides and proteins. Give examples of some important peptides. 33
7. What are domains, folds, motifs and supersecondary structures? 33
8. What is the physiological function of myoglobin? 43
9. Describe the role of haemoglobin in the action of nitric oxide. 44

CHAPTER 3
Enzymes   46

1. Describe enzyme classification. 46
2. Differentiate between co-factor, co-enzyme and prosthetic group. 47
3. Enumerate various mechanisms of catalysis. 47
4. Differentiate between general and specific acid-base catalysis. 47
5. Give examples of enzyme functioning by covalent catalysis. 48
6. Differentiate between Fischer's 'lock and key model' and Koshland's 'induced fit model' of enzyme action. 48
7. What are conserved residues in enzymes? 48
8. How can enzymes be used to measure blood glucose in lab? 49
9. Give examples of functional enzymes of blood. 49
10. How is measurement of levels of non-functional enzymes of blood useful? 49
11. What are ribozymes? Give examples of ribozymes. 49
12. What are irreversible and reversible reactions? 50
13. How reactions can become functionally irreversible under physiological conditions? 50
14. What is the relation between ΔG, K_{eq} and speed of reaction? 50
15. What are the factors on which reaction rate depends? 50
16. Describe how changes in temperature affect rate of enzyme catalysed reaction. 51
17. How change in pH can affect rate of enzyme catalysed reactions? 51
18. Why is the V_i or the initial rate/velocity of reaction used to study effect of substrate concentration on enzyme activity? 51
19. Describe how can we study the effect of substrate concentration on reaction rate of a multi-substrate reaction. 52
20. Enumerate the different types of graphs used to study the relation of V_i versus substrate concentration. 52
21. Describe organophosphate poisoning. 54
22. What are allosteric enzymes? 54
23. What is passive regulation of enzyme activity? 56
24. Why metabolite flow in most metabolic pathways tends to be unidirectional? 57
25. How can compartmentation/separation of anabolic and catabolic pathways involving same metabolites can be achieved? 57
26. What is rate limiting enzyme of a pathway? 57
27. How are intracellular enzymes degraded? 58
28. In what ways can hormones regulate metabolic enzymes? 58
29. Give examples of different covalent modifications that can regulate enzyme activity. 58
30. What are the advantages of activation by selective proteolysis of pro-enzyme? 58
31. What are the advantages of covalent modification by phosphorylation? 58
32. What are isoenzymes? Describe with examples the significance of isoenzymes in our body. ... 59

CHAPTER 4
Bioenergetics and Oxidative Phosphorylation   60

1. What reaction is catalysed by myokinase and what is its advantage? 60
2. What is the difference between $\Delta G°$, $\Delta G°'$ and ΔG? Elaborate with an example. 61
3. How both catabolic and anabolic reactions are made spontaneous or favourable in our body? 62
4. Why the 'high energy phosphate bond' is misnomer or why ATP acts as energy currency molecule? 63

5. How ATP provides energy for endergonic reactions? 64
6. What is the advantage of activation reactions such as acyl CoA synthetase converting ATP to AMP rather than ADP? 65
7. Classify the enzymes involved in oxidation-reduction reactions giving example of each. 68
8. Why names homogentisate oxidase and aldehyde dehydrogenase are misnomers? 68
9. What is hydroxylase cycle? 68
10. Why 2,4-DNP or 2,4-dinitrophenol is a banned drug? 69
11. Describe agents which interfere with oxidative phosphorylation. What is the difference between uncouples and inhibitors of electron transport chain? 69
12. What is the mechanism and features of cyanide toxicity? 71
13. What are conditions which limit the rate of cellular respiration during exercise? 72
14. What are the different states of respiratory control? 72
15. NADPH is required in synthetic reactions in cytosol. Give examples of some intramitochondrial reactions requiring NADPH. 73
16. What are the sources of intramitochondrial NADPH? 73
17. Enumerate some oxidants and free radicals that are produced in mitochondria. 73
18. Differentiate between glycerophosphate and malate aspartate shuttle. 73
19. Where else besides inner mitochondrial membrane is glutamate aspartate exchanger found and what is its function there? 74
20. Enumerate some of the transporters present in inner mitochondrial membrane. 74
21. What is the irreversible step in electron transport and how is its rate controlled? 75
22. Oxidative phosphorylation requires the transfer of electrons donated by NADH. (a) Is NADH imported directly into the mitochondria? Explain. (b) Enumerate two import mechanisms that transfer cytosolic electrons from NADH into the mitochondrion. (c) Why is it important to maintain a relatively constant level of cytosolic NAD^+? 75
23. Explain how 1 NADH produces 2.5 ATP and 1 $FADH_2$ produces 1.5 ATP and what is P/O ratio? 76

CHAPTER 5
Carbohydrate Chemistry and Metabolism 77

1. Enumerate the causes responsible for 'withdrawal' of carbohydrate from blood. 77
2. Enumerate the causes for the 'release' of glucose by liver to the blood. 78
3. Give the biochemical basis of muscular cramps and pain associated with vigorous exercise. 78
4. Major source of energy in RBCs is anaerobic glycolysis although oxygen is present. Comment. 78
5. What is 'curd' formation? 78
6. Why are many adults intolerant to milk? 79
7. Galactose is highly toxic if transferase enzyme is missing. How? 80
8. What are the important compounds derived from galactose? How can a galactosaemic child with galactose-free diet cope up? 80
9. How anaerobic exercise training affects glycolysis in athletes? 80
10. Gluconeogenesis in most of the tissues ends at glucose-6-PO_4 rather than glucose apart from liver. Explain. 81
11. Enlist the proteins required to convert glucose-6-PO_4 to glucose. 81
12. Differentiate between (a) lactulose and lactose; (b) dextrose and dextrin. 81
13. Differentiate between glycolysis inhibition by arsenite and arsenate. 82
14. Differentiate between glycogen metabolism in liver and muscle. 83
15. Discuss the clinical significance of (a) enolase, (b) transketolase, (c) D-xylose, (d) 2-deoxyfluoroglucose (FDG), (e) glucagon-like peptide (GLP). 87

16. Enumerate the vitamins that play a key role in citric acid cycle. 90
17. Discuss the biochemical basis of anaemias due to defect in enzymes involved in RBC
    metabolism. 91
18. Differentiate between the different isoenzymes of hexokinase. 93
19. Why anaerobic metabolism leads to lactic acidosis? Describe the biochemistry behind lactic
    acidosis and the different types of lactic acidosis. Explain the significance of plasma lactate
    levels in emergency patients. 95
20. What is D-lactic acidosis? 99
21. What are Pasteur and Warburg effects? Why cancer tissues have increased rate of glycolysis
    even when sufficient oxygen is available? 100
22. What is metabolic budgeting by pyruvate kinase? Describe the role of its feed forward
    activation in glycolysis. 102
23. What are anaplerotic, or "Filling Up", reactions? Why fats are said to be burning in a flame
    of carbohydrates? 103
24. Explain how excess consumption of sweetened beverages is harmful to health. 106
25. What is the mechanism for hyperuricemia in Von Gierke's disease? 109
26. Describe the unique structure of glycogen and its advantages. 110

CHAPTER 6
Lipid Metabolism   114

1. Differentiate between 'ketone' and 'ketone bodies'. 114
2. Which produces more ATP: cis-Δ^9 C18:1 or cis-Δ^6 C18:1? 114
3. What is the role of beta oxidation of fatty acids in gluconeogenesis? 114
4. Why is beta oxidation an aerobic process? 116
5. Which organ can produce ketone bodies and which organs can consume ketone bodies? 116
6. Explain how ketone body synthesis is regulated? 116
7. How many ATPs are produced from 1 mol of palmitate when 3-β-hydroxybutyrate is end
   product? 116
8. What is the clinical manifestation of in-born error with deficiency of HMG CoA synthase? 117
9. Which ketone bodies can be detected by Rothera's test? 117
10. Out of measurement of ketone bodies in urine or blood, which is the preferred test in a patient
    of ketoacidosis? 117
11. Why drugs which inhibit fatty acid oxidation are used in treatment of chronic angina? 117
12. In a newborn screening programme dried filter paper blood spot collected for a neonate was
    found to have elevated C8 acyl carnitine levels. Testing also revealed decreased free carnitine
    levels. What is the most likely diagnosis? What will be the clinical manifestations? What will
    be the biochemical basis of treatment? 118
13. Why is coconut oil beneficial for an 8-year-old boy with cystic fibrosis who develops mal-
    absorption? 118
14. Comment on the dietary therapy used for refractory seizures. 119
15. What are the various uses of ketogenic diet? 119
16. A 3-month-old male infant had facial dysmorphism, hypotonia, psychomotor retardation and
    hepatomegaly. He had a brother with same facial features and hypotonia who died of hepatic
    failure at 4 months of age. Biochemical studies (Tandem Mass Spectrometry – TMS) revealed
    elevation of blood pipecolic acid and VLCFAs. What is the likely diagnosis? 120
17. What is the role of lysolecithin in atherosclerosis? 121
18. Enumerate the useful compounds synthesized during cholesterol synthesis pathway. 121

19. Why is Butylated hydroxyanisole (BHA)/E320 added to packed food items? 122
20. Give examples of drugs for which liposomes are used for delivery. 124
21. What are the various factors regulating fatty acid synthesis? 124
22. Enumerate the essential fatty acids. 124
23. Which unsaturated fatty acids can be synthesized in human body? 124
24. How can diagnosis of essential fatty acid deficiency be confirmed by lab tests? 125
25. Explain giving examples the difference between suicide enzyme and suicide inhibition. 125
26. How is fish oil protective against myocardial infarction (MI)? 126
27. Describe the beneficial actions of ω_3 and ω_6 fatty acids. 126
28. What is the role of liver X receptors in regulation of cholesterol metabolism? 127
29. How are apo B100 and apo B48 are produced from the same gene? 127
30. Which lipoprotein fraction does not move towards charged end in electrophoresis? 127
31. How do adipose tissue obtain glycerol-3-phosphate for TG synthesis? 128
32. Which phospholipase is involved in production of prostaglandins? 128
33. Which compounds contain ceramide? 128
34. Intravenous imiglucerase or recombinant glucocerebrosidase is used in treatment of which disease? 128
35. Which lipid storage disease causes severe demyelination? 129
36. An 8-year girl was admitted for heart/liver transplant.
    History: CHD in family; xanthomas appeared on legs when she was 2 years old; xanthomas appeared on elbows when she was 4 years old; admitted with MI symptoms when she was 7 years old (Total cholesterol = 1240 mg/dl; Triglycerides = 350 mg/dl; Total cholesterol of father = 355 mg/dl; Total cholesterol of mother = 310 mg/dl); 2 weeks after MI she had coronary bypass surgery; past year she had severe angina and second bypass; despite low-fat diet, cholestyramine and lovastatin therapy, total cholesterol = 1000 mg/dl.
    What is the likely diagnosis and biochemical explanation for these features? 130
37. Describe briefly the function and consequences of defects in various apolipoproteins and enzymes involved in lipoprotein/lipid transport. Explain with suitable examples the role of LDL and HDL in atherosclerosis. Which is more important – LDL or HDL? 135

CHAPTER 7
Amino Acid and Heme Metabolism   143

1. What are nutritionally essential and non-essential amino acids? 143
2. How can nitrogen balance or protein balance be measured? 143
3. Describe glycine metabolism and associated clinical implications. 144
4. Describe the unique characteristics of branched-chain amino acids metabolism. 149
5. Explain the biochemical basis of maple syrup urine disease and its management. 149
6. How is arginine synthesized in body? 154
7. How is nitrogen transported from tissues for its disposal? 155
8. How many ATPs are required to produce 1 molecule of urea? 156
9. How are amino acids transported across cell membranes? 157
10. Describe the biochemical basis of clinical features of urea cycle defects. 159
11. Explain biochemical basis of management of urea cycle defects. 161
12. What are the causes and effects of tetrahydrobiopterin deficiency? Explain the biochemical basis of management. 163
13. What are the biological functions of heme degradation products – carbon monoxide and bilirubin/biliverdin? 166

CHAPTER 8
Nucleotide Metabolism — 168

1. Why pyrimidines and purines are called 'Bases'? 168
2. What is the fate of nucleic acids and nucleotides consumed in diet? 169
3. What are the different biological functions of nucleotides? 171
4. What is salvage pathway and what is its importance? 171
5. Which reactions use PRPP and how its levels are regulated? 172
6. What is tumor lysis syndrome? 173
7. Describe regulation of purine synthesis and its clinical implications. 174
8. Classify the different causes of hyperuricemia and explain the underlying biochemical basis. 176
9. Discuss renal handling of uric acid and its clinical implications. 177
10. What is the role of alcohol in gout? 178
11. Why is hypouricemic therapy not given during attacks of acute gout? 179
12. What is the difference in action of allopurinol in gout and Lesch-Nyhan syndrome (HGPRT deficiency)? 179
13. What is the physiological significance of β-alanine and β-aminoisobutyric acid (BAIBA)? 180
14. What is the difference between xanthine oxidase and xanthine dehydrogenase? 181

CHAPTER 9
Nutrition, Vitamins and Minerals — 182

1. What is thermic effect of food? 182
2. How are nutritional recommendations on quantities of different nutrients to be consumed daily made? 183
3. What is FIGLU test? What are the functions of folate in body and why daily intake is required if it is a coenzyme? Which other tests are used to detect folate deficiency? 184
4. What is folate trap? Explain its biochemical basis. 186
5. Excessive intake of vitamin D can cause toxicity but excessive exposure to sunlight does not, why? 187
6. What are the different actions of vitamin D? 190
7. What is glycemic index and glycemic load? 191
8. What is protein quality and how is protein quality assessed? 192
9. What is the pharmacological application of niacin and its biochemical basis? 195
10. Enumerate nutritional/dietary factors related to risk of metabolic syndrome and cardiovascular diseases. 196
11. What are goitrogenic factors? How selenium deficiency affects thyroid function? 197
12. What are the different consequences of Iodine deficiency and their biochemical basis? .. 198
13. What are the different consequences of iodine excess and their biochemical basis? 204

CHAPTER 10
Genetics — 207

1. What is DNA tautomerization and what is its significance? 207
2. What is DNA damage and mutation? What are differences between them? 209
3. Describe the different types of DNA damages and their causes. 210
4. What are the consequences of DNA damage/mutations? 215
5. What is photoreactivation? 217
6. Why combination therapy is required in HIV treatment? 218

7. What is proofreading by DNA polymerase and how does it occur? 219
8. Why primer is required for DNA replication? 220
9. What is end replication problem? 220
10. What are the similarities and differences between eukaryotes and prokaryotes in DNA replication? 223
11. A 3-year-old male child presented with brownish-black pigmentation on the sun exposed part of the body like face, hands and neck at the age of 2 years. Dry skin was also evident. He also complained of burning sensation on exposure to sunlight. There were no other findings. What is the probable diagnosis? How can it be confirmed and managed? 226

CHAPTER 11
Membrane and Transport   230

1. What are the different types of lipids present in membranes and their significance? 230
2. Describe the role and functions of cholesterol in plasma membranes. 234
3. How are proteins held in the plasma membrane? 236
4. What is asymmetric distribution of lipids? How is it maintained and what is its significance? 239
5. What are lipid rafts and caveolae and what is their significance? 241
6. What are the factors which affect membrane fluidity? 246
7. How are transport proteins classified? 248
8. What are the similarities between transporters and enzymes? 249
9. What are pore-forming toxins and ionophores? 249
10. What are ABC transporters and describe their clinical significance. 252

CHAPTER 12
Integration of Metabolism and Endocrinology   255

1. How is eating behaviour regulated in humans? 255
2. Describe the changes in metabolism in starve–feed cycle and with different phases of glucose homeostasis. 260
3. What is the significance of AMP-activated protein kinase? 269
4. What is the biochemical basis of harmful effects of obesity? 272
5. Why there is hyperlipoproteinemia in DM when there is lack of insulin (or insulin resistance) as insulin increases lipid synthesis? What are the differences in metabolic abnormalities in type 1 DM and type 2 DM? 277
6. What are calcimimetics? What is their mechanism of action and use? 280
7. Explain how teriparatide (recombinant PTH 1-34) can be used for treatment of osteoporosis. 282
8. How hormones effect gene expression? What are HREs? What are nuclear receptors and nuclear receptors with special ligands? Describe their characteristic structural features. 284

CHAPTER 13
Glycoproteins, ECM and Protein Trafficking   290

1. What is sugar code of life or how carbohydrates can carry biological information? 290
2. Describe the general structure and classification of proteoglycans and their functions. 293
3. Differentiate between heparin and heparan sulphate. 304
4. Describe role of oligosaccharides in protein folding. 305
5. What are lectins, their significance and applications? 308

CHAPTER 14
Organ Function Tests — 313

1. What is serum–ascites albumin gradient? 313
2. What is the biochemical basis of development of ascites in cirrhosis? 314
3. How to distinguish pleural or other fluids as transudate or exudate by biochemical tests? 315
4. Describe the utility of different biochemical tests in liver diseases. 316
5. Describe the cell-based model of coagulation. Describe its advantages over the cascade/waterfall model. 327

CHAPTER 15
Immunology — 338

1. Describe the antiviral defence of innate immune system. 338
2. Explain the biochemical basis of tolerance. Give some therapeutic applications of the phenomena of tolerance. 342
3. Explain biochemical basis of autoimmunity, give examples of some autoimmune diseases. 348
4. How are transplant grafts rejected? Explain the immune mechanisms and describe the methods used to prevent graft rejection. 354
5. What are superantigens? 365
6. What are isotypes, allotypes and idiotypes? 367
7. What are cryoglobulins and cold agglutinins? 369

CHAPTER 16
Xenobiotic Metabolism, Antioxidants and Biochemistry of Ageing — 373

1. What are xenobiotics? How are they metabolized and what is the importance of their biotransformation? 373
2. What can be the harmful effects of xenobiotics? 376
3. How are xenobiotics metabolized? 376
4. Give examples of the reactions of xenobiotic metabolism participating in metabolism of endogenous compounds. 384
5. Give examples of some xenobiotics activated during their metabolism. 384
6. What is the effect of caloric restriction on longevity? 386
7. Describe the relative importance of various antioxidants. Why exogenous antioxidant supplements have little effect or may even be harmful? 388

Index 391

Water, Amino Acids and Peptides

Chapter 1

Q. 1. Describe the properties of water that make it most fit solvent in biological systems.

Ans. Water is the predominant chemical component of living organisms as:
- Water is an ideal biologic solvent/universal solvent
- It determines the 3-dimensional structure of all macromolecules
- Takes part in many metabolic reactions
- Slight tendency to dissociate
- High boiling point and viscosity.

Universal solvent

- The two hydrogen and the unshared electrons of the remaining two sp^3-hybridized orbitals of oxygen occupy the corners of the tetrahedron. Water is a **dipole**, a molecule with electrical charge distributed asymmetrically about its structure. This leads to a high dielectric constant (the dielectric constant for vacuum is unity; hexane is 1.9; ethanol – 24.3; water – 78.5) as the dipoles of water decrease the force of attraction between ion pairs. Thus, crystalline substances/salts like NaCl, $MgCl_2$, KCl having ionic bonds easily separate into individual atoms and dissolve in water.
- Water molecules form hydrogen bonds: Hydrogen bonding favours the self-association of water molecules into ordered arrays and profoundly influences the physical properties of water and accounts for its exceptionally high viscosity, surface tension, and boiling point. Each molecule in liquid water associates through hydrogen bonds with 3.5 other water molecules. Organic molecules having O, N, P, S and H atoms easily form hydrogen bonds with O and H of water allowing them to dissolve.

It determines the 3-dimensional structure of all macromolecules – interacts with a solvated biomolecule influencing their structure.

- Most biomolecules are **amphipathic** – possess regions rich in charged or polar functional groups as well as regions with hydrophobic character. The common theme is that macromolecules tend to assume 3D structure so as to keep the polar regions on surface and hide the hydrophobic regions from water minimizing their interaction with water.
- When phospholipids interact with water they form cell membranes/liposomes/micelles. The hydrophobic fatty acid chain is kept inside the micelle/bilayer or liposome while the polar phosphate head groups interact with water on outside by hydrogen and ionic interactions (Figs. 1.1 and 1.2).

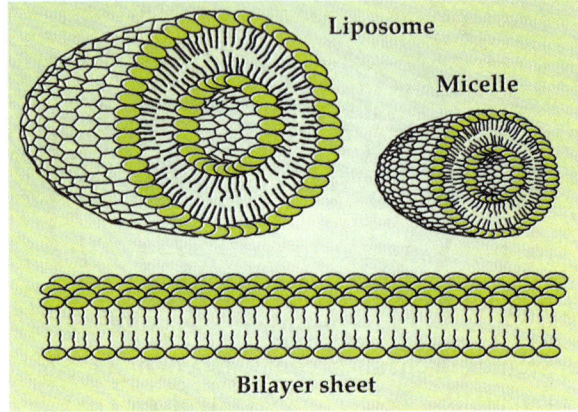

Fig. 1.1. Membrane bilayer, liposome and micelle.

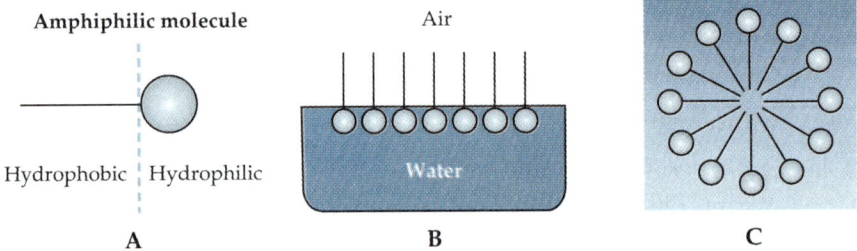

Fig. 1.2. Interaction of amphiphatic phospholipid molecules with water.

- When single-stranded DNA interacts with water it leads to base stacking – the nitrogenous bases of the DNA have aromatic structure and are hydrophobic while the sugar phosphate backbone is hydrophilic. The bases arrange in a parallel fashion over each other like a stack of coins to maximize the surface area exposed to other bases and minimize area exposed to water (Fig. 1.3).
- When two complementary DNA strands interact with water in presence of Mg ions, the dsDNA helix is formed. The phosphate groups have negative charge and two DNA strands will repel each other unless the charge is neutralized by association with divalent Mg atoms. Then just like the lipid bilayer, when two strands come together the bases face themselves avoiding interaction with water and sugar phosphate backbone stays on outside. The hydrophobic interaction of bases is the main force keeping two strands of DNA together in a duplex while the complementary hydrogen bonding between A-T and G-C also contributes though by itself is not sufficient to maintain the double-stranded structure (Fig. 1.4).

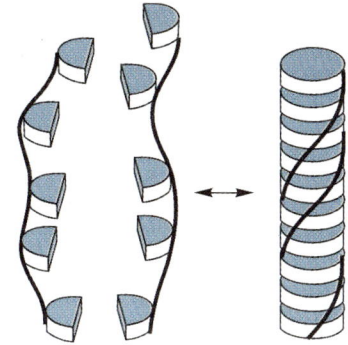

Fig. 1.3. Base stacking in ssDNA on interaction with water.

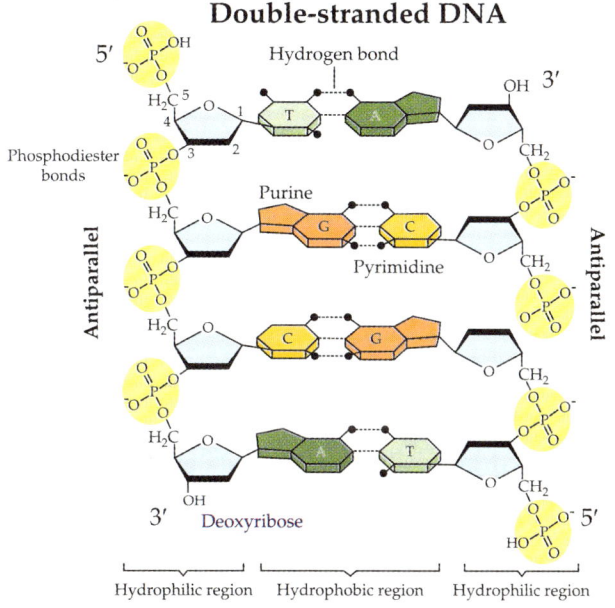

Fig. 1.4. Double-stranded DNA.

- When polypeptides interact with water tertiary structure of globular proteins is formed. Proteins tend to fold with the R-groups of amino acids with hydrophobic side chains in the interior (Figs. 1.5 and 1.6).

Excellent nucleophile (takes part in metabolic reactions)
- Metabolic reactions often involve the attack by lone pairs of electrons residing on electron-rich molecules termed **nucleophiles** upon electron-poor atoms called **electrophiles**. Two lone pairs of sp^3 electrons bear a partial negative charge and make water strong nucleophile. Nucleophilic attack by water generally results in the cleavage of the amide, glycoside, or ester bonds that hold biopolymers together. This process is termed hydrolysis. Conversely, when monomer units are joined together to form biopolymers such as proteins or glycogen, water is a product.

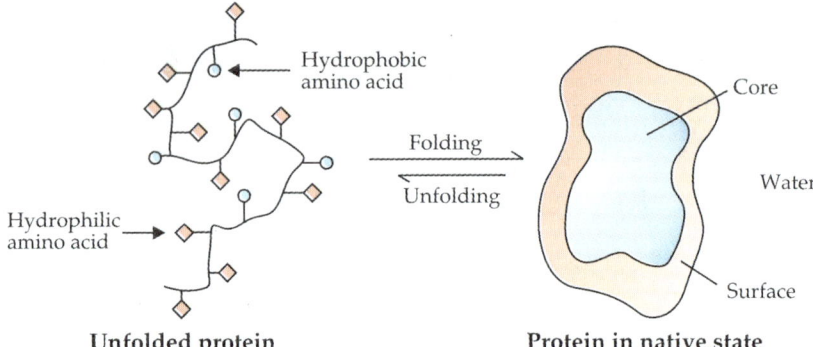

Fig. 1.5. Folding of a polypeptide due to interaction with water.

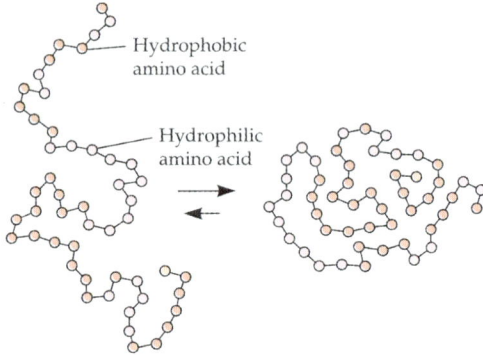

Fig. 1.6. Protein folding: Hydrophilic amino acids are on the surface, while hydrophobic amino acids get buried in the core.

- While hydrolysis is a thermodynamically favoured reaction, the amide and phosphoester bonds of polypeptides and oligonucleotides are still stable in the aqueous environment of the cell. This is because even though favourable, the rate of reaction is extremely slow making DNA stable for millions of years. Thermodynamics governing the equilibrium of a reaction do not determine the rate at which it will proceed. Breakdown rate is accelerated in presence of enzymes like proteases, nucleases, amylase which do not need any energy or ATP for action.
- The reverse process i.e. formation of peptide and phosphodiester bonds requires expenditure of ATP to occur.

Slight tendency to dissociate

- The ability of water to ionize, while slight, is of central importance for life. Water can act both as an acid and as a base. The removal and addition of hydrogen i.e. oxidation and reduction are a central concept of many metabolic reactions, e.g. shuttling of $NADH^+$/NADPH and NAD/NADP serves to transfer energy released from catabolism for ATP synthesis and anabolism.

Q. 2. What are pH and pKa? What are their physiological and clinical significance?

Ans. In pure water, molecules exist in equilibrium with hydrogen ions and hydroxide ions.

$$H_2O \leftrightarrow H^+ + OH^-$$

The water equilibrium constant is written as:

$$K = [H^+][OH^-] / [H_2O]$$

$[H_2O] = 55.5$ M and can be ignored as it is $>>> [H^+][OH^-]$. Experimentally, it has been found that the concentration of:

$$H^+ = OH^- = 10^{-7}$$
$$K_w = [H^+][OH^-].$$

Therefore, $K_w = [10^{-7}][10^{-7}] = [10^{-14}]$

The values for K_w, H^+, OH^- concentration all indicate that the equilibrium favours the reactant (water molecules). In other words, only very small amounts of H^+ and OH^- ions are present. If an acid (H^+) is added to the water, the equilibrium shifts to the left and the OH^- ion concentration decreases (Water equilibrium: $H_2O \leftrightarrow H^+ + OH^-$). If base ($OH^-$) is added to water, the equilibrium shifts to left and the H^+ concentration decreases. The multiplication product of H^+ and OH^- ion concentration must always be equal to 10^{-14}. Both H^+ and OH^- ions are always present in any solution. A solution is acidic if the H^+ are in excess. A solution is basic, if the OH^- ions are in excess. The concentrations of hydrogen ions and indirectly hydroxide ions are given by a pH number. pH is defined as the negative logarithm of the hydrogen ion concentration. 'p' stands for 'power' of H ions. The equation is:

$$pH = -\log[H^+]$$

Similarly, $pOH = -\log[OH^-]$

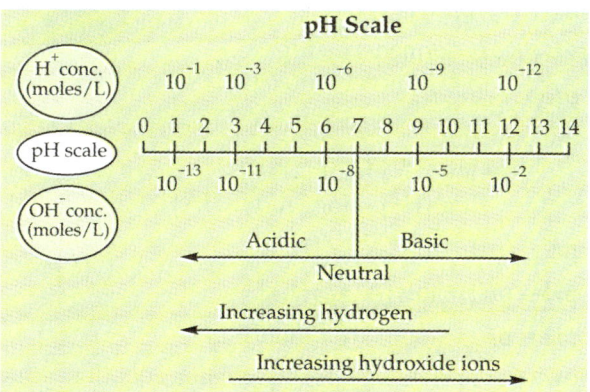

Fig. 1.7. The pH scale.

Low pH values correspond to high concentrations of H^+ and high pH values correspond to low concentrations of H^+. The pH scale, (0–14), is the full set of pH numbers which indicate the concentration of H^+ and OH^- ions in water (Fig. 1.7).

But the scale is limited from 0 to 14. pH is measured by a glass electrode which detects the electrochemical activity of H^+ ions. For acids with concentration above 1 M the calculated pH will come negative, which is never measurable on the electrode. At very high concentrations strong bases and acids do not dissociate completely and neither are all H^+ ions able to produce the complete activity on the electrode. Thus, the scale is limited for concentrations less than 1 M for acids as well as bases.

pH in living systems	
Compartment	pH
Gastric acid	1–2
Lysosomes	4.5
Granules of chromaffin cells	5.5
Human skin	5.5
Urine	6.0
Pure H_2O at 37°C	6.81
Cytosol	7.2
Cerebrospinal fluid (CSF)	7.5
Blood	7.34–7.45
Mitochondrial matrix	7.5
Pancreas secretions	8.1

While strong acids dissociate completely in water and concentration of H and pH can be easily calculated, most organic or biomolecules in living systems are weak acids which don't dissociate completely. Their dissociation at different pH of the solvent can be clinically relevant in many cases.

The equilibrium of acid dissociation can be written symbolically as:

$$HA \leftrightarrow H^+ + A^-$$
$$K_a = [H^+][A^-]/[HA]$$

Just like pH, pK_a is defined as $-\log(K_a)$.

$$pK_a = -\log K_a$$

Then,
$$pK_a = -\log K_a$$
$$= -\log [H^+][A^-]/[HA]$$
$$= -\log [H^+] - \log [A^-]/[HA]$$

Or, $pK_a = pH - \log [A^-]/[HA]$

Or, $pH = pK_a + \log [A^-]/[HA]$

Or, $pH = pK_a + \log [\text{salt}]/[\text{acid}]$

This is known as the Henderson–Hasselbalch equation, which describes the dissociation of any weak acid at a particular pH. If $pH = pK_a$, $\log [A^-]/[HA] = 0$, or $[A^-]/[HA] = 1$, implying that equal amount of undissociated and dissociated acid is present or that acid will be 50% or half dissociated. A weak acid has a pK_a value in the approximate range –2 to 12 in water. Acids with a pK_a value of less than about –2 are said to be strong acids; a strong acid is almost completely dissociated in aqueous solution, to the extent that the concentration of the undissociated acid becomes undetectable. Also when both HA and A^-, the weak acid and salt, are present in a solution, addition or removal of H^+ will shift the dissociation equilibrium ($HA \leftrightarrow H^+ + A^-$) to left or right respectively and H^+ will be consumed or generated minimizing or buffering the change in H^+ conc. or the pH! This accounts for the useful buffering activity of the combination of a weak acid and its salt. As it has to resist both addition or removal of acid or base it works best when HA (acid) = A^- (salt) or at pH =

pK_a! Thus, buffers work best at pH = pK_a of the buffer system. Further, they work maximally between pH range of ±1 of the pK_a as when pH is pK_a ± 1, [salt] / [acid] becomes equal to 100/1 or 1/100, then the ability to resist change in concentration of H or pH decreases greatly.

At pH > pK_a dissociated or ionized species will be greater and at pH < pK_a dissociated species or unionized acid will be predominant. This can be important in biological systems as the chemical reactivity, solubility, ability to cross lipid membranes, colour, electrophoretic mobility (mobility under electric field) and interaction with other compounds of the ionized anion and dissociated weak acid can be very different.

Significance of pH and pK_a

1. Most biochemical compounds possess functional groups that are weak acids or bases. Carboxyl groups, amino groups, sulfhydryl and phosphate esters, whose pK_a falls within the physiologic pH range, are present in proteins, enzymes and nucleic acids, most coenzymes, and most intermediary metabolites. Change in pH will alter their ionization and thus change drastically their 3-dimensional structures, catalytic activity of active centres of enzymes and interaction with other compounds (like enzyme – substrate, hormone – receptor, antibody – antigen, haemoglobin – oxygen, etc.).
2. Biological systems need to maintain pH in narrow range as:
   (a) Alteration in pH will alter 3D structures of proteins, enzymes, nucleic acids, etc. making them lose their biological activity.
   (b) It will affect the metabolic reactions that are accompanied by the release or uptake of protons.
   (c) The H^+ gradient of electron transport chain essential for ATP synthesis will be disturbed.
   (d) Oxidative metabolism produces CO_2, the anhydride of carbonic acid, which if not buffered would produce severe acidosis.
   (e) Change in H^+ ion concentration will affect the distribution of K^+ in cells and ECF, symporters, antiporters and pumps using H^+ and hence the fluid and electrolyte balance in the body.
   (f) As pH is a logarithmic scale, slight change in pH values mean a large change in H^+ concentration.
   (g) Change in pH alters the proportion of ammonia present as NH_3 and NH_4^+ ion in blood. As only NH_3 can cross blood-brain barrier and cause toxicity to CNS, change in pH alters the fraction of total ammonia present as NH_3 and hence ammonia entry into brain.
   (h) Both H^+ and Ca^{2+} (ionized calcium) in blood competitively bind with albumin. Changes in H^+ concentration thus can cause increased binding or release of Ca^{2+} from albumin altering the ionized Ca levels while total calcium remains the same. This affects many physiological processes needing Ca^{2+} and decrease in ionized Ca^{2+} can cause tetany.
3. Biological systems use weak acids as buffers. Intracellular pH is 6.8. Thus, the phosphate buffer ($H_2PO_4^-$ – acid / HPO_4^{2-} – salt, pK_a 7.2) and R (imidazole) group of histidine with pK_a 6.0 act as the best buffers. Of all the R groups of different amino acids only the pK_a of histidine is closest to physiological pH, making His present in proteins a very good buffering system.

4. Solubility and the ability of compounds to distribute through an organism: Charged compounds are most soluble in polar solvents, like water, and are much less soluble in non-polar substances, like lipids or fats. Thus, a charged molecule will distribute only to watery fluids in an organism and will be blocked by lipid layers (like cell walls), whereas uncharged compounds will have the possibility of distributing across cell membranes.
5. Uric acid stones: Uric acid has 4 ionizable hydrogen ions (positions 1, 3, 7, and 9). Only the hydrogen ion on position 9 ($pK_a = 5.8$) is ionizable at physiologic pH. Sodium urate is 15 times more soluble than uric acid. When urine pH levels equal the pK_a (5.8), uric acid and sodium urate are present in equal quantities. As pH levels increase, the ratio of sodium urate to uric acid increases. At a pH level of 6.8, 10 times more sodium urate is present than uric acid; whereas, at a pH level of 7.8, 100 times more sodium urate is present than uric acid. Thus alkanization of urine dissolves stones and prevents further formation.
6. Kidney uses NH_3 generated from glutamine to excrete H as shown in Fig. 1.8. The NH_4^+ being polar cannot re-enter the tubular cell.

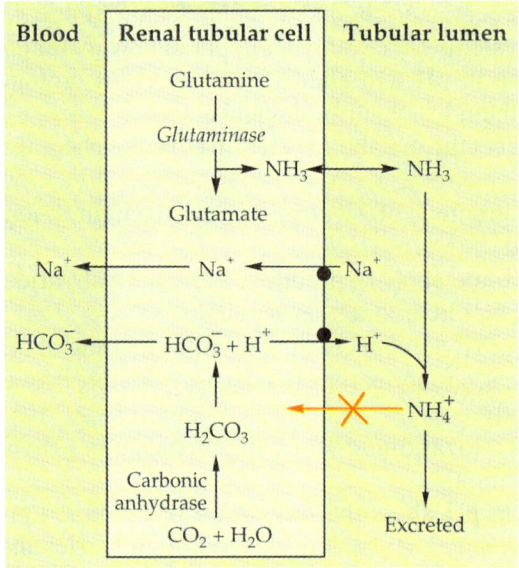

Fig. 1.8. Use of NH_3 generated from Gln to excrete H^+.

7. During ammonia toxicity to decrease absorption of NH_3 produced by bacteria in GIT lactulose is given to decrease the pH. At lower pH equilibrium ($NH_3 + H^+ \leftrightarrow NH_4^+$) shifts to right converting NH_3 to polar NH_4^+ which cannot cross cell membrane and hence is not absorbed. Similarly, changes in pH affects movement of NH_3 across blood-brain barrier (BBB). Normally, at pH of 7.4, only 2% of total ammonia is present as NH_3, remaining is NH_4^+. Only NH_3 crosses blood-brain barrier. If pH changes to 7.6, NH_3 increases by 67% to 5% of total blood ammonia.
8. Absorption of drugs across GIT and their entry into cells across the lipid cell membrane depends on the pK_a of drugs, e.g., acetylsalicylic acid is a weak acid with a pK_a of 3.5 and is rapidly absorbed and hydrolysed to salicylic acid and acetic acid. It is better absorbed

from the acid environment of the stomach (when it is undissociated and unionized and crosses lipid membrane easily) than from the alkaline small intestine. Further, it is better absorbed empty stomach when pH < 3.5 and the undissociated species predominates.
9. Charge-based separations such as electrophoresis, ion exchange chromatography, isoelectric focusing also are best understood in terms of the dissociation behaviour of functional groups.

Q. 3. What are viscosity and hyperviscosity syndromes ?

Ans. **Viscosity** is a measure of the resistance of a fluid which is being deformed by either shear or tensile stress. Blood viscosity is a measure of the thickness of blood. The thinner the blood, the less it resists flow, moving smoothly throughout the body. Several factors affect blood viscosity:
- Composition of blood – cells, proteins and fats
- Temperature

This is a concern with frostbite, when chilling of the extremities can make the blood so viscous that it does not circulate and the tissue dies as a result of lack of oxygen and nutrients. When the flow of blood is slow, cellular reactions that lead to adhesions and clotting can take place. Cells in the blood will start to stick together, forming clumps that thicken the blood. Blood viscosity also tends to increase in narrow blood vessels. High blood viscosity also forces the heart to work harder to pump the blood increasing the blood pressure.

Hyperviscosity syndrome (HVS) refers to the clinical effects of increased blood viscosity. Increased serum viscosity usually results from increased circulating:
- Serum immunoglobulins – Waldenström macroglobulinemia and multiple myeloma;
- Increased cellular blood components (typically white or red blood cells) – leukemias, polycythemia, and the myeloproliferative disorders.

Clinical effects are:
- The tendency to bleed is the most common symptom of hyperviscosity syndrome – Spontaneous gum bleeding, bruises, epistaxis, rectal bleeding, menorrhagia, persistent bleeding after minor procedures, visual changes ranging from blurred vision to vision loss.
- Ophthalmic examination may reveal decreased visual acuity, dilated retinal veins, "sausage-linked" or "boxcar segmentation" of the retinal veins, or retinal haemorrhages.
- Neurologic manifestations are frequent and varied. The neurologic symptoms of hyperviscosity have been referred to as the Bing-Neal syndrome – vertigo, hearing loss, paresthesias, ataxia, headaches, seizures, somnolence progressing to stupor and coma.
- Other manifestations may include congestive heart failure, volume overload (rales, lower extremity edema, elevated JVP), shortness of breath, hypoxia, fatigue, and anorexia.

Q. 4. What is selenocysteine? How is it incorporated into proteins?

Ans. Selenocysteine (abbreviated as Sec or U) is the 21st proteinogenic amino acid. It exists naturally in all kingdoms of life as a building block of selenoproteins. Selenocysteine is a structural analog of cysteine with selenium atom replacing the sulphur atom. The pK_a of selenocysteine, 5.2, is three units lower than that of cysteine. Unlike other unusual amino acids, selenocysteine is not the product of a post-translational modification. Rather, it is inserted directly into a growing polypeptide during translation. Selenocysteine, thus, is commonly referred to as the "21st amino acid". However, unlike other 20 genetically encoded amino acids, selenocysteine is specified by a much larger and more complex genetic element than the basic three-letter codon.

Proteins that contain one or more selenocysteine residues are called selenoproteins and those with catalytic activities which depend on selenocysteine's biochemical activity are called selenoenzymes. Twenty-five human proteins contain selenocysteine (selenoproteins). Human selenoproteins include:
- Iodothyronine deiodinases 1-3: DIO1, DIO2, DIO3
- Glutathione peroxidases: GPX1, GPX2, GPX3, GPX4, GPX6
- Selenoproteins: SelH, SelI, SelK, SelM, SelN, SelO, SelP, SelR, SelS, SelT, SelV, SelW, Sel15
- Selenophosphate synthetase 2 (SPS2)
- Thioredoxin reductases 1-3: TXNRD1, TXNRD2, TXNRD3

Unlike other amino acids present in biological proteins, selenocysteine is not coded for directly in the genetic code. Instead, it is encoded in a special way by a UGA codon, which is normally a stop codon. Such a mechanism is called translational recoding and its efficiency depends on the selenoprotein being synthesized and on translation initiation factors. When cells are grown in the absence of selenium, translation of selenoproteins terminates at the UGA codon, resulting in a truncated, nonfunctional enzyme. The UGA codon is made to encode selenocysteine by the presence of a selenocysteine insertion sequence (SECIS) in the mRNA. The SECIS element is defined by characteristic nucleotide sequences and secondary structure base-pairing patterns. In bacteria, the SECIS element is typically located immediately following the UGA codon within the reading frame for the selenoprotein. In eukaryotes, the SECIS element is in the 3' untranslated region (3' UTR) of the mRNA, and can direct multiple UGA codons to encode selenocysteine residues (Fig. 1.9).

Again unlike the other amino acids, no free pool of selenocysteine exists in the cell. Its high reactivity would cause damage to cells. Instead, cells store selenium in the less reactive selenide form (H_2Se). Selenocysteine synthesis occurs on a specialized tRNA, which also functions to incorporate it into nascent polypeptides. The selenocysteine tRNAs are initially charged with serine by seryl-tRNA ligase, but the resulting Ser-tRNASec is not used for translation because it is not recognised by the normal translation factor (EF-Tu in bacteria, eEF1A in eukaryotes). Rather, the tRNA-bound seryl residue is converted to a selenocysteine residue by the pyridoxal phosphate-containing enzyme selenocysteine synthase. Finally, the resulting Sec-tRNASec is specifically bound to an alternative translational elongation factor (SelB or mSelB (or eEFSec)), which delivers it in a targeted manner to the ribosomes translating mRNAs for selenoproteins. The specificity of this delivery mechanism is brought about by the presence of an extra protein domain (in bacteria, SelB) or an extra subunit (SBP2 for eukaryotic mSelB/eEFSec) which bind to the corresponding RNA secondary structures formed by the SECIS elements in selenoprotein mRNAs (Fig. 1.9).

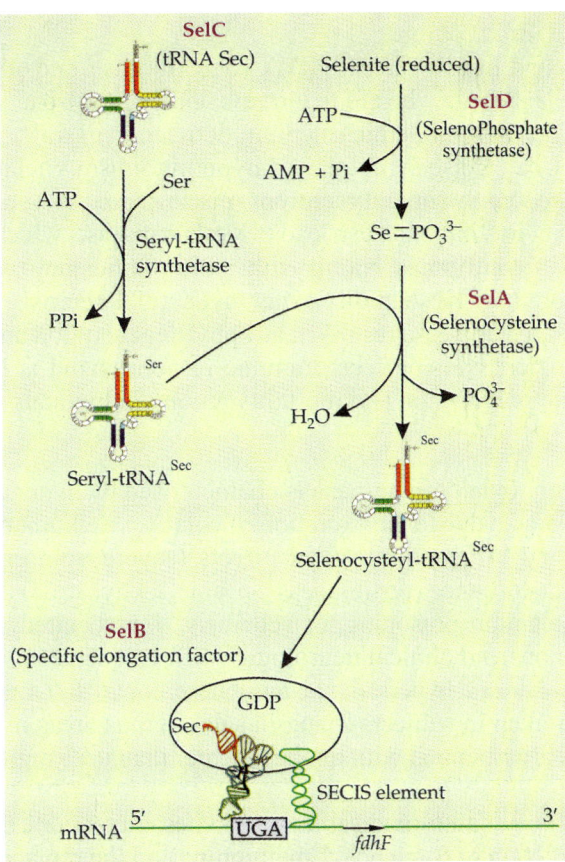

Fig. 1.9. Insertion of selenocysteine during translation.

Selenium is present in foods particularly fish (0.32 mg/kg), offal (0.42 mg/kg), brazil nuts (0.25 mg/kg), eggs (0.16 mg/kg) and cereals (0.02 mg/kg). In foods, selenium is generally present as the amino acid derivatives selenomethionine and selenocysteine. Selenium is present in several licensed medicines both alone and in combination with other substances, and is present in a number of food supplements at doses up to 0.3 mg/daily dose.

Recommended nutritional intake is 0.075 and 0.060 mg selenium/day for males and females respectively, and 0.075 mg selenium/day for lactating women. The lower limit of the WHO safe range to meet requirements is 0.040 mg selenium/day.

Selenium compounds are readily absorbed from the small intestine. The extent of absorption depends on the nature of the compound, with soluble selenate and selenomethionine being most readily absorbed.

Due to its incorporation in the selenoproteins, it is essential for:
- Protection against oxidative damage – glutathione peroxidase, selenoprotein P (which is involved in antioxidant and transport functions), thioredoxin reductases (maintenance of the intracellular redox state)
- Selenium is necessary for the conversion of the thyroid hormone thyroxine (T_4) into its more active counterpart, triiodothyronine (T_3).

Deficiency

Some health conditions – such as HIV, Crohn's disease, and others – are associated with low selenium levels. People who are fed intravenously are also at risk for low selenium. Certain regions in Africa have endemic selenium deficiency in soil.

Deficiency can cause symptoms of hypothyroidism, including extreme fatigue, mental slowing, goitre, cretinism and recurrent miscarriage. Selenium deficiency in combination with Coxsackievirus infection can lead to Keshan disease, which is potentially fatal. Selenium deficiency also contributes (along with iodine deficiency) to Kashin-Beck disease. The primary symptom of Keshan disease is myocardial necrosis, leading to weakening of the heart. Kashin-Beck disease results in atrophy, degeneration and necrosis of cartilage tissue. Selenium deficiency also affects immune responses and is linked to lower CD4+ T cell counts, disease progression and mortality among individuals infected with HIV-1.

Toxicity

Acute selenium toxicity in humans is characterised by hypersalivation, emesis and a garlic aroma on the breath due to the excretion of volatile selenium metabolites. These effects may be accompanied by gastrointestinal effects (severe vomiting and diarrhoea), hair loss, neurological disturbance (restlessness, spasms, tachycardia) and fatigue.

Chronic selenium poisoning, or selenosis, is associated with changes to the hair and nails, skin lesions and clinical neurological effects such as peripheral hypoaesthesia, acroparasthaesiae, pain and hyperreflexia; numbness, convulsions and paralysis may then develop. Studies undertaken in subjects living in seleniferous areas of the USA and China indicate that selenosis is associated with intakes greater than 0.91 mg/day (0.015 mg/kg bw for a 60 kg adult).

Redox cycling of auto-oxidisable metabolites, glutathione depletion, inhibition of protein synthesis, depletion of S-adenosyl-methionine and the replacement of sulphur by selenium in critical sulphydryl groups are possible mechanisms of toxicity.

Q. 5. Which is the 22nd amino acid?

Ans. Pyrrolysine (abbreviated as Pyl or O) is a naturally occurring, genetically coded amino acid used by some methanogenic archaea and one known bacterium in enzymes that are part of their methane-producing metabolism. It is similar to lysine, but with an added pyrroline ring linked to the end of the lysine side chain. It forms part of an unusual genetic code in these organisms, and is considered the 22nd proteinogenic amino acid. Pyrrolysine is synthesized in vivo by joining two molecules of L-lysine. It is present at active site of several methyl-transferases.

Unlike post-translational modifications of lysine, such as hydroxylysine and methyllysine, pyrrolysine is incorporated during translation (protein synthesis) as directed by the genetic code, just like the standard amino acids. It is encoded in mRNA by the UAG codon, which in most organisms is the 'amber' stop codon. This requires only the presence of the pylT gene, which encodes an unusual transfer RNA (tRNA) with a CUA anticodon, and the pylS gene, which encodes a class II aminoacyl-tRNA synthetase that charges the pylT-derived tRNA with pyrrolysine. The UAG codon is followed by a PYLIS downstream sequence, which forms a stem-loop structure and directs insertion of pyrrolysine in the translating protein.

Water, Amino Acids and Peptides

Q. 6. What is isoelectric point or isoelectric pH? How to calculate isoelectric pH of amino acids?

Ans. Amino acids have –COOH and –NH_3 functional groups which are weak acid and base as it can form –COO^- and NH_4^+. This ionization, however, depends on their pK_a and pH of the medium. Further some amino acids have ionisable acidic or basic functional group in their side chains.

For nomenclature: pK_{a1} = pK_a of α-carboxyl group, pK_{a2} = pK_a of α-ammonium ion, and pK_{a3} = pK_a of side chain group.

Isoelectronic point (pI) or **isoionic point** is the pH at which the amino acid does not migrate in an electric field. This means it is the pH at which the amino acid has equal number of positive and negative charges and thus is neutral, i.e. the zwitterion form is dominant.

There are 3 cases to consider:

1. Amino acids with neutral side chains: These amino acids are characterised by two pK_as – pK_{a1} and pK_{a2} – for the carboxylic acid and the amino group, respectively. The isoelectronic point will be halfway between, or the average of these two pK_as, i.e. **pI = 1/2 (pK_{a1} + pK_{a2})**.

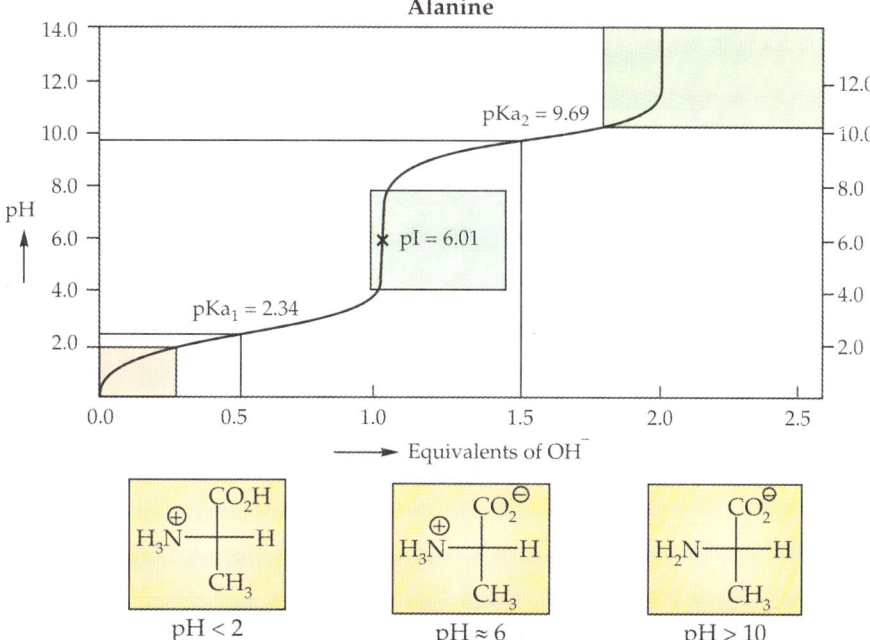

The titration curve for alanine (Fig. 1.10) demonstrates this relationship. At a pH lower than 2.34, both the carboxylate and amino functional groups are protonated, so the alanine

Fig. 1.10. Titration curve for alanine.

molecule has a net positive charge. At a pH greater than 9.69, the amino group exists as a neutral base and the carboxyl group as its conjugate base, so the alanine molecule has a net negative charge. At intermediate pHs the zwitterion concentration increases, and at a characteristic pH, called the **isoelectric point (pI)**, the negatively and positively charged molecular species are present in equal concentration.

2. Amino acids with acidic side chains: If the side chain is acidic (asp and glu), then average the side chain pK_a (pK_{a3}) with the α-COOH (pK_{a1}) to calculate pI.

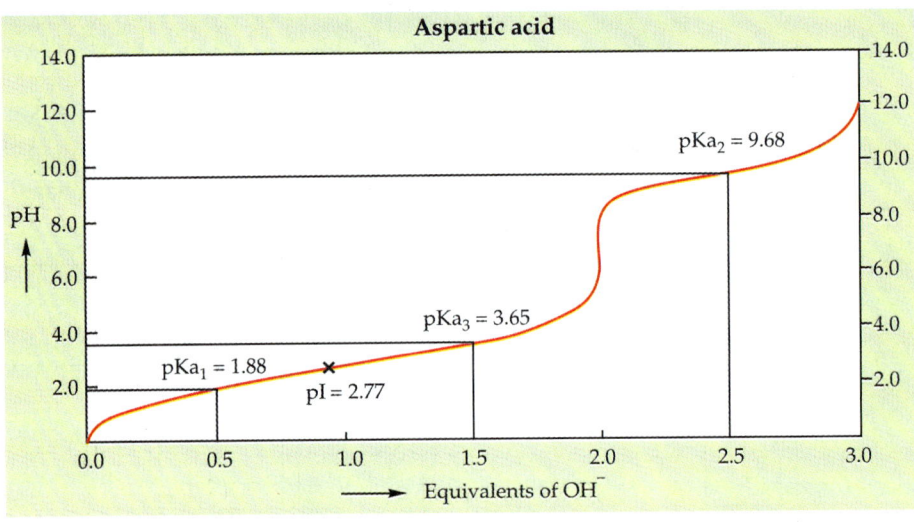

For example, for aspartic acid, the neutral form is dominant between pH 1.88 and 3.65, pI is halfway between these two values, i.e. **pI = 1/2 (pK_{a1} + pK_{a3})**, so pI = 2.77 (Fig. 1.11).

Fig. 1.11. Titration curve of aspartic acid.

3. Amino acids with basic side chains: If the side chain is basic (his, arg, and lys), then average the side chain pK_a (pK_{a3}) with the α-NH_3 pK_a (pK_{a2}). For example, for histidine, the neutral form is dominant between pH 6.00 and 9.17, pI is halfway between these two values, i.e. **pI = 1/2 (pK_{a2} + pK_{a3})**, so pI = 7.59 (Fig. 1.12).

Water, Amino Acids and Peptides

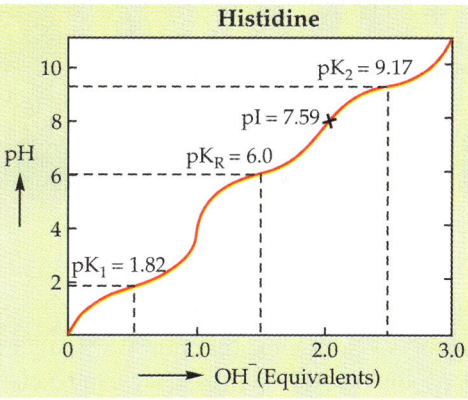

Fig. 1.12. Titration curve of histidine.

The pKa values and the isoelectronic point, pI, are given below for the 20 α-amino acids.

pKa values and the isoelectronic point, pI, for the 20 α-amino acids				
Amino acid	*pKa₁*	*pKa₂*	*pKa₃*	*pI*
Glycine	2.34	9.60	—	5.97
Alanine	2.34	9.69	—	6.00
Valine	2.32	9.62	—	5.96
Leucine	2.36	9.60	—	5.98
Isoleucine	2.36	9.60	—	6.02
Methionine	2.28	9.21	—	5.74
Proline	1.99	10.6	—	6.30
Phenylalanine	1.83	9.13	—	5.48
Tryptophan	2.83	9.39	—	5.89
Asparagine	2.02	8.80	—	5.41
Glutamine	2.17	9.13	—	5.65
Serine	2.21	9.15	—	5.68
Threonine	2.09	9.10	—	5.60
Tyrosine	2.2	9.11	—	5.66
Cysteine	1.96	8.18	—	5.07
Aspartic acid	1.88	9.60	3.65	2.77
Glutamic acid	2.19	9.67	4.25	3.22
Lysine	2.18	8.95	10.53	9.74
Arginine	2.17	9.04	12.48	10.76
Histidine	1.82	9.17	6.00	7.59

Protein Chemistry, Structure and Function

Chapter 2

Q. 1. What are the biological functions of proteins?

Ans. Proteins are the agents of biological function. Virtually every cellular activity is dependent on one or more particular proteins. Thus, they can be classified according to the biological functions (Fig. 2.1). Proteins can carry out almost every biological role – structural, source of energy, catalysts, transporters, muscle contraction, signalling and communication, vision, etc. with the exception of information storage (function of DNA). Thus, they are the molecules of primary importance (*'proteos'* = the most important one). All proteins function through specific recognition and binding of some target molecule. Proteins generally bind with targets (other proteins, lipids, sugars, nucleic acids) by non-covalent interaction. Some examples of functions of proteins are:

- Transport proteins include membrane proteins that transport substances across membranes, as well as soluble proteins that deliver specific nutrients or waste products throughout the body.
- Catalytic proteins (enzymes) mediate almost every metabolic reaction.
- Regulatory proteins that bind to specific nucleotide sequences within DNA control gene expression.
- Hormones are another kind of regulatory protein in that they convey information about the environment and deliver this information to cells when they bind to specific receptors.
- Switch proteins such as G-proteins can switch between two conformational states – an "on" state and an "off" state – and act via this conformational switching, as regulatory proteins.
- Structural proteins give form and shape to cells and subcellular structures.
- Scaffold proteins are a class of binding proteins that use protein–protein interactions to recruit other proteins into multimeric assemblies whose purpose is to mediate and coordinate the flow of information in cells.

Protein Chemistry, Structure and Function

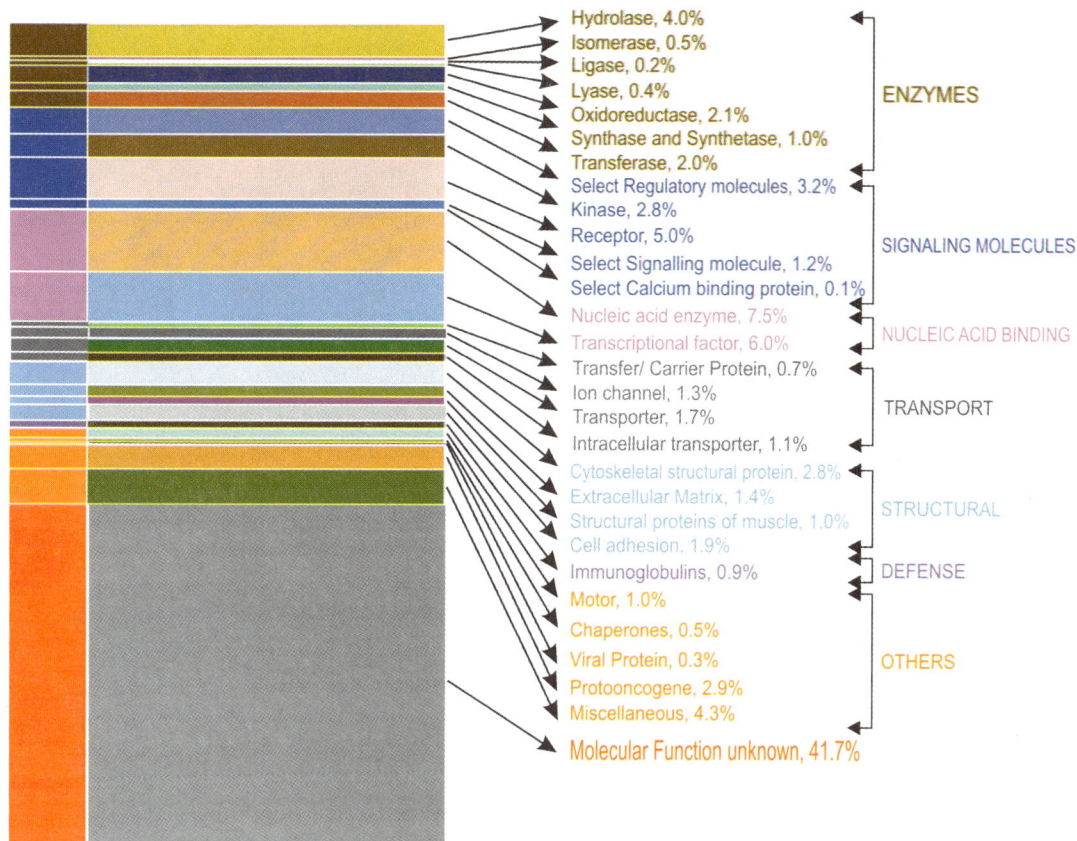

Fig. 2.1. Human proteins and their functions.

The function of more than 40% of the proteins encoded by the human genome remains unknown. Enzymes (including kinases and nucleic acid enzymes) account for about 20% of the total number of proteins and nucleic acid-binding proteins of various kinds for about 14%, out of which almost half are gene-regulatory proteins (transcription factors). Transport proteins collectively constitute about 5% of the total; and structural proteins another 5% (Fig. 2.1).

Based on their general shape and solubility proteins can be grouped broadly into three classes (Fig. 2.2):

1. **Fibrous proteins:** These tend to have relatively simple, regular linear structures. Often serve structural roles in cells. They are usually insoluble in water or in dilute salt solutions.
2. **Globular proteins:** These are roughly spherical in shape. The polypeptide chain is compactly folded so that hydrophobic amino acid side chains are in the interior of the molecule and the hydrophilic side chains are on the outside exposed to the solvent, water. Thus, they are usually very soluble in aqueous solutions. Most soluble proteins of the cell, such as the cytosolic enzymes, are globular in shape.

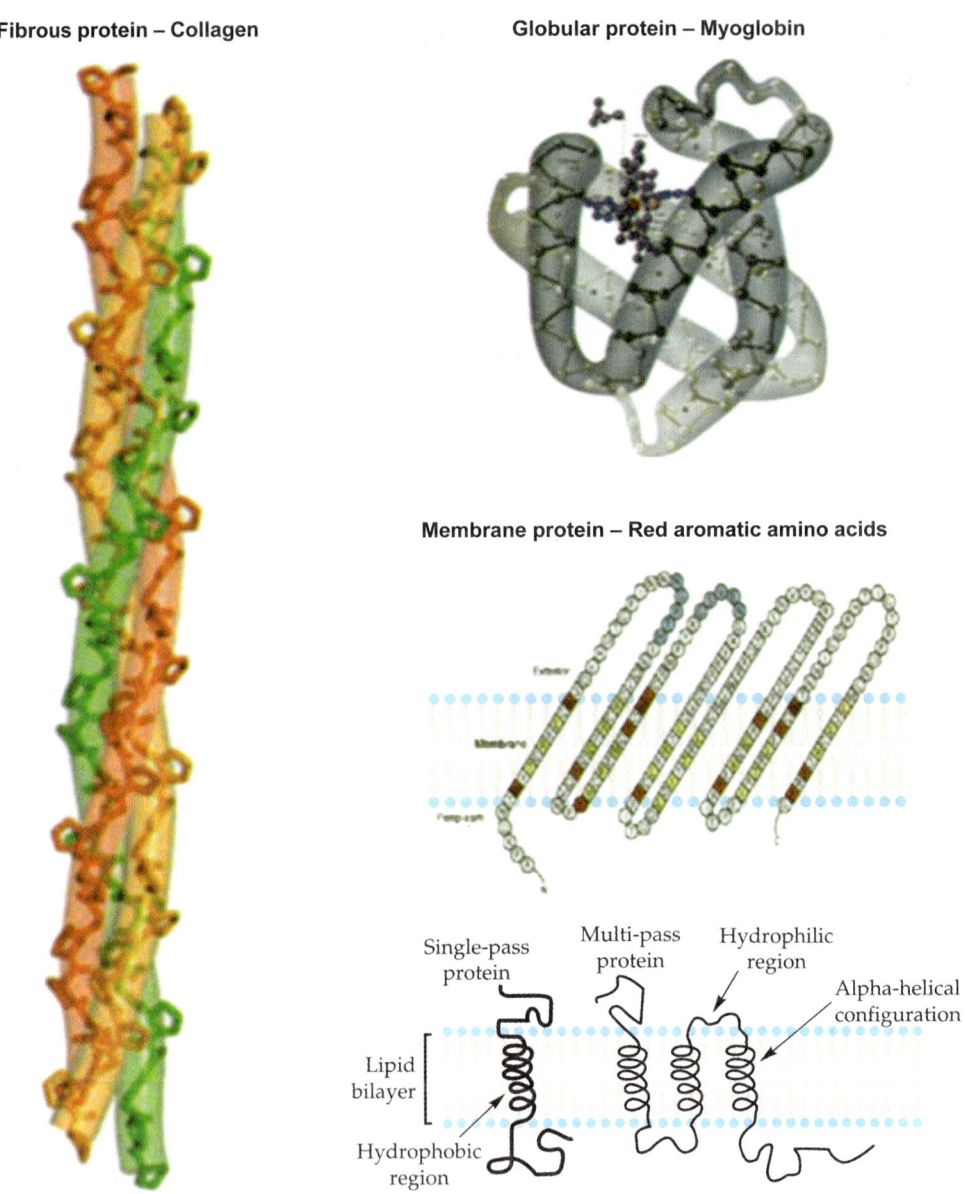

Fig. 2.2. Fibrous, globular and membrane proteins.

3. **Membrane proteins:** These are found in association with the various membrane systems of cells. They have hydrophobic amino acid side chains oriented outward for interaction with the hydrophobic membrane core. The cytoplasmic and cytosolic extensions have hydrophilic amino acids and aromatic amino acids tend to form the interface/junction between hydrophobic and hydrophilic regions of the lipid bilayer. As such membrane proteins are insoluble in aqueous solutions but can be solubilized in solutions of detergents, they have fewer hydrophilic amino acids than cytosolic proteins.

Q. 2. Differentiate between configuration and conformation.

Ans. The overall three-dimensional architecture of a protein is called its conformation. Configuration denotes the geometric arrangements or possibilities for a particular set of atoms. Different configurations give rise to d/l, D/L, R/S, cis/trans isomers.

For changing configuration, covalent bonds must be broken and rearranged. In contrast, the different conformations of a molecule are achieved without breaking any covalent bonds (Fig. 2.3).

In proteins, rotations about each of the single bonds along the peptide backbone have the potential to alter the course of the polypeptide chain in three-dimensional space. These rotational possibilities create many possible orientations for the protein chain, referred to as its conformational possibilities (Fig. 2.3).

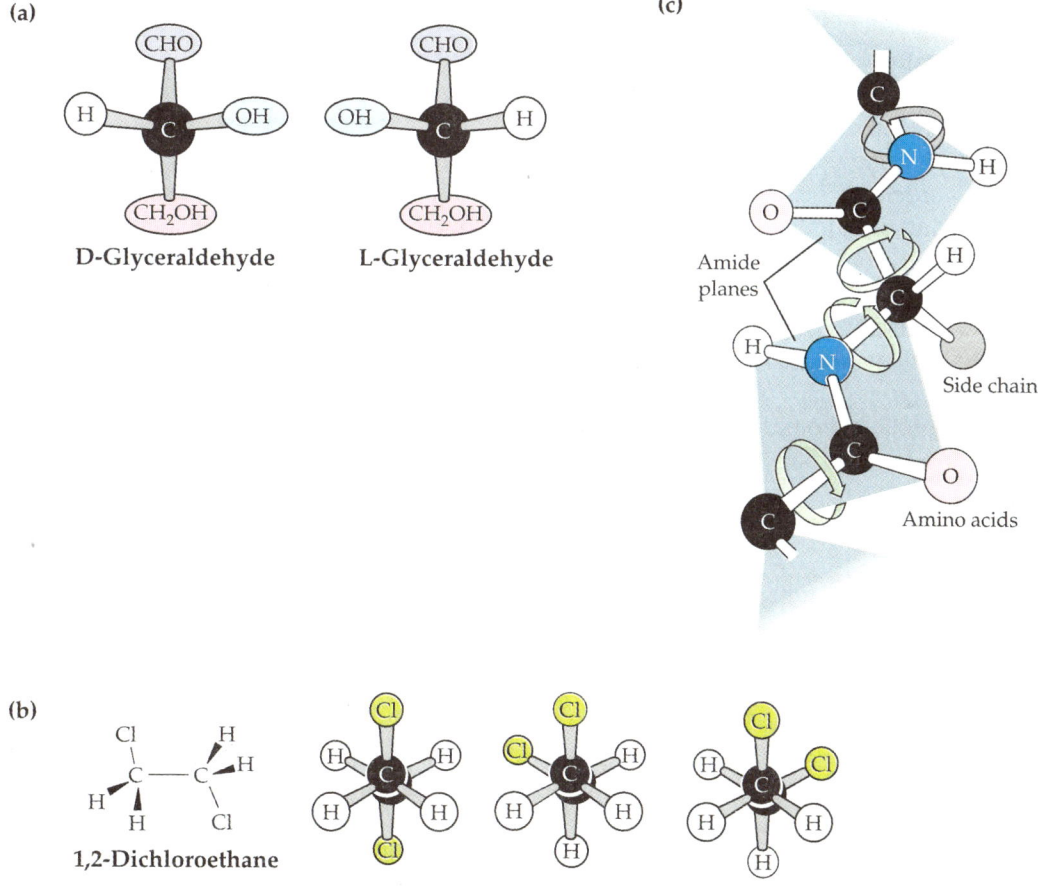

Fig. 2.3. Configuration and conformation. Rearrangements between configurational alternatives of a molecule can be achieved only by breaking and remaking bonds, as in the transformation between the D- and L-configurations of glyceraldehyde. The intrinsic free rotation around single covalent bonds creates a great variety of three-dimensional conformations, for a relatively simple molecule 1,2-dichloroethane or in proteins where rotation about the C–Cα and C–N bonds can create many possible conformations.

Q. 3. What are unstructured proteins?

Ans. Even though traditionally specific protein function has been attributed to the specific three-dimensional structure of protein, many proteins exist and function normally in a partially or completely unfolded state at physiological temperature. Such proteins are termed intrinsically unstructured proteins (IUPs) or natively unfolded proteins. These proteins have an extended conformation with high intramolecular flexibility and almost complete absence of folding. Some proteins are disordered throughout their length, whereas others may contain stretches of 30 to 40 residues or more that are disordered and embedded in an otherwise folded protein (partially unfolded conformations, PUFs). Unstructured protein domains resemble the molten globule intermediate seen in protein folding pathways.

Many gene sequences in eukaryotic genomes encode entire proteins or large segments of proteins that lack a well-structured three-dimensional structure. Like structured domains, disordered regions can be highly conserved between species in both composition and sequence.

Existence of unfolded proteins is not very energetically unfavourable as folded proteins are only 21–42 kJ/mol (5–10 kcal/mol) more stable than unfolded ones. Unstructured proteins lack the features which lead to stabilization of the folded state. However, compared with ordered proteins, IUPs have higher levels of polar or charged amino acids – E, K, R, G, Q, S, and proline (which tends to disrupt secondary structures), and low amounts of hydrophobic and aromatic amino acids – I, L, V, W, F, Y, C, and N. So, they have a unique combination of high net charge and low overall hydrophobicity (lack a hydrophobic core). Thus they interact with water to form hydrogen bonds and polar interactions helping to achieve stability despite lack of secondary and tertiary structure. Based on these characteristic sequences, unstructured regions can be predicted in the genome with more than 80% accuracy. Predictive analysis of whole genomes indicates that 2% of archaeal, 4.2% of bacterial, and 33% of eukaryotic proteins probably contain long regions of unfolded state.

Properties

- Flexible.
- High net charge.
- Large binding surface area: Intrinsically unstructured proteins contact their targets over a large surface area, e.g., the p27 protein complexed with cyclin-dependent protein kinase 2 (Cdk2) and cyclin A shows that p27 is in contact with its binding partners across its entire length (Fig. 2.4).
- Can bind multiple targets because of high flexibility, larger interacting surface and weaker binding with ligands than folded proteins. IUPs and PUFs often function by binding to DNA/RNA and other proteins. Binding may induce structure in the unfolded polypeptide. This production of a defined structure means decrease in entropy and would thus require energy and hence weakens the force of interaction between the unfolded polypeptide and ligand. This weak binding to ligand is often advantageous as weak and transient interactions are required for many biological processes. Also, it allows binding with greater number of ligands. This is because of the unfolded state providing them plasticity or flexibility to assume different conformations on binding as well as the weak nature of interaction. For example:

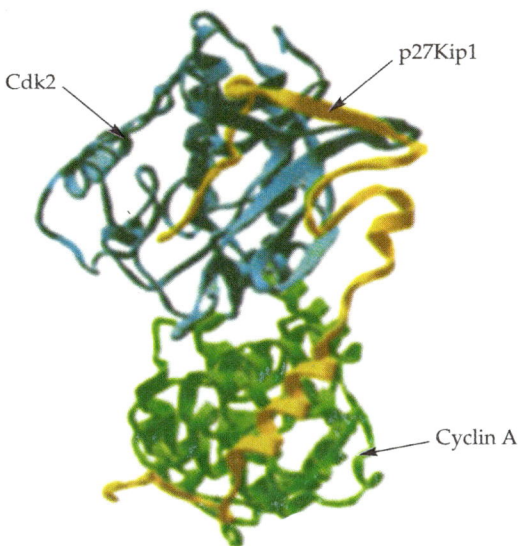

Fig. 2.4. Intrinsically unstructured proteins (IUPs) contact their target proteins over a large surface area. p27Kip1 (yellow) complexed with cyclin-dependent kinase 2 (Cdk2, blue) and cyclin A (CycA, green).

- p53 – unstructured region in carboxy terminal end can interact with 4 different partners (cyclin A, sirtulin, CBP, s100B) and assumes a different conformation in each complex.
- The cyclin-dependent kinase inhibitor p21 has ability to bind to different cyclin-dependent kinases (CDKs) and thus regulate multiple CDKs present in different stages of cell cycle.
• Many unstructured proteins undergo transitions to more ordered states upon binding to their targets. Many disordered segments fold or assume different well-defined 3D structure on binding to different biological targets (coupled folding and binding).
• Can bind multiple ligands simultaneously due to larger binding area and thus act as scaffolds for assembly of multi-protein complexes (Fig. 2.5).

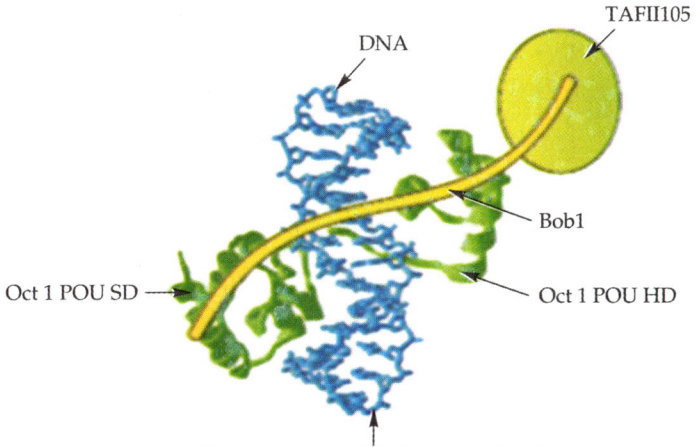

Fig. 2.5. Bob 1 transcriptional coactivator (yellow) in contact with its four partners: TAFII105 (green oval), the Oct 1 domains POU SD and POU HD (green), and the Igκ promoter (blue).

- Some IUPs act to inhibit other proteins by an unusual mechanism (Figs. 2.4 and 2.6) by wrapping around multiple target protein. Example: IUP p27, which controls cell cycle, lacks a definable structure in solution but inhibits action of multiple cyclin-dependent kinases (CDKs) by wrapping around them. Tumor cells have decreased p27. Lower levels of p27 imply poorer prognosis.
- Disorder in the bound state (fuzzy complexes): Intrinsically disordered proteins can retain their conformational freedom even when they bind specifically to other proteins. This can be further modified by post-translational and covalent modifications. Also, alternative splicing can alter the length of fuzzy/unstructured regions altering the specificity of binding of certain DNA binding proteins.

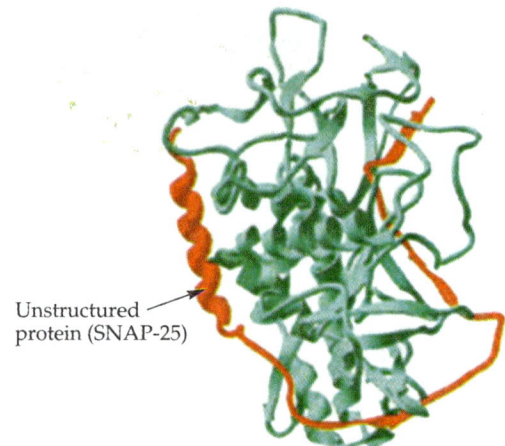

Fig. 2.6. SNAP-25 bound to BoNT/A. The unstructured proteins (SNAP-25) binds to the target (BoNT/A) by wrapping around it. Then the botulinum neurotoxin (BoNT/A) cleaves SNAP-25 by protease action. As SNAP-25 is required for vesicle fusion and neurotransmitter exocytosis, BoNT/A blocks release of neurotransmitters particularly acetylcholine causing toxicity.

The IUPs and PUFs include scaffold proteins, hormones, activation domains of transcription factors, cyclin-dependent kinases and their inhibitors, proteins in cellular signal transduction, and amino terminal segments of histone proteins.

Significance of IUPs

- Act as flexible linkers: Unstructured or unfolded regions in proteins act as flexible linkers allowing the connected domains to freely twist and rotate through space to recruit their ligands and allow large scale interdomain conformation changes on binding of ligands.
- Because of structural disorder and high charge density, function as spacers, insulators or linkers in larger structures.
- Help limit cell, genome and protein size: Compared with compact, folded proteins, disordered segments in proteins have larger intermolecular interfaces to which ligands, such as other proteins, could bind. Folded proteins will have to be two to three times larger to produce similar sized binding surface area as of a disordered protein. Such large proteins would increase cellular crowding or could increase cell size by 15% to 30%. The flexibility of disordered proteins may thus reduce protein, genome, and cell sizes.

- Can serve multiple functions: Interaction with different ligands could provide different functions in the cell.
- Scavengers and reservoirs: Because of high charge density, can act as scavengers, binding up small ions and molecules in solute and as reservoir or garbage dumps.
- Scaffold proteins having unfolded conformation and hence a large ligand binding surface area allows them to group or bring together many proteins into a complex and permit changes in group members as per physiological needs.
- Certain disordered regions might serve as "molecular switches" in regulating biological function by switching to ordered conformation upon molecular recognition, i.e., binding to DNA/RNA/ions, etc.
- Assembly of complexes involved in the transcription of DNA into RNA – large number of proteins must be recruited in such macromolecular complexes. For example, as shown in Fig. 2.5, Bob 1 transcriptional coactivator (yellow) is in contact with its four partners: TAFII105 (green oval), the Oct 1 domains POU SD and POU HD (green), and the Igκ promoter on DNA (blue).

Disorder and disease

- Intrinsically unstructured proteins have been implicated in a number of diseases. The aggregation of the intrinsically unstructured protein α-Synuclein is thought to be responsible for synucleinopathies. The structural flexibility of this protein together with its susceptibility to modification leads to misfolding and aggregation. Genetic changes, oxidative and nitrative stress can modify the structural flexibility of the unstructured α-Synuclein protein causing aggregation.
- Many key oncogenes have large intrinsically unstructured regions, for example p53 and BRCA1. These regions of the proteins are responsible for mediating many of their interactions.

Q. 4. What are salting in and salting out? Why ammonium sulphate is most commonly used for this purpose?

Ans. A protein contains multiple ionised groups. The ionic charges are counterbalanced by presence of cations and anions in the solution maintaining electroneutrality. The ionised groups on protein are also solvated by water or have hydration shells just like free ions. The entire surface of the protein exposed to water has a layer of water molecules around it which is more ordered than the free water molecules of the solvent. This is known as the hydration shell of the protein. These water molecules are more ordered or have decreased entropy. The ionic and dipole interaction of polar residues on protein surface with water and the interaction of hydrophobic residues inside the core away from water compensates for the decreased entropy of the hydration shell water molecules as compared to free water molecules, keeping the globular protein soluble. The hydration shell also decreases coulombic attraction forces between protein molecules. Further, net charge on protein molecules repels them from other protein molecules preventing aggregation. Indeed at isoelectric pH when protein molecules have 0 net charge and regions of both positive and negative charges they are least soluble and tend to aggregate with each other and precipitate out (Fig. 2.7). Thus, globular proteins are kept soluble by charge, polarity and hydration shell.

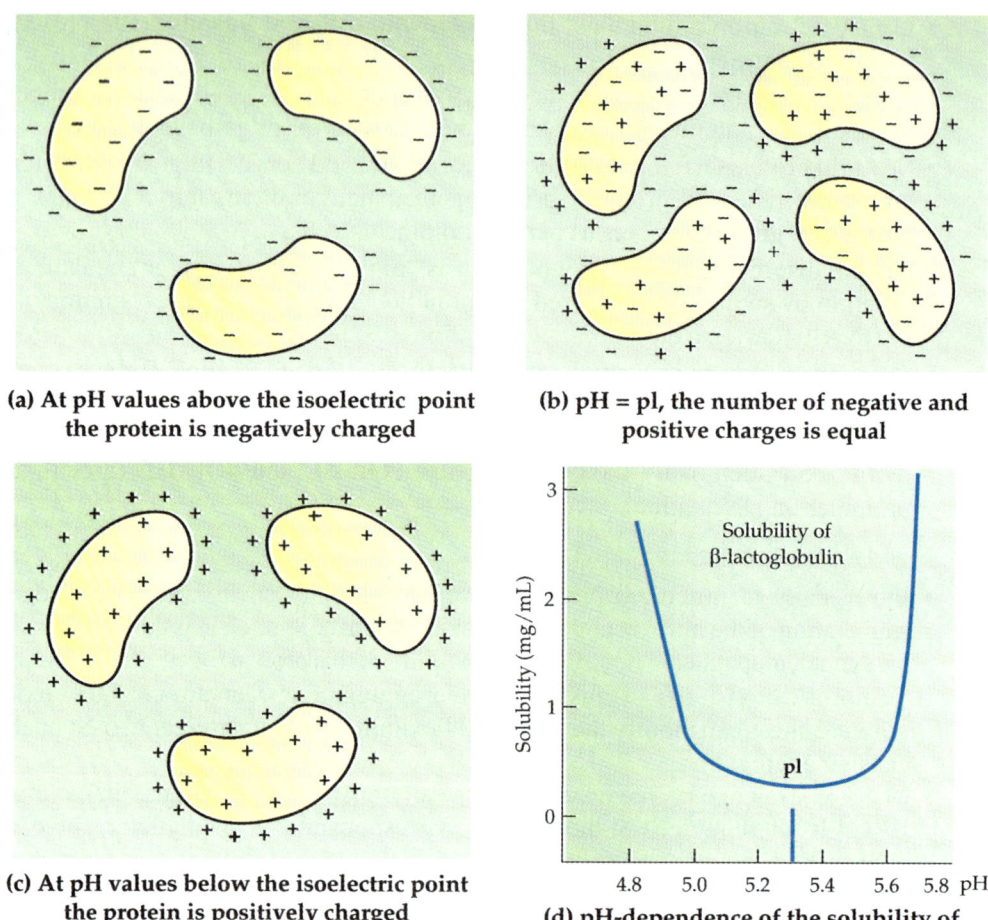

(a) At pH values above the isoelectric point the protein is negatively charged

(b) pH = pI, the number of negative and positive charges is equal

(c) At pH values below the isoelectric point the protein is positively charged

(d) pH-dependence of the solubility of the β-lactoglobulin protein

Fig. 2.7. Effect of pH on protein solubility

The solubility of a protein thus depends on the pH, polarity of the solvent, concentration of other ions or salts and temperature.

The solubility of a protein at low ion concentration increases as more salt is added. This is called SALTING IN. The additional ions shield the protein's multiple ionic charges and thus weaken the attractive forces between individual protein molecules, which tend to aggregate and precipitate them (Fig. 2.8).

But as more salt is added the total ion concentration of water increases and solubility of protein starts decreasing, and ultimately with addition of more salt proteins precipitate out. This is SALTING OUT. This is because of competition between ions for water molecules to form hydration shell. The salt ions due to smaller size exert higher attractive force on the partially charged water molecules (dipoles) as force is inversely proportional to square of distance. Thus, when they compete for the limited number of water molecules with the salt ions, the proteins lose their hydration shell decreasing their solubility and ultimately they precipitate out. As the hydration shell is lost, proteins can aggregate because of dipole interactions or interactions of small hydrophobic patches on their surface (Figs. 2.9 and 2.10).

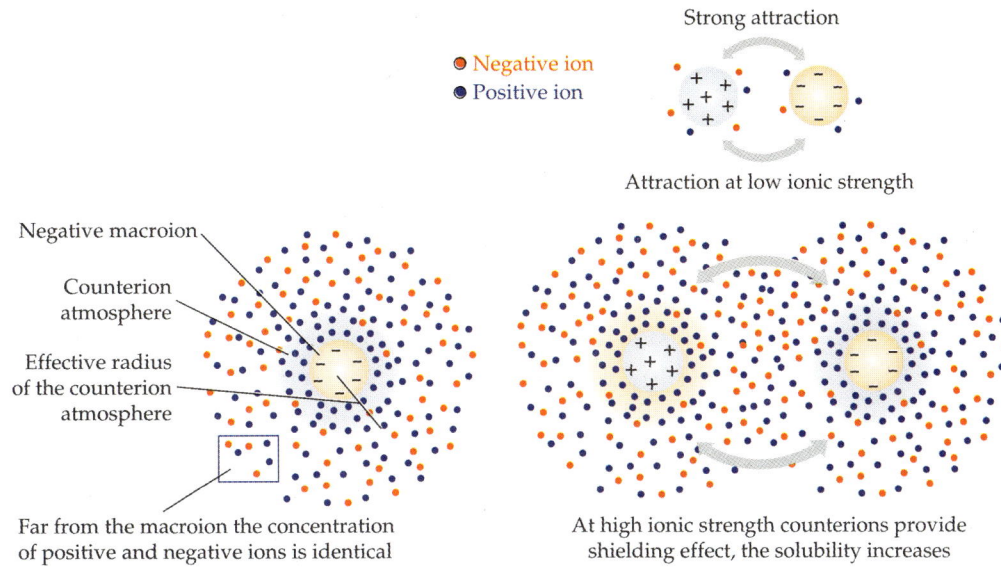

Fig. 2.8. The 'salting-in' effect. The solubility of proteins is usually low in deionised water, but it increases with increasing ionic strength of the solution, up to a certain point. Dissolved salt (ions) facilitates solvation of proteins by shielding the exposed charges of protein molecules. This shielding effect hinders intermolecular attracting interactions between opposite charges of individual protein molecules and, by doing so, it prevents protein aggregation.

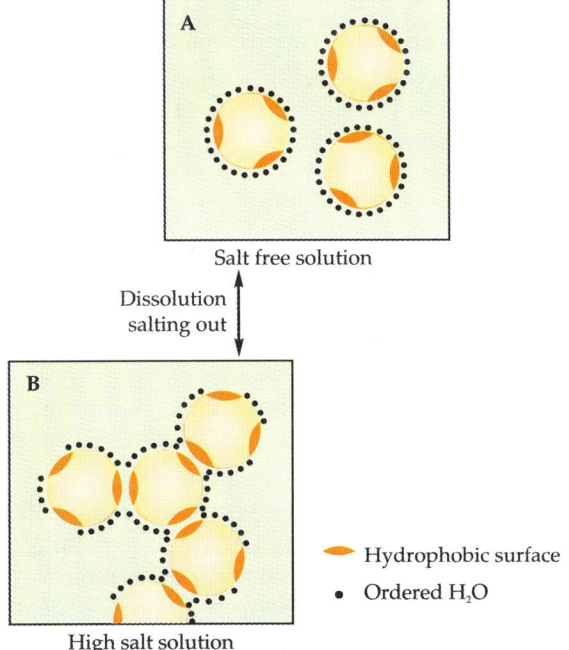

Fig. 2.9. Salting out. As hydration shell is lost the hydrophobic patches on surface are exposed and interact with other such patches on other protein molecules leading to aggregation.

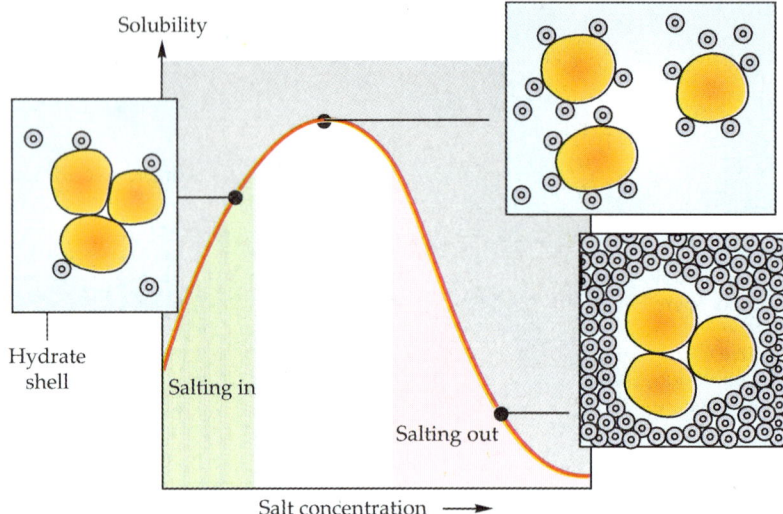

Fig. 2.10. Salting in and out, dependence of protein solubility on salt concentration.

Different proteins have different ionic and hydrophobic composition and hence require different amounts of salt concentration for salting out. This can help separate or purify proteins. Adjustment of salt concentration to just below the precipitation point for the desired protein results in precipitation of many other unwanted proteins. Then the supernatant is separated and salt concentration raised slightly to precipitate out the desired protein.

Ammonium sulphate, $(NH_4)_2SO_4$, is a preferred and most commonly used salt for salting out. A salt's ability to induce selective precipitation is dependent on many interactions with the water and solutes. Research by Franz Hofmeister in the early 20th century organized various anions and cations by their ability to salt out proteins. The ordering of cations and anions is called the Hofmeister Series.

The cations are arranged as follows:

$$NH_4^+ > K^+ > Na^+ > Li^+ > Mg^{2+} > Ca^{2+}$$

where ammonium has the highest ability to precipitate proteinacious solutes. Likewise, the order for anions is:

$$F^- \geq SO_4^{2-} > H_2PO_4^- > H_3CCOO^- > Cl^- > NO_3^- > Br^- > ClO_3^- > I^- > ClO^-$$

Between cations and anions in solution the concentration of the anion typically has the greatest effect on protein precipitation. Ammonium sulfate is preferentially used because:
- The ions produced in an aqueous solution are very high on the Hofmeister Series, and their direct interaction with the protein itself is relatively low.
- Other ions such as iodide are very good at precipitating proteins, but are not used due to their propensity to denature or modify the protein.
- It has high solubility in water (3.9 M at 0°C); large amounts can be added before saturation.
- Each mole provides 3 moles of ions to remove hydration shell of proteins.
- The pH can be simultaneously adjusted to isoelectric point of proteins to further decrease their solubility (proteins are least soluble at isoelectric pH).

Q. 5. What are disulfide bonds? How are they formed and what are their significance in protein structure?

Ans. A disulfide bond is a covalent bond, derived by the coupling of two thiol (–SH) groups. The linkage is also called an SS bond or disulfide bridge. The overall connectivity is therefore C–S–S–C. The disulfide bond is a strong bond (dissociation energy being 60 kcal/mole). It is about 40% weaker than C–C and C–H bonds. The disulfide bond is about 2.05 Å in length, about 0.5 Å longer than a C–C bond. Rotation about the S–S axis is easily possible. Disulfide bonds in proteins are formed between the thiol groups of cysteine residues. The other sulfur-containing amino acid, methionine, cannot form disulfide bonds. The prototype of a protein disulfide bond is the two-amino-acid peptide, cystine, which is composed of two cysteine amino acids joined by a disulfide bond (Fig. 2.11). The bond angle between the two sulphur atoms shows preference for angles near 90°. When the angle approaches 0° or 180°, then the disulfide becomes a significantly better oxidant.

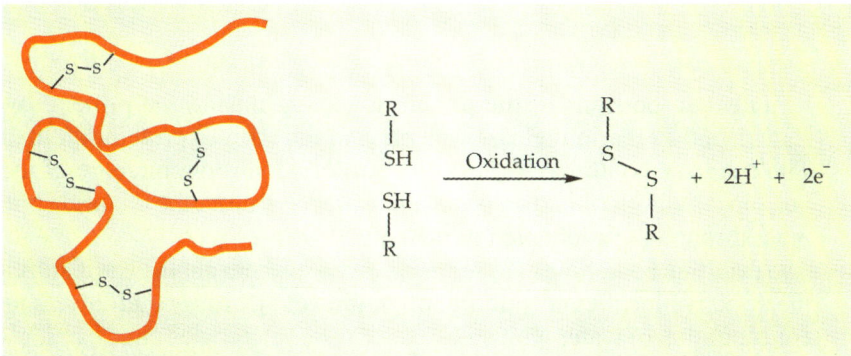

Fig. 2.11. Disulfide bond and its formation between two thiol (SH) groups of cysteine.

The conversion of two sulfhydryl groups to a disulfide linkage is an oxidation reaction. It involves removal of two hydrogens ($H^+ + e^-$) from each thiol (by an oxidizing agent), and concomitant formation of a new covalent bond – the disulfide bond. The oxidizing agent can be another disulfide linkage, in which case the net redox reaction would be a disulfide exchange: $2\,Cys + R–S–S–R \rightarrow cystine + 2\,RSH$. Conversely, disulfide bonds can be reduced to yield two thiols.

As the formation of disulfide requires oxidation and the environment within most cells is highly reducing, it precludes the formation of –S–S– bonds. Since most cellular compartments have reducing environments, in general, disulfide bonds are unstable in the cytosol, unless a sulfhydryl oxidase enzyme is present. In eukaryotes, disulfide bonds are found primarily in secreted and extracellular proteins (for example, the hormone insulin). Disulfide bonds are also uncommon in bacterial proteins.

In eukaryotic cells, in general, stable disulfide bonds are formed in the lumen of the RER (rough endoplasmic reticulum) and the mitochondrial intermembrane space but not in the cytosol. This is due to more oxidizing environment of these compartments and more reducing environment of the cytosol. Thus, disulfide bonds are mostly found in secretory proteins, lysosomal proteins, and the exoplasmic domains of membrane proteins. Notable exceptions to this rule include a number of cytosolic proteins which have cysteine residues in proximity to each other that function as oxidation sensors or redox catalysts; when the reductive potential of the cell decreases, their –SH groups oxidize to –S–S– and trigger cellular response mechanisms.

Not all disulfide/thiol exchange in biochemistry involves cysteine residues. An enzyme-linked prosthetic group, lipoamide, alternates between an internal five-membered ring disulfide form and a reduced ring-opened thiol pair form, dihydrolipoamide, as it participates in oxidative decarboxylation of α-keto acids and pyruvate.

Disulfide linkages are rare in hyper-thermostable proteins, presumably because they are chemically labile at high temperatures.

Disulfide bonds can occur in two ways: intramolecularly and intermolecularly. Intramolecular disulfide bonds occur within a polypeptide chain and are usually responsible for stabilizing tertiary structures of proteins. Intermolecular disulfide bonds occur between two polypeptide subunits and play a role in stabilizing quaternary protein structures. For example, disulfide bonds play very important role in the structure of antibody molecules.

Significance of disulfide bonds

- The disulfide bond stabilizes the folded form of a protein in several ways:
  - It holds two portions of the protein together, biasing the protein towards the folded state. Bond formation releases energy and thus drives protein folding.
  - The disulfide bond may form the centre of a hydrophobic core of the folded protein, i.e., local hydrophobic residues may condense around the disulfide bond and onto each other through hydrophobic interactions.
  - The disulfide bond links two segments of the protein chain. The disulfide bond increases the effective local concentration of amino acid residues and lowers the effective local concentration of water molecules. Since water molecules attack amide–amide hydrogen bonds and break up secondary structure, a disulfide bond stabilizes secondary structure in its vicinity.
- Glutathione (GSH) cycles between GSH (reduced form) and GSSG (oxidized form with disulfide bond between two glutathione molecules) to carry out its functions.
- Thioredoxin has two close cysteines (–C–X–X–C–) and their SH groups are normally kept in reduced state by thioredoxin reductase (a selenoprotein) with the help of NADPH. Thioredoxin in turn provides reducing equivalents (electrons) to peroxidases and ribonucleotide reductase. It helps in keeping SH group of cytosolic proteins in reduced state like glutathione. It also helps in reduction of H_2O_2 like GSH. For these functions it cycles between the reduced (Trx–SH) and oxidized state (Trx–S_2, having intramolecular disulfide bond). It can stimulate or inhibit different transcription factors like NF-κB and Ref-1-dependent AP1 (depends on Trx for DNA binding) depending on whether it is present in reduced or oxidized state, thus acting as a redox sensor of oxidative stress. Trx-SH inhibits apoptosis by complexing with ASK1 (Activation of Apoptosis Signal-Regulating Kinase 1) while Trx-S_2 cannot inhibit apoptosis. Thus, during oxidant stress, when TrX-SH converts to TrX-S2, balance shifts in favour of apoptosis.
- Disulfide bonds play an important protective role for bacteria as a reversible switch that turns a protein on or off when bacterial cells are exposed to oxidation reactions and oxidant stress. Hydrogen peroxide (H_2O_2) in particular could severely damage DNA and kill the bacterium at low concentrations if not for the protective action of the SS-bond.

During oxidative stress formation of disulfide bonds in cytosolic proteins serves many functions like:
- Activation of transcription factor OxyR induces enzymes for degradation of peroxides, many regulatory proteins and small non-coding regulatory RNA OxyS.
- Activation of chaperone function of heat shock protein (HSP33).
- Activation of transcription factor Yap1p and its migration into nucleus where it causes expression of many genes.
- Activation of RsrA transcription factor, which induces Trx and thioredoxin reductases expression.

- As disulfide bonds can be reversibly reduced and re-oxidized, the redox state of these bonds has evolved into a signalling element. In eukaryotes, changes in disulfide bond formation occur following reactive oxygen species exposure in cytosol. Such cytosolic disulfide-bonded proteins (DSBP) include peroxiredoxins, thioredoxin reductase, nucleoside-diphosphate kinase, and ribonucleotide-diphosphate reductase. Many other DSBP proteins are involved in molecular chaperoning, translation, glycolysis, cytoskeletal structure, cell growth, and signal transduction. These include:
  - Molecular chaperones – HSP70, HSP90, HSC70.
  - Translation factors – EF1α1, eEF-2γ, eEF2, cysteinyl tRNA synthetase, glycyl TRNA synthetase.
  - Glycolysis – enolase, lactate dehydrogenase, pyruvate kinase m2, 3-phosphoglyceraldehyde dehydrogenase.
  - Cell growth – ribonucleotide diphosphate reductase m1, NDP kinase B.
  - Antioxidant – peroxiredoxin 1 & 2, Trx reductase.
  - Cytoskeleton – tubulin.
  - Signal transduction – NFκB2, p21 activated kinase 2.
  - Others – histone acetyltransferase, ubiquitin thiolesterase 5.

  As oxidative stress increases these proteins form disulfide bond with glutathione or intra-/intermolecular disulfide bonds under more severe oxidant stress. E.g., HSP70 can form mixed disulfide bond with β4 spectrin and APC. This leads to their activation or inactivation (molecular switching and signalling).

  The protein mutated and inactivated in the inherited aplastic anaemia, Fanconi anaemia type C (FANCC, Fanconi anaemia type C protein) normally functions to:
  - increase the survival of hematopoietic progenitor cells by preventing disulfide bond formation in cytosolic proteins;
  - prevent formation of inactivating disulfide bonds in glutathione S-transferase P1 (which prevents apoptosis by protecting from oxidant damage); and
  - prevent H_2O_2-induced activation of the redox-sensitive kinase ASK1 (involved in apoptosis).

  Thus, its inactivation due to mutation leads to increased disulfide bond formation in cytosolic proteins and increases apoptosis leading to death of hematopoietic progenitor/stem cells and aplastic anemia.

- In chloroplasts, the enzymatic reduction of disulfide bonds has been linked to the control of numerous metabolic pathways as well as gene expression. The reductive signalling activity is carried out by the ferredoxin thioredoxin system, channeling electrons from the light reactions of photosystem I to catalyse reduction of disulfides in regulatory proteins in a light-dependent manner. In this way chloroplasts adjust the activity of key processes such as the Calvin-Benson cycle, starch degradation, ATP production and gene expression according to light intensity.

- Over 90% of the dry weight of hair comprises of proteins called keratins, which have a high disulfide content, from the amino acid cysteine. Different parts of the hair have different cysteine levels, leading to harder or softer material. Manipulating disulfide bonds in hair is the basis for the making of permanent wave in hairstyling. Reagents that cause the making and breaking of S–S bonds are used, e.g., ammonium thioglycolate (Fig. 2.12) or heat (of curling iron) can break existing disulfide bonds. Once bonds are broken curling or straightening is done and disulfide bonds are then allowed to form again in new shape by cooling or chemicals. Such styling is not permanent as when new hair grows the natural shape and pattern of disulfide bonds is restored. The high sulfur content of hair contributes to the disagreeable odour that results when they are burned (Fig. 2.12).

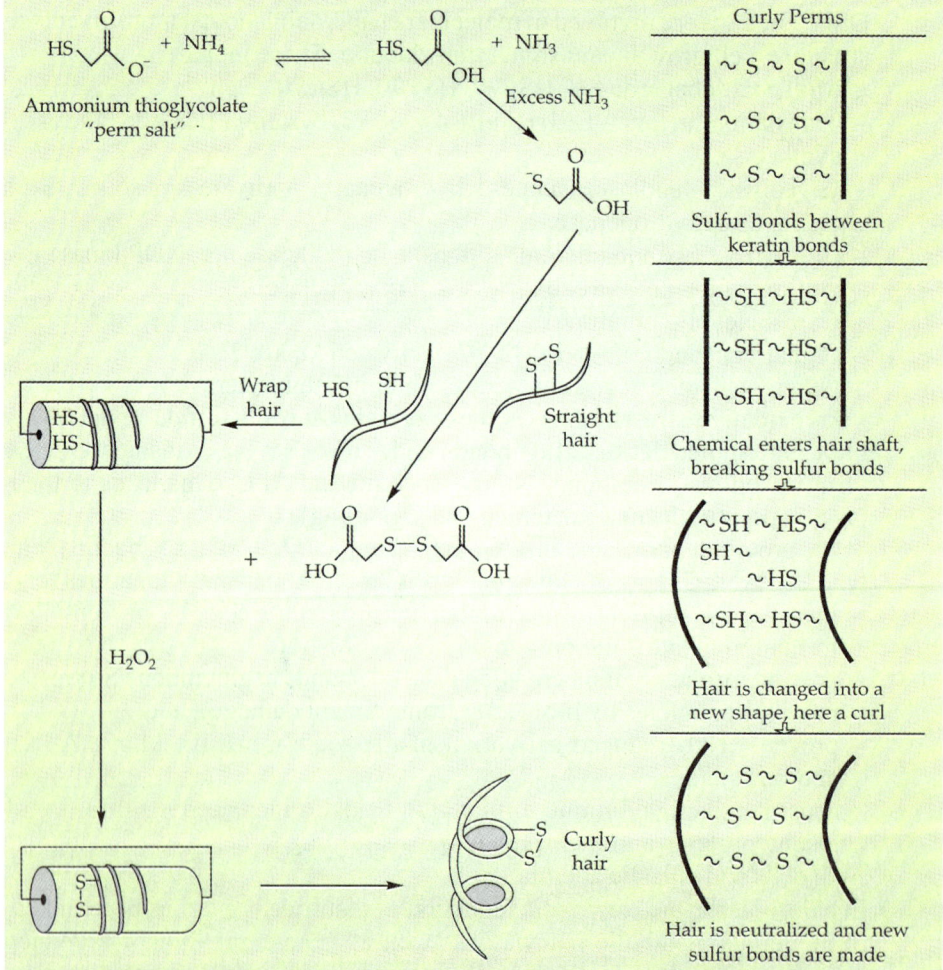

Fig. 2.12. Role of disulfide bond in hair curling and straightening.

- **Proteomics:** In order to analyze the structure of proteins, it is often necessary to break disulfide bonds. This reduction of disulfide bonds can be accomplished by treatment with 2-mercaptoethanol, dithiothreitol, or tris(2-carboxyethyl)phosphine.

Pathway for disulfide bond formation in the endoplasmic reticulum (ER) of eukaryotic cells (Figs. 2.13 & 2.14)

Oxidizing equivalents flow from the ER membrane protein Ero1p to proteins via protein disulfide isomerase (PDI) for the formation of disulfide bonds. Disulfides are formed in the presence of enzymes of the protein disulfide isomerase (PDI) family. If the cysteines are close to one another they will form a disulfide bond even if the protein is not properly folded. If a disulfide bond forms when the protein is not properly folded, it is called a non-native disulfide. This could be a misfolded protein, or it could be one of the intermediates before the protein folds into its native state. PDIs help non-native disulfides become native disulfides by acting as a catalyst to the isomerization process (they help brake the non-native disulfide bond so that the protein can finish folding properly before they can form the native disulfide bond). PDI can catalyze both formation and reduction (breakage) of disulfide bonds.

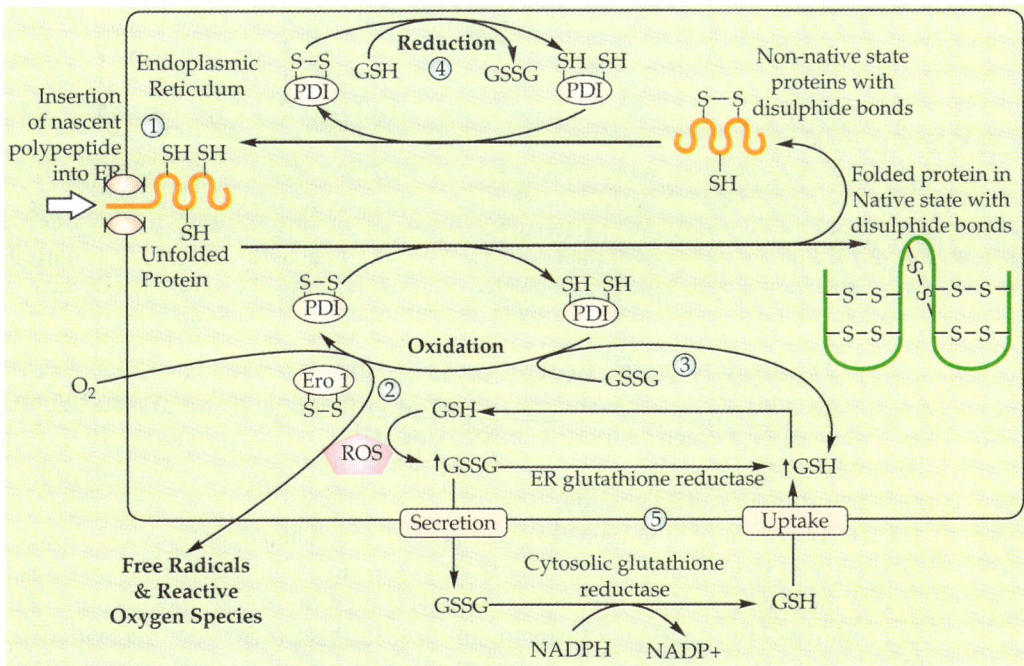

Fig. 2.13. Production of disulfide bonds in proteins – role of PDI, Ero1 and GSH. (1) Newly synthesized polypeptide with cysteines is inserted into the ER. (2) Disulfide bonds are formed by PDI, which gets reduced. PDI is oxidized by Ero1, which is oxidized by O_2, a process that generates reactive oxygen species (ROS). Detoxification of ROS can lead to an increase in GSSG. (3) PDI might also be oxidized by GSSG leading to an increase in GSH. (4) PDI is reduced by GSH, which leads to an increase in GSSG. (5) Influx and efflux of GSH or GSSG from the ER may control their ratio. Cytosolic GSSG is reduced by glutathione reductase. Similar activity might occur in the ER lumen.

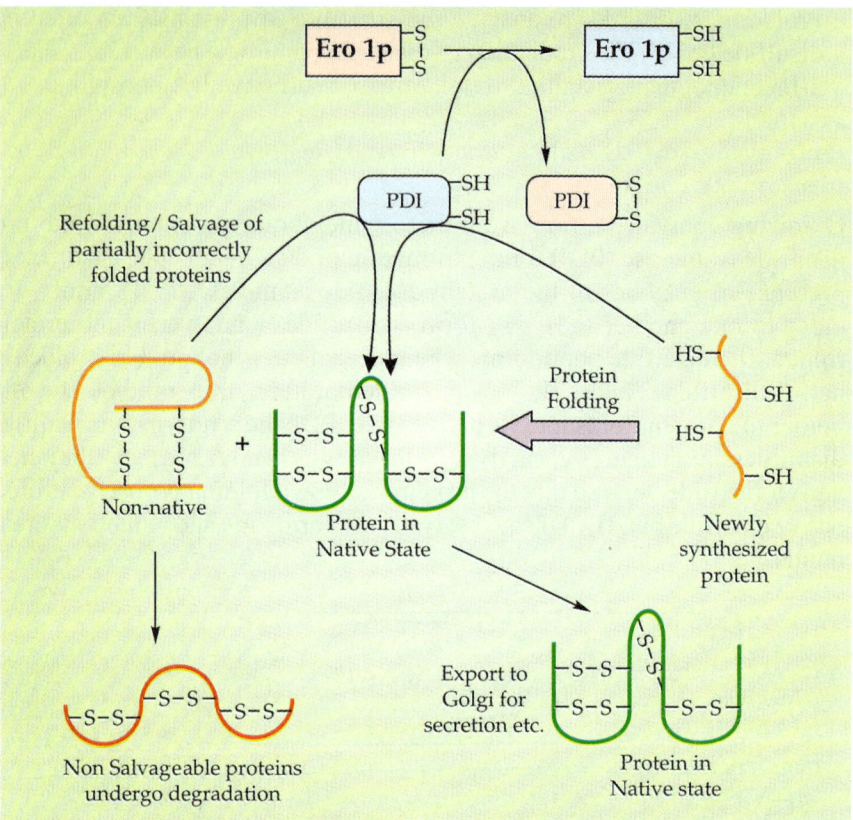

Fig. 2.14. Primary pathway of native disulfide bond formation in the ER. PDI transfers oxidizing equivalents from Ero1p to reduced, unfolded proteins. Non-native disulfide bonds must isomerize to the native state. Those proteins that do not attain the native state are degraded rather than secreted.

Ero1 (ER oxidoreductin, Ero1p): Ero1p and the mammalian homologues ERO1(alpha) and ERO1(beta) are able to catalyze oxidation by coupling de novo disulfide formation to the reduction of oxygen to hydrogen peroxide (H_2O_2). Ero1p oxidizes PDI, which allows PDI to exchange disulfides on the protein. In higher eukaryotes there are other pathways also for forming disulfide bonds.

PRDX4: Because hydrogen peroxide is produced when disulfides are formed via ERO1 catalysis, and H_2O_2 can cause damage to biomolecules, there are other proteins in order to remove the H_2O_2. Perodoxiredoxin (PRDX4) is a group of enzymes located in the ER that both removes H_2O_2 and also forms disulfides. In this process the peroxidatic cysteine in PRDX4 takes an oxygen from H_2O_2 to make water and a –SOH group, this then reacts with the adjacent –SH group to form a disulfide bond. This can now be exchanged with the –SH groups on some PDI proteins so it can in turn exchange it with substrate proteins.

Glutathione: GSH acts as a net reductant in the ER, either by maintaining ER oxidoreductases in a reduced state or by directly reducing non-native disulfide bonds in the folding proteins. Glutathione has a main role not only in allowing native disulfide bonds to form, but also in balancing redox reactions and thereby protecting the cell from oxidative stress.

Production of eukaryotic proteins in bacteria by recombinant DNA technology: Eukaryotic proteins may have disulfide bonds which are not usually formed in bacterial cytoplasm. Modulation of the redox environment in the bacterial cytoplasm, co-production of a disulfide isomerase and Ero1p in endoplasmic reticulum or DsbA and DsbB (involved in disulfide bond production) in the periplasm allows the formation of disulfide bonds in the proteins made by recombinant DNA technology.

Q. 6. Distinguish between peptides and proteins. Give examples of some important peptides.

Ans. Both are polymers of amino acids, i.e. chains of amino acids linked by peptide bonds. Peptides contain less than 40 amino acids, while proteins contain > 40 amino acids. 40 residues appear to be near the minimum required for a polypeptide chain to fold into a discrete and stable 3-dimensional shape that allows it to carry out particular functions. The largest protein is titin having 34,350 amino acids. Most proteins have 100 to 1000 amino acids.

When a few (2–20) amino acids are joined by peptide bonds, the structure is called an oligopeptide. Although the terms "protein" and "polypeptide" are sometimes used interchangeably, molecules referred to as polypeptides generally have molecular weights below 10,000, and those called proteins have higher molecular weights.

Peptides are short polymers of amino acids (< 40 amino acids). Shorter a peptide, greater are the chances that it exists as a linear unfolded polypeptide. However, they still serve many important biological functions. For example:

1. Peptide hormones – β-Corticotropin (ACTH), β-MSH, Gastrin, Glucagon, Secretin, Oxytocin, Vasopressin, TRH.
2. Antibiotics – Bacitracins, Penicillin, Polymyxins, Gramicidin S, Chloramphenicol.
3. Anticancer drug – Bleomycin.
4. Muscle relaxants – Kallidin, Bradykinin.
5. Vasoconstrictors – Angiotensins (Angiotensin I, Angiotensin II, Angiotensin III), Vasopressin.
6. Neuromodulators – Endorphins, Enkephalin.
7. Toxic peptides – Microcystin, Nodularin.
8. Biological reductant – Glutathione.
9. Artificial sweetener – Aspartame.
10. Muscle peptides – Creatine, Carnosine, Anserine.

Table 2.1 lists the common peptides and their biological significance.

Q. 7. What are domains, folds, motifs and supersecondary structures?

Ans. Domain

Proteins range in molecular weight from a thousand to more than a million. Proteins composed of about 250 amino acids or less often have a simple, compact globular shape. However, larger globular proteins are usually made up of two or more recognizable and distinct structures or modules.

Domains are individually or independently folding compact regions or units connected by short segments in the overall tertiary structure of proteins. Proteins can have just one or

Table 2.1. Some important peptides and their functions

Name	No. of amino acids	Significance
Hormones		
Angiotensin I	10	Renin from the juxtaglomerular cells converts angiotensinogen to angiotensin I. Angiotensin converting enzyme (ACE), a glycoprotein found in lung, endothelial cells, and plasma, removes two carboxyl terminal amino acids from angiotensin I to form angiotensin II.
Angiotensin II	8	Stimulates aldosterone release; vasoconstrictor.
Angiotensin III	7	Stimulates aldosterone release, formed from angiotensin II.
Aspartame	2	Used as artificial sweetener.
Bradykinin	9	Smooth muscle relaxant.
Bacitracin	Cyclic polypeptide	Commercially manufactured by growing the bacteria *Bacillus subtilis*; is used as a topical antibiotic.
β-Corticotropin (ACTH)	39	Stimulates secretion of glucocorticoid hormone from adrenal cortex cells, especially in the zona fasciculata.
β-MSH	18	Cleavage product of a large precursor peptide called pro-opiomelanocortin (POMC). Stimulates the production and release of melanin by melanocytes in skin and hair. Neurotransmitter in hypothalamus.
Bleomycin		Produced by the bacterium *Streptomyces verticillus*. Acts as an anti-cancer drug used in the treatment of Hodgkin's lymphoma, testicular tumors and squamous cell carcinoma.
Creatine	3	Stored as creatine-P in skeletal muscles; a high energy compound.
Carnosine	2	Highly concentrated in muscle and brain tissues. Anserine is methylated carnosine. Acts as a pH buffer.
Dynorphin	13	Endogenous opioid peptide has been shown to be a modulator of pain response. Also called superopiate since it is highly potent.
Endorphins	5–40	Endorphins ("endogenous morphine") are endogenous opioid peptides and act as neuromodulators, associated with pain or pleasure. Resemble the opiates in their abilities to produce analgesia and mood elevation.
Gastrin		Gastrin stimulates parietal cells of the stomach to secrete hydrochloric acid (HCl)/gastric acid.
Big gastrin	34	
Little gastrin	17	
Mini Gastrin	14	
Pentagastrin	5	Artificially synthesized (5 amino acids).

(Contd.)

Table 2.1 (Contd.)

Name	No. of amino acids	Significance
Glutathione (GSH)	3	Removal of hydrogen peroxide in the reaction catalyzed by glutathione peroxidase. Important intracellular antioxidant reductant, helping to maintain essential SH groups of enzymes in their reduced state. Also helps in the transport of certain amino acids across membranes in the kidney (Meister's cycle).
Gramicidin S	10	Cyclodecapeptide, an antibiotic effective against some Gram-positive and negative bacteria as well as some fungi.
Glucagon	29	Stimulates glycogenolysis, gluconeogenesis, lipolysis and reduces protein synthesis.
Kallidin	10	A bioactive kinin formed in response to injury from kininogen precursors through the action of kallikreins. It is converted to bradykinin by the aminopeptidase enzyme by removal of amino terminal lysine.
Leuenkephalin	5	Produces opioid effects, such as analgesia and mood elevation.
Metencephalin	5	Endogenous opioid peptide.
Microcystin		Cyclic peptide; hepatotoxic.
Nodularin	5	Potent hepatotoxin.
Oxytocin	9	Milk ejection from the lactating mammary glands, uterine contractions, during the second and third stage of labor.
Penicillin	3	Group of antibiotics derived from *Penicillium* fungi, e.g. benzylpenicillin (penicillin G), procaine benzylpenicillin (procaine penicillin), benzathine benzylpenicillin (benzathine penicillin), and phenoxymethylpenicillin (penicillin V).
Polymyxins		Cyclic, positively charged peptides, antibiotics. Used in the treatment of Gram-negative bacterial infections, relatively neurotoxic and nephrotoxic.
Secretin	27	Stimulates the release of watery bicarbonate-rich fluid from pancreatic and bile duct epithelium.
TRH	3	Thyrotropin-releasing hormone, stimulates TSH release in pituitary.
Vasopressin	9	Arginine vasopressin (AVP), or antidiuretic hormone (ADH), controls the reabsorption of water in the tubules of the kidney, causes vasoconstriction and hence increases BP.

many domains. These individual domains can be isolated by gentle proteolysis; they may retain not only their structure, but even their catalytic or other function like ligand binding. For example, the chaperone Hsc70 has three domains: an ATPase, a peptide-binding and a regulatory domain. Gentle treatment with chymotrypsin will digest the links between those domains. The isolated ATPase domain will still hydrolyse ATP.

Domains vary in length from about 25 amino acids to 500 amino acids. The shortest domains such as zinc fingers are stabilized by metal ions and disulfide bridges. Domains often form functional units, such as the calcium-binding EF hand domain of calmodulin.

Typical domain structures consist of hydrophobic cores with hydrophilic surfaces.

Individual domains often possess unique functional behaviours (for example, the ability to bind a particular ligand with high affinity and specificity), and an individual domain from a larger protein often expresses its unique function within the larger protein in which it is found. Multidomain proteins typically possess the sum total of functional properties and behaviours of their constituent domains.

The organisation of large proteins by structural domains represents an advantage for protein folding, with each domain being able to individually fold, accelerating the folding process and reducing a potentially large number of non-native or incorrect conformations.

One domain may appear in a variety of different proteins. Molecular evolution uses domains as building blocks and these may be recombined in different arrangements to create proteins with different functions. Thus, protein domains are nature's modular strategy for protein design. Further, as they are independently stable, domains can be "swapped" by genetic engineering between one protein and another to make chimeric proteins!

It is likely that proteins consisting of multiple domains (and thus multiple functions) evolved by the fusion of genes that once coded for separate proteins. Thus, evolution by gene duplication is very common and approximately 90% of domains in eukaryotes have been duplicated. Thus, the protein domain is a fundamental unit in evolution. Many proteins have been "assembled" by duplicating domains and then combining them in different ways. Fig. 2.15 shows the tertiary structures of nine domains that are frequently duplicated, and Fig. 2.16 presents several proteins that contain multiple copies of one or more of these domains.

Bioinformatic or computerized assessment of sequence and structural data from several million proteins in both protein and genome databases has shown that there is a relatively limited number of structurally distinct domains in proteins. According to their folding pattern, protein domains may be hierarchically classified into groups. One commonly used scheme is the **Structural Classification of Proteins (SCOP)** database (http://scop.mrc-lmb.cam.ac.uk/scop/) (Fig. 2.17).

The following taxa are used in SCOP:

Class

Coarse classification according to the relative content of α-helix and β-strand. Class is determined from the overall composition of secondary structure elements in a domain. Classes include:

- All-α proteins – which contain only α-helices, or where the content of β-strands is insignificant.
- All-β proteins – which contain only β-strands, or where the content of α-helices is insignificant.
- α/β proteins – which contain alternating or interspersed α-helices and β-strands. Mainly parallel β-sheets (beta-alpha-beta units).
- α + β proteins – which contain segregated α-helices and β-strands. Mainly antiparallel β-sheets.

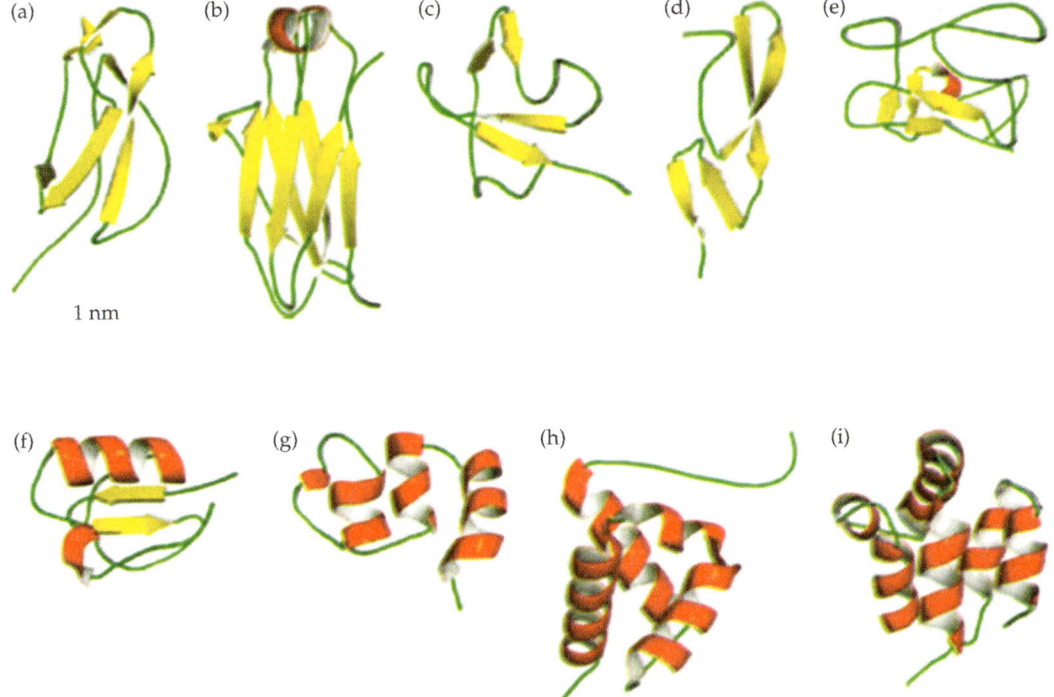

Fig. 2.15. Examples of some domains or modules: (a) Complement control protein module. (b) Immunoglobulin module. (c) Fibronectin type I module. (d) Growth factor module. (e) Kringle module. (f) GYF module. (g) γ-Carboxyglutamate module. (h) FF module. (i) DED domain.

- Multi-domain proteins – Folds consisting of two or more domains belonging to different classes.
- Membrane and cell surface proteins (excluding proteins from the immune system) – Usually the transmembrane domains are α-helical, but β-barrels may also occur.
- Small proteins – Usually dominated by metal ligand, haeme, and/or disulfide bridges.
- Coiled coil proteins – α-helices wound around each other.

All the classes together include 1086 types of folds, e.g. all-α protein class has 284 folds.

Fold

A fold describes the number, arrangement, and connections of various secondary structure elements. It describes a major structural similarity; the protein domains have identical secondary structure elements (at least in part) and the same 3D or topological connections. However, there may be considerable variation in peripheral regions of a domain. Similarities may arise from common origin or from convergent evolution. For example:

- **Rossman fold** – Structural motif/pattern found in proteins that bind nucleotides, especially the cofactor NAD.
- **Globin fold** – The globin fold is a common three-dimensional fold in proteins. This fold typically consists of eight alpha helices, although some proteins have additional helix extensions at their termini. The globin fold is found in proteins hemoglobin and myoglobin.

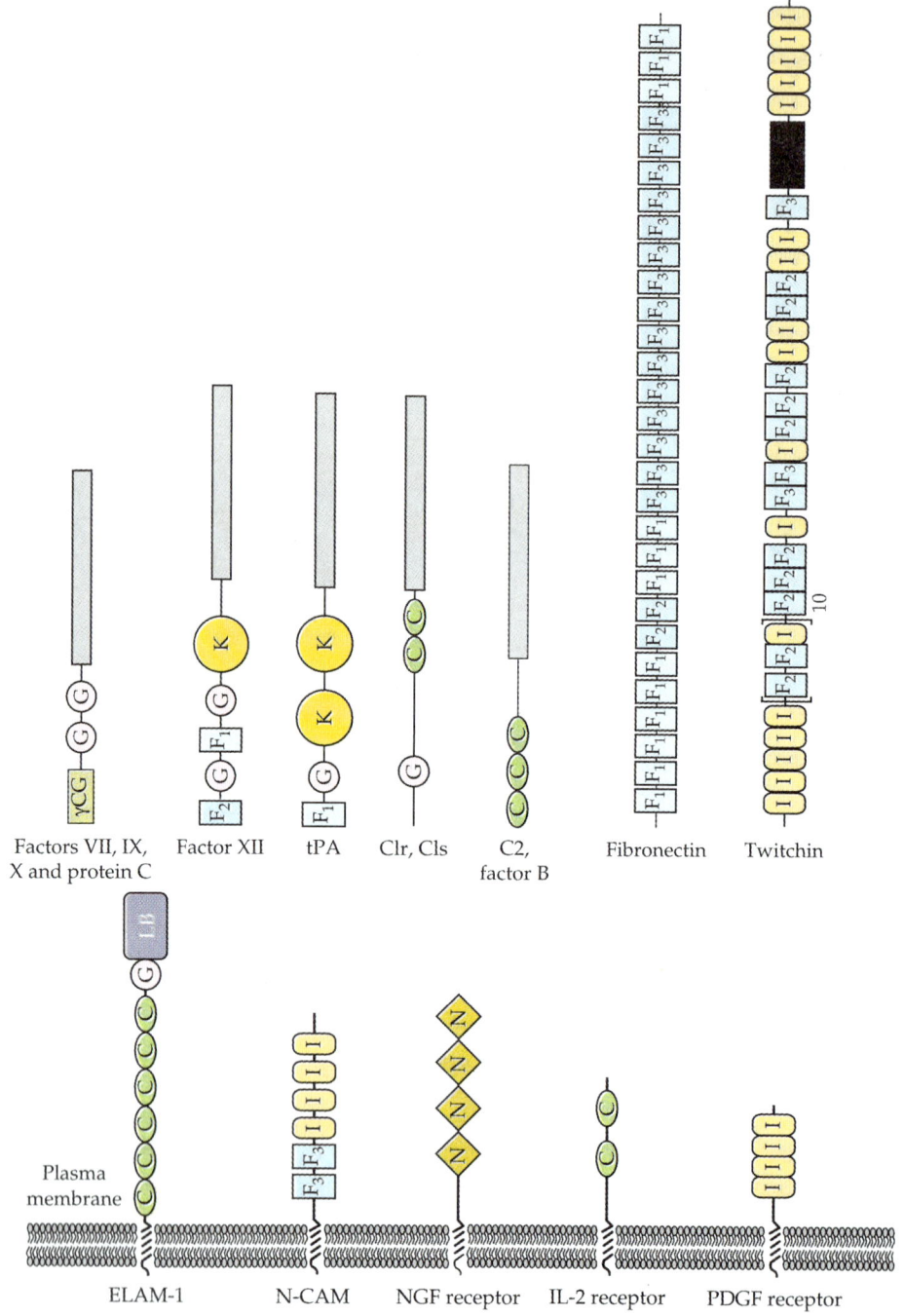

Fig. 2.16. Examples of some proteins made up of combination of individual domains. The domains are labelled as γCG – a module containing γ-carboxyglutamate residues; G – an epidermal growth factor-like module; K – the "kringle" domain; C – complement module; F_1, F_2, and F_3 – first found in fibronectin domains; I – immunoglobulin superfamily domain; LB – a lectin module found in some cell surface proteins, etc.

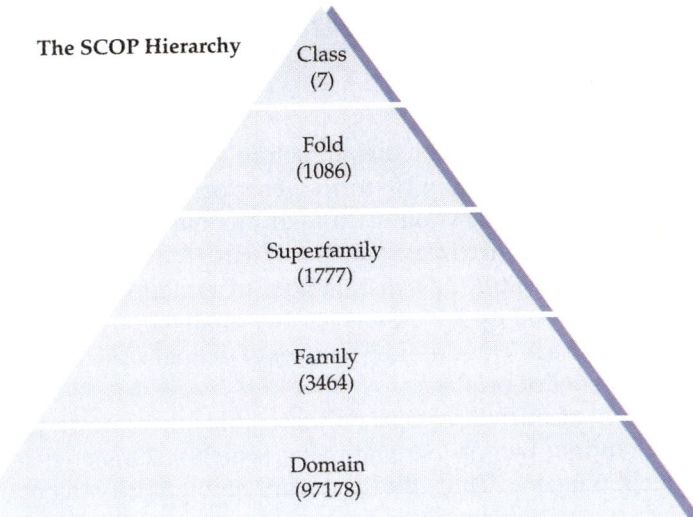

Fig. 2.17. SCOP classification: The Structural Classification of Proteins database. Protein domains are grouped into families, superfamilies, folds and classes in a hierarchical fashion according to structural and functional similarities.

- **Death fold** – Tertiary structure motif/pattern commonly found in proteins involved in apoptosis or inflammation-related processes. Death fold domains are an evolutionarily conserved superfamily of domains that mediate apoptotic signalling. Examples of death fold domains include the death domain (DD), death effector domain (DED), Caspase Recruitment Domain (CARD), and pyrin domain (PYD).

The 1086 folds together include 1777 superfamilies, e.g the globin fold has two superfamilies – the globin-like and the α-helical ferredoxin (containing two Fe4-S4 clusters).

Superfamily

A superfamily includes domains of similar folding pattern and usually similar functions, thus suggesting a common evolutionary ancestry. Domains of a superfamily have a common folding pattern and their functions are similar, but sequence identity may be low. The ATPase domains of actin, hexokinase and Hsc70 are an example for a superfamily. 1777 superfamilies together have 3464 families. For example, the globin-like superfamily has four families:

1. Truncated haemoglobin
2. Neural globin
3. Globins (heme binding proteins)
4. Phycocyanin-like proteins.

Family

A family usually includes domains with closely related amino acid sequences (in addition to folding similarities). Protein domains with high sequence homology (> 30% identity) and/or similar function are included. Proteins clearly have an evolutionary relationship. 3464 families together include 97178 domains. The domains are further divided into species, e.g. the globin (heme-binding proteins) family has 81 domains like legohemoglobin, haemoglobin α-chain, non-symbiotic plant haemoglobin, etc. Under each domain entry, like under the haemoglobin α-chain entry the Hb-α chains of all species are listed. The 3-D structure of all these domains is stored as PDB or protein database images. The images shown in Fig. 2.18 are examples of PDB images.

The number of protein domains in nature is large but limited and are depicted in Fig. 2.17. There are approximately 10^3 to 10^5 genes per organism and approximately 13.6 million species of living organisms on earth (and this latter number is likely an underestimate). Thus, there may be approximately ($10^3 \times 1.36 \times 10^7$) or 10^{10} to 10^{12} different proteins in all organisms on earth. Still, this vast number of proteins may consist of limited number of domains as shown in Fig. 2.17, a remarkably small number compared to the total number of protein coding genes. Thus, limited number of domains/modules are used as building blocks of the vast number of proteins.

Most newly identified proteins will resemble other known proteins and most structures can be broken into two or more domains, which resemble tertiary structures observed in other protein domains. Thus, the secondary and tertiary structure, possible functions and ligands of any newly identified protein sequence can often be predicted by identifying the possible domains and their comparison with known domains of proteins using computers without any experimentation – the field of Bioinformatics! It may not always tell the actual function but does narrow down possibilities saving lot of precious time and expenditures on the number of experiments required to find the 3D structure, protein–protein interactions and functions of newly sequenced/identified proteins.

Because structure depends on sequence, and because function depends on structure, proteins with similar sequences and/or similar structure should share a common function, but this is not always true in nature.

Homologous proteins – similar structure but different functions

The TIM barrel is a common protein fold consisting of eight α-helices and eight β-strands that alternate along the peptide backbone to form a doughnut-like tertiary structure. The TIM barrel is named for triose phosphate isomerase, an enzyme that interconverts ketone and aldehyde substrates in the breakdown of sugars. However, other TIM barrel proteins carry out very different functions, including the reduction of aldose sugars and hydrolysis of phosphate esters. These are homologous proteins having similar structure; they have evolved by gene duplications and have developed different functions by mutations during evolution.

Analogous proteins – different structures but similar functions

These are the proteins carrying out same function but having very different structures. For example, in Fig. 2.18, yeast aspartate aminotransferase and D-aminotransferase catalyse the same aminotransferase reaction, but they bear little structural similarity to each other.

Orthologous

'Same' protein in different species, e.g. cytochrome *c* of different species.

Paralogous

'Same' protein in same species – arise by gene duplication, e.g. beta globin proteins, embryonic, fetal and adult beta-globin proteins, two of these have arisen by gene duplication of the original beta globin gene.

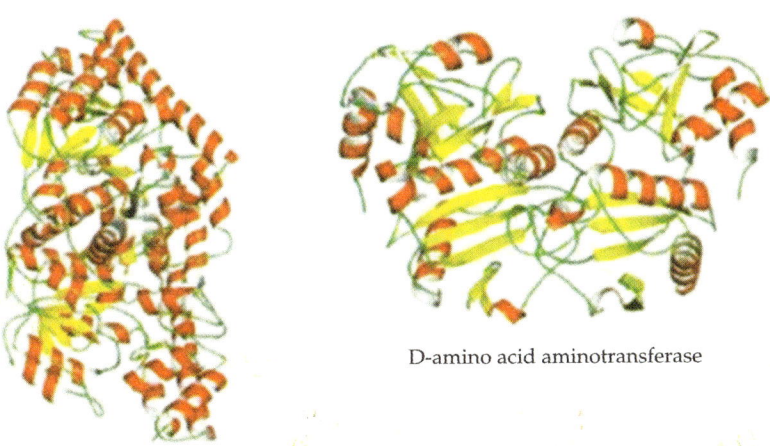

Fig. 2.18. (a) Homologous proteins – share similar structural features but carry out different functions (triose phosphate isomerase, aldose reductase, phosphotriesterase). (b) Analogous proteins – different structures but carrying out similar functions (yeast aspartate aminotransferase; D-amino acid aminotransferase).

Motifs (folding patterns found in many proteins) / Supersecondary structures

A motif is simply a recognizable folding pattern involving two or more elements of secondary structure and the connection(s) between them. The terms motif, and supersecondary structure are generally used interchangeably. A supersecondary structure is a compact three-dimensional protein structure of several adjacent secondary structure elements, that is smaller than a protein domain. Supersecondary structures can act as nucleation site centres in the process of protein folding.

A motif or supersecondary structure can be very simple, such as two elements of secondary structure folded against each other, example – a β-α-β loop. Or it can be a very complex and elaborate structure involving many secondary structure elements folded together, such as the β barrel. Motifs are much more stable during evolution than amino acid sequences. Some proteins can be shown to be homologous by their folding patterns, even though they no longer have significant similarity in their amino acid sequence (for example, the muscle protein actin, the enzyme hexokinase and the chaperone Hsc70).

Examples of motifs (Fig. 2.19)

- **Beta hairpin:** Extremely common. Two antiparallel beta strands connected by a tight turn of a few amino acids between them.
- **Greek key:** 4 beta strands folded over into a sandwich shape.
- **Omega loop:** A loop in which the residues that make up the beginning and end of the loop are very close together.
- **Helix-loop-helix:** Consists of alpha helices bound by a looping stretch of amino acids. This motif is seen in transcription factors.
- **Zinc finger:** Two beta strands with an alpha helix end folded over to bind a zinc ion. Important in DNA binding proteins.
- **Helix-turn-helix:** Two α-helices joined by a short strand of amino acids. Capable of binding to DNA and present in DNA-binding proteins.
- **Nest:** Extremely common. Just three consecutive amino acid residues form an anion-binding concavity.
- **Niche:** Extremely common. Just three consecutive amino acid residues form a cation-binding feature.

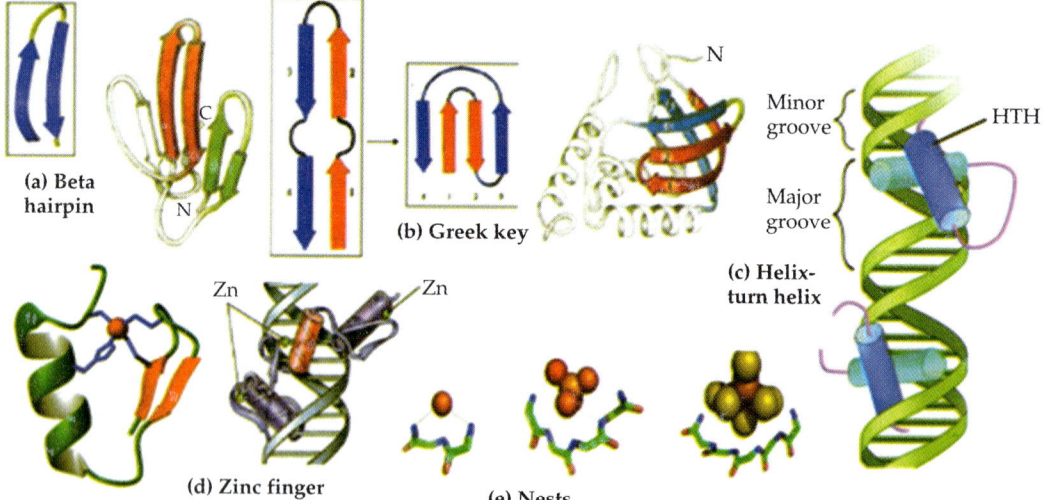

Fig. 2.19. Supersecondary structures or motifs. (a) Beta-Hairpin – beta-hairpin in the snake venom erabutoxin, (b) Greek Key – contained in a nuclease enzyme, (c) Helix-turn-helix binding to DNA, (d) Zinc finger and Zinc finger bound to DNA, (e) Nests – nest-bound to an oxygen atom; three overlapping nests belonging to a P-loop in the G-protein P21ras bound to a phosphate; four overlapping nests bound to an Fe_3S_4 centre in ferredoxin.

Q. 8. What is the physiological function of myoglobin?

Ans. Myoglobin was considered an O_2 storage protein in red muscle fibre. However, now its major physiological role is considered as to facilitate oxygen diffusion in muscles. Diffusion of O_2 from capillaries to tissue is limited due to its low solubility in blood (10^{-4} M). Myoglobin binds to O_2, acting as its carrier or a molecular bucket. Because of high affinity of Mb for O_2 and its hyperbolic O_2 dissociation curve it has P_{50} of 2.8 mmHg (Fig. 2.20). The pO_2 of blood varies from 100 mmHg in arteries to 30 mmHg in veins. Over this entire range Mb is almost fully saturated with O_2. Thus, it efficiently attracts O_2 from capillaries to muscle creating a strong gradient towards it. It efficiently relays O_2 from capillaries to muscle cells, boosting the diffusion of O_2 from capillaries to muscles.

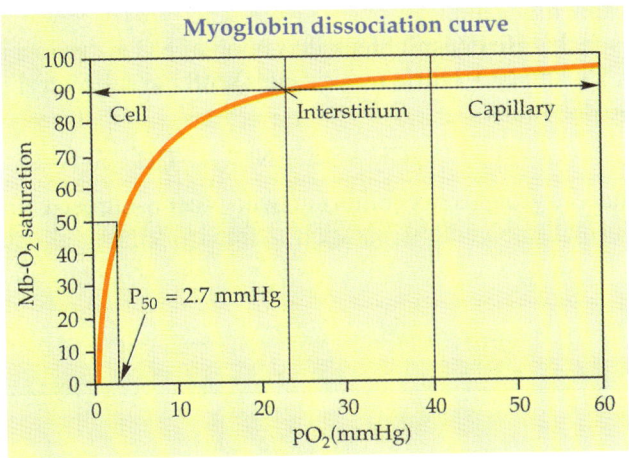

Fig. 2.20. Oxygen dissociation curve of myoglobin

The pO_2 in human quadriceps femoris working at 50–100% of capacity has pO_2 of 3.1 ± 0.4 mmHg, which is still higher than P_{50} of Mb. The oxygen storage function of Mb is significant probably only in aquatic animals like whales and seals who have muscle myoglobin concentration ten times higher than terrestrial animals. Mice with Mb gene knocked out are normal indicating that Mb is not essential for muscles under normal metabolic conditions either as store of O_2 or facilitator of diffusion. In human heart, left ventricle, depending on Mb concentration, Mb-facilitated O_2 transport maintains O_2 supply to the left ventricle wall during first 22–34 milliseconds of the total 150 milliseconds systole, while Mb storage function accounts for a further 12–17 milliseconds. When Mb is completely absent, anoxia begins to develop after 99–116 milliseconds. While Mb plays no significant role during diastole, it supplies O_2 to the left ventricular wall for ≤ 50 milliseconds of the total 150 milliseconds systole, whereas capillary haemoglobin is responsible for approximately 80 milliseconds. Slight increases in haemoglobin concentration, blood flow, or capillary density can compensate for the absence of Mb, a finding which agrees well with the observations using Mb knockout mice.

Neuroglobin, a myoglobin-like protein in brain, may be essential for boosting O_2 concentrations in neural tissues which are metabolically highly active. Forming only 2% mass of whole body they consume 20% of the body's oxygen supply.

Q. 9. Describe the role of haemoglobin in the action of nitric oxide.

Ans. Nitric oxide (NO) is a simple gaseous molecule with many physiological functions. These are:

- Neurotransmitter.
- Second messenger in signal transduction.
- Acts as the endothelial relaxing factor (ERF, also known as endothelium-derived relaxing factor, or EDRF), it acts to relax the musculature of the walls of blood vessels and lower blood pressure acting through cGMP as second messenger.

NO is a high-affinity ligand for Hb, binding to its heme-Fe^{2+} atom with an affinity 10,000 times greater than that of O_2. Still Hb does not prevent its action and rather acts as the carrier of this unstable molecule.

The reason that Hb doesn't block the action of NO is due to a unique interaction between Cys 93β of Hb and NO. Nitric oxide reacts with the sulfhydryl group of Cys 93β, forming an S-nitroso derivative.

$$-CH_2-SH + NO \rightarrow -CH_2-S-N=O$$

This S-nitroso group is in equilibrium with other S-nitroso compounds formed by reaction of NO with small-molecule thiols such as free cysteine or glutathione.

$$H_3^+N-\underset{COO^-}{CH}-CH_2-CH_2-\underset{O}{\overset{\|}{C}}-NH-\underset{\underset{N=O}{|}}{\underset{S}{|}}{\underset{CH_2}{|}}{CH}-\overset{O}{\overset{\|}{C}}-NH-CH_2-COO^-$$

S-nitrosoglutathione

These small-molecule thiols serve to transfer NO from erythrocytes to endothelial receptors, where it acts to relax vascular tone. NO itself is a reactive free-radical compound whose biological half-life is very short (1–5 sec). S-nitrosoglutathione and Hb-NO have a half-life of several hours.

The reactions between Hb and NO are complex. NO forms a ligand with the heme-Fe^{2+} that is quite stable in the absence of O_2. However, in the presence of O_2, NO is oxidized to NO_3^- and the heme-Fe^{2+} of Hb is oxidized to Fe^{3+}, forming methemoglobin. The interaction of Hb with NO is controlled by the allosteric transition between R-state Hb (oxyHb) and T-state Hb (deoxyHb). Cys 93β is more exposed and reactive in R-state Hb than in T-state Hb, and binding of NO to Cys 93β prevents reaction of NO with heme iron and oxygen to form methemoglobin.

Upon release of O_2 from Hb in tissues, Hb shifts conformation from R state to T state, and binding of NO at Cys 93β is no longer favoured. Consequently, NO is released from Cys 93β and transferred to small-molecule thiols for delivery to endothelial receptors, causing capillary vasodilation. In the T state O_2 is absent preventing the conversion of NO to NO_3^- and subsequent methemoglobin formation. In the T state NO is bound to the Fe^{2+} as Hb-NO.

This mechanism also explains the puzzling observation that free Hb produced by recombinant DNA methodology for use as a whole-blood substitute causes a transient rise of 10–12 mmHg in diastolic blood pressure in experimental clinical trials. The synthetic Hb (which has no bound NO) binds the NO present in the blood, blocking its vasoregulatory function.

During hemoglobin evolution, the only invariant/unchanged amino acid residues in globin chains are His F8 (the obligatory heme ligand) and a Phe residue helping to wedge the heme into its pocket. However, in mammals and birds, Cys 93β is also invariant, due to its vital role in NO delivery.

NO is bound as Hb-NO (HbFe^{2+}-NO) in T state and is transferred to Cys 93β in R (oxy Hb) state by allosteric transfer. NO bound to Cys 93β in R state (SNO-Hb) inhibits polymerization of HbS in sickle cell disease patients by stabilizing R state Hb. Hydroxyurea which acts by increasing HbF in long term is beneficial in sickle cell disease in short term by increasing NO levels 30–1. SNO-Hb decreases HbS polymerization even at high concentrations of HbS, while also leading to vasodilatation and increased oxygen affinity, beneficial in sickle cell disease. HbNympheas (Cys 93β → Ser mutation) produced artificially by site directed mutagenesis shows slightly increased oxygen affinity, decreased co-operativity and slightly reduced alkaline Bohr effect.

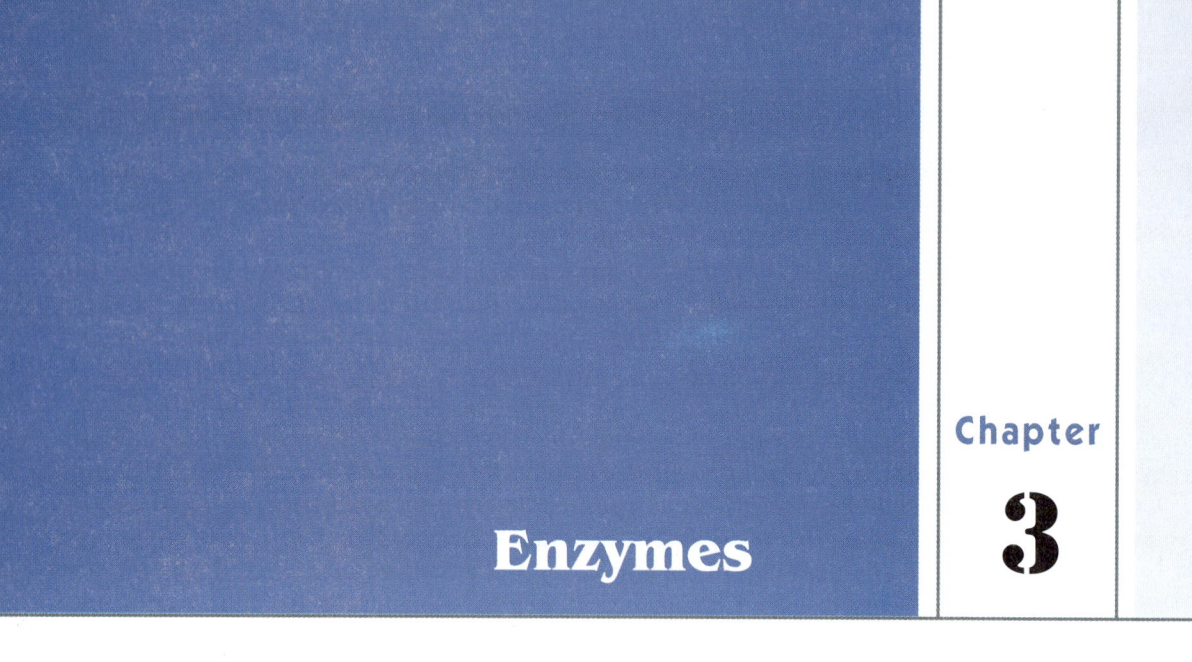

Chapter 3

Enzymes

Q. 1. Identify the correct pairs and describe enzyme classification.

1. DNA polymerase   a. oxidoreductase
2. Hydratase   b. transferase
3. Aminopeptidase   c. hydrolase
4. Helicase   d. lyase
5. Topoisomerases   e. isomerase
6. 21-Hydroxylase   f. ligase

Ans. 1-b, 2-d, 3-c, 4-c, 5-e, 6-a

Enzyme classification

1. **Oxidoreductases:** Catalyse oxidations and reductions; include oxidases, dehydrogenases, hydroperoxidases, oxygenases (mono- and dioxygenase), superoxide dismutase.
2. **Transferases:** Catalyse transfer of functional group or a part of one molecule like moieties such as glycosyl, methyl, or phosphoryl groups from donor to acceptor. DNA polymerase transfers the base-sugar-P moiety from a nucleotide (base-sugar-P-P-P) to the 3′ phosphate end of growing DNA.
3. **Hydrolases:** Catalyse *hydrolytic* cleavage of C—C, C—O, C—N, and other bonds, or break bonds by addition of water (H and OH).
4. **Lyases:** Catalyse cleavage of C—C, C—O, C—N, and other bonds by atom *elimination*, leaving double bonds). In other words they break bonds by means other than hydrolysis and oxidation. Dehydratases (or hydratase in reverse direction) remove H and OH atoms producing double bonds. E.g. fumarase, enoyl CoA hydratase, aldolase, decarboxylase. Lyases (often also referred to as "synthases") can also catalyse reactions involving either the cleavage or formation of chemical bonds without use of ATP (adenylyl cyclase, enolase, citrate synthase, glycogen synthase, ALA synthase).
5. **Isomerases:** Catalyse geometric or structural changes within a molecule.
6. **Ligases:** Catalyse the joining together of two molecules with the use of ATP; are thus synthetases.

Q. 2. Differentiate between co-factor, co-enzyme and prosthetic group.

Ans. Prosthetic groups are tightly and stably incorporated into protein's structure by covalent or non-covalent forces. Can be removed by denaturation only. May be organic like heme, PLP, TPP, FMN, FAD or inorganic metal ions like Co, Cu, Mn, Zn. Enzymes with metal ions as prosthetic groups are called metalloenzymes.

Co-factors serve functions similar to prosthetic groups but are present freely in solution and not tightly bound to the enzymes. Enzymes that require metal ion in solution as co-factor are called metal-activated enzymes.

Role of metal ions as prosthetic group or co-factors

- As super acids: Stronger than H^+, introduce positive charge into substrate or accept negative charge, interact with substrates to render them more electrophilic (electron-poor) or nucleophilic (electron-rich).
- As template: Coordinate more than 2 ligands, can bring them together. Metals also may facilitate the binding and orientation of substrates by the formation of covalent bonds with reaction intermediates (Co^{2+} in coenzyme B_{12}).
- As redox catalysts: Accept/donate electrons. Metal ions that participate in redox reactions generally are complexed to prosthetic groups such as heme or iron-sulfur clusters.

Coenzymes: Function of cofactor and prosthetic groups is similar while co-enzymes are group transfer agents/substrate shuttles. E.g. NADH for H, coenzyme A for acetate, folate for methyl, dolichol for oligosaccharides. Cofactors and prosthetic groups are regenerated in the same catalytic cycle while coenzymes are regenerated in another reaction by another enzyme elsewhere and, thus, can also be called co-substrates. Co-enzymes are recyclable shuttles moving substrates from one part of a cell to another. They also facilitate recognition and binding of small chemical groups like acetate and stabilize the reactive hydrogen atoms or hydride ions. NADH and NADPH act as carriers of H^+ in a cell.

Q. 3. Enumerate various mechanisms of catalysis.

Ans. Catalysis can occur by:
A. Proximity
B. Strain
C. Acid base catalysis
D. Covalent catalysis

Q. 4. Differentiate between general and specific acid-base catalysis.

Ans. Acid base catalysis involves transfer (addition/removal) of protons.

Specific acid base catalysis: Proton is transferred from the protonated solvent (H_3O^+). Proton from solvent diffuses into active site, hence reaction is affected by change in pH of medium. Water is proton donor or acceptor. Proton is transferred before the slow step of reaction involving the transition state. Occurs in strong acidic medium and hence not affected by concentration of other weak acids or buffers.

General acid base catalysis: Proton is transferred during the transition state from a proton donor or acceptor. Ionisable buffer molecule present in solution or at active site of enzyme transfers or accepts proton. As proton is transferred by an ionisable acid/base other than the H^+ of the medium (water) it is affected by all acid or bases or buffers present, so affected by pH as well by buffer concentrations. E.g. Carbonic anhydrase, serine proteases – trypsin, chymotrypsin, elastase, thrombin, plasmin, TPA, serine proteases (have mixture of covalent and general acid catalysis), aspartate proteases – pepsin, renin, HIV protease.

Q. 5. Give examples of enzyme functioning by covalent catalysis.

Ans.
1. Chymotrypsin
2. Fructose-2,6-bisphosphatase
3. Transaminases

Q. 6. Differentiate between Fischer's 'lock and key model' and Koshland's 'induced fit model' of enzyme action.

Ans. According to Fischer's 'lock and key model' enzyme and substrate have rigid complementary structure like a key and lock and as each lock fits only one key each enzyme acts on a specific substrate. However, Koshland's model is more dynamic model which says that approach and binding of substrate induces conformational change in enzyme like a hand introduces in a glove and makes the enzyme bind specifically to the substrate. By allowing conformational change it explains the mechanism of catalysis like catalysis by strain which cannot be justified by Fischer's model (Fig. 3.1).

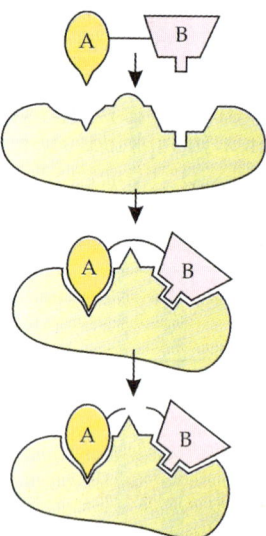

Fig. 3.1. Koshland's induced fit model of enzyme action.

Q. 7. What are conserved residues in enzymes?

Ans. Conserved residues are specific amino acids at similar positions in different enzymes having similar function in terms of binding to similar substrates or having similar catalytic action. These are usually present at the active sites or sites of substrate binding. For example, all aspartate proteases (pepsins, cathepsins, renin, etc.) have a highly conserved sequence of

Asp-Thr-Gly at active site. They have two highly conserved aspartates in the active site. They are optimally active at acidic pH (use general acid catalysis) and tend to clone dipeptide bonds that have hydrophobic amino acids as well as a beta-methylene group.

Q. 8. How can enzymes be used to measure blood glucose in lab?

Ans. Glucose-6-phosphate dehydrogenase converts glucose-6-phosphate to 6-phosphogluconolactone and simultaneously converts NADP to NADPH (Fig. 3.2). NADPH absorbs light at 340 nm and its rate of production is proportional to glucose concentration and is measured. All substrates besides glucose and enzymes are taken in large excess in reagent to ensure that only glucose concentration is the limiting factor to determine rate of reaction which is measured by measuring rate of NADPH production.

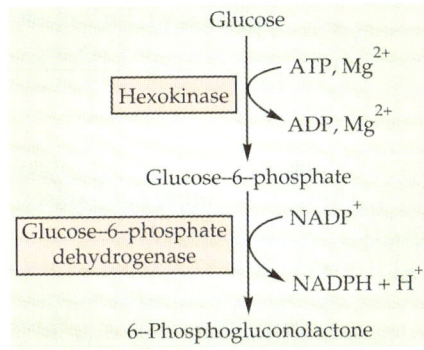

Fig. 3.2. Reactions used for measurement of glucose.

Q. 9. Give examples of functional enzymes of blood.

Ans.
1. LCAT
2. Lipoprotein lipase
3. Pseudocholinesterase

Q. 10. How is measurement of levels of non-functional enzymes of blood useful?

Ans. Non-functional enzymes and proteins of blood enter blood from broken or dead cells in which they are normally present. Thus, they are markers of death or injury of particular cells. Increased levels are diagnostic of injury or diseases in their parent or source tissue. Levels depend on magnitude of cell damage in the tissue containing the enzyme as well as the rate of removal from blood by kidney and proteolytic destruction. Some of the common non-functional plasma enzymes and their diagnostic uses are given in Table 3.1.

Q. 11. What are ribozymes? Give examples of ribozymes.

Ans. While enzymes are usually proteins by nature, some rRNAs also possess catalytic properties. These are called ribozymes. Examples of ribozymes are:
1. Peptidyl transferase
2. Hepatitis delta virus RNA
3. Hammerhead
4. SNURPS

Table 3.1. Non-functional enzymes in blood and their diagnostic uses

Serum Enzyme	Major Diagnostic Use
Aminotransferases	
• Aspartate aminotransferase (AST, or SGOT)	Myocardial infarction
• Alanine aminotransferase (ALT, or SGPT)	Viral hepatitis
Amylase	Acute pancreatitis
Ceruloplasmin	Hepatolenticular degeneration (Wilson's disease)
Creatine kinase	Muscle disorders and myocardial infarction
γ-Glutamyl transferase	Various liver diseases
Lactate dehydrogenase isozyme 5	Liver diseases
Lipase	Acute pancreatitis
Phosphatase, acid	Metastatic carcinoma of the prostate
Phosphatase, alkaline (isozymes)	Various bone disorders, obstructive liver diseases

Q. 12. What are irreversible and reversible reactions?

Ans. Irreversible reactions are those in which at equilibrium the product concentration >>>> substrate concentration. Thus, the equilibrium constant (K_{eq} = [P] / [S]) is very large for irreversible reactions. K_{eq} for reversible reactions is closer to 1. Enzymes cannot make reactions reversible or irreversible as enzymes cannot alter K_{eq}, the equilibrium constant.

Q. 13. How reactions can become functionally irreversible under physiological conditions?

Ans. Reactions (including reversible reactions) can be made 'functionally irreversible' in body. Functionally irreversible reactions are those which appear to be occurring in only one direction in the body. This can be achieved by rapid removal of product by a subsequent reaction, which prevents the reverse reaction. Thus, they occur in non-equilibrium condition and equilibrium is never reached.

Q. 14. What is the relation between ΔG, K_{eq} and speed of reaction?

Ans. For a reaction, A + B ↔ C + D.

$$K_{eq} = C \times D / A \times B$$
$$\Delta G^0 = - RT \ln K_{eq}$$

Thermodynamics, free energy change and K_{eq} do not affect rate or speed of reactions and enzymes cannot alter thermodynamics, free energy change and K_{eq}. Reactions are 'irreversible' due to large K_{eq} or large negative ΔG. $\Delta G^0 = - RT \ln K_{eq}$ describes relation between ΔG and K_{eq}.

Q. 15. What are the factors on which reaction rate depends?

Ans. Rate of reactions depends on:

1. Concentration of reactants and products
2. Temperature
3. Presence of enzymes

Q. 16. Describe how changes in temperature affect rate of enzyme catalysed reaction.

Ans. Increasing the temperature increases collision force and frequency between substrates and enzymes increasing the rate of reaction. But high temperature can decrease rate by denaturing protein enzymes. Most enzymes have optimal temperature of action at 37°C. Increasing the temperature from lower temperatures till 42°C increases the reaction rate. Beyond 45–50°C rate decreases due to denaturation of enzymes.

Q. 17. How change in pH can affect rate of enzyme catalysed reactions?

Ans. pH can affect reaction rate by:
1. Denaturing enzymes
2. Altering charge of substrate
3. Altering charge of active site amino acids

The rate of almost all enzyme-catalysed reactions exhibits a significant dependence on hydrogen ion concentration. Most intracellular enzymes exhibit optimal activity at pH values between 5 and 9 (Fig. 3.3). For enzymes whose mechanism involves acid-base catalysis, the residues involved must be in the appropriate state of protonation for the reaction to proceed. The binding and recognition of substrate molecules with dissociable groups also typically involves the formation of salt bridges with the enzyme. The most common charged groups are carboxylate groups (negative) and protonated amines (positive). Gain or loss of critical charged groups adversely affects substrate binding and thus will retard or abolish catalysis.

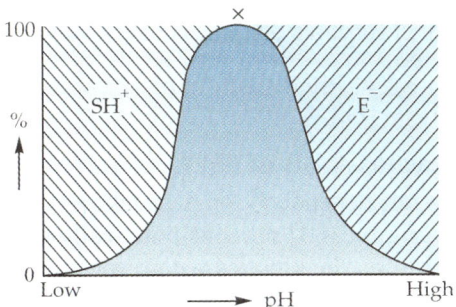

Fig. 3.3. Effect of pH on enzyme activity.

Q. 18. Why is the V_i or the initial rate/velocity of reaction used to study effect of substrate concentration on enzyme activity?

Ans. For a reaction A + B ↔ P, reaction rate can be measured as rate of disappearance of A or appearance of P on addition or mixing of the substrates A and B. With the elapse of time the rate of forward reaction decreases as concentration of A and B decreases and rate of reverse reaction increases. When equilibrium is reached, rates of forward and reverse reactions become same and rate of disappearance of A or appearance of P becomes 0! (Fig. 3.4). To study the dependence of reaction rate (forward reaction) on [A] measurements of the rates of enzyme-catalyzed reactions use relatively short time periods, conditions that approximate initial rate conditions. Under these conditions, only traces of product accumulate, making the rate of the reverse reaction negligible. Hence, rate of production of P or disappearance of

A in the initial period over which V_i is measured is not affected by the reverse reaction. The initial velocity (V_i) of the reaction thus is essentially that of the rate of the forward reaction. Then a graph of V_i versus [A] is plotted. If measured over longer period when backward reaction becomes significant the rate of disappearance of A will be affected by both forward and backward reaction and rates of forward and backward reaction cannot be measured separately.

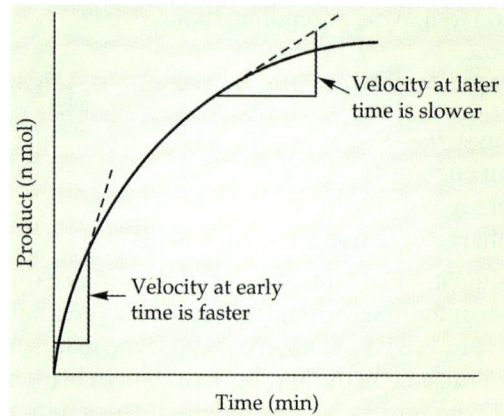

Fig. 3.4. Measurement of Vi: The velocity is not necessarily the same at all times after you start the reaction. The depletion of substrate, inhibition by the product, or instability of the enzyme can cause the velocity to change with time. The initial velocity is measured early, before the velocity changes. Initial velocity measurements also lets you assume that the amount of substrate has not changed and is equal to the amount of substrate that was added.

Q. 19. Describe how can we study the effect of substrate concentration on reaction rate of a multi-substrate reaction.

Ans. For example, the reaction A + B ↔ C + D.

To study reaction rate dependence on A we take [B] >>>>> [A] so that when V_i is measured change in [B] is negligible, [B] remains practically constant and rate effectively becomes k × [A]. In the laboratory, the kinetics with respect to a particular reactant (A in this case), referred to as the variable reactant or substrate, can be determined by maintaining the concentration of the other reactants constant by taking concentrations in large excess over the variable reactant. Then the rate is effectively dependent on [A] only and the reaction is called pseudo-first-order. The concentration of the fixed reactant(s) remains virtually constant. The rate of reaction will depend exclusively on the concentration of the variable reactant, sometimes also called the limiting reactant. Under pseudo-first-order conditions the behaviour of a multisubstrate enzyme will be like one having a single substrate.

Q. 20. Enumerate the different types of graphs used to study the relation of V_i versus substrate concentration.

Ans.
1. Michaelis–Menten equation (Vi vs. [S]) (Fig. 3.5)
2. Lineweaver–Burk plot (1/v vs. 1/[S])
3. Hanes equation ([S]/v vs. [S])
4. Eadie–Hofstee equation (v vs. v/[S])
5. Hill equation (for allosteric enzymes) (Fig. 3.6)

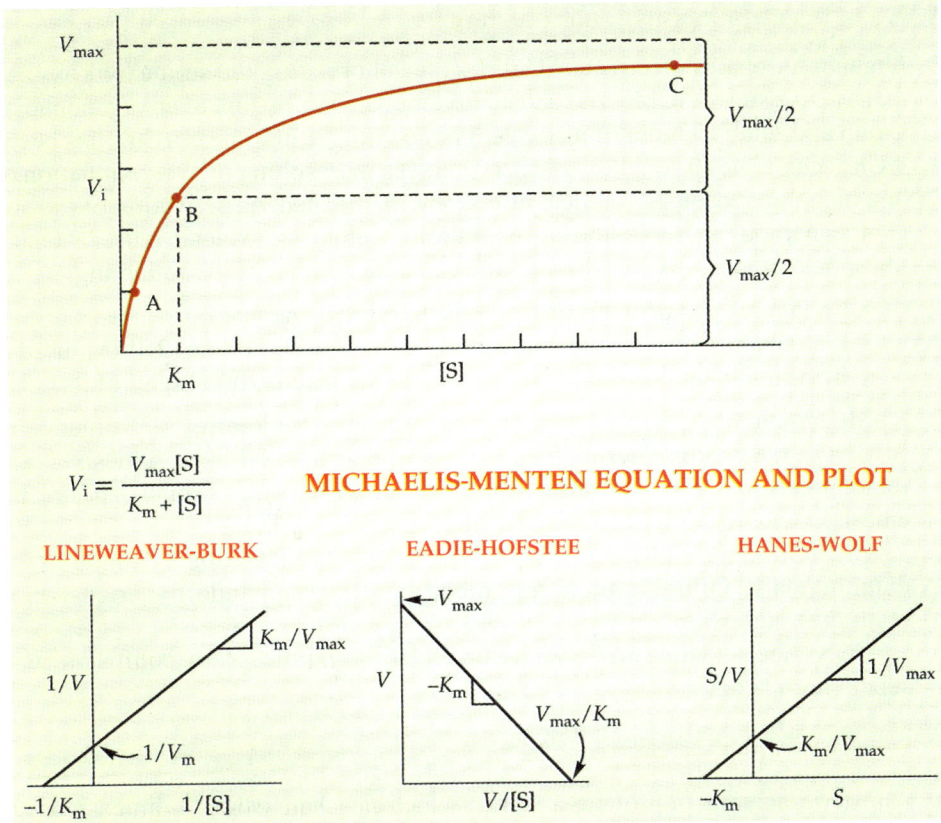

Fig. 3.5. Linear alternatives of Michaelis–Menten equation and plot.

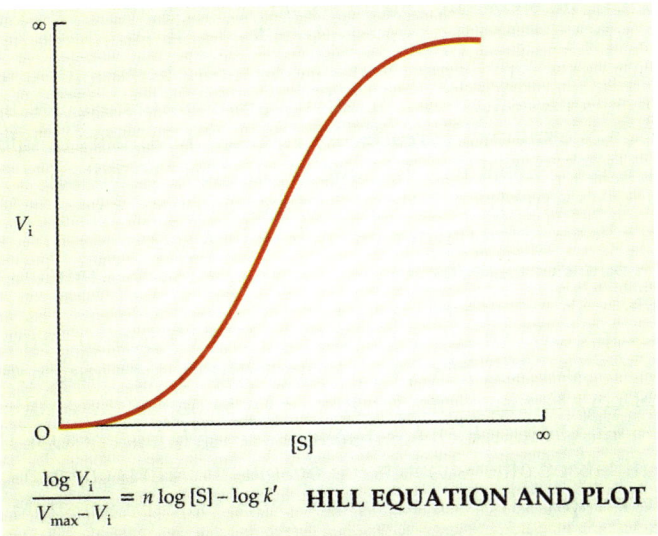

Fig. 3.6. Hill equation and plot.

Q. 21. Describe organophosphate poisoning.

Ans. Organophosphates inactivate AChE by phosphorylating the serine hydroxyl group located at the active site of AChE. The phosphorylation occurs by loss of an organophosphate leaving group and establishment of a covalent bond with AChE. Once AChE has been inactivated, ACh accumulates throughout the nervous system, resulting in overstimulation of muscarinic and nicotinic receptors. Clinical effects are manifested via activation of the autonomic and central nervous systems and at nicotinic receptors on skeletal muscle. Once an organo-phosphate binds to AChE, the enzyme can undergo one of the following:

- Endogenous hydrolysis of the phosphorylated enzyme by esterases or paraoxonases.
- Reactivation by a strong nucleophile such as pralidoxime (2-PAM, used as antidote).
- Irreversible binding and permanent enzyme inactivation (ageing).

Mnemonic devices used to remember the muscarinic effects of organophosphates are SLUDGE (salivation, lacrimation, urination, diarrhea, GI upset, emesis) and DUMBELS (diaphoresis and diarrhea; urination; miosis; bradycardia, bronchospasm, bronchorrhea; emesis; excess lacrimation; and salivation).

Nicotinic signs and symptoms include muscle fasciculations, cramping, weakness, and diaphragmatic failure. Autonomic nicotinic effects include hypertension, tachycardia, mydriasis, and pallor.

CNS effects include anxiety, emotional lability, restlessness, confusion, ataxia, tremors, seizures, and coma.

Q. 22. What are allosteric enzymes?

Ans. Allosteric enzymes or proteins are those which can change their 3-dimensional conformation on binding an effector molecule or modulator and the conformational change modifies the affinity of the enzyme/protein for its main substrate or ligand or its activity. This "action at a distance" or "allostery" i.e. binding of a modulator affecting affinity at a separate binding site is the essence of the allosteric concept. The modulator binds at the 'allosteric site'. Such enzymes are usually multimeric i.e. having multiple subunits or domains coupled to each other. The subunits show co-operativity amongst themselves as the binding of ligand/modulator on one subunit increases or decreases the affinity of interaction of other subunits with their ligands/substrates. Binding of allosteric modulator can affect enzyme activity positively or negatively. Allosteric enzymes can be K-class or V-class based on whether binding of allosteric modulator changes only K_m or V_{max}. In some enzymes binding of allosteric modulator changes both K_m and V_{max}. Allosteric modulators can be homotropic or heterotropic.

Homotropic: When the substrate/ligand itself acts as a modulator (i.e. ligand and modulator are same), it increases binding affinity for substrate/ligand on other subunits (positive effect). For example, binding of O_2 to one of the 4 subunits increases affinity of others in haemoglobin which has 4 subunits (each binds one O_2). Binding of 2nd O_2 further increases affinity on other subunits (co-operativity). Hb is one non-enzyme allosteric protein.

In **heterotropic effect**, a modulator other than the substrate positively or negatively affects binding of enzyme and substrate. For example, feedback inhibition of hexokinase by Glu-6P.

Biochemical basis for co-operativity: Each subunit exists in a conformational state that has either a low affinity (T or tense state) or a high affinity (R or relaxed state) for substrate. The T and R states coexist in the absence of substrate. An effector that binds preferentially to the T state decreases the already low concentration of the R state and makes it even more difficult for the substrate to bind. These effectors decrease the velocity of the overall reaction and are referred to as allosteric inhibitors (Fig. 3.7). An example is the effect of ATP or citrate on the activity of phosphofructokinase. Effectors that bind specifically to the R state shift the T–R equilibrium toward the more active (higher-affinity) R state. Now all the sites are of the high-affinity R type, even before the first substrate binds. Effectors that bind to the R state increase the activity (decrease the $S_{0.5}$) and are known as allosteric activators. An example is the effect of AMP on the velocity of the phosphofructokinase reaction.

Because of co-operativity such proteins/enzymes do not follow normal Michaelis–Menten kinetics, rather display a sigmoidal dependence on the concentration of their substrates in positively cooperative systems (Fig. 3.8). Enzymes that are positively cooperative are very sensitive to changes of substrate near the $S_{0.5}$ (concentration at half max velocity). This makes the enzyme behave more like an on–off switch and is useful metabolically to provide a large change in velocity in response to a small change in substrate concentration. In the presence of an allosteric activator, the v versus [S] plot looks more hyperbolic and less sigmoidal – consistent with shifting the enzyme to all R-type active sites (Fig. 3.9).

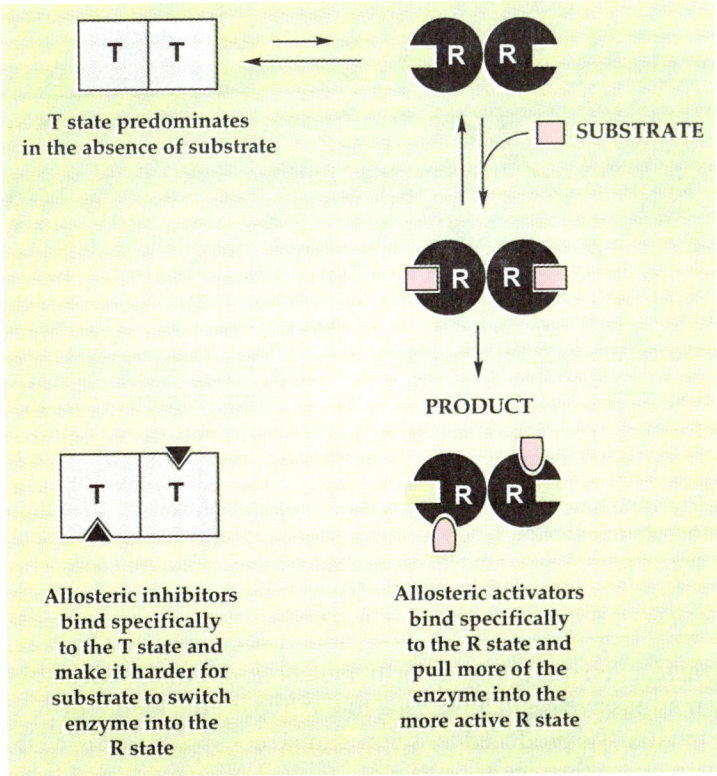

Fig. 3.7. Biochemical basis of co-operativity.

Hemoglobin and aspartate carbamoyltransferase (ATCase) are classical examples of allosteric protein and enzyme. Ribonucleoside diphosphate reductase and pyruvate UDP N-acetylglucosamine transferase are examples of exceptional allosteric enzymes which are monomeric (only 1 subunit).

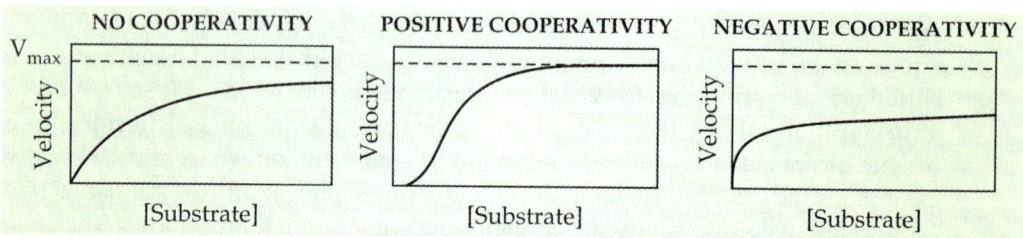

Fig. 3.8. Co-operative enzymes do not show a hyperbolic dependence of the velocity on substrate concentration. If the binding of one substrate increases the affinity of an oligomeric enzyme for binding of the next substrate, the enzyme shows positive co-operativity. If the first substrate makes it harder to bind the second substrate, the enzyme is negatively co-operative.

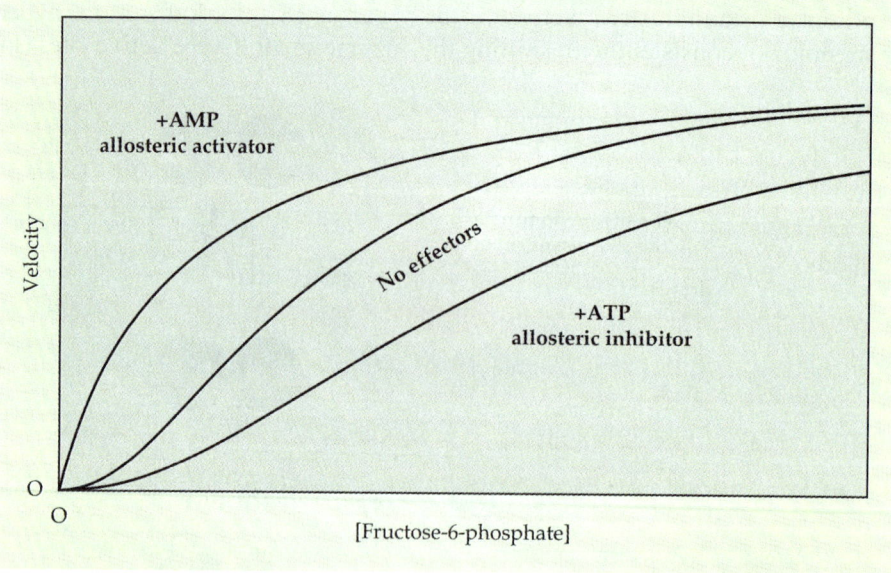

Fig. 3.9. Phosphofructokinase shows positive co-operativity with fructose-6-phosphate as the substrate. ATP, an allosteric inhibitor, binds to the T state and decreases the velocity. AMP, a signal for low energy, binds to the R state and increases the velocity of the reaction.

Q. 23. What is passive regulation of enzyme activity?

Ans. Change in reaction rate or regulation of metabolic enzymes activity by substrate concentration is known as passive regulation. Due to the hyperbolic nature of V_i vs [S] curve, maximum change in V (ΔV) is produced for same change in [S] (ΔS) when [S] is near K_m. The K_m value of most enzymes thus tends to be close to their average intracellular concentration of their substrate in a cell making passive regulation a significant process (Fig. 3.10).

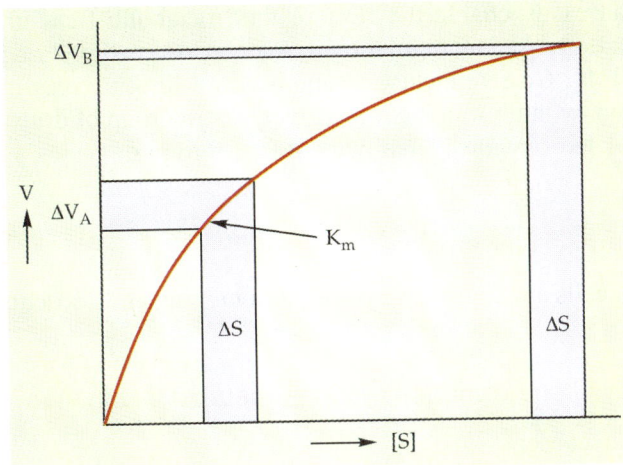

Fig. 3.10. Curve showing V_i vs [S] relation. Change in ∆V is much greater for same ∆S when [S] is near the K_m.

Q. 24. Why metabolite flow in most metabolic pathways tends to be unidirectional?

Ans. This is because few reactions have very large negative ∆G, making them irreversible. They pull the whole pathway in one direction making the net ∆G of the complete pathway sufficiently negative.

For example, in the following pathway:

A → B ↔ C ↔ D ↔ E → F ↔ G

A → B and E → F make the whole pathway unidirectional acting as valves. These reactions are irreversible as they have large negative ∆G.

Q. 25. How can compartmentation/separation of anabolic and catabolic pathways involving same metabolites be achieved?

Ans. Compartmentalization can be achieved by:
1. Different subcellular locations.
2. Segregation of pathways in different specialized cells.
3. Use of NADH and NADPH for alternative pathways.
4. Presence of one or more unique intermediates and enzymes.

Fatty acid biosynthesis from acetyl CoA occurs in cytosol and oxidation to acetyl CoA occurs in mitochondria. Biosynthetic pathways use NADPH and catabolism produces NADH. Glycolysis and gluconeogenesis proceed via few different steps and intermediates (the three most energetically disfavoured steps of glycolysis are replaced by new reactions). Gluconeogenesis enzymes are present only in liver and kidney cells while glycolysis enzymes are present in all cells. This helps to regulate anabolism and catabolism to occur at different times or places and avoid futile cycles.

Q. 26. What is rate limiting enzyme of a pathway?

Ans. Rate limiting enzyme is the slowest step in a pathway due to low enzyme levels or low catalytic efficiency or both. It acts as a bottleneck or checkpost causing traffic jam. Regulating this step can easily enable the flow or the 'metabolic flux' in the whole pathway to be increased or decreased by regulating it. Acetyl CoA carboxylase in fatty acid synthesis is an example. HMG CoA reductase is another rate limiting enzyme involved in cholesterol synthesis and by inhibiting it competitively statin group of drugs can effectively inhibit the whole cholesterol synthesis pathway. Rate limiting enzymes are thus very efficient drug targets.

Q. 27. How are intracellular enzymes degraded?

Ans. Enzymes in cells are degraded by ubiquitin tagging and subsequent degradation in proteasomes.

Q. 28. In what ways can hormones regulate metabolic enzymes?

Ans. Hormone can cause:
- Covalent modification: Phosphorylation by protein kinase
- Allosteric regulation: By second messengers like Ca^{2+}, etc.
- Induction and repression at genetic level.

Q. 29. Give examples of different covalent modifications that can regulate enzyme activity.

Ans. Methylation, acetylation, ADP-ribosylation, phosphorylation are reversible and partial proteolysis is irreversible covalent modification used to regulate enzyme activity.

Q. 30. What are the advantages of activation by selective proteolysis of pro-enzyme?

Ans. Advantages are:
1. Used when enzymes are required intermittently but rapidly.
2. Provides very rapid response required in conditions such as clotting.
3. Digestive enzymes can be stored in harmless forms.

Q. 31. What are the advantages of covalent modification by phosphorylation?

Ans.
1. Allows hormonal and neural control.
2. Once need has passed enzyme can be converted back to original inactive form.
3. Phosphoryl group have high tendency to form salt bridges.
4. Enables control of same enzyme by different stimuli/signals.
5. Multiple enzymes/pathways can be regulated together.

Covalent modification allows hormonal and neural control. Once need has passed enzyme can be converted back to original form. High charge density of phosphoryl group (–2 at physiological pH) and their tendency to form salt bridges with arginyl and lysyl residues help them alter protein conformation and hence catalytic activity of enzymes. Phosphorylation can be done by multiple kinases on same enzyme and at multiple sites enabling control of same enzyme by different stimuli/signals or fine modulation of activity. Same protein kinases and phosphatases can act on multiple enzymes enabling same signal to co-ordinately increase or decrease activity of many enzymes and pathways.

Q. 32. What are isoenzymes? Describe with examples the significance of isoenzymes in our body.

Ans. Isoenzymes are different enzymes catalysing same reactions. They are coded by different genes and arise by gene duplication. They exhibit differences in isoelectric pH, optimal temp, pH, K_m, V_{max} and sensitivity to inhibitors.

Significance of isoenzymes in our body
1. Different locations and metabolic roles for isoenzymes in the same cell: The isocitrate dehydrogenase isozymes of the cytosol and the mitochondrion are an example.
2. Different regulation and kinetics as per metabolic requirements of the tissue:
    Hexokinase IV (glucokinase) of liver and the hexokinase isozymes of other tissues differ in their K_m for glucose and this difference is responsible for their different metabolic roles. The K_m of muscle hexokinase II is only 0.1 mM (1.8 mg/dL) and thus it is saturated at even very low glucose concentrations, continuously processing glucose irrespective of blood glucose levels to provide the cells with energy. Hexokinase IV (glucokinase) of liver has K_m of 10 mM (180 mg/dL) and functions to remove glucose from the blood following a meal, providing glucose 6-phosphate in excess of requirements for glycolysis, which is used for glycogen synthesis and lipogenesis. Glucokinase in pancreatic cells acts as a glucose sensor activating glycolysis and ATP production only when glucose is sufficiently high to cause insulin release (ATP inhibits K channel leading to depolarization). Muscle hexokinase I and II are feedback inhibited by glucose-6-phosphate while glucokinase is not, while glucokinase is inducible by insulin which promotes glucose uptake and storage as lipids or glycogen in liver.
    The different LDH isozymes have significantly different values of V_{max} and K_m, particularly for pyruvate. The properties of LDH 4 favour rapid reduction of very low concentrations of pyruvate to lactate in skeletal muscle, whereas those of isoenzyme LDH 1 favour rapid oxidation of lactate to pyruvate in the heart.
    For glycogen phosphorylase the isoenzymes in skeletal muscle and liver have different regulatory properties (regulation by glucagon, epinephrine and Ca^{2+}) reflecting the different roles of glycogen breakdown in the two tissues. Muscle phosphorylase also has much higher V_{max} than the liver enzyme to supply glucose at a very high rate.
3. Different stages of development in embryonic or fetal tissues and in adult tissues: For example, the fetal liver has a characteristic isozymes distribution of LDH, which changes as the organ develops into its adult form. Some enzymes of glucose catabolism in malignant (cancer) cells occur as their fetal, not adult, isozymes.

Bioenergetics and Oxidative Phosphorylation

Chapter 4

Q. 1. What reaction is catalysed by myokinase and what is its advantage?

Ans. Myokinase or adenylyl kinase enzyme is present in most cells. It catalyzes the following reaction:

$$ATP + AMP \leftrightarrow 2ADP$$

This reaction is reversible and allows:
- High-energy phosphate in ADP to be used for the synthesis of ATP.
- When muscle is contracting vigorously ADP accumulates and interferes with ATP dependent muscle contraction. This reaction lowers ADP and salvages some ATP.
- AMP, formed as a consequence of several activating reactions converting ATP to AMP, to be recovered by rephosphorylation to ADP, which can be converted to ATP in mitochondria.
- Normally, cells have a far higher concentration of ATP (5 to 10 mM) than of AMP (< 0.1 mM). When some process (muscle contraction, etc.) consumes ATP, AMP is produced in two steps. First, hydrolysis of ATP produces ADP, then the myokinase reaction produces AMP. If ATP is consumed such that its concentration drops 10%, the relative increase in [AMP] is much greater (600%) than that of [ADP] because of the myokinase reaction (Table 4.1). This large relative (600%) change in AMP concentration makes it a very sensitive indicator of a cell's energy state. Therefore many regulatory processes are keyed to changes in AMP concentration. Probably the most important mediator of regulation by AMP is AMP-activated protein kinase (AMPK). It signals to increase the rate of catabolic reactions, which in turn lead to the generation of more ATP and it also inhibit the energy requiring processes.

Deficiency of myokinase in RBC causes haemolytic anemia; some cases have mental retardation also. Myokinase has two isoenzymes – AK1 is cytosolic and AK2 is located in the mitochondria. Adenylate kinase 2 (AK2) deficiency in humans causes hematopoietic defects associated with sensorineural deafness.

Table 4.1. Relative changes in ATP, ADP and AMP concentration in muscle cell after exercise

Adenine nucleotide	Concentration before ATP depletion (mM)	Concentration after ATP depletion (mM)	Relative change
ATP	5.0	4.5	10%
ADP	1.0	1.0	0
AMP	0.1	0.6	600%

Q. 2. What is the difference between $\Delta G°$, $\Delta G°'$ and ΔG? Elaborate with an example.

Ans. ΔG is the free energy change for any chemical reaction. It depends on the equilibrium constant of the reaction and the actual concentrations of the reactants in the system. The standard Gibbs free energy of formation of a compound is the change of Gibbs free energy that accompanies the formation of 1 mole of that substance from its component elements, at their standard states (the most stable form of the element at 25 degrees Celsius and 101.3 kilopascals). $\Delta G°$ is the standard free energy change when reactants are present in concentration of 1.0 mol/L (including H^+ ions) while $\Delta G°'$ is the standard free energy change defined for biological system where standard state is defined as having pH of 7.0. However, in reactions inside the cells the concentrations of reactants and products are different than the standard conditions. Also, free energy changes depend on the pH, temperature, total ionic strength and Mg^{2+} concentrations which are not apparent from the usual reaction equations written in metabolic pathways.

$$A + B \rightleftharpoons C + D$$

$$\Delta G = \Delta G° + RT \ln \frac{[C][D]}{[A][B]}$$

The free energy change for a reaction can be very different from the standard-state value if the concentrations of reactants and products differ significantly from unit activity (1 M for solutions). The effects can often be dramatic. Consider the hydrolysis of phosphocreatine:

$$\text{Phosphocreatine} + H_2O \rightarrow \text{Creatine} + P_i$$

This reaction is strongly exergonic and $\Delta G°'$ at 37°C is –42.8 kJ/mol. Physiological concentrations of phosphocreatine, creatine, and inorganic phosphate are normally between 1 mM and 10 mM. Assuming 1 mM concentrations the ΔG for the hydrolysis of phosphocreatine is:

$$\Delta G = -42.8 \text{ kJ mol}^{-1} + (8.314 \text{ J mol}^{-1} K^{-1})(310 K) \ln \frac{[0.001][0.001]}{[0.001]}$$

$$\Delta G = -60.5 \text{ kJ/mol}$$

At 37°C, the difference between standard-state and 1 mM (actual) concentrations for such a reaction is thus approximately –17.7 kJ/mol.

In addition, the standard Gibbs free energy changes aren't very useful when dealing with charged molecules and the ATP hydrolysis reactions have charged molecules – even when some of the negative charges are neutralized by Mg^{2+} ions. Standard Gibbs free energy changes are at 25°C (298 K) and pH 7.0. For reactions like ATP hydrolysis, actual free energy changes occur at physiological concentrations of ATP, ADP, P_i, 3 mM of Mg^{2+} and ionic strength of 0.25 M. In a muscle cell concentration of ATP is 8.1 mM, ADP is 0.93 mM and of P_i is 8.1 mM, then for hydrolysis of ATP with $\Delta G^{\circ\prime}$ of –32.1 KJ/mol the actual ΔG will be –49.6 kJ/mol and this much energy will also be required to synthesize ATP from ADP in physiological condition. Thus, the maintenance of high concentration of ATP with low concentration of ADP in the cells contributes to large negative free energy change when ATP is converted into ADP.

Q. 3. How both catabolic and anabolic reactions are made spontaneous or favourable in our body?

Ans. Spontaneous or favoured reactions have negative ΔG. At equilibrium, $\Delta G = 0$ and [C][D] / [A][B] = K_{eq}. We have $\Delta G^\circ = -RT \ln K_{eq}$. Freely reversible reactions have ΔG near 0 and are at equilibrium and can proceed in both forward and backward directions equally. Most reactions of anabolic and catabolic pathways are of such type, but there are few 'irreversible' steps which drive the whole pathway and regulate the metabolic flux in one direction. The 'irreversible' reactions are non-equilibrium reactions with concentrations of reactants and products far from equilibrium. They have net large negative ΔG and are spontaneous and exergonic. The heat released is not wasted but helps in maintaining body temperature. Reactions with large negative ΔG are coupled with those reactions having positive ΔG and as free energy changes are additive, the net negative ΔG ensures that overall reaction is favoured. All irreversible reactions have sufficiently large $-\Delta G$. In catabolic pathways fuel breakdown is coupled to synthesis of ATP, NADH or NADPH (compounds with high group transfer potential) which are then used to drive the anabolic reactions (Table 4.2 and Figs. 4.1 and 4.2).

Table 4.2. Types of transfer potential (used to couple exergonic and endergonic reactions)

	Proton Transfer Potential (Acidity)	Standard Reduction Potential (Electron Transfer Potential)	Group Transfer Potential (High-Energy Bond)
Simple equation	$AH \rightleftharpoons A^- + H^+$	$A \rightleftharpoons A^+ + e^-$	$A \sim P \rightleftharpoons A + P_i$
Equation including acceptor	$AH + H_2O \rightleftharpoons A^- + H_3O^+$	$A + H^+ \rightleftharpoons A^+ + \tfrac{1}{2}H_2$	$A \sim PO_4^{2-} + H_2O \rightleftharpoons A{-}OH + HPO_4^{2-}$
Measure of transfer potential	$pK_a = \dfrac{\Delta G^\circ}{2.303\,RT}$	$\Delta ?_0 = \dfrac{-\Delta G^\circ}{n?}$	$\ln K_{eq} = \dfrac{-\Delta G^\circ}{RT}$
Free energy change of transfer is given by	ΔG° per mole of H^+ transferred	ΔG° per mole of e^- transferred	ΔG° per mole of phosphate transferred

Examples of coupling of exergonic and endergonic reactions

Production of ATP in glycolysis:

$\ $ PEP + $H_2O \rightarrow$ Pyruvate + P_i $\qquad \Delta G = -78$ kJ/mol
$+\ $ ADP + $P_i \rightarrow$ ATP + H_2O $\qquad \Delta G = +55$ kJ/mol
$=\ $ PEP + ADP $\rightarrow$ Pyruvate + ATP $\quad$ Total $\Delta G = -23$ kJ/mol

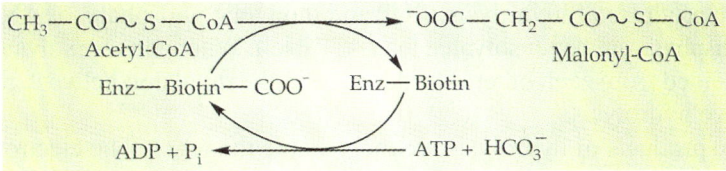

Fig. 4.1. ATP can be used to drive synthetic reactions.

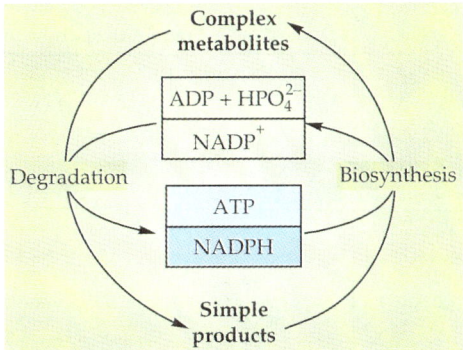

Fig. 4.2. Coupling of catabolism (exergonic) and anabolism (endergonic).

Q. 4. Why the 'high energy phosphate bond' is misnomer or why ATP acts as energy currency molecule?

Ans. Those phosphorylated compounds having a relatively high free energy of hydrolysis, such as ATP, phosphocreatine and phosphopyruvate, are often spoken of as having high-energy phosphate bonds, and such bonds are universally designated by the symbol ~P. These expressions have been very useful and handy to biochemists, but they can be very misleading. The term "high-energy phosphate bond" is an unfortunate misnomer because it implies that the energy spoken of is in the bonds and that when the bond is split, energy is set free. This is quite wrong. Bond energy is defined as the energy required to break a given bond between two atoms. Actually relatively enormous energies are required to break chemical bonds, which would not exist if they were not stable. The term "phosphate bond energy" thus does not refer to the true bond energy of the covalent linkages between the phosphorus atom and the oxygen or nitrogen atom. The term "high energy phosphate bond" means only that the difference in energy content between the reactants and the products of hydrolysis is relatively high: the free energy of hydrolysis is not localized in the actual chemical bond itself (Fig. 4.3).

$$ATP + H_2O \to ADP + P_i \qquad \Delta G° = -32 \text{ kJ mol}^{-1}$$

Several factors contribute to the large amount of energy released during hydrolysis of the phosphoanhydride linkages of ATP.

1. Electrostatic repulsion among the negatively charged oxygen atoms of the phosphoanhydride groups of ATP is less after hydrolysis. (In cells, $\Delta G°$ hydrolysis is actually increased [made more positive] by the presence of Mg^{2+} which partially neutralizes the charges on the oxygen atoms of ATP and diminishes electrostatic repulsion.)

2. The products of hydrolysis, ADP and inorganic phosphate, or AMP and inorganic pyrophosphate, are better solvated than ATP itself. When ions are solvated, they are electrically shielded from each other. The decrease in the repulsion between phosphate groups helps drive hydrolysis.
3. The products of hydrolysis are more stable than ATP. The electrons on terminal oxygen atoms are more delocalized than those on bridging oxygen atoms. Hydrolysis of ATP replaces one bridging oxygen atom with two new terminal oxygen atoms.

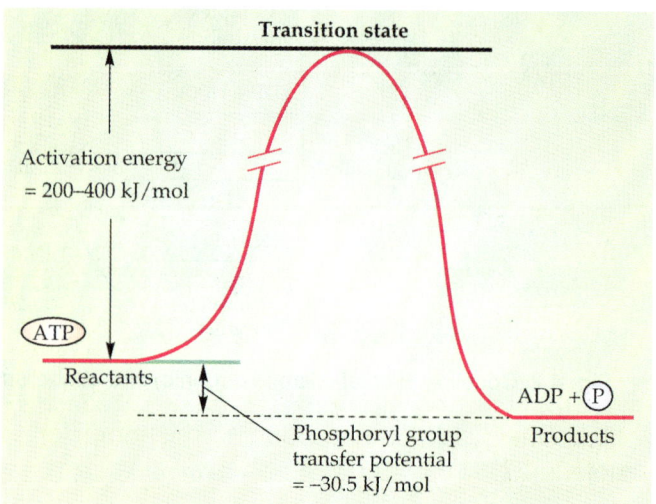

Fig. 4.3. Release of energy from 'high energy phosphate bond'.

Q. 5. How ATP provides energy for endergonic reactions?

Ans. In the chemical reactions in our body ATP rarely undergoes 'hydrolysis' to release its energy to drive endergonic reactions. Reactions or processes usually depict with a single arrow showing the conversion of ATP to ADP and P_i (or, in some cases, of ATP to AMP and pyrophosphate). When written this way, these reactions of ATP seem to be simple hydrolysis reactions in which water displaces P_i, (or PP_i), and one is tempted to say that an ATP-dependent reaction is "driven by the hydrolysis of ATP". This is not the case as ATP hydrolysis per se usually accomplishes nothing but the liberation of heat, which cannot drive a chemical process in an isothermal system. Actually reactions are a two-step process as shown in Fig. 4.4.

A part of the ATP molecule, a phosphoryl or pyrophosphoryl group or the adenylate moiety (AMP), is first transferred to a substrate molecule or to an amino acid residue in an enzyme, becoming covalently attached to the substrate or the enzyme and raising its free-energy content. Then, in a second step, the phosphate-containing moiety transferred in the first step is displaced generating P_i, PP_i, or AMP. Thus ATP participates covalently in the enzyme-catalysed reaction to which it contributes free energy.

Some processes do involve direct hydrolysis of ATP (or GTP). For example, non-covalent binding of ATP (or GTP), followed by its hydrolysis to ADP (or GDP) and P_i, can provide the energy to cycle some proteins between two conformations producing mechanical motion.

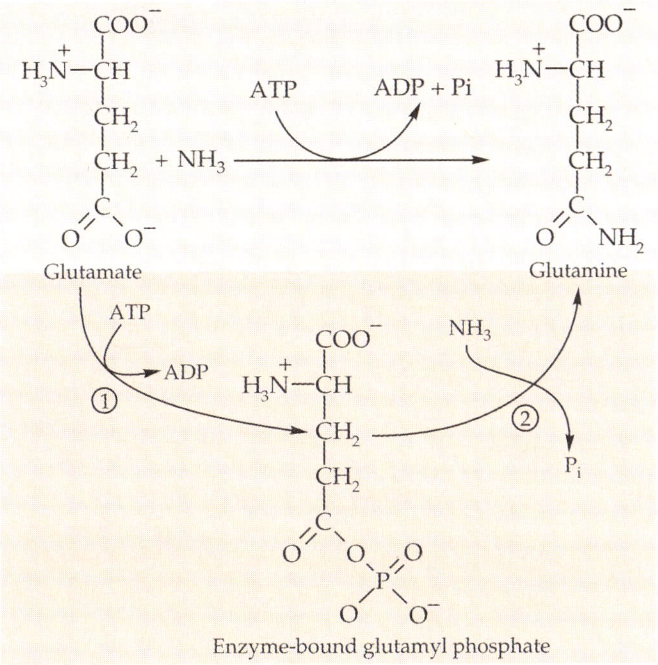

Bioenergetics and Oxidative Phosphorylation

Fig. 4.4. How ATP actually transfers energy.

This occurs in muscle contraction and in the movement of enzymes along DNA or of ribosomes a long messenger RNA. The energy-dependent actions catalyzed by helicases, RecA protein, and some topoisomerases also involve direct hydrolysis of phosphoanhydride bonds. The AAA family ATPases involved in DNA replication and other processes use ATP hydrolysis to cycle associated proteins between active and inactive forms. GTP-binding proteins that act in signaling pathways directly hydrolyze GTP to drive conformational changes that terminate signals triggered by hormones or by other extracellular factors.

Q. 6. What is the advantage of activation reactions such as acyl CoA synthetase converting ATP to AMP rather than ADP?

Ans. Many reactions convert ATP to AMP and PP_i (pyrophosphate rather than ADP and P_i (inorganic phosphate). $\Delta G^{\circ\prime}$ for ATP to AMP conversion is –32.2 kJ/mol and for ATP to ADP is –30.5 kJ/mol. Thus there is not much benefit in terms of gain of extra Gibbs free energy for driving endergonic reactions. Neither can the PP_i transfer any group or energy in subsequent reaction as being very unstable it is rapidly split to $2P_i$. $\Delta G^{\circ\prime}$ for PP_i to $2P_i$ is –19.2 kJ/mol and this is a spontaneous reaction. It is this hydrolytic splitting of PP_i that drives or shift equilibrium of the first reaction to right constantly removing the product and driving the reaction forward, not allowing equilibrium to reach. Consider the reaction catalysed by acyl CoA synthetase, which takes place in 2 steps (Figs. 4.5 and 4.6).

The two combined reactions have a net $\Delta G^{\circ\prime}$ of about –0.8 kJ/mol, so that the reaction is easily reversible (equilibrium constant near 1). However the splitting of PP_i with its large negative ΔG makes the overall reaction highly favourable with net large negative ΔG (Fig.

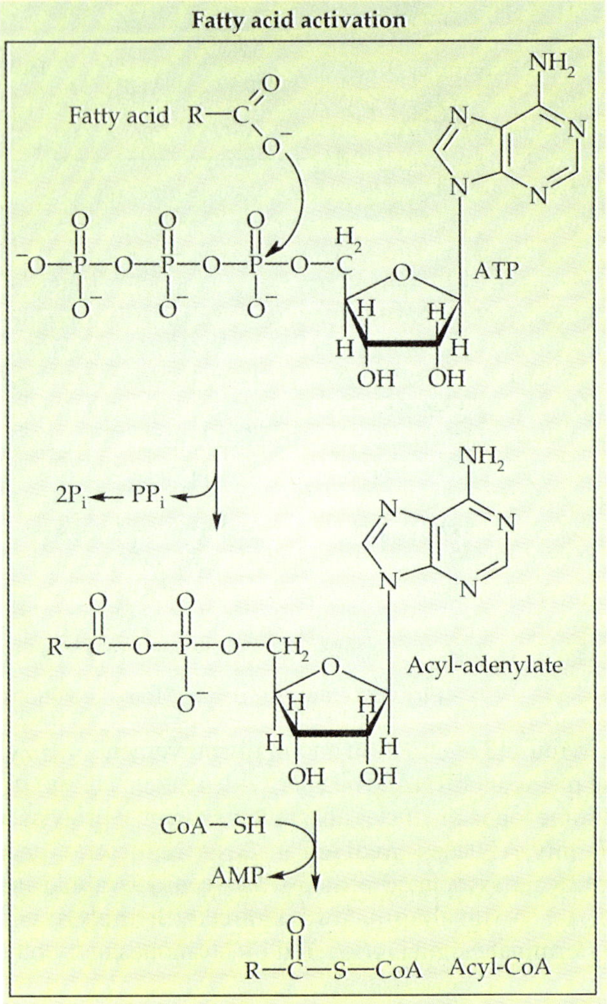

Fig. 4.5. Reaction of acyl CoA synthetase.

4.7). The splitting of PP_i makes the activation reaction irreversible (non-equilibrium) under physiological conditions. Some other reactions which use similar principles of driving reaction forward by hydrolysis of PP_i are:

- UDPGlc pyrophosphorylase – synthesis of UDP-glucose and other such enzymes synthesizing nucleotide sugars like UDPN-acetylglucosamine, etc.
- Synthesis of CDP choline during phospholipid synthesis
- Synthesis of CDP – DAG during triacylglycerol synthesis
- Adenylate cyclase and guanylate cyclase
- Arginosuccinate synthase of urea cycle
- Synthesis of benzoyl CoA from benzoate and addition of CoA to other compounds
- Aminoacyl tRNA synthetase
- Ubiquitin ligase

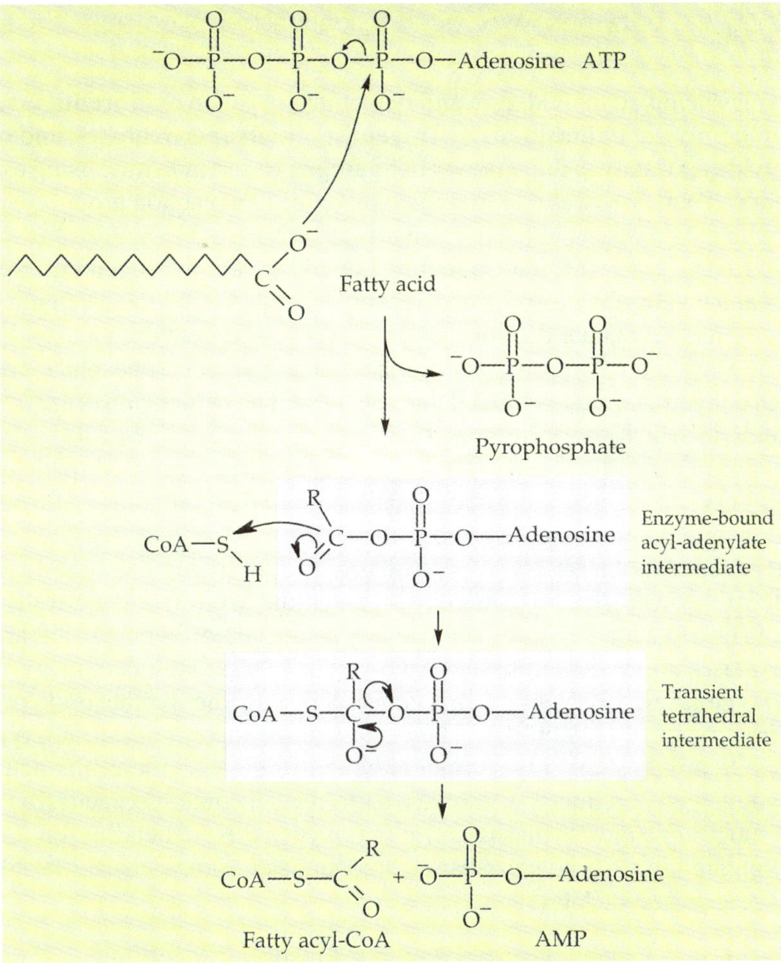

Fig. 4.6. Actual steps of acyl CoA synthetase reaction.

$\Delta G^{\circ\prime}$ for ATP $\rightarrow$ AMP + PPi = $-32.3 \frac{kJ}{mol}$

$\Delta G^{\circ\prime}$ for acyl-CoA synthesis = $+31.5 \frac{kJ}{mol}$

Net $\Delta G^{\circ\prime}$ = $-0.8 \frac{kJ}{mol}$

$\Delta G^{\circ\prime} = -33.6$ kJ/mol

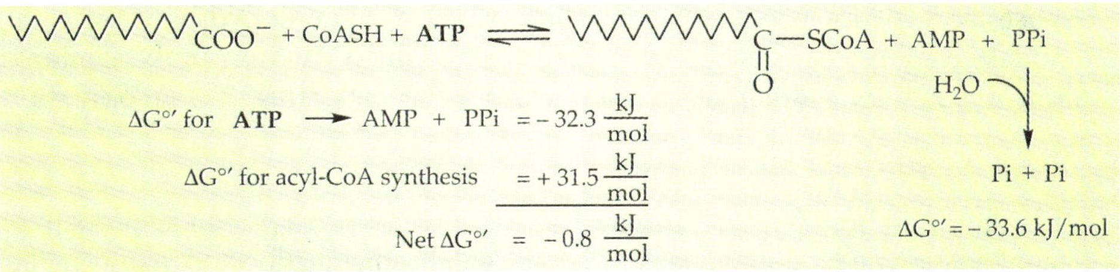

Fig. 4.7. Energetics of acyl CoA synthetase reaction.

- Asparagine synthetase
- DNA ligase
- DNA polymerase, RNA polymerase
- mRNA capping enzyme
- Firefly luciferase

Q. 7. **Classify the enzymes involved in oxidation-reduction reactions giving example of each.**

Ans. Enzymes involved in oxidation and reduction are called **oxidoreductases** and are classified into four groups: **oxidases, dehydrogenases, hydroperoxidases,** and **oxygenases**.

Oxidase: Catalyze the removal of hydrogen from a substrate using oxygen as a hydrogen acceptor. They form water or hydrogen peroxide as a reaction product, e.g. xanthine oxidase, L-amino acid oxidase, aldehyde dehydrogenase.

Dehydrogenases: Catalyse removal or addition of hydrogen but use carriers like NAD, FMN and FAD as donors or acceptors of H, e.g. NADH-linked dehydrogenases – isocitrate dehydrogenase, malate dehydrogenase; FAD-linked dehydrogenases – acyl CoA dehydrogenase, succinate dehydrogenase, mitochondrial glycerol 3-phosphate dehydrogenase; FMN-linked dehydrogenase – NADH dehydrogenase. The **cytochromes** are iron-containing hemoproteins in which the iron atom oscillates between Fe^{3+} and Fe^{2+} during oxidation and reduction. Except for cytochrome oxidase, they are classified as dehydrogenases. In the respiratory chain, they are involved as carriers of electrons from flavoproteins on the one hand to cytochrome oxidase on the other.

Hydroperoxidases: Hydroperoxidases include peroxidases and catalase. Peroxidases reduce peroxides using various electron acceptors, while catalase uses H_2O_2 as both electron donor and acceptor. They protect the body against harmful peroxides, are found in RBC and peroxidases are present in tissues involved in eicosanoid metabolism.

Oxygenases: Oxygenases are concerned with the synthesis or degradation of many different types of metabolites. They catalyze the incorporation of oxygen into a substrate molecule in two steps: (1) oxygen is bound to the enzyme at the active site; and (2) the bound oxygen is reduced or transferred to the substrate. Oxygenases may be divided into two subgroups, dioxygenases and monooxygenases, depending on 2 or 1 oxygen atoms incorporated, e.g. dioxygenases – homogentisate dioxygenase, tryptophan dioxygenase; monoxygenases – CYP450 enzymes.

Q. 8. **Why names homogentisate oxidase and aldehyde dehydrogenase are misnomers?**

Ans. Homogentisate oxidase is a dioxygenase which incorporates both atoms of oxygen into the substrate, hence it is actually an oxygenase. Aldehyde dehydrogenase is an FAD-linked oxidase enzyme present in mammalian livers, which contains molybdenum and nonheme iron and acts upon aldehydes and N-heterocyclic substrates. It is an oxidase by action.

Q. 9. **What is hydroxylase cycle?**

Ans. It is the cycle used by cytochrome P450 enzymes which are an important superfamily of heme-containing monooxygenases. These cytochromes are located mainly in the endoplasmic reticulum in the liver and intestine, but are also found in the mitochondria in some tissues. Both NADH and NADPH donate reducing equivalents for the reduction of these cytochromes, which in turn are oxidized by substrates in a series of enzymatic reactions collectively known as the **hydroxylase cycle**. The enzyme adds one atom of O_2 to the bound substrate and other atom is used to make water with the help of 2 H^+ from NADPH + H^+ as shown in the cycle. The enzyme gets oxidized during the addition of O atom to substrate and is subsequently reduced by NADPH + H^+ (Fig. 4.8).

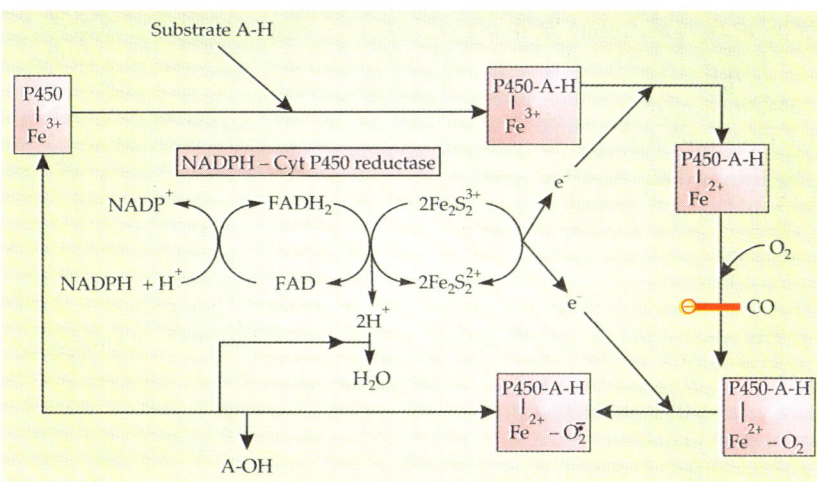

Fig. 4.8. The hydroxylase cycle. The cycle involves reduction of oxygen to water, monooxygenation of substrates like morphine and oxidation of NADPH + H⁺ to NADP⁺.

In the endoplasmic reticulum of the liver, cytochromes P450 are found together with cytochrome b5 and have an important role in detoxification. The rate of detoxification of many medicinal drugs by cytochromes P450 determines the duration of their action. Benzpyrene, aminopyrine, aniline, morphine, and benzphetamine are hydroxylated, increasing their solubility and aiding their excretion. Many drugs such as phenobarbital have the ability to induce the synthesis of cytochromes P450.

Q. 10. Why 2,4-DNP or 2,4-dinitrophenol is a banned drug?

Ans. It is a proton ionophore which uncouples respiratory chain from phosphorylation leading to excessive heat production, shortage of ATP and increased O_2 consumption. Toxicity causes heavy breathing and fatal hyperthermia. It was earlier tried as a slimming agent as it wastes body's ATP and energy as heat. It is sold mostly over the internet under a number of different names as a rapid weight loss/slimming aid. Many people have died while using it as unlicensed weight-reducing pill. It was earlier used as a pesticide also. Exposure to farmers while spraying caused toxicity.

Q. 11. Describe agents which interfere with oxidative phosphorylation. What is the difference between uncouples and inhibitors of electron transport chain?

Ans. *Inhibitors of ETC*

Complex I	Complex II	Complex III	Complex IV
Rotenone	Carboxin	Antimycin	Cyanide, H_2S
Amobarbital	TTFA	BAL (Dimercaprol)	& azide
Secobarbital	Malonate	Phenformin	CO
Piericidin A (comp. COQ)	Naphthoquinone		
Chlorpromazine			
Guanethidine			

Uncouplers of oxidative phosphorylation
- 2,4-Dinitrophenol
- 2,4-Dinitrocresol
- CCCP (most active) chlorocarbonyl cyanide phenyl hydrazone
- Dicoumarol (vit. K analogue)
- Valinomycin
- Calcium

Physiological uncouplers
- UCP1 (thermogenin) activation of fatty acid oxidation; heat production in brown adipose tissue
- Excessive thyroid hormone
- EFA deficiency
- Long-chain fatty acids in adipose tissue
- Conjugated hyperbilirubinemia

Rotenone is an odourless, colourless, crystalline ketonic chemical compound used as a broad-spectrum insecticide, piscicide, and pesticide. It occurs naturally in the seeds and stems of several plants, such as the jicama vine plant, and the roots of several members of Fabaceae family. Amobarbital is a barbiturate drug used as a sedative-hypnotic. Barbiturates such as amobarbital inhibit electron transport via Complex I by blocking the transfer from Fe-S to Q. At sufficient dosage, they are fatal in vivo. Antimycin A and dimercaprol inhibit the respiratory chain at Complex III. The classic poisons H_2S, carbon monoxide, and cyanide

Table 4.3. Mechanism of action of inhibitors and uncouplers of ETC

Type of interference	Compound	Target/mode of action
Inhibition of electron transfer	Cyanide Carbon monoxide	Inhibit cytochrome oxidase
	Antimycin A	Blocks electron transfer from cytochrome b to cytochrome c_1
	Myxothiazol Rotenone Amytal Piericidin A	Prevent electron transfer from Fe-S centre to ubiquinone
	DCMU	Competes with Q_B for binding site in PSII
Inhibition of ATP synthase	Aurovertin	Inhibits F_1
	Oligomycin Venturicidin	Inhibit F_o and CF_o
	DCCD	Blocks proton flow through F_o and CF_o
Uncoupling of phosphorylation from electron transfer	FCCP DNP	Hydrophobic proton carriers
	Valinomycin	H^+ ionophore
	Thermogenin	In brown adipose tissue, forms proton-conducting pores in inner mitochondrial membrane
Inhibition of ATP-ADP exchange	Atractyloside	Inhibits adenine nucleotide translocase

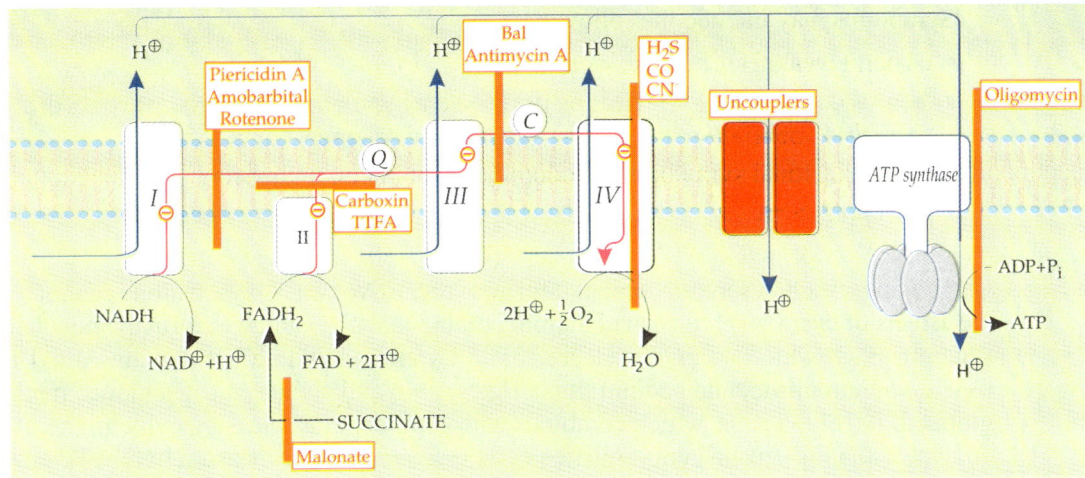

Fig. 4.9. Inhibitors and uncouplers of ETC: site of action.

inhibit Complex IV and can therefore totally arrest respiration. Malonate is a competitive inhibitor of Complex II. Atractyloside inhibits oxidative phosphorylation by inhibiting the transporter of ADP into and ATP out of the mitochondrion.

Difference between inhibitors and uncouplers

Inhibitors cause inhibition of ETC and decrease ATP production, oxygen consumption and cause hypothermia and histotoxic hypoxia. Atractyloside, an inhibitor of ATP/ADP exchanger and oligomycin (inhibitor of ATP synthase), has similar effects. However, uncouplers dissipate the proton gradient without ATP production causing decreased ATP, increased electron flow in ETC, hyperthermia, increased oxygen consumption (shortage of ATP drives ETC) and increased rate of breathing.

Q. 12. What is the mechanism and features of cyanide toxicity?

Ans. The cyanide ion halts cellular respiration by inhibiting cytochrome c oxidase. It binds to Fe^{3+} of cytochrome a_3. Cyanide toxicity is generally considered to be a rare form of poisoning; however, cyanide exposure occurs relatively frequently in patients with smoke inhalation from residential or industrial fires. Cyanide poisoning also may occur in industry, particularly in the metal trades, mining, electroplating, jewellery manufacturing, and radiographic film recovery. It is also encountered in fumigation of ships, warehouses, and other structures. Cyanides are also used as suicidal agents, particularly among healthcare and laboratory workers, and they can potentially be used in a terrorist attack. Numerous forms of cyanide exist, including gaseous hydrogen cyanide (HCN), water-soluble potassium and sodium cyanide salts, and poorly water-soluble mercury, copper, gold, and silver cyanide salts. In addition, a number of cyanide-containing compounds, known as cyanogens, may release cyanide during metabolism. These include, but are not limited to, cyanogen chloride and cyanogen bromide (gases with potent pulmonary irritant effects), nitriles (R—CN), and sodium nitroprusside, which may produce iatrogenic cyanide poisoning during prolonged or high-dose intravenous (IV) therapy (> 10 mcg/kg/min).

Symptoms may include the following:
- General weakness, malaise, and collapse
- Neurologic symptoms (reflecting progressive hypoxia) – Headache, vertigo, dizziness, giddiness, inebriation, confusion, generalized seizures, coma
- Gastrointestinal symptoms – Abdominal pain, nausea, vomiting
- Cardiopulmonary symptoms – Shortness of breath, possibly associated with chest pain, apnea

Treatment includes hydroxocobalamin and supportive care. Oxygen alone cannot reverse the effects of cyanide. Hydroxocobalamin combines with cyanide to form cyanocobalamin (vitamin B_{12}), which is renally cleared. The Cyanide Antidote Kit contains amyl nitrite pearls, sodium nitrite, and sodium thiosulfate. Amyl and sodium nitrites induce methemoglobin in red blood cells, which combines with cyanide, thus releasing cytochrome oxidase enzyme. Inhaling crushed amyl nitrite pearls is a temporizing measure before IV administration of sodium nitrite. Sodium thiosulfate enhances the conversion of cyanide to thiocyanate, which is renally excreted. Thiosulfate has a somewhat delayed effect and thus is typically used with sodium nitrite for faster antidote action.

Q. 13. What are conditions which limit the rate of cellular respiration during exercise?

Ans. Conditions limiting the rate of cellular respiration:
- A. Capacity of respiratory chain
- B. Availability of oxygen
- C. ATP/ADP transporter may become rate limiting

Q. 14. What are the different states of respiratory control?

Ans. **Limiting factor/states of respiratory control**

State 1	Availability of ADP and substrate
State 2	Availability of substrate only
State 3	The capacity of the respiratory chain itself, when all substrates and components are present in saturating amounts
State 4	Availability of ADP only
State 5	Availability of oxygen only

Most cells in the resting state are in state 4, and respiration is controlled by the availability of ADP. When work is performed, ATP is converted to ADP, allowing more respiration to occur, which in turn replenishes the store of ATP. Under certain conditions, the concentration of inorganic phosphate can also affect the rate of functioning of the respiratory chain. As respiration increases (as in exercise), the cell approaches state 3 or state 5 when either the capacity of the respiratory chain becomes saturated or the pO_2 decreases below the K_m for heme a_3. There is also the possibility that the ADP/ATP transporter, which facilitates entry of cytosolic ADP into and ATP out of the mitochondrion, becomes rate-limiting.

Q. 15. NADPH is required in synthetic reactions in cytosol. Give examples of some intramitochondrial reactions requiring NADPH.

Ans. Intramitochondrial NADPH is required for:
- A. Steroid synthesis enzymes
- B. Glutamate dehydrogenase
- C. NO synthase
- D. Glutathione reductase
- E. Beta oxidation of unsaturated FA

Q. 16. What are the sources of intramitochondrial NADPH?

Ans. Proton translocating transhydrogenase and NADH, glutamate dehydrogenase and isocitrate dehydrogenase are the sources of intramitochondrial NADPH.

Q. 17. Enumerate some oxidants and free radicals that are produced in mitochondria.

Ans.
1. Superoxide (O_2^-) produced from ubisemiquinone.
2. Hydrogen peroxide (H_2O_2) from O_2^- by superoxide dismutase.
3. Nitric oxide (NO) from NO synthase.
4. Peroxynitrate ($ONOO^-$) from NO.

Q. 18. Differentiate between glycerophosphate and malate aspartate shuttle.

Ans. NADH produced in glycolysis by glyceraldehyde-3-P dehydrogenase is transported from cytosol to mitochondrial matrix by use of these two shuttle systems (Figs. 4.10 and 4.11).
1. Malate shuttle is the more common and present in all tissues, while glycerophosphate shuttle is present in brain and white skeletal muscle.
2. Malate shuttle works across outer membrane and glycerophosphate shuttle works across inner mitochondrial membrane.
3. Malate shuttle is reversible and glycerophosphate shuttle is irreversible.

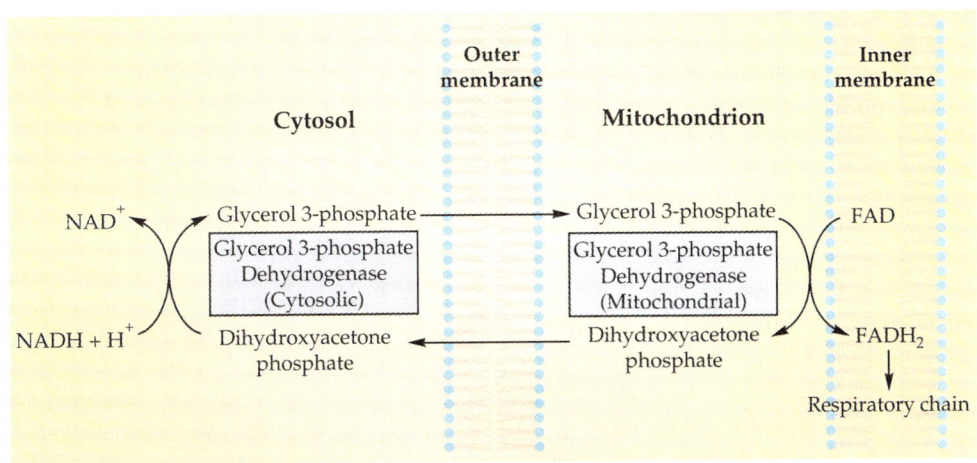

Fig. 4.10. Glycerophosphate shuttle.

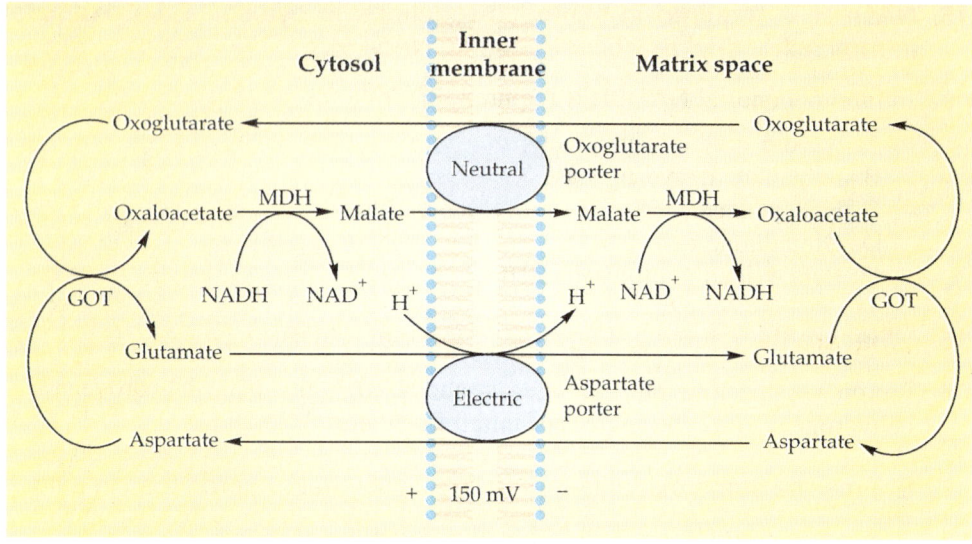

Fig. 4.11. Malate shuttle.

4. Malate shuttle operates only when NADH/NAD ratio is higher in cytosol than in mitochondrial matrix but glycerophosphate shuttle can operate even when this ratio is very low in cytosol.
5. Malate shuttle leads to production of 2.5 ATP from 1 NADH, while glycerophosphate shuttle leads to production of only 1.5 ATP as mitochondrial glycerol-3-phosphate dehydrogenase uses FAD.

Q. 19. Where else besides inner mitochondrial membrane is glutamate aspartate exchanger found and what is its function there?

Ans. GLutamate ASpartate Transporter (GLAST) mediates the transport of glutamic and aspartic acid with the cotransport of three Na^+ and one H^+ cations and counter transport of one K^+ cation and can work against concentration gradient. It is a part of the malate shuttle on inner mitochondrial membrane (Fig. 4.11). GLAST is expressed throughout the CNS, and is highly expressed in astrocytes. Glutamate aspartate antiporter is present on plasma membrane. This co-transport coupling (or symport) allows the transport of glutamate into cells against a concentration gradient, allowing it to remove glutamate from the extracellular space. Defect of this exchanger causes type 6 episodic ataxia.

Q. 20. Enumerate some of the transporters present in inner mitochondrial membrane.

Ans. The inner mitochondrial membrane limits the permeability and transport of intermediates, nucleotides and substrates to maintain the proton gradient. Different transporters allow the required selective movement of various compounds. While it is freely permeable to unchanged small molecules such as O_2, H_2O, CO_2, NH_3, monocarboxylic acids, 3OH-butyric acid, acetoacetic acid and acetic acid, transporters are required for pyruvate, ADP, ATP, malate, citrate, alpha-ketoglutarate, carnitine, long-chain fatty acids, etc. (Fig. 4.12).

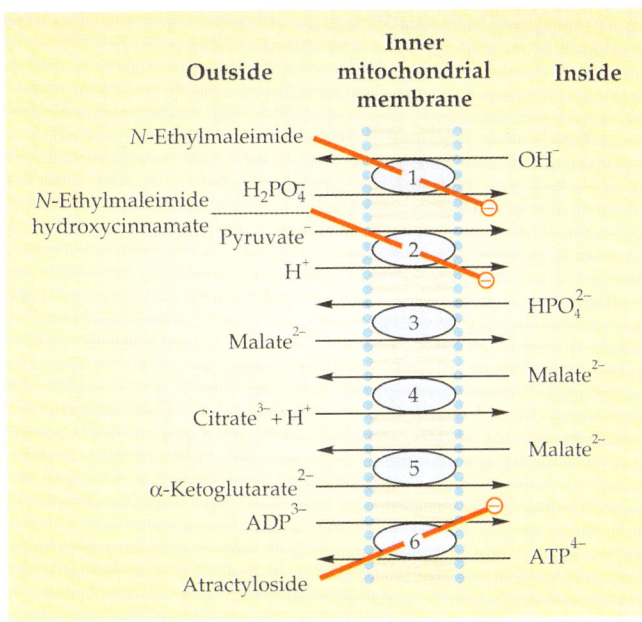

Fig. 4.12. Transporters in inner mitochondrial membrane.

Q. 21. What is the irreversible step in electron transport and how is its rate controlled?

Ans. The irreversible step in electron transport is the formation of water from oxygen. The rate of cytochrome *c* oxidase reaction is controlled by the ratio of reduced to oxidized cytochrome *c*, which is in turn controlled by the [NADH]/[NAD$^+$] and [ATP]/[ADP][P$_i$] ratios. Electron transfer from NADH to cytochrome *c* is nearly at equilibrium. In contrast, the cytochrome *c* oxidase reaction is irreversible and hence its rate depends on the concentration of its substrate, reduced cytochrome *c*. Increased NADH concentrations and decreased ATP concentrations lead to the production of more reduced cytochrome *c* and hence to increased electron transfer rates. Thus, the overall rate of oxidative phosphorylation depends on the ratios [NADH]/[NAD$^+$] and [ATP]/[ADP][P$_i$], which in turn may depend on the activities of the respective mitochondrial transporters and their concentrations in cytosol.

Q. 22. Oxidative phosphorylation requires the transfer of electrons donated by NADH. (a) Is NADH imported directly into the mitochondria? Explain. (b) Enumerate two import mechanisms that transfer cytosolic electrons from NADH into the mitochondrion. (c) Why is it important to maintain a relatively constant level of cytosolic NAD$^+$?

Ans. (a) The negatively charged phosphate groups of NADH prevent its diffusion across the inner mitochondrial membrane, and there are no NADH transport proteins to facilitate its transport.
(b) The malate–aspartate and glycerophosphate shuttles (Figs. 4.10 and 4.11) allow the indirect import of NADH reducing equivalents.
(c) Cytosolic NAD$^+$ is required for the glyceraldehyde-3-phosphate dehydrogenase reaction of glycolysis. Limited [NAD$^+$] would shut down glycolysis.

Q. 23. Explain how 1 NADH produces 2.5 ATP and 1 $FADH_2$ produces 1.5 ATP and what is P/O ratio?

Ans. The ratio of the amount of ATP produced to the amount of substrate oxidized (measured as oxygen consumed) is called the P/O ratio. The P/O ratio refers to atomic oxygen, O, rather than molecular oxygen, O_2, because each substrate (NADH or $FADH_2$) transfers two electrons, not four. Depending on where a substrate's electrons enter the electron-transport chain, the P/O ratio is ~2.5 or ~1.5. Production of 1 ATP by ATP synthase requires 4 H^+ (3 for rotation of F_1 and 1 for transport of P_i). For example, the two electrons transferred from NADH through Complexes I, III, and IV pump 10 protons, which would yield 2.5 ATP, whereas the two electrons transferred from $FADH_2$ through Complexes II, III, and IV pump 6 protons, which would yield 1.5 ATP (Fig. 4.13). However, actual numbers are lower due to leakage of protons, P_i transport and use of proton gradient to drive some transporters present in the inner mitochondrial membrane. The P/O ratio is not necessarily a whole number, because protons are contributed to the gradient by more than one process and some protons leak back into the matrix or are used for other processes than ATP synthesis.

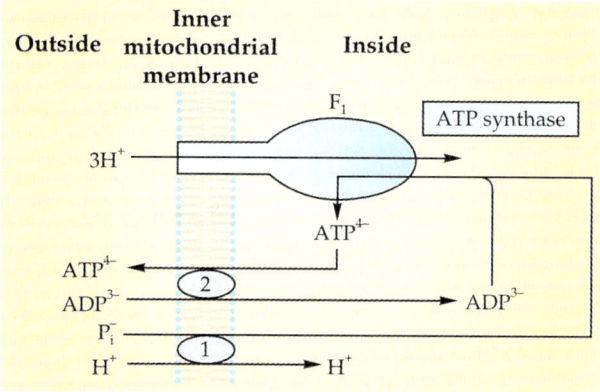

Fig. 4.13. ATP synthesis on inner mitochondrial membrane.

Carbohydrate Chemistry and Metabolism

Chapter 5

Q. 1. Enumerate the causes responsible for 'withdrawal' of carbohydrate from blood.

Ans.
- Utilization of glucose by oxidation (glycolysis) for energy production and by oxidation in HMP and uronic acid pathway.
- Conversion of glucose to glycogen (glycogenesis) for storage in liver and muscles.
- Uptake of hexoses by the liver cells such as galactose and fructose and their conversion to glucose by liver cells.
- Utilization of glucose for synthesis of other compounds like fatty acids, certain amino acids, etc. (Fig. 5.1).

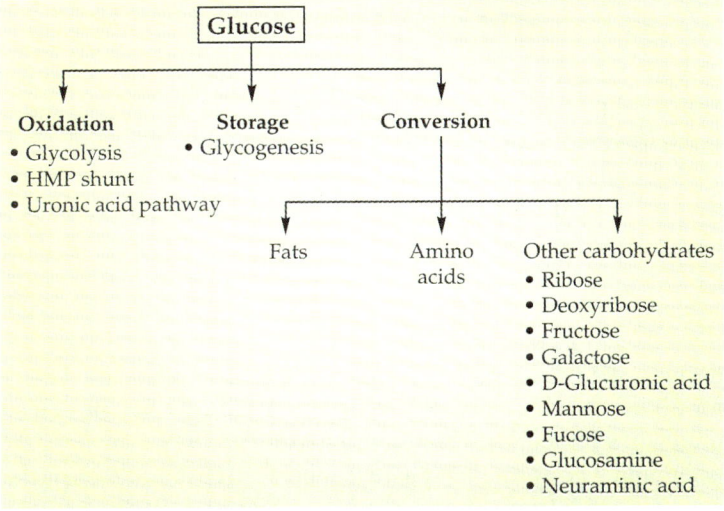

Fig. 5.1. Utilization of glucose by various processes.

Q. 2. Enumerate the causes for the 'release' of glucose by liver to the blood.

Ans.
- Conversion of liver glycogen to blood glucose i.e. "glycogenolysis".
- Formation of blood glucose by the liver from non-carbohydrate sources i.e. gluconeogenesis (from glucogenic amino acids, lactate, glycerol and propinoyl-CoA from odd chain fatty acids).
- Formation of blood glucose from other hexoses by liver.

Q. 3. Give the biochemical basis of muscular cramps and pain associated with vigorous exercise.

Ans. In vigorously contracting skeletal muscles anaerobic glycolysis becomes the main source of energy. Lactate is the end product of anaerobic glycolysis. So, during strenuous muscular activity (e.g. during a sprint) lactate accumulates in skeletal muscles resulting in lactic acidosis which in turn is responsible for muscular cramps and pain. Depletion of glycogen leads to depletion of ATP which is required for dissociation of myosin from actin. Depletion of ATP means that myosin remains attached to actin not allowing the muscle to relax and causing cramps. Other causes of cramps include electrolyte imbalance (low sodium/low potassium/low magnesium/low ionized calcium).

Q. 4. Major source of energy in RBCs is anaerobic glycolysis although oxygen is present. Comment.

Ans. RBCs do not have mitochondria. So, in spite of presence of oxygen, pyruvate cannot be aerobically oxidised and therefore anaerobic oxidation is the main source of energy in RBCs. Similar is the case seen with leukocytes, cells of renal medulla, testes, eye lens and cornea which have no or few mitochondria.

Q. 5. What is 'curd' formation?

Ans. In the Indian subcontinent, the word "curd" is widely used to refer to what is known as "yoghurt". Lactobacilli anaerobically oxidise lactose (glucose + galactose) to lactic acid which lowers the pH of milk. This leads to precipitation of milk protein 'casein' at its isoelectric pH of 4.6 and this forms the basis of curd formation. Milk is actually a colloid or an emulsion with pH around 6.7 and casein protein is present in the form of micelles.

Yoghurt gels are formed by the fermentation of milk with thermophilic starter bacteria consisting of a mixture of *Streptococcus thermophilus* and *Lactobacillus delbrueckii* subsp. *bulgaricus*. When incubated with lactobacilli, production of lactic acid causes drop in pH and the sour taste. In yogurt production, milk is normally heated at a high temperature (e.g., 85°C for 30 min.), which causes the denaturation of whey proteins (i.e., β-lactoglobulin). Denatured whey proteins interact with κ-casein on the surface of casein micelles and cross-link caseins and whey proteins. There is increased casein–casein attraction as the pH of milk decreases from ~6.6 (typical milk pH) to ~4.6 during yogurt fermentation, which results in gelation as caseins approach their isoelectric point. The decrease in pH causes changes in the casein micelle structure due to the solubilization of colloidal calcium phosphate (CCP), i.e. conversion of colloidal calcium to Ca^{2+}.

- At pH 6.6–5.9: When the milk and culture begin incubating, there is no change in casein micelle, size is about 0.1 μm and its casein is homogenously distributed. The net negative charge of the casein is slowly decreasing, causing decreasing electrostatic repulsion. Only a small amount of CCP is solubilized at this point, there is no gel formation yet.
- At pH 5.5–5.2: Partial micellar disintegration occurs and casein particles aggregate to form structures with empty spaces between them. At this stage, milk gel should not be disturbed. The net negative charge of casein micelles greatly decreases, dramatically reducing the electrostatic repulsion and steric stability. The increasing rate of CCP solubilization also weakens the internal structure of the casein micelles and increases electrostatic repulsion between the exposed phosphoserine residues, encouraging the formation of a structural network at the solution's margin.
- At isoelectric pH of 4.6: As casein approaches the isoelectric point (pH 4.6, the point at which casein precipitates), the negative charge decreases to zero, decreasing the electrostatic repulsion between charged groups. The hydrophobic and electrostatic interactions cause aggregation. The acidification process causes the formation of a three-dimensional network of casein chains, creating the natural gel-like structure that gives yoghurt the traditional, rich velvety texture. The hairy strucute is due to κ-casein macromolecule retaining steric repulsions.

Curds are a dairy product obtained by curdling (coagulating) milk with rennet (rennin enzyme which converts casein into calcium paracaseinate) or any edible acidic substance such as lemon juice or vinegar, and then allowing it to set. The increased acidity causes the milk proteins (casein) to denature and tangle into solid masses, or curds. The remaining liquid, which contains only whey proteins, is the whey. In cow's milk, 80% of the proteins are caseins. Milk that has been left to sour (raw milk alone or pasteurized milk with added lactic acid bacteria or yeast) will also naturally produce curds. Boiling milk to 100°C (scalded milk) before cooling and curdling with acid/lemon, etc. causes coagulation of milk proteins, producing thicker and more solid 'curds'. These are referred to as 'paneer' in India.

Q. 6. Why are many adults intolerant to milk?

Ans. Many adults are unable to metabolise milk sugar (lactose) and experience gastrointestinal disturbances if they drink milk. Lactose intolerance or hypolactesia is most commonly caused due to deficiency of lactase (lactase activity normally starts declining after the infant is weaned). Mucosal damage in small intestine due to giardiasis, infections, chronic diarrhoea, etc. can damage the brush border enzymes causing lactose intolerance.

Normally

$$\text{Lactase} \xrightarrow{\text{Lactase}} \text{Glucose} + \text{Galactose}$$

In lactase deficiency

$$\text{Lactose} \xrightarrow{\text{Intestinal bacteria}} \text{Lactic acid} + CH_4 + H_2 \text{ gas}$$

The gas so produced causes flatulence and abdominal distention. The lactate so produced is osmotically active, resulting in diarrhoea. Treatment includes avoiding consumption of milk, and lactase enzyme can be taken orally with milk products.

Q. 7. Galactose is highly toxic if transferase enzyme is missing. How?

Ans. Disruption of galactose metabolism is referred to as galctosemia and most commonly occurs due to inherited deficiency of galactose-1-PO_4 uridyl transferase. It causes accumulation of Gal-1-PO_4 and thus phosphate (Pi) trapping, decreasing levels of inorganic phosphate (Pi) and ATP. Decreased Pi decreases glycogen phosphorylase action causing hypoglycaemia as well as hepatomegaly due to decreased glycogen breakdown. Accumulated Gal-1-PO_4 inhibits galctokinase causing galactose levels to rise causing galactosuria. Accumulated galactose is converted to galactitol by alodose reductase causing cataract in lens due to osmotic damage and CNS damage leading to mental retardation. Gal-1-PO_4 also damages renal tubules causing aminoaciduria. Depletion of Pi and ATP in liver causes damage to hepatocytes causing jaundice, coagulation abnormalities and accumulation of ammonia (liver failure). Early diagnosis and removal of galactose from diet prevents irreversible damage in CNS, liver and lens of eye.

Symptoms

Vomiting and diarrhoea after consuming milk.

Signs

- Jaundice.
- Enlargement of liver; sometimes progressing to cirrhosis.
- Cataract formation.
- CNS malfunction like delayed acquisition of language skills.

Q. 8. What are the important compounds derived from galactose? How can a galactosaemic child with galactose-free diet cope up?

Ans. Galactose is an important constituent of sugar nucleotide (UDP-galactose) which is used for synthesis of important glycoproteins, glycolipids and proteoglycans. These are essential for protein function, CNS and ECM. The galactosemic child will convert glucose-1-PO_4 to UDP-galactose by the following reaction.

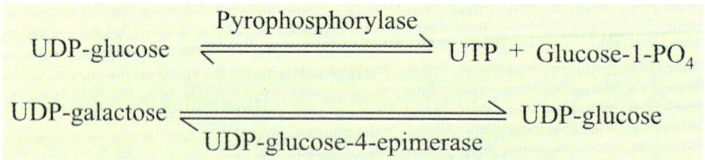

Q. 9. How anaerobic exercise training affects glycolysis in athletes?

Ans. Anaerobic exercise training activates HIF-1 (Hypoxia inducible transcription factor-1).

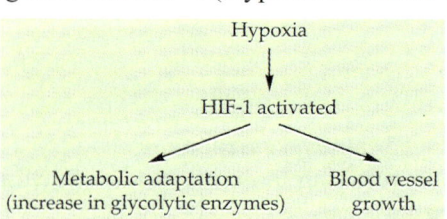

Carbohydrate Chemistry and Metabolism

These biochemical effects are responsible for improving athletic performance that results from training. Under hypoxic conditions, the enzyme prolyl hydroxylase (heme-containing protein, requires O_2 for action) is not able to hydroxylate HIF-1 protein. Hydroxylation of HIF-1 causes binding to ubiquitin E3 ligase and degradation. Lactate/pyruvate inhibit prolyl hydroxylase activity while α-ketoglutarate from TCA stimulates it. HIF-1 upregulates transcription of GLUT2 (for glucose uptake), glycolytic enzymes and VEGF (vascular endothelial growth factor).

Q. 10. Gluconeogenesis in most of the tissues ends at glucose-6-PO_4 rather than glucose apart from liver. Explain.

Ans. Generation of free glucose is an important end point. In most of the tissues gluconeogenesis ends at glucose-6-PO_4 which is further processed in some other fashion.

The enzyme required to convert G-6-PO_4 to glucose i.e. glucose-6-phosphatase is regulated and is present in the tissue whose metabolic duty is to maintain blood glucose i.e. liver.

Q. 11. Enlist the proteins required to convert glucose-6-PO_4 to glucose.

Ans. Five proteins are required to convert glucose-6-PO_4 to glucose in ER in liver cells.
- Three transport proteins:
  - One to transport Glu-6-PO_4 from cytoplasm to lumen of ER (Glu-6-PO_4 translocase)
  - Second and third for transport of glucose and inorganic phosphate back to cytoplasm (GLUT 7 and microsomal Pi transporter).
- Ca^{2+} binding protein to stabilise glucose-6-phosphatase.
- Glucose-6-phosphatase enzyme.

Q. 12. Differentiate between (a) lactulose and lactose; (b) dextrose and dextrin.

Ans.

Lactulose	Lactose
• Disaccharide of fructose and galactose.	• Disaccharide of glucose and galactose.
• Cannot be digested in intestine but is fermented by intestinal bacteria.	• Acted upon by lactase and broken into glucose and galactose.
• Synthetic compound.	• Natural compound.
Clinical significance:	*Clinical significance:*
• Used as a laxative.	• Deficiency of lactase enzyme is associated with lactose intolerance.
• Used in hepatic encephalopathy to decrease absorption of ammonia from gut.	

Dextrose	Dextrin
• It is D-glucose.	• These compounds are formed during partial hydrolysis of starch.
Clinical significance:	*Clinical significance:*
• Available in various concentrations – 5%, 10%, 25%, and used in hypoglycaemia and for parenteral nutrition.	• Used as plasma expander in treatment of hypovolemic shock.

Q. 13. Differentiate between glycolysis inhibition by arsenite and arsenate.

Ans.

Inhibition of glycolysis by arsenite	Inhibition of glycolysis by arsenate
• A chemical compound containing an arsenic oxoanion where arsenic has oxidation state +3 (AsO_3^{3-}). • Combines with lipoic acid of PDH complex and inhibits the conversion of pyruvate to acetyl CoA. • Trivalent arsenic inhibits numerous other cellular enzymes through sulfhydryl group binding. Trivalent arsenic inhibits cellular glucose uptake, gluconeogenesis, fatty acid oxidation, and further production of acetyl CoA; it also blocks the production of glutathione, which prevents cellular oxidative damage. • Arsenic prevents use of thiamine resulting in a clinical picture resembling thiamine deficiency. Poisoning with arsenic can raise lactate levels and lead to lactic acidosis. Low potassium levels in the cells increase the risk of experiencing a life-threatening heart rhythm problem from arsenic trioxide. • Arsenic in cells stimulates the production of hydrogen peroxide (H_2O_2). When the H_2O_2 reacts with certain metals such as iron or manganese it produces a highly reactive hydroxyl radical. • Inorganic arsenic trioxide found in ground-water particularly affects voltage-gated potassium channels, disrupting cellular electrolytic balance resulting in neurological disturbances, cardiovascular episodes such as prolonged QT interval, neutropenia, high blood pressure, central nervous system dysfunction, anemia, and death.	• It is AsO_4^{3-}. Arsenic atom in arsenate has a valency of 5 and is also known as pentavalent arsenic or As[V]. • Arsenate can replace inorganic phosphate in the step of glycolysis that produces 1,3-bisphosphoglycerate from glyceraldehyde-3-phosphate. This yields 1-arseno-3-phosphoglycerate instead, which is unstable and quickly hydrolyzes, forming the next intermediate in the pathway, 3-phosphoglycerate. Therefore, glycolysis proceeds, but the ATP molecule that would be generated from 1,3-bisphosphoglycerate is lost – arsenate is an uncoupler of glycolysis. • Like arsenite, arsenate can also inhibit the conversion of pyruvate into acetyl-CoA, blocking the Krebs cycle and therefore resulting in further loss of ATP. • Effects of pentavalent inorganic arsenic occur partially because of its transformation to trivalent arsenic. • Main effect is, however, by uncoupling of oxidative phosphorylation which occurs in glycolysis leading to loss of ATP.

- The trivalent forms are more toxic and react with thiol groups, while the pentavalent forms are less toxic but uncouple oxidative phosphorylation.
- Arsenic exposure is usually suicidal, malicious, homicidal, or occupational.
- Clinical effects of arsenic toxicity depend on the chronicity (e.g., acute, chronic) and type of poisoning (e.g., arsenic, trivalent arsenic, arsine gas).
- Frequently, patients exposed to arsenic have a garlic smell to their breath and tissue fluids.
- Acute severe arsenic poisoning manifests with the following signs and symptoms:
  – Tachycardia, hypotension, and even shock.
  – Altered mental status, delirium, coma, seizures (acute encephalopathy).
- In trivalent arsenic poisoning, clinical effects depend on the chronicity of exposure.
  – Acute exposures generally manifest with the cholera-like gastrointestinal symptoms of vomiting (often times bloody) and severe diarrhea (which may be rice-watery in character and often bloody); these patients will experience acute distress, dehydration (often), and hypovolemic shock.
  – Chronic toxicity is more insidious and may manifest as a classical dermatitis (hyperkeratosis with a classical "dew drops on a dusty road" appearance) or peripheral neuropathy (usually a painful paresthesia that is symmetrical and stocking-glove in distribution).
  – Whitish lines (Mees lines) that look much like traumatic injuries are found on the fingernails.
  – Cardiac arrhythmias. Prolongation of the QT and ventricular fibrillation after acute arsenic intoxication can occur.
  – Chronic hepatic and renal damage is common with chronic exposure.

- Arsine gas exposure manifests with an acute hemolytic anemia and striking chills.
- Treatment of acute arsenic toxicity is supportive. Chelation therapy is imperative in all symptomatic patients; however, the use of chelators in patients exposed to arsine gas is controversial.
- Chelators include Dimercaprol (BAL in Oil), Succimer (DMSA), and Dimerval (DMPS).

Q. 14. Differentiate between glycogen metabolism in liver and muscle.

Ans.

Muscle	Liver
• Muscle glycogen provides energy to muscles during aerobic or anaerobic exercise in red and white muscle fibres. Muscles do not contribute directly to blood glucose levels in post-absorptive state. However, in prolonged fasting (2 days or more) and some defects of liver glycogen metabolism it can indirectly contribute to blood glucose by Cori and glucose alanine cycles. Muscle glycogen synthesis is more significant than liver glycogenesis in clearing the glucose from blood after a carbohydrate-rich meal. • Glycogen is the main energy substrate during high intensity exercises when oxygen uptake rate is 70% or more of the maximal oxygen uptake rate possible in a subject. Fatigue develops when the glycogen stores are depleted in the active muscles.	• Liver glycogen is a critical source of blood glucose for brain and other tissues in the post-absorptive state/fasting state when dietary glucose is not available. Liver concentration of glycogen is equivalent to about 450 mM glucose after a meal, falls to 200 mM after overnight fast to almost total depletion after 12–18 hours of fasting. Though the total amount of energy stored as glycogen (1000 kcal in a 70-kg man) is far less than the amount stored as fat (141,000 kcal in a 70-kg man), it is critically important as fats cannot be converted to glucose to maintain supply to brain.
Allosteric regulation: • 5′ AMP: ADP + ADP → ATP + AMP (Myokinase). AMP is a potent indicator of low energy state of muscle and forms as the concentration of ADP begins to increase to indicate the need for increased ATP formation. It can allosterically activate the dephosphorylated b (inactive) form of muscle phosphorylase. • Glucose-6-phosphate and ATP can inhibit phosphorylase a (active form) overriding the hormonal control and inhibiting glycogenolysis. ATP blocks the allosteric site where AMP binds.	Allosteric regulation: • Glucose, glucose-6-phosphate and ATP can inhibit active phosphorylase a overriding the hormonal control and inhibiting glycogenolysis. Liver phosphorylase a acts as a glucose receptor as glucose has hormone-independent effect on glycogen breakdown and synthesis in liver. • Glucose inhibits glycogenolysis by inhibiting phosphorylase a (binding of glucose to phosphorylase a makes it a better substrate for protein phosphatase by causing a conformational change to expose the phosphorylated serine residues). • Glucose also stimulates glycogen synthesis as it relieves inhibition of glycogen synthase by phosphorylase a (phosphorylase a can inhibit dephosphorylation of glycogen synthase b by protein phosphatase).

Muscle	Liver
Regulation by calcium: Calcium release from sarcoplasmic reticulum causes muscle contraction and stimulates glycogenolysis as well, synchronizing the two processes. It inhibits glycogen synthesis. Glycogenolysis: Muscle phosphorylase kinase is a tetramer of four different subunits α, β, γ and δ. The α and β subunits contain serine residues that are phosphorylated by cAMP-dependent protein kinase. The δ subunit is identical to the Ca^{2+}-binding protein calmodulin, and binds four Ca^{2+}. The binding of Ca^{2+} activates the catalytic site of the α subunit even while the enzyme is in the dephosphorylated *b* state. The phosphorylated *a* form is also fully activated in the presence of high concentrations of Ca^{2+} only. Glycogen synthesis: Ca^{2+} stimulates phosphorylase kinase, calmodulin-dependent protein kinase and protein kinase *C* through calmodulin. All of these phosphorylate and inhibit glycogen synthase.	

Hormonal:
• Epinephrine and norepinephrine mediate the 'fear, flight or fight' response and effect of sympathetic activity. Both increase cAMP through β receptors to stimulate glycogenolysis and inhibit glycogen synthesis.
• Insulin: Increases glucose entry (by GLUT4) and subsequent glycolysis increasing the glucose-6-phosphate levels. Glucose-6-phosphate binds and makes glycogen synthase a better substrate for protein phosphatase, thus promoting its dephosphorylation (activation).
	Hormonal regulation:
	• Glucagon increases cAMP leading to stimulation of glycogenolysis and inhibition of glycogen synthesis.
	• Epinephrine and norepinephrine act by α1 receptors to increase Ca^{2+} release in cytosol which stimulates calmodulin-sensitive phosphorylase kinase to increase glycogenolysis. Ca^{2+} also mediates the effects of vasopressin, oxytocin, and angiotenisongen II to stimulate cAMP-independent glycogenolysis.
	• Insulin
	  1. Inhibits glycogen synthase kinase-3 through protein kinase B. GSK3 is an inhibitor of glycogen synthase.
	  2. Stimulate protein phosphatase-1 by promoting dephosphorylation of its G subunit and degrades cAMP by activating phosphodiesterase. Protein phosphatase-1 activates glycogen synthase and inactivates phosphorylase and phosphorylase kinase.
	  3. It increases glucose-6-phosphate levels which binds and makes glycogen synthase a better substrate for protein phosphatase.
	  4. Induces glycogen synthase.

Muscle and liver glycogen phosphorylase are isoenzymes, other isoenzyme is brain type.

The disorders of liver and muscle glycogen metabolism are summarised in Table 5.1.

Table 5.1. Disorders of liver and muscle glycogen metabolism

Disorder	Defect	Manifestations	Comments
LIVER GLYCOGENOSES			
DISORDERS WITH HEPATOMEGALY AND HYPOGLYCEMIA			
Ia/Von Gierke	Glucose-6-phosphatase	Growth retardation, enlarged liver and kidney, hypoglycemia, elevated blood lactate, cholesterol, triglycerides, and uric acid, impaired platelet adhesion	Common, severe hypoglycemia. Complications in adulthood include hepatic adenomas, hepatic carcinoma, renal failure
Ib	Glucose-6-phosphate translocase	As for Ia, with additional findings of neutropenia and neutrophil dysfunction	10% of type I
Ic	Microsomal Pi transporter	Same as Ia	
IIIa/Cori or Forbes	Liver and muscle debranching enzyme	Childhood: Hepatomegaly, growth retardation, muscle weakness, hypoglycemia, hyperlipidemia, elevated liver transaminases; liver symptoms improve with age Adulthood: Muscle atrophy and weakness; onset: third to fourth decades; variable cardiomyopathy	Common, intermediate severity of hypoglycemia; hepatic adenomas, liver cirrhosis, and hepatic carcinoma can occur, glycogen resembling limit dextrin accumulates
IIIb	Liver debranching enzyme (normal muscle debrancher activity)	Liver symptoms same as in type IIIa; no muscle symptoms	15% of type III
VI/Hers	Liver phosphorylase	Hepatomegaly, variable hypoglycemia, hyperlipidemia and ketosis, post-prandial lactic academia; symptoms may improve with age	Rare, often a "benign" – glycogenosis, severe cases being recognized
IX/phosphorylase kinase deficiency	Liver phosphorylase kinase *a* subunit	As for VI	Common, X-linked, typically less severe than autosomal forms; clinical variability within and between subtypes; severe cases being recognized
0/glycogen synthase deficiency	Glycogen synthase	Fasting hypoglycemia and ketosis, elevated lactic acid and hyperglycemia after glucose load	Decreased glycogen stores
XI/Fanconi-Bickel	Glucose transporter-2	Failure to thrive, rickets, hepatomegaly, proximal renal tubular dysfunction, impaired glucose and galactose utilization	Rare, consanguinity in 70%

(Contd.)

Table 5.1 (*Contd.*)

Disorder	Defect	Manifestations	Comments
DISORDERS WITH LIVER CIRRHOSIS			
IV/Andersen/ amylopectinosis	Branching enzyme	Failure to thrive, hypotonia, hepatomegaly, splenomegaly, progressive liver cirrhosis and failure (death usually before fifth year); some without progression. Prenatal diagnosis by enzyme assay in cultured amniocytes/chorionic villi sample or by mutation analysis	One of the rarer glycogenoses; other neuromuscular variants (adult polyglucosan body disease) exist, glycogen structure is abnormal and resembles amylopectin
MUSCLE GLYCOGENOSES			
DISORDERS WITH MUSCLE-ENERGY IMPAIRMENT			
V/McArdle	Muscle phosphorylase	Exercise intolerance, muscle cramps, myoglobinuria and low lactate on strenuous exercise, increased CK, moderate exercise can be performed by most patients for long duration, second wind phenomena	Common, male predominance
VII/Tarui	Phosphofructokinase – M subunit	As for type V, with additional findings of a compensated hemolysis	Prevalent in Ashkenazi Jews and Japanese
Phosphoglycerate kinase deficiency	Phosphoglycerate kinase	As for type V, with additional findings of a hemolytic anemia and CNS dysfunction	Rare, X-linked
Phosphoglycerate mutase deficiency	Phosphoglycerate mutase – M subunit	As for type V	Rare; most patients are African American
Lactate dehydrogenase deficiency	Lactic acid dehydrogenase – M subunit	As for type V, with additional findings of erythematous skin eruption and uterine stiffness resulting in childbirth difficulty in female	Rare
Muscle phosphorylase kinase deficiency	Muscle-specific phosphorylase kinase	As for type V, some patients may have muscle weakness and atrophy	Rare, autosomal recessive

(*Contd.*)

Table 5.1 (Contd.)

Disorder	Defect	Manifestations	Comments
DISORDERS WITH PROGRESSIVE SKELETAL MYOPATHY AND/OR CARDIOMYOPATHY			
II/Pompe Infantile	Lysosomal acid α-glucosidase	Hypotonia, muscle weakness, cardiac enlargement and failure, fatal by 2 years age	Common, undetectable, or very low level of enzyme activity
Pompe Juvenile	Lysosomal acid α-glucosidase	Progressive skeletal muscle weakness and atrophy, proximal muscle and respiratory muscle are seriously affected, cardiomyopathy, respiratory insufficiency	Residual enzyme activity
Pompe Adult	Lysosomal acid α-glucosidase	-do-	-do-
Danon disease	Lysosome-associated membrane protein 2 (LAMP2)	Heterotrophic cardiomyaopathy	Rare X-linked
PRKAG2 deficiency	AMP-activated protein kinase γ	Heterotrophic cardiomyopathy	Autosomal dominant
Cardiac phosphorylase kinase deficiency	Cardiac-specific phosphorylase kinase	Severe cardiomyopathy and early heart failure	Very rare

Q. 15. Discuss the clinical significance of (a) enolase, (b) transketolase, (c) D-xylose, (d) 2-deoxyfluoroglucose (FDG), (e) glucagon-like peptide (GLP).

Ans. **(a) Enolase**

- Fluoride is a competitor of enolase's substrate 2-phosphoglycerate (2-PG). Fluoride forms a complex with magnesium and phosphate, which binds in the active site instead of 2-PG. Thus, it inhibits conversion of 2-phosphoglycerate to PEP, inhibiting glycolysis.
- For estimation of blood glucose, NaF along with K_2EDTA is added to blood. While EDTA chelates calcium preventing blood clotting, fluoride ions inhibit enolase and thus glycolysis, preventing the blood cells – RBCs and WBCs from continuing to use glucose which will lead to a fall in glucose by as much as 10 mg/dL/hour when sample is waiting to be analysed in a lab or being transported. This prevents false low values.
- Drinking fluoridated water provides fluoride at a level that inhibits oral bacteria's enolase activity without harming humans. Disruption of the bacteria's glycolytic pathway – and, thus, its normal metabolic functioning – prevents dental caries from forming.
- There are three subunits of enolase, α, β, and γ, each encoded by a separate gene that can combine to form five different isoenzymes: αα, αβ, αγ, ββ, and γγ. Three of these isoenzymes (all homodimers) are more commonly found in adult human cells than the others:

- αα or non-neuronal enolase (NNE), which is found in a variety of tissues, including liver, brain, kidney, spleen and adipose tissue. Also known as enolase 1.
- ββ or muscle-specific enolase (MSE). Also known as enolase 3.
- γγ or neuron-specific enolase (NSE). Also known as enolase 2.
- Higher concentrations of neuron-specific enolase in cerebrospinal fluid are indicative of low-grade astrocytoma. Patients with fast rate of tumor growth have the highest levels of CSF enolase.
- Detection of NSE with antibodies can be used to identify neuronal cells and cells with neuroendocrine differentiation. It can confirm the neuroendocrine origin of undifferentiated tumor cells, helping predict the cause of tumor or metastasis. NSE is produced by small cell carcinomas which are of neuroendocrine origin. NSE is therefore a useful tumor marker for lung cancer patients.
- Alpha-enolase has been identified as an autoantigen in Hashimoto's encephalopathy.
- It has also been identified as an autoantigen associated with severe asthma and a putative target antigen of anti-endothelial cell antibody in Behçet's disease.

(b) Transketolase

- It causes transfer of two carbon units comprising carbon 1 and 2 of a ketose to the aldehyde carbon of an aldose sugar in the HMP pathway. Thus, it converts a keto-sugar to aldo-sugar with 2 carbons less and simultaneously an aldo-sugar into a keto-sugar with two carbons more. In mammals, transketolase connects the pentose phosphate pathway to glycolysis, feeding excess sugar phosphates into the main carbohydrate metabolic pathways. It requires thiamine pyrophosphate (TPP) as its prosthetic group and calcium for activity. Thus, thiamine deficiency can be assessed by measuring transketolase activity in RBCs. Decreased activity is seen in beri-beri, chronic alcoholism, Wernicke's encephalopathy and other states of thiamine deficiency.
- The erythrocyte transketolase test requires a sample of hemolyzed blood to be incubated with excess ribose 5-phosphate (or xylulose 5-phosphate), in the presence of excess added thiamine pyrophosphate (matched with a control that has no added TPP). After the incubation period, one then measures the amount of substrate remaining and the amount of product formed. These concentrations are measured by using high performance liquid chromatography (HPLC). Any enhancement in enzyme activity resulting from the added thiamine pyrophosphate indicates that the sample was originally deficient in thiamine. The extent of deficiency in thiamine is expressed in percent stimulation over the control value.

Classification of thiamine deficiency	TPP stimulation
Acceptable (low risk)	0–15%
Low (medium risk)	16–20%
Deficient (high risk)	> 20%

(c) D-Xylose

- It is a five carbon monosaccharide, used clinically to detect carbohydrate malabsorption. The urinary D-xylose test for carbohydrate absorption provides an assessment of proximal small-intestinal mucosal function. D-Xylose, a pentose, is absorbed almost exclusively in the proximal small intestine. The test is performed by giving 25 g D-xylose and collecting urine for 5 h. An abnormal test (< 4.5 g excretion) reflects the presence of duodenal/jejunal mucosal diseases like Whipple's disease, small intestinal bacterial overgrowth and malabsorption. Treatment with antibiotic in bacterial overgrowth leads to normalization. The D-xylose test can also be abnormal in patients with blind loop syndrome and, can be false positive in patients with ascites, pleural fluid, edema, etc. The ease of obtaining a mucosal biopsy of the small intestine by endoscopy and the high false-negative rate of the D-xylose test have led to diminished use of this test.

(d) 2-Deoxyfluoroglucose (FDG)

- It is an artificial analogue of glucose that is labelled with fluorine-18 (^{18}F) which is substituted for the normal hydroxyl group at the 2' position in the glucose molecule. This radioisotope is clinically used in Positron emission tomography (PET scan) in oncology and neurology. It is taken up by high-glucose-using cells such as brain, kidney, and cancer cells, where it is phosphorylated by hexokinase (whose mitochondrial form is greatly elevated in rapidly growing malignant tumors). No further reactions take place due to the missing 2' hydroxyl (–OH) group of normal glucose. Thus, like 2-deoxy-D-glucose, FDG cannot be further metabolized in cells. The phosphorylated form cannot leave the cell either and thus accumulates resulting in intense radio-labelling of tissues with high glucose uptake such as brain, liver and most cancer tissues.
- The radioisotope undergoes positron emission decay (also known as positive beta decay). It emits a positron. The emitted positron travels in tissue for a short distance (typically less than 1 mm), after which it collides with an electron and annihilates both electron and positron, producing a pair of gamma photons moving in approximately opposite directions. These are detected when they reach a scintillator in the scanning device (like CT scan), creating a burst of light which is detected by photomultiplier tubes or silicon avalanche photodiodes.

Applications

- Thus, FDG–PET scans can be used to detect, image and locate cancers. It is helpful in staging and monitoring cancer treatment and detecting metastasis as well.
- The concentrations of tracer imaged will indicate tissue metabolic activity and can be used as important research tool to map normal human brain function. PET neuroimaging is based on an assumption that areas of high radioactivity are associated with high brain activity (glucose consumption) and high blood flow rate (which is thus measured indirectly).
- In clinical cardiology, FDG–PET can identify so-called "hibernating myocardium".

After ^{18}F–FDG decays radioactively, its 2'-fluorine is converted to $^{18}O^-$, and after picking up a proton H^+ from a hydronium ion in its aqueous environment, the molecule becomes glucose-6-phosphate labelled with harmless non-radioactive "heavy oxygen" in the hydroxyl group at the 2' position. The new presence of a 2' hydroxyl now allows it to be metabolized normally in the same way as ordinary glucose, producing non-radioactive end-products.

(e) Glucagon Related Peptide (GLP)

- GLP-1 is a peptide hormone secreted by the L cells throughout the lining of the intestines as a gut hormone (incretin). It is derived by proteolytic cleavage of proglucagon (also a source of GLP-2).

- GLP-1 secretion by ileal L cells is stimulated by the presence of nutrients (carbohydrates, proteins and lipids) in the lumen of the small intestine. GLP-1 has a half-life of less than 2 minutes, due to rapid degradation by the enzyme dipeptidyl peptidase-4.
- The functions of GLP-1 are:
  - Increases glucose-dependent insulin secretion from the pancreas (Fig. 5.2).
  - Decreases glucagon secretion from the pancreas (Fig. 5.2).
  - Increases insulin-sensitivity in both alpha cells and beta cells.
  - Inhibits acid secretion and gastric emptying in the stomach, this delays and protracts carbohydrate absorption and contributes to a satiating effect.
  - Decreases food intake by increasing satiety in brain.
  - Promotes insulin sensitivity.
  - Inhibits pancreatic β-cell apoptosis and stimulates the proliferation and differentiation of insulin-secreting β-cells.
  - Increases beta cells' mass, insulin gene expression and post-translational processing.

GLP-1 agonists or analogues (drugs mimicking function of GLP-1) are used for the treatment of diabetes type 2 combined with other anti-diabetic drugs. Their main advantage over older insulin secretagogues, such as sulfonylureas or meglitinides, is that they have a lower risk of causing hypoglycaemia as they stimulate insulin release in glucose-dependent manner i.e. only when glucose (food) is present in GIT. Approved GLP-1 agonists include exenatide, liraglutide, lixisenatide, albiglutide and dulaglutide. Sitagliptin, competitive inhibitor of the enzyme dipeptidyl peptidase 4 (DPP-4) which breaks down GLP-1, is also used similarly (Fig. 5.2).

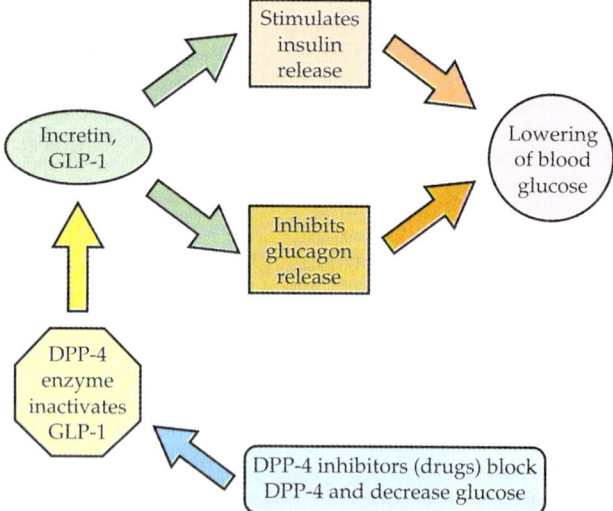

Fig. 5.2. Action of GLP-1 and related drugs.

Q. 16. Enumerate the vitamins that play a key role in citric acid cycle.

Ans.
1. **Riboflavin:** In the form of FAD, it is a co-factor in α-ketoglutarate dehydrogenase complex and succinate dehydrogenase.
2. **Niacin:** In the form of NADH, it is the co-enzyme for isocitrate dehydrogenase, α-ketoglutarate dehydrogenase complex, succinate dehydrogenase and malate dehydrogenase.

3. **Thiamine:** As TPP, it is prosthetic group for decarboxylation in α-ketoglutarate dehydrogenase complex.
4. **Pantothenic acid:** It is a part of coenzyme A in acetyl CoA and succinyl CoA.
5. **Lipoic acid:** Present in α-ketoglutarate dehydrogenase complex.

PDH complex also uses riboflavin, niacin, thiamine and lipoic acid. Glycogen phosphorylase requires pyridoxal phosphate (vitamin B_6). Thus the vitamins – thiamine, riboflavin and niacin – play a major role in catabolism and energy generation from glucose and fats as TPP, FAD and FAD. So their recommended daily allowance is many times specified in terms of the calories consumed. RDA for thiamine is 0.5 mg/1000 Cal consumed, for niacin it is 6.6 mg/1000 Cal and for riboflavin – 0.6 mg/1000 Cal consumed.

Q. 17. Discuss the biochemical basis of anaemias due to defect in enzymes involved in RBC metabolism.

Ans. Haemolytic anemias due to enzymopathies include (Table 5.2):

1. Abnormalities of the glycolytic pathway
- RBCs rely exclusively on the anaerobic glycolysis for producing energy in the form of ATP. Shortage of ATP hampers the functioning of Na^+-K^+ ATPase which continuously pumps three Na^+ out for exchange with two K^+. Thus, it causes net outward movement of ion and water by osmosis to counteract the net movement of water into RBC due to higher protein concentration (Gibbs–Donnan effect). Failure of Na^+-K^+ ATPase causes failure to pump out cations and maintain water balance causing osmotic damage and haemolysis. Accumalation of Na and water causes cellular swelling. This swelling causes rigidity of the RBC and eventually splenic hemolysis from an inability to distort through splenic sinusoids.
- Pyruvate kinase deficiency: Pyruvate kinase (PK) deficiency is the most common cause of haemolytic anemia due to enzyme defect of glycolytic pathway (prevalence – 1 : 10,000) and second most common anemia due to enzyme defect after G-6-PD deficiency. It often presents in the newborn with neonatal jaundice; the jaundice persists, and it is usually associated with a very high reticulocytosis. The anemia is of variable severity; sometimes it is so severe as to require regular blood transfusion treatment; sometimes it is mild, bordering on a nearly compensated hemolytic disorder. The anemia is remarkably well tolerated, because the metabolic block at the last step in glycolysis causes an increase in bisphosphoglycerate (or DPG), which causes the hemoglobin–oxygen dissociation curve to shift to right and decreases affinity of Hb for oxygen; thus, the oxygen delivery to the tissues is enhanced.
- Other defects in enzymes leading to shortage of ATP are shown in Table 5.2.
- Diphosphoglycerate mutase (DPGM) deficiency causes decreased levels of 2,3-BPG causing decreased oxygen delivery, hypoxia and thus moderately increased RBC count due to increased erythropoietin. Despite increased ATP and Hb levels, there is still an anaemic state as oxygen delivery is hampered! Thus, the basic definition of anemia is a decrease in oxygen delivery capacity rather than simply reduced Hb content in blood.

Table 5.2. Defects in enzymes leading to hemolytic anemias

Enzyme (Acronym)	Prevalence of enzyme deficiency (Rank)	Other tissues affected	Comments
GLYCOLYTIC PATHWAY (Shortage of ATP)			
Hexokinase (HK)	Very rare		Other isoenzymes known
Glucose-6-phosphate isomerase (G6PI)	Rare	Nerve muscle, CNS	
Phosphofructokinase (PFK)	Very rare	Myopathy	
Aldolase	Very rare		
Triose phosphate isomerase (TPI)	Very rare	CNS (severe), nerve muscle	
Glyceraldehyde-3-phosphate dehydrogenase (GAPD)	Very rare	Myopathy	
Diphosphoglycerate mutase (DPGM)	Very rare		Erythrocytosis rather than hemolysis
Phosphoglycerate kinase (PGK)	Very rare	CNS, nerve muscle	May benefit from splenectomy
Pyruvate kinase (PK)	Rare		May benefit from splenectomy
REDOX			
Glucose-6-phosphate dehydrogenase (G6PD)	Common	Very rarely granulocytes	In almost all cases only anaemia occurs due to exogenous oxidant trigger
Glutathione synthase	Very rare	CNS	
Glutamylcysteine synthase	Very rare	CNS	
Cytochrome b5 reductase	Rare	CNS	Methemoglobinemia rather than hemolysis
NUCLEOTIDE METABOLISM			
Adenylate kinase (AK)	Very rare	CNS	
Pyrimidine 5′-nucleotidase (P5N)	Rare		May benefit from splenectomy

2. Abnormalities in redox systems

- GSH is very important intracellular antioxidant in the defence against oxidative stress. Inherited defects of GSH metabolism are exceedingly rare, but all can give rise to chronic hemolytic anemia. Even acquired selenium deficiency leads to decreased activity of glutathione peroxidase and hence haemolytic anemia.
- Of these, G6PDH deficiency is the most common cause of anemia due to enzymopathy. Others are shown in Table 5.2.
- G6PDH is an enzyme of HMP pathway which generates NADPH which supplies reducing equivalents required to regenerate oxidized glutathione (GSSH). RBCs do not have any other source of NADPH besides HMP pathway. Thus, shortage of NADPH hampers availability of reduced GSH and ability of RBC to protect against oxidant damage. Oxidant

damage to RBC lipid membrane and cytoskeleton proteins causes loss of flexibility and haemolysis when they pass through the spleen. Oxidant damage is caused by exogenous agents which increase oxidant load. Thus, a kind of acquired haemolytic anemia occurs due to exposure to three types of triggers: (1) fava beans, (2) infections, and (3) drugs. Severe oxidant damage can cause intravascular haemolysis, hemoglobinuria and renal failure (Fig. 5.3).

3. Pyrimidine 5´-Nucleotidase (P5N) Deficiency

- P5N is a key enzyme in the catabolism of nucleotides arising from the degradation of nucleic acids that takes place in the final stages of erythroid cell maturation. The mechanism of anemia is not known but a highly distinctive feature of this condition is a morphologic abnormality of the red cells known as basophilic stippling. The condition is rare, but it ranks third in frequency among red cell enzyme defects (after G6PD deficiency and PK deficiency). The anemia is lifelong, of variable severity, and may benefit from splenectomy.

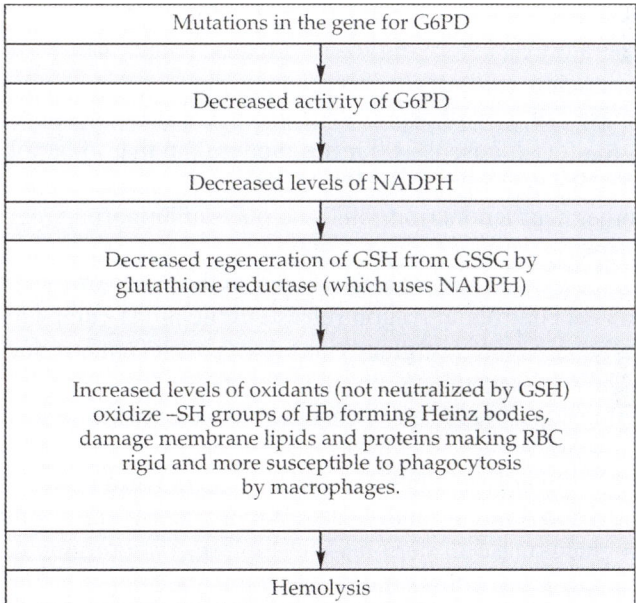

Fig. 5.3. Haemolysis in G6PDH deficiency.

Q. 18. Differentiate between the different isoenzymes of hexokinase.

Ans. There are four main hexokinase isozymes that vary in subcellular locations and kinetics with respect to different substrates and conditions. They are designated hexokinases I, II, III, and IV or hexokinases A, B, C, and D.

Hexokinases I, II, and III

- Hexokinases I, II, and III ("low K_m" isozymes) have very low K_m (< 5 mg/dL) (Fig. 5.4).
- Have high affinity for glucose even at low concentrations (below 20 mg/dL).
- Hexokinases I and II follow Michaelis–Menten kinetics at physiologic concentrations of substrates (Fig. 5.4).

- All three are strongly feedback inhibited by their product, glucose-6-phosphate, in an allosteric way.
- All are made of two similar 50 kD halves, but only in hexokinase II, both halves have functional active sites.
- Hexokinase I is found in all mammalian tissues, and is always expressed or is a "housekeeping enzyme". It is thus not unaffected by most physiological, hormonal, and metabolic changes.
- Hexokinase II is the main regulated isoenzyme and is increased in many cancers.
- Hexokinase III is substrate-inhibited by glucose at physiologic concentrations.

Hexokinase IV/Glucokinase

- Hexokinase IV is monomeric but shows positive cooperativity with glucose (Hill coefficient = 1.7).
- It is the only regulatory enzyme with only one subunit and single binding site but still shows cooperativity for glucose. Does not follow Michaelis–Menten kinetics. Its K_m or more accurately $S_{0.5}$ is 72 mg/dL for glucose (Fig. 5.4).
- Not allosterically inhibited by its product, glucose-6-phosphate.
- Glucokinase can only phosphorylate glucose if the concentration of this substrate is high enough. K_m for glucose is 100 times higher than that of hexokinases I, II, and III.
- Hexokinase IV is present in the liver, pancreas, hypothalamus, small intestine, and perhaps certain other neuroendocrine cells, and plays an important regulatory role in carbohydrate metabolism.
- Serves as the glucose sensor in the β-cells of the pancreatic islets, to control insulin release, and similarly controls glucagon release in the alpha cells. Only when glucose levels are sufficiently high (> K_m of glucokinase) glycolysis and production of enough ATP occurs to close the ATP-sensitive K^+ channels to cause depolarization and insulin release.
- In liver, glucokinase responds to changes of ambient glucose levels by increasing or reducing glycogen synthesis.
- Its activity in liver is regulated by GKRP-glucokinase regulatory protein which competes with glucose to bind to glucokinase. When glucose and insulin are low (fasting), GKRP binds to glucokinase in peripheral cytoplasm (where glucokinase is found mainly and glycogen synthesis occurs) and moves it into the nucleus where it is held in inactive form. When glucose and insulin levels rise glucokinase is released from GKRP and moves back to cytoplasm. GKRP is found in excess of glucokinase and GKRP – glucokinase ratio varies with diet, insulin, etc.
- Glucokinase mutation causes a monogenic form of DM (MODY2).

Metabolic significance of isoenzymes of hexokinase

- The difference in K_m of hexokinase and glucokinase ensures that non-hepatic tissues (which contain hexokinase) rapidly and efficiently trap blood glucose within their cells by converting it to glucose-6-phosphate even at low blood glucose levels.
- One major function of the liver is to deliver glucose to the blood and this is ensured by having a glucose phosphorylating enzyme (glucokinase) whose K_m for glucose is sufficiently higher than the normal circulating concentration of glucose (60 mg/dL). Phosphorylation of glucose traps it in the cell preventing transport back to blood.

- After meals, when postprandial blood glucose levels are high, liver glucokinase is significantly active, which causes the liver preferentially to trap and to store circulating glucose.
- When blood glucose falls to very low levels, tissues such as liver and kidney, which contain glucokinase but are not highly dependent on glucose, do not continue to use the meagre glucose supplies that remain available.
- At the same time, tissues, such as the brain, which are critically dependent on glucose, continue to scavenge blood glucose using their low K_m (much lower than blood glucose levels).
- Under various conditions of glucose deficiency, such as long periods between meals, the liver is stimulated to supply the blood with glucose through the pathway of gluconeogenesis. The levels of glucose produced during gluconeogenesis are insufficient to activate glucokinase, allowing the glucose to pass out of hepatocytes into the blood.
- The regulation of hexokinase and glucokinase activities is also different. Hexokinases I, II, and III are allosterically inhibited by product (G6P) accumulation, whereas glucokinase is not. This further ensures liver accumulation of glucose stores during times of glucose excess.

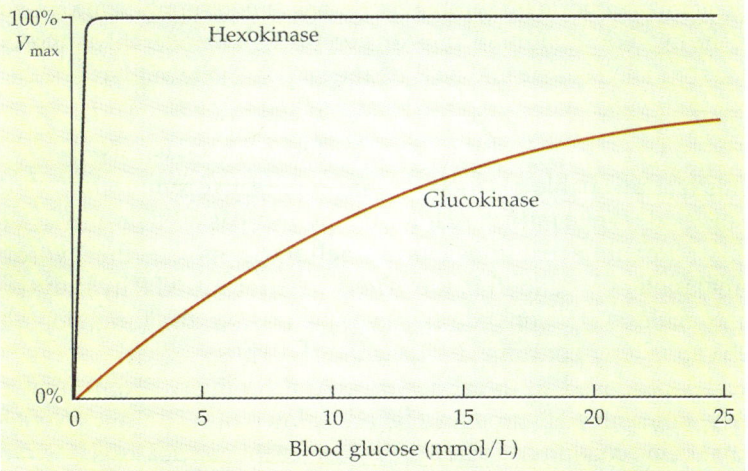

Fig. 5.4. Kinetics and K_m of hexokinase and glucokinase.

Q. 19. Why anaerobic metabolism leads to lactic acidosis? Describe the biochemistry behind lactic acidosis and the different types of lactic acidosis. Explain the significance of plasma lactate levels in emergency patients.

Ans. It is the anaerobic metabolism or ATP production from glycolysis alone which generates both H^+ and excess lactate, rather than lactic acid being responsible for acidosis itself.

Aerobic metabolism

Cells require a continuous supply of energy. This energy is stored as the phosphate bonds of the ATP molecule. ATP is produced mainly in mitochondria and some amount in glycolysis (substrate level phosphorylation). The hydrolysis of ATP results in the following reaction, where ADP is adenosine diphosphate and Pi is inorganic phosphate.

$$ATP = ADP + Pi + H^+ + energy$$

With an adequate supply of oxygen, the cells use ADP, Pi, and H^+ in the mitochondria to reconstitute ATP. This process requires reducing equivalents (NADH). These are supplied by glycolysis and TCA. Pyruvate produced by glycolysis can enter mitochondria and is used by pyruvate dehydrogenase to form acetyl CoA which runs the TCA. Mitochondrial ETC uses NADH produced in glycolysis and TCA to generate ATP and supplies back NAD^+ required for glycolysis and TCA. Thus pyruvate and NADH are end products of glycolysis which are consumed by mitochondria to make ATP and regenerate NAD for glycolysis (aerobic conditions). When mitochondria are functioning the H^+ released from ATP break down and are reused for ATP production.

Anaerobic metabolism

Mitochondrial metabolism (PDH, TCA and ETC) requires oxygen. In conditions of decreased tissue oxygen supply, mitochondrial metabolism cannot occur and pyruvate is not consumed but is converted to lactic acid by lactate dehydrogenase which also converts NADH to NAD^+. This allows regeneration of NAD^+ so that glycolysis can continue even in lack of oxygen to generate some ATP for cell. 32 ATPs are generated per glucose (2 from glycolysis and 30 in mitochondria) in aerobic conditions, but to supply same amount of ATP by glycolysis alone in hypoxic condition rate of glycolysis considerably increases along with lactate production. Then lactate and ATP are the end products of glycolysis. Lactate is formed in the cytosol catalyzed by the enzyme lactate dehydrogenase, as shown below:

$$\text{Pyruvate} + \text{NADH} \leftrightarrow \text{Lactate} + NAD^+$$

This is a reversible reaction that favours lactate synthesis with the lactate-to-pyruvate ratio of 25 : 1. When mitochondria work pyruvate is used up and lactate converts to pyruvate by this reversible reaction. During cellular hypoxia, the hydrolysis of ATP leads to accumulation of H^+ and Pi in the cytosol. Therefore, ATP hydrolysis is the actual source of cellular acidosis (H^+ ions) during hypoxia and not the formation of lactate from glucose, which can neither consume nor generate H^+. Thus:

- The H^+ produced by breakdown of ATP produced from mitochondria is recycled in mitochondria but H^+ produced by breakdown of ATP from glycolysis is not recycled.
- In anaerobic conditions source of H^+ responsible for acidosis is hydrolysis of ATP produced in glycolysis (substrate level phosphorylation) rather than lactate itself.
- Rate of glycolysis is much higher in anaerobic conditions to produce sufficient ATP and so more lactate is generated.
- Second source of H^+ in anaerobic conditions: A second cellular source of anaerobic ATP is the adenylate kinase reaction, also called the myokinase reaction, where 2 molecules of ADP join to form ATP and adenosine monophosphate (AMP). This reaction leads to increased intracellular levels of AMP, Pi, and H^+. Thus, H^+ can increase during hypoxemia without the notable increase in cellular lactate concentration also.
- It is the anaerobic metabolism which generates both H^+ and excess lactate, rather than lactic acid being responsible for acidosis.
- Even if the oxygen supply is adequate, lactate concentrations can rise without acidosis if rate of glycolysis is much higher than normal. The metabolites of ATP (ADP + Pi + H^+) are recycled in the mitochondria and the cytosolic lactate concentration rises without H^+ accumulation (acidosis). This is seen in malignancies where rate of glycolysis is very much increased even in aerobic conditions.

Cellular transport of lactate

Intracellular accumulation of lactate creates a concentration gradient favouring its release from the cell. Lactate leaves the cell in exchange for a hydroxyl anion (OH^-) by a membrane-associated, pH-dependent, antiport system. The source of extracellular OH^- is the dissociation of water into OH^- and H^+. Extracellular H^+ combines with lactate leaving the cell, forming lactic acid, while intracellular OH^- binds to H^+ generated during the hydrolysis of ATP to form water. Therefore, cellular transport of lactate helps to moderate the increase in cytosolic H^+ resulting from hydrolysis of anaerobically generated ATP.

Utilization of blood lactate

The heart, liver, and kidneys use lactate from blood by converting it to pyruvate which undergoes aerobic metabolism to carbon dioxide and ATP. Alternatively, hepatic and renal tissues can use lactate to produce glucose via gluconeogenesis.

Normal lactate balance (Fig. 5.5)

- The arterial concentration of lactate depends on the rates of its production and use by various organs.
- Blood lactate concentration is normally maintained below 2 mmol/L, although lactate turnover in healthy, resting humans is approximately 1300 mmol every 24 hours.
- Lactate producers are skeletal muscle, brain, gut, and erythrocytes.
- Lactate metabolizers are liver, kidneys, and heart.
- Lactate is cleared from blood, primarily by the liver, with the kidneys (10–20%) and skeletal muscles doing so to a lesser degree.
- The ability of the liver to consume lactate is concentration-dependent and progressively decreases as the level of blood lactate increases. Lactate uptake by the liver also is impaired by several other factors, including acidosis, hypoperfusion, and hypoxia.
- When lactate blood levels exceed 4 mmol/L, the skeletal muscle becomes a net consumer of lactate.
- The metabolism of glucose to lactate by one tissue, such as red blood cells, and conversion of lactate to glucose by another tissue, such as the liver, is termed the Cori cycle (Fig. 5.5).

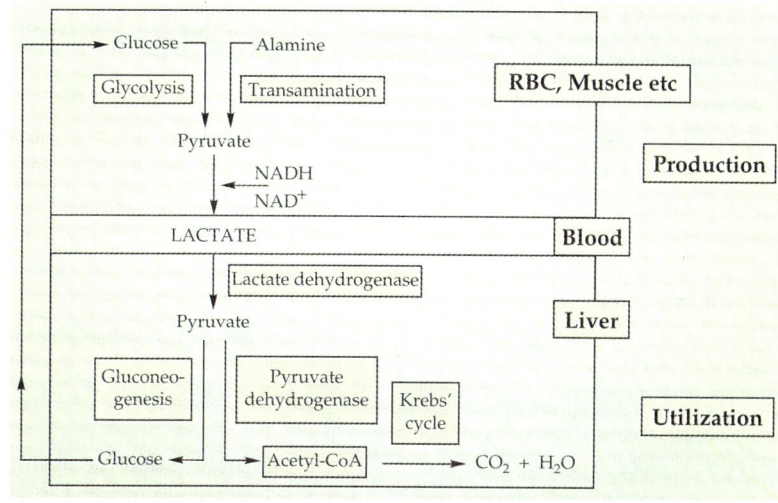

Fig. 5.5. Lactic acid production and utilization (Cori cycle).

Hyperlactatemia and lactic acidosis

- The normal blood lactate concentration in unstressed patients is 0.5–1 mmol/L.
- Patients with critical illness can be considered to have normal lactate concentrations of less than 2 mmol/L.
- Hyperlactatemia is defined as a persistent, mild to moderate (2–4 mmol/L) increase in blood lactate concentration without metabolic acidosis, whereas lactic acidosis is characterized by persistently increased blood lactate levels (usually > 5 mmol/L) in association with metabolic acidosis.
- Hyperlactatemia can occur in the setting of adequate tissue perfusion, intact buffering systems, and adequate tissue oxygenation.
- Increased blood lactate may not necessarily produce acidemia in a patient. The development of lactic acidosis depends on the magnitude of hyperlactatemia, the buffering capacity of the body, and the coexistence of other conditions that produce tachypnea and alkalosis (e.g., liver disease, sepsis). Thus, hyperlactatemia may be associated with acidemia, a normal pH, or even alkalemia.

Biochemical basis of causes of hyperlactatemia and lactic acidosis

- Increased lactic acid generation
    - Reduced oxygen delivery – Hypotension, shock, reduced arterial oxygen content, hypoxemia, anemia, carbon monoxide poisoning.
    - Increased tissue glycolysis – Exercise, seizures, sepsis, catecholamines, alkalosis, malignancy.
- Decreased lactic acid utilization – Liver dysfunction.
    - Reduced perfusion, reduced mass, cellular dysfunction, enzymatic or cofactor deficiency (inherited or acquired).
- Combination of increased generation and decreased utilization – Malignancy, diabetes, alcohol, drugs.

Types of lactic acidosis

Cohen and Woods divided lactic acidosis into 2 categories, type A and type B.

- Type A lactic acidosis occurs in association with clinical evidence of poor tissue perfusion or oxygenation of blood (e.g., hypotension, cyanosis, cool and mottled extremities). It can be caused by the overproduction of lactate or the underutilization of lactate. In cases of overproduction, circulatory, pulmonary, and hemoglobin transfer disorders are commonly responsible. In cases of underutilization of lactate, liver disease, gluconeogenesis inhibition, thiamine deficiency, and uncoupled oxidative phosphorylation are responsible.
- Type B lactic acidosis occurs when no clinical evidence of poor tissue perfusion or oxygenation exists. However, in many cases of type B lactic acidosis, occult tissue hypoperfusion is now recognized to accompany the primary etiology. Type B is divided into 3 subtypes based on underlying etiology.
    - Type B1 occurs in association with systemic disease, such as renal and hepatic failure, diabetes and malignancy.
    - Type B2 is caused by several classes of drugs and toxins – acetaminophen, alcohols and glycols (ethanol, ethylene glycol, methanol, propylene glycol), antiretroviral nucleoside analogs (zidovudine, didanosine, lamivudine), beta-adrenergic agents (epinephrine,

ritodrine, terbutaline), biguanides (phenformin, metformin), cocaine, cyanogenic compounds (cyanide, aliphatic nitriles, nitroprusside), diethyl ether, 5-fluorouracil, halothane, iron, isoniazid, propofol, sugars and sugar alcohols (fructose, sorbitol, and xylitol), salicylates, strychnine, sulfasalazine, valproic acid.
- Type B3 is due to inborn errors of metabolism. These include:
  - Glucose-6-phosphatase deficiency (von Gierke disease), fructose-1,6-diphosphatase deficiency and pyruvate carboxylase deficiency due to decreased gluconeogenesis from lactate.
  - Pyruvate dehydrogenase deficiency, oxidative phosphorylation defects, and methylmalonic aciduria – decreased mitochondrial metabolism of pyruvate.
  - Lactic acidosis may be present in the MELAS syndrome (mitochondrial encephalopathy, lactic acidosis, and stroke-like episodes).

Significance of plasma lactate in adults
- Just like for estimation of blood glucose sample for lactate levels is taken in fluoride-containing tubes to inhibit glycolysis and hence the production of lactate by RBC from blood glucose. Delay in analysing a sample kept without fluoride leads to decrease in glucose and increase in lactate levels due to RBC glycolysis.
- Lactate acidosis as a metabolic monitor of shock: The amount of lactate produced is believed to correlate with the total oxygen debt, the magnitude of hypoperfusion, and the severity of shock. Serial lactate determinations may be helpful in patients resuscitated from shock to assess the adequacy of treatment.
- Hyperlactemia and lactic acidosis in sepsis: Patients who develop severe sepsis or septic shock commonly demonstrate hyperlactemia and lactic acidosis. Patients with septic shock have lactate levels of more than 5 mmol/L, a lactate-to-pyruvate ratio greater than 10–15 : 1, and arterial pH of less than 7.35.
- Mortality and morbidity: Patients who have an arterial lactate level of more than 5 mmol/L and a pH of less than 7.35 are critically ill and have a very poor prognosis. Multicenter trials have shown a mortality rate of 75% in these patients.

Q. 20. What is D-lactic acidosis?

Ans. D-lactic acidosis

L-lactate is the optical isomer of lactate involved in carbohydrate metabolism and substrate for the lactate dehydrogenase found in our body. D-lactate is generated from:
- Glucose and carbohydrate by bowel bacteria in short bowel syndromes.
- Methyl-glyoxal pathway.
- Dietary intake – fermented fruits and vegetables such as pickles, yogurt, and sauerkraut.
- Administration for medical use – ringer lactate.
- Propylene glycol (anti-freeze) poisoning.

Normal humans metabolize d-lactate efficiently – a person weighing 70 kg can metabolize about 2,500 mEq of d-lactate per day. Since mammals lack d-LDH, the enzyme responsible for metabolism of d-lactate in mammals is d-2-hydroxy-acid-dehydrogenase, a mitochondrial enzyme that converts d-lactate to pyruvate. It is a nonspecific flavoprotein, and its substrates include d-lactic acid as well as other d-2-hydroxy acids.

Pathogenesis of d-lactic acidosis

D-lactic acidosis occurs with:

- Carbohydrate malabsorption with increased delivery of nutrients to the colon.
- Abnormal colonic bacterial flora of a type that produces d-lactic acid – gram-positive anaerobes (*Lactobacillus* species).
- Ingestion of large amounts of carbohydrate.
- Diminished colonic motility, allowing time for nutrients in the colon to undergo bacterial fermentation.
- Impaired d-lactate metabolism.

Only d-lactate accumulates because of its slower metabolism. Clinically it presents as unexplained high anion gap metabolic acidosis, malabsorption and neurological symptoms – confusion, ataxia, slurred speech and weakness.

Q. 21. What are Pasteur and Warburg effects? Why cancer tissues have increased rate of glycolysis even when sufficient oxygen is available?

Ans. **Pasteur effect**

Due to this effect aerobic oxidation (via the citric acid cycle) inhibits the anaerobic degradation of glucose. It is the inhibition of glycolysis by occurrence of aerobic metabolism of mitochondria (i.e. use of acetyl CoA generated from β-oxidation of fatty acids and glycolysis itself).

Mechanism

- The inhibition of phosphofructokinase-1 by citrate and ATP.
- The inhibition of phosphofructokinase-1 leads to accumulation of glucose-6-phosphate that, in turn, inhibits further uptake of glucose in extrahepatic tissues by allosteric inhibition of hexokinase.

Warburg effect

It is the observation that most cancer cells predominantly produce energy by a high rate of glycolysis followed by lactic acid fermentation in the cytosol even in presence of oxygen, rather than by a comparatively low rate of glycolysis followed by oxidation of pyruvate in mitochondria (aerobic metabolism) as in most normal cells. Malignant, rapidly growing tumor cells typically have glycolytic rates up to 200 times higher than those of their normal tissues of origin; this occurs even if oxygen is plentiful. The Warburg effect has important medical applications as high aerobic glycolysis by malignant tumors is used clinically to diagnose and monitor treatment responses of cancers by imaging uptake of 2-18F-2-deoxy-glucose (FDG) with positron emission tomography (PET).

Mechanism and Advantages

- Damage to the mitochondria in cancer cells.
- Result of cancer genes shutting down the mitochondria because they are involved in the cell's apoptosis program which would otherwise kill cancerous cells.
- Adaptation to low-oxygen environments within tumors. Hypoxia in parts of large tumors with poor blood supply enhances tumor growth by activating hypoxia-induced transcription factor (HIF-1). HIF-1 induces expression of GLUT 1 and 3 (which increase glucose uptake) and VEGF (vascular endothelial growth factor) which increases growth of new vessels.

- Association with cell proliferation. Since glycolysis provides most of the building blocks required for cell proliferation, cancer cells (and normal proliferating cells) have need to activate glycolysis, despite the presence of oxygen, to proliferate.
- High aerobic glycolytic rates occur due to an overexpressed form of mitochondrially-bound hexokinase responsible for driving the high glycolytic activity. The upregulation of hexokinase II expression in tumor cells is thought to provide both a metabolic benefit and an apoptosis suppressive capacity that gives the cell a growth advantage and increases its resistance to chemotherapy. Hexokinase competes with Bcl2 family proteins for binding to VDAC (voltage-dependent anion channels) to influence the balance of pro- and anti-apoptotic proteins that control outer membrane permeabilization of mitochondria (a process involved in apoptosis) and thus inhibits apoptosis.
- In kidney cancer, this effect could be due to the presence of mutations in the Von Hippel–Lindau tumor suppressor gene upregulating glycolytic enzymes, including the M2 splice isoform of pyruvate kinase. This enzyme form is not usually found in healthy tissue, though it is apparently necessary when cells need to multiply quickly, e.g. in healing wounds or hematopoiesis. The dimeric form of pyruvate kinase M2 (PK-M2) is less active and slows conversion of PEP to pyruvate allowing the intermediates of glycolysis to be channelled into synthetic pathways for ribose, NADPH, glycerol and amino acid (serine, glycine and cysteine from 3-phosphoglycerate) production. PK-M2 also has pro-proliferative and anti-apoptotic effects. PKM2 contains an inducible nuclear translocation signal in its C-domain. Nuclear PKM2 participates in the phosphorylation of histone 1 by direct phosphate transfer from PEP to histone 1.
- Increased glycolysis leads to increased formation of Glu-6-PO_4 which increases HMP pathway which generates reducing equivalents (NADPH) required for biosynthetic pathways (lipid synthesis, etc.) and ribose required for nucleotide, RNA and DNA synthesis and cell proliferation.
- Generation of excess lactic acid from glycolysis due to the Warburg effect provides acidic environment. Lactic acid and acidic environment favours tumor invasion, metastasis and evasion of immune system. Excess lactic acid is generated even under aerobic conditions due to mitochondrial damage. Lactic acid can also be produced by hypoxic tumor cells and stromal cells which are away from capillaries in the tumor (see Lactate shuttle, Fig. 5.6). Lactate promotes inflammation by increasing IL-23/IL-17 production. Lactate efflux through MCT4 increases IL-8 production. Lactate entry through the monocarboxylate transporter MCT-1 leads to increased formation of NADH (which promotes reactive oxygen species formation by NADH oxidase) and increases formation of pyruvate by LDH-1. Pyruvate inhibits prolyl hydroxylase (PHD) which normally causes degradation of HIF-1. Inhibition of PHD triggers the stimulation of NF-kB/IL-8 pathway and VEGF production (by active HIF) driving cell migration and tube formation. Thus lactate promotes inflammation, cell migration and angiogenesis.
- CO_2 produced from HMP pathway, malic enzyme and TCA (Fig. 5.6) adds to the acidity. Low pH can induce apoptosis in normal cells, but not in cancer cells due to p53 mutations. Low pH activates HIF-1 signalling and increases VEGF and IL-8 production which increase angiogenesis. Low pH also favours extracellular matrix degradation by activation of matrix metalloproteinases, proteases, plasminogen activator and cathepsin B and also inhibits immune response against tumor cells.

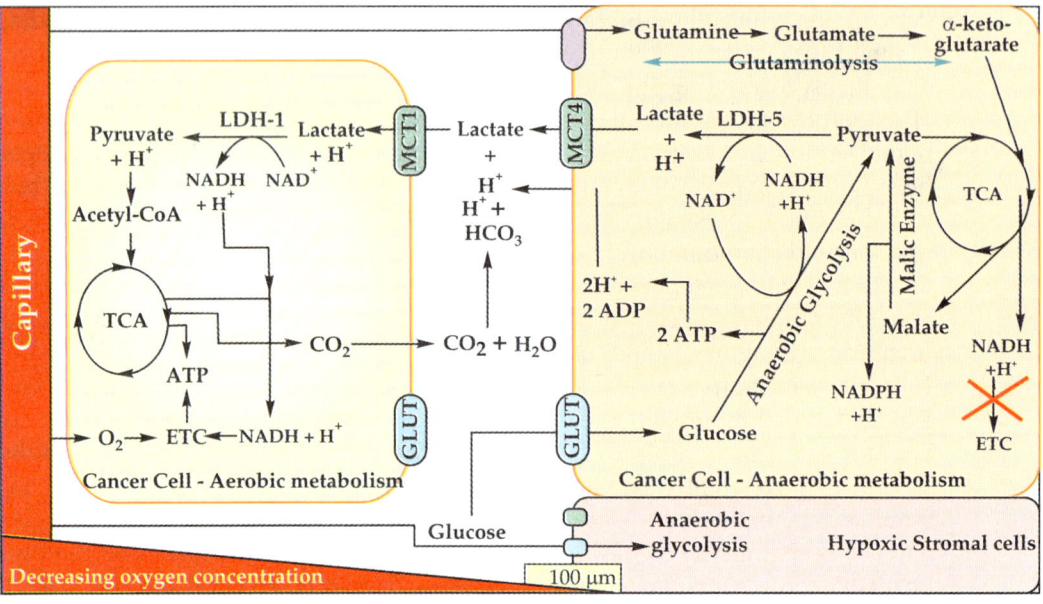

Fig. 5.6. Model of lactate shuttles in cancer. Solid tumors typically comprise oxygenated tumor cells close to blood vessels and hypoxic cells at distance from blood vessels. Hypoxic cells produce energy from glucose using glycolysis uncoupled from oxidative phosphorylation of the tricarboxylic acid (TCA) cycle, which requires high-rate glucose import by glucose transporters (GLUT) to produce 2 ATPs per molecule of glucose. Pyruvate, produced either from glycolysis or generated by the malic enzyme (ME) from malate from TCA, is reduced to lactate by lactate dehydrogenase-5 (LDH-5). NADH is oxidized to NAD$^+$, which is a substrate of glyceraldehyde-3-P dehydrogenase (GAPDH) and therefore maintains glycolysis at high rate. α-ketoglutarate from glutaminolysis enters TCA to form malate which generates NADPH and pyruvate and then lactate from malic enzyme contributing to Warburg effect. Glucose-6-PO$_4$ through HMP and malic enzyme provides NADPH for anabolic reactions. Lactate is exported together with a H$^+$ by monocarboxylate transporters (MCT), primarily MCT4. Oxidative tumor cells have a preference for lactate compared to glucose to fuel their oxidative metabolism. Lactate together with a H$^+$ is taken up by MCT1, oxidized to pyruvate by LDH-1, and pyruvate is incorporated into the TCA cycle to yield up to 18 ATPs per molecule of lactate. CO$_2$ is produced and exported to the extracellular space where it generates bicarbonate and additional H$^+$. Thus tumors are metabolic symbionts in which lactate as a preferential oxidative fuel increases rate of glycolysis and glucose availability.

Q. 22. What is metabolic budgeting by pyruvate kinase? Describe the role of its feed forward activation in glycolysis.

Ans. Pyruvate kinase reaction has a large negative free energy change and is irreversible. Pyruvate kinase activity is regulated by:
- Feed forward activation by its own substrate PEP and fructose 1,6-bisphosphate, an intermediate in glycolysis. Thus, glycolysis is driven to operate faster when more substrate is present.
- ATP, acetyl-CoA and alanine are inhibitors.

Puruvate kinase has two isoenzymes – PK-M (PK-muscle) and PK-L,R (PK-liver, erythrocyte). The PK-M gene further produces the isoenzymes PK-M1 and PK-M2 by alternate splicing, using exon 9 for PK-M1 and exon 10 for PK-M2. Depending upon the different metabolic functions of the tissues, different isoenzymes of pyruvate kinase are expressed. The pyruvate kinase isoenzyme type M2 is expressed in some differentiated tissues, such as lung, fat tissue, retina, and pancreatic islets, as well as in all cells with a high rate of nucleic acid synthesis, such as normal proliferating cells, embryonic cells, and especially tumor cells.

Pyruvate kinase isozymes M1/M2 are also known as pyruvate kinase muscle isozyme (PKM), pyruvate kinase type K, cytosolic thyroid hormone-binding protein (CTHBP), thyroid hormone-binding protein 1 (THBP1), or opa-interacting protein 3 (OIP3).

Unlike pyruvate kinase M1 which exists only in tetrameric form PK-M2 exists in both tetrameric and dimeric forms. The tetrameric form of M2-PK has a high affinity to its substrate phosphoenolpyruvate (PEP), and is highly active at physiological PEP concentrations. When M2-PK is mainly in the highly active tetrameric form, which is the case in differentiated tissues and most normal proliferating cells, glucose is converted to pyruvate for production of energy.

The dimeric form of M2-PK is characterized by a low affinity to its substrate PEP and is nearly inactive at physiological PEP concentrations. When M2-PK is mainly in the less active dimeric form, which is the case in tumor cells, all glycolytic intermediates above pyruvate kinase accumulate and are channelled into synthetic processes, which branch off from glycolytic intermediates, such as for nucleic acid, phospholipid, and amino acid synthesis.

Due to the key position of pyruvate kinase within glycolysis, the tetramer : dimer ratio of PKM2 determines whether glucose carbons are converted to pyruvate and lactate for the production of energy (tetrameric form) or channelled into synthetic processes (dimeric form).

The tetramer : dimer ratio of PKM2 is not fixed. High levels of the fructose 1,6-diphosphate induce the re-association of the dimeric form of M2-PK to the tetrameric form (feed forward activation). As a consequence, glucose is converted to pyruvate and lactate with the production of energy until fructose 1,6-diphosphate levels drop below a critical value to allow the dissociation to the dimeric form. This regulation is termed metabolic budget system.

Another activator of M2-PK is the amino acid serine. The thyroid hormone 3,3′,5-triiodo-L-thyronine (T3) binds to the monomeric form of M2-PK and prevents its association to the tetrameric form.

Q. 23. What are anaplerotic, or "Filling Up", reactions? Why fats are said to be burning in a flame of carbohydrates?

Ans. TCA acts as an amphibolic pathway – it is involved in both catabolism and anabolism. Carbon skeletons of many amino acids and propionyl-CoA from odd chain fatty acids are converted to intermediates of TCA for catabolism. As shown in Fig. 5.7, intermediates of the TCA cycle also are required or used for a variety of biosynthetic processes. α-Ketoglutarate, succinyl-CoA, fumarate, oxaloacetate and citrate are all precursors of important cellular compounds. Oxaloacetate is taken away by gluconeogenesis also. Thus, many processes consume TCA intermediates. It is important to maintain the level of TCA intermediates so as to ensure that acetyl-CoA from β-oxidation of fats and PDH can be efficiently metabolised for ATP production. This is especially important in starved state when oxaloacetate leaves for gluconeogenesis and can quickly deplete TCA intermediates. The cell

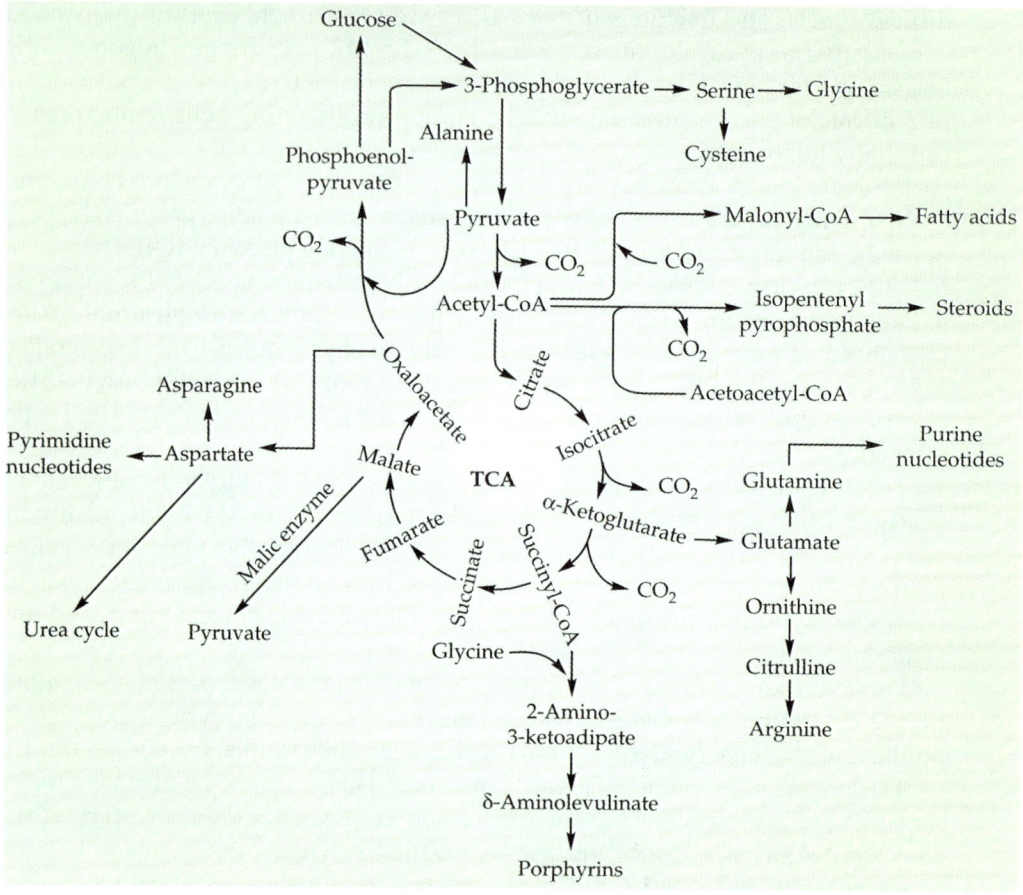

Fig. 5.7. Intermediates of TCA are important anabolic precursors.

feeds many intermediates back into the TCA cycle from other reactions. Such reactions replenish the TCA cycle intermediates and are called Anaplerotic, or "Filling Up", reactions (Fig. 5.8). These include:

- Phosphoenolpyruvate (PEP) carboxylase, pyruvate carboxylase, and malic enzyme (Fig. 5.9).
- Pyruvate carboxylase is the most important of the anaplerotic reactions. It exists in the mitochondria of animal cells but not in plants, and it provides a direct link between glycolysis and the TCA cycle.
- Pyruvate carboxylase has an absolute allosteric requirement for acetyl-CoA. Thus, when acetyl-CoA levels exceed the oxaloacetate supply, allosteric activation of pyruvate carboxylase by acetyl-CoA raises oxaloacetate levels, so that the excess acetyl-CoA can enter the TCA cycle.
- PEP carboxylase occurs in yeast, bacteria, and higher plants, but not in animals. The enzyme is specifically inhibited by aspartate, which is produced by transamination of oxaloacetate. Thus, organisms utilizing this enzyme control aspartate production by regulation of PEP carboxylase.

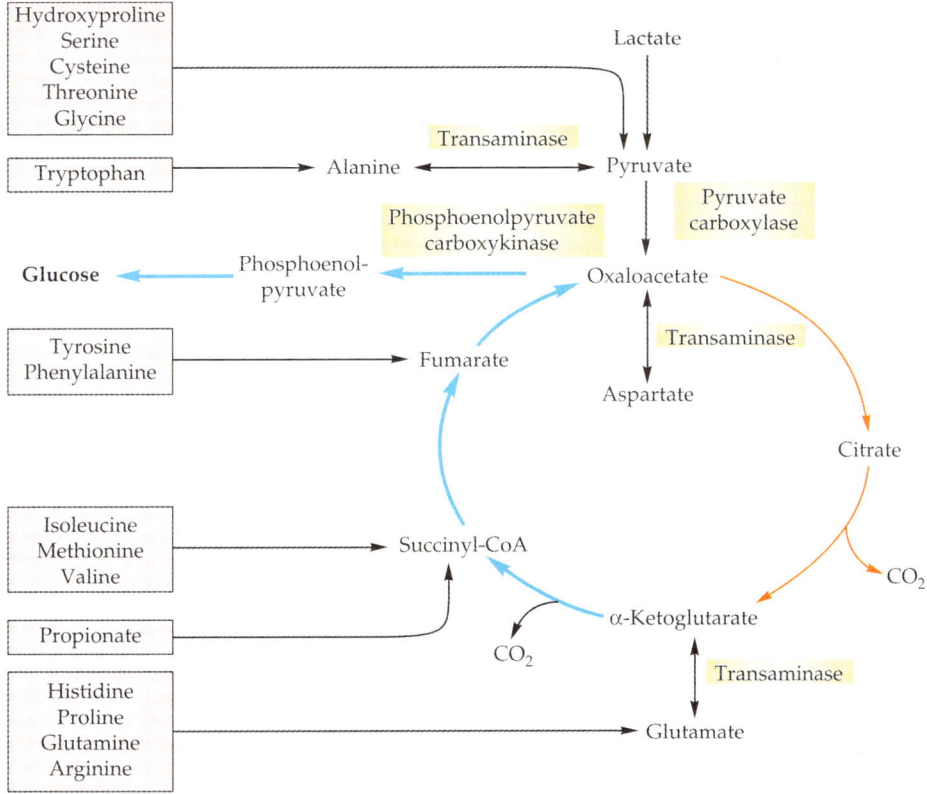

Fig. 5.8. The anapleuritic reactions: Gluconeogenesis removes oxaloacetate. Pyruvate carboxylase maintains levels of oxaloacetate by conversion from pyruvate.

- Malic enzyme is found in the cytosol or mitochondria of many animal and plant cells and is an NADPH-dependent enzyme.
- Reaction catalyzed by PEP carboxykinase could also function as an anaplerotic reaction, were it not for the particular properties of the enzyme. CO_2 binds weakly to PEP carboxykinase, whereas oxaloacetate binds very tightly ($K_D = 2 \times 10^{-6}$ M), and, as a result, the enzyme favours formation of PEP from oxaloacetate rather than oxaloacetate from PEP.

β-oxidation of fatty acids produces acetyl-CoA which is consumed by TCA to produce 2 CO_2 molecules. Thus, the whole TCA acts like an enzyme complex as its intermediates are neither produced nor consumed in the process of burning of acetyl-CoA from fats. However, the concentration of its intermediates tends to diminish with time. This can hamper β-oxidation due to accumulation of acetyl-CoA. The intermediates are restored by pyruvate carboxylation reaction which requires pyruvate from glycolysis. Thus, a minimum amount of glycolysis is required to supply pyruvate to maintain concentration of TCA intermediates or that fats burn in the flame (TCA) provided by carbohydrate glucose.

Hence, skeletal muscles cannot use fatty acid oxidation for energy once the supply of glucose is diminished or glycogen is depleted even while adipose tissue continues to supply fatty acids. Thus, even long distance marathon runners consume glucose intermediately to ensure that muscles can continue β-oxidation.

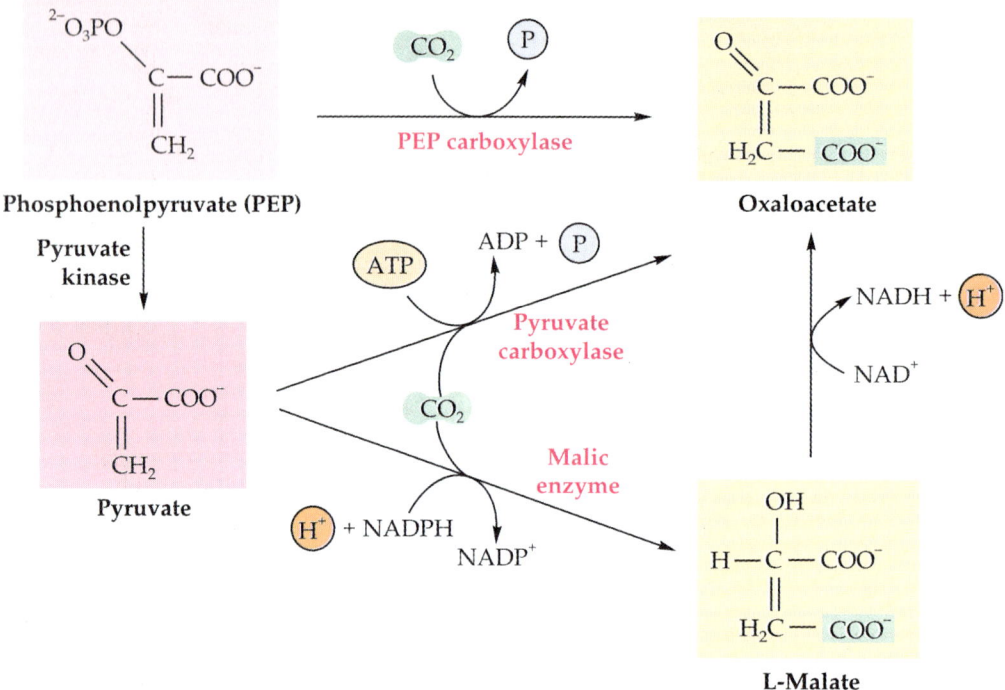

Fig. 5.9. The 3 main anapleurotic reactions.

Q. 24. Explain how excess consumption of sweetened beverages is harmful to health.

Ans. Food items containing large amount of sucrose or high-fructose syrups (HFS) or 'invert syrup' (a mixture of fructose and glucose) which are used in manufactured foods and beverages lead to large amounts of fructose (and glucose) entering the hepatic portal vein. Sucrose-based diet containing 20% fructose can upregulate the GLUT5 transporter suggesting that diets high in added sugars may increase the absorption of fructose and hence its metabolic effects. Fructose enters hepatocytes by GLUT2.

Fructose metabolism (Fig. 5.10)

A specific kinase, fructokinase, in liver, kidney, and intestine, catalyzes the phosphorylation of fructose to fructose-1-phosphate. It does not act on glucose, and, unlike glucokinase, its activity is not affected by fasting or by insulin. Fructose-1-phosphate is cleaved to D-glyceraldehyde and dihydroxyacetone phosphate by aldolase B, an enzyme found in the liver, by cleaving fructose-1,6-bisphosphate. D-Glyceraldehyde enters glycolysis via phosphorylation to glyceraldehyde-3-phosphate catalyzed by triokinase.

Intracellular ATP and citrate exert a negative feedback on phosphofructokinase, so that hepatic glucose catabolism is tuned to the energy status of the liver cells, and insulin regulates glucokinase expression and the activity of key glycolytic enzymes. Thus, in liver cells, as in other cells of the body, the breakdown of glucose is matched to meet energy requirements. By contrast, fructose metabolism is not tuned to energy needs. These two, fructokinase and aldolase B acting specifically on fructose and fructose-1-phosphate, respectively, are regulated

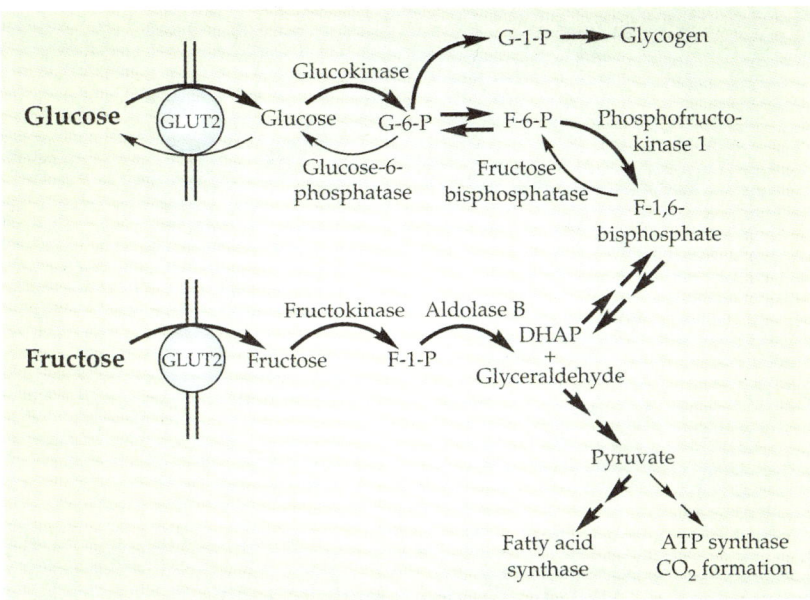

Fig. 5.10. Fructose metabolism.

neither by insulin nor by the energy status of the cell. As a consequence most fructose in portal blood is rapidly converted into triose-phosphate in hepatocytes. Fructose undergoes more rapid glycolysis in the liver than does glucose as it bypasses the regulatory step catalyzed by phosphofructokinase (Fig. 5.10). This leads to the following:

1. A high consumption rate of hepatic ATP for the initial phosphorylation of fructose, which can lead, when fructose intake is high, to transient ATP depletion, formation of AMP and degradation of adenosine to uric acid (Fig. 5.11). Rapid phosphorylation of fructose without any feedback regulation causes sequestration of inorganic phosphate in fructose-1-phosphate and diminished ATP synthesis. As a result, there is less inhibition of de novo purine synthesis by ATP, and uric acid formation is increased.
2. An overflow of triose-phosphates, which are secondarily converted into lactate (glycolysis) or glucose (gluconeogenesis) to be released into the circulation. These are the main fate of most of the fructose metabolized in the liver.
3. Stimulation of glycogen synthesis.
4. Stimulation of the synthesis of fatty acids from the carbons of fructose, through de novo lipogenesis. In the fed state glycolysis from fructose leads to flooding of acetyl-CoA production which leads to increased fatty acid and triglyceride synthesis and secretion of VLDL, which will raise serum triacylglycerols and ultimately LDL cholesterol concentrations which promote atherosclerosis.
5. Fructose ingestion acutely decreases VLDL-triglyceride (VLDL-TG) clearance in adipose tissue, thus increasing VLDL-TG residence time in the blood.

In the 1980s, the use of pure fructose as a sweetener for type 2 diabetic patients was recommended on the grounds that fructose might be less harmful than sucrose or glucose because, unlike glucose, it causes little hyperglycemia after eating (postprandial hyper-

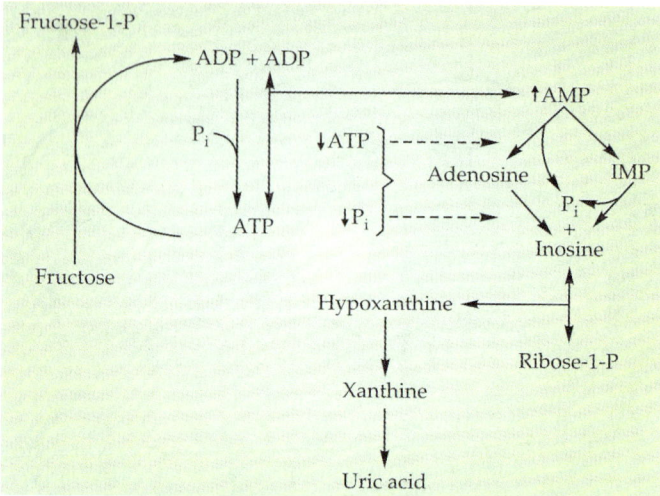

Fig. 5.11. How fructose leads to ATP depletion and urate production. Dotted lines indicate inhibition.

glygemia), and is metabolized independently of insulin. Furthermore, it enhances energy expenditure compared to similar doses of glucose, which was thought to help prevent weight gain. However, many short-term studies showed that substituting fructose for starch in the diet of type 2 diabetic patients was associated with an increase in plasma triglyceride concentrations (both fasting and postprandial), raising the possibility that any beneficial effect on glycemic control may be counterbalanced by pro-atherogenic effects of hypertriglyceridemia and increased VLDL and LDL levels.

Excess fructose consumption in diet is harmful as (Fig. 5.12):
- Fructose or sucrose exerts less satiating effects than starch or glucose due to a lower insulin response. A meal containing 30% energy as fructose, compared with a similar meal containing 30% glucose, elicits lower postprandial concentrations of glucose, insulin and leptin, and higher concentrations of ghrelin in the blood. Since high blood glucose, insulin and leptin are known as satiating signals to the brain, while ghrelin stimulates food intake, fructose would exert lower satiating effects than other carbohydrates.
- Fructose intake more than 60–100 g/day raises plasma triglyceride levels and even with moderate amounts of fructose (40 g/day) that do not change fasting plasma triglycerides, one can observe a shift from large to more atherogenic small, dense LDL particles. More than half the population in developed nations have consumption higher than 50–75 g of fructose/day. High fructose consumption can cause fatty liver due to increased TG synthesis. Increased diacylglycerol produced causes protein kinase C activation and insulin resistance.
- Fructose causes hyperuricemia as describes above. Uric acid has been shown to enter cells via specific transporters such as URAT-1 where it can induce pro-inflammatory and prooxidative effects. Uric acid production by xanthine oxidase also generates reactive oxygen species. Uric acid also causes endothelial dysfunction and hypertension by decreasing NO (leading to vasoconstriction).

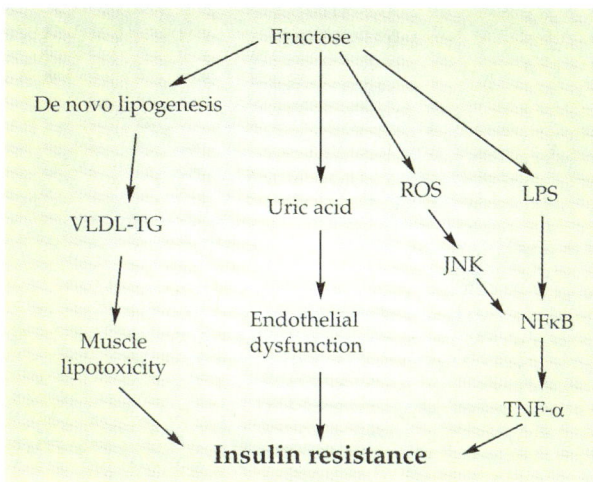

Fig. 5.12. Mechanisms that may link excessive fructose intake to the development of metabolic disorders in the long term.

- Fructose can increase the translocation of bacterial endotoxin (lipopolysaccharide, LPS) into the portal blood, causing endotoxin-mediated stimulation of inflammation. Tumor necrosis factor (TNF) produced in this process increases insulin resistance in the body.
- Since fructose is absorbed from the small intestine by (passive) carrier-mediated diffusion, high oral doses may lead to osmotic diarrhoea.

All these effects cause development of obesity, metabolic syndrome, insulin resistance and ultimately type 2 DM and increased cardiovascular risk.

Q. 25. What is the mechanism for hyperuricemia in Von Gierke's disease?

Ans. Von Gierke's diseases is characterized by deficiency of glucose-6-phospahtase, so Glu-6-PO_4 cannot be converted to glucose in liver leading to postprandial hypoglycaemia. Mechanisms of increased uric acid production include:

- Hypoglycaemia causes glucagon release and this activates glycogen phosphorylase to degrade glycogen to glucose-6-phosphate. There results an increased intracellular concentration of Glu-6-PO_4, fructose-6-phosphate and fructose-1,6-bisphosphate produced from glucose-6-phosphate by glycolysis. Glucose-6-phospahtase which frees the PO_4 group is absent. Hence, while ATP is depleted during production of phorphorylated sugars, trapping of P_i also hampers regeneration of ATP from ADP. These events lead to a depletion of ATP and inorganic P_i concentration, and thus activation of purine nucleotide degradation and increased synthesis of uric acid (Fig. 5.13).
- The increased accumulation of phosphorylated sugars also leads to hyparlacticacidemia by glycolysis and this decreases the renal excretion of urate as lactate competes with uric acid for excretion.
- Excess Glu-6-PO_4 is diverted to HMP pathway which produces ribose which in turn produces PRPP (phosphoribosylpyrophosphate) which increases de novo purine synthesis. Excess purines are degraded to uric acid.

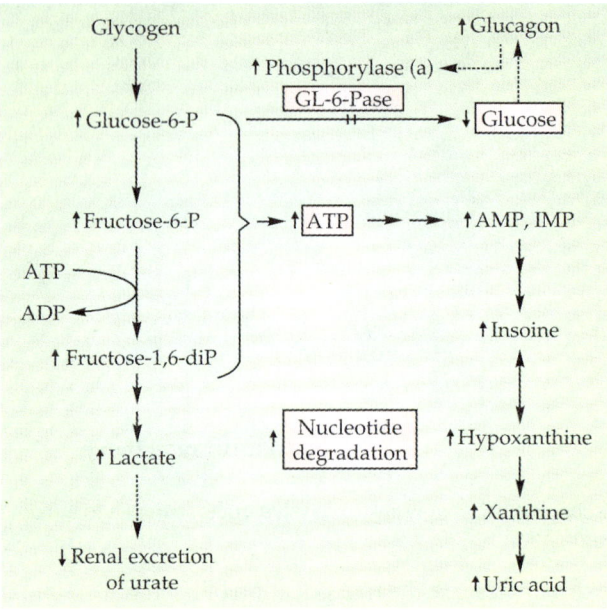

Fig. 5.13. Mechanisms for hyperuricemia in glucose-6-phosphatase deficiency.

Q. 26. Describe the unique structure of glycogen and its advantages.

Ans. **Glycogen structure (Whelan's model)**

Glycogen molecule is made of chains of an average length of 13 α-D-glucose molecules joined to each other by α-1 → 4 glycosidic linkages (Fig. 5.14). There are 2 types of chains: (A) unbranched, and (B) branched chains. Each B chain has 2 branches creating further A or B chains. Branch points have α-1 → 6 bonds (Fig. 5.14). There are 4 glucose residues between two branch points and a short tail after the 2nd branch in B chains (Fig. 5.15). All except the innermost chain originate as branches. The chains are thus arranged in 12 concentric layers or tiers making the entire molecule a sphere of 21 nM radius (Fig. 5.16). The number of chains in each tier is twice as much in previous. All the A chains are in the last tier and the total number of A and B chains are equal. The first carbon (C1, anomeric carbon or reducing carbon) of the first glucose of each chain is attached to sixth carbon atom (C6) of the branch point glucose. Thus, the last glucose (free end) of all the chains has 4th carbon free. This is known as the non-reducing end. The C1 of the first glucose of the innermost chain is also not free as it is covalently bound to OH group of a tyrosine of a protein known as glycogenin (Fig. 5.16). Glycogenin is present in the centre at glycogen molecules and acts as an starting point for the glycogen synthesis.

Glycogen molecule has a molecular mass of 10^7 Da, containing around 55,000 glucose residues with about 2100 nonreducing ends. This molecule can be seen under an electron microscope and is referred to as the β particle. Muscle glycogen granules are β particles while in liver α-rosettes are also present. α-rosettes are aggregates of 20–40 β particles. They can be seen with optical microscope in liver tissue samples from a well fed animal.

Carbohydrate Chemistry and Metabolism 111

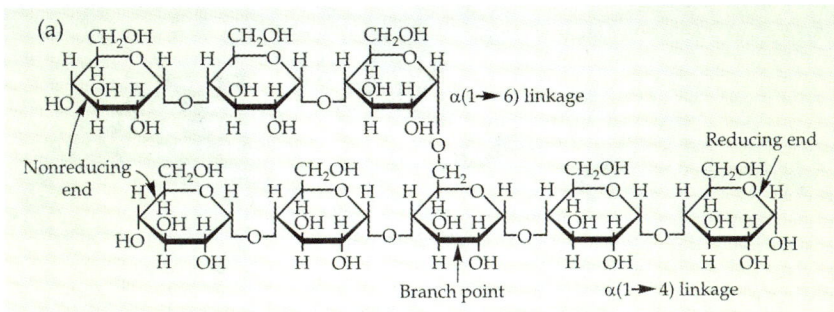

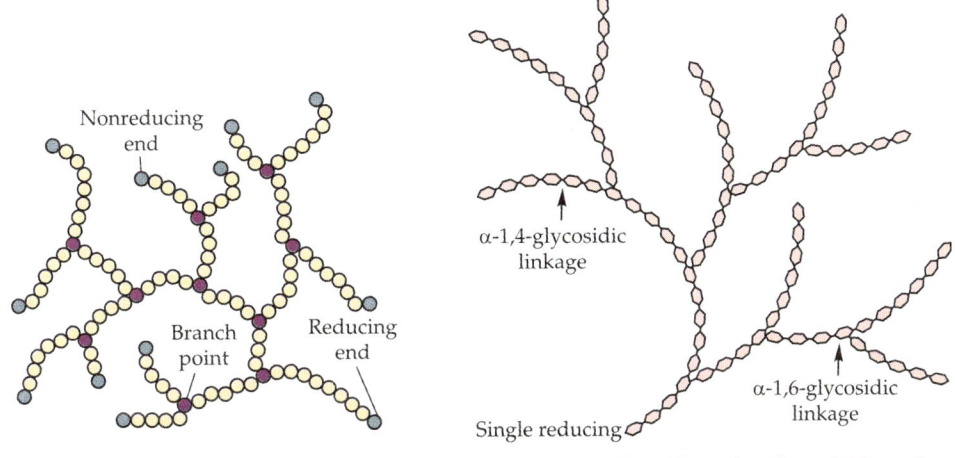

Structure of glycogen

Structure of amylopectin, a branched starch

Fig. 5.14. Structure of glycogen.

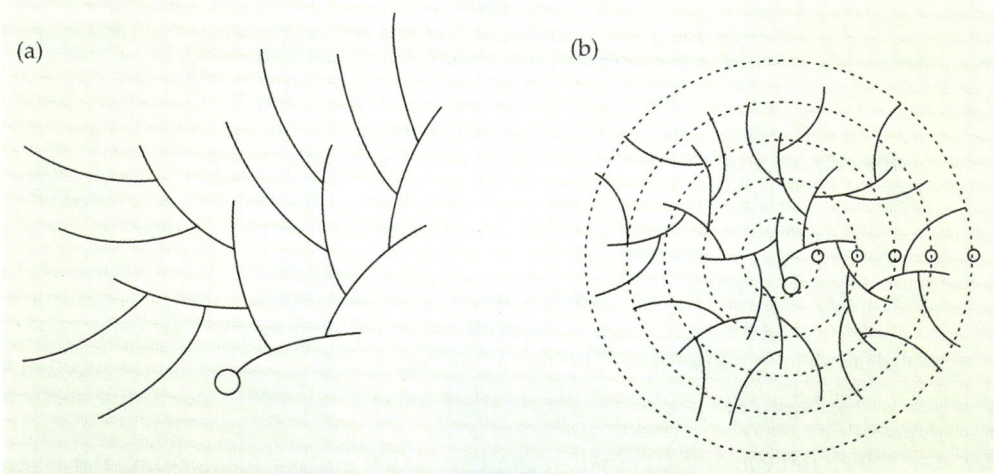

Fig. 5.15. Branched (B) and unbranched (A) chains of glycogen and the spherical structure made of 12 tiers (only 5 are shown here).

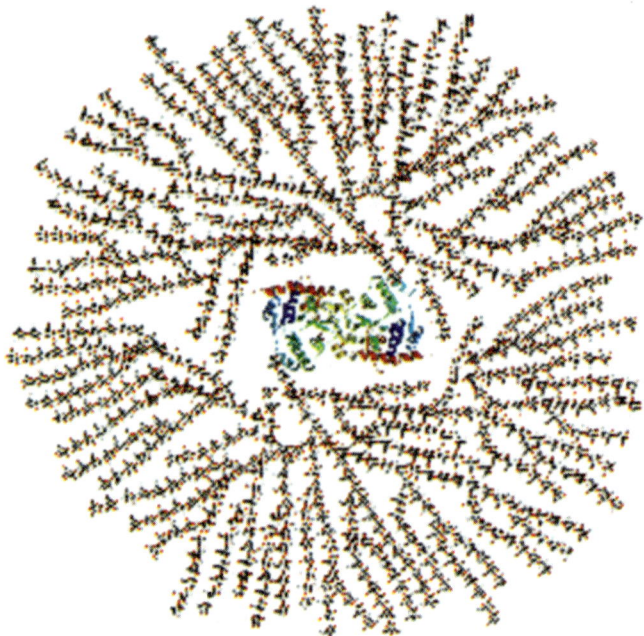

Fig. 5.16. The spherical β particle of glycogen with glycogenin in centre.

Advantages of the structure of glycogen

The structure of glycogen is beautifully optimized for its function of supplying glucose at the maximum possible rate in rapidly exercising muscles. In conditions of strenuous or rapid exercise, rate of aerobic glycolysis is limited by rate of oxygen and pyruvate transport into mitochondria. Not involving the TCA and ETC, anaerobic glycolysis is a much shorter pathway, reaching steady state very quickly. Anaerobic glycolysis of glucose-6-phosphate derived locally from glycogen can generate ATP at a much higher maximal speed. It produces ATP at a maximum rate of 40 mmol of ATP/second as compared to the maximum possible rate of ATP production from aerobic glycolysis of 17 mmol of ATP/second. For example, in a 100 m sprint glycogen breakdown supplies 68% of the total energy, 29% coming from phosphocreatine. Under maximal rates of exercise phosphocreatine lasts only for 30 seconds, while anaerobic glycolysis from glycogen can provide energy for up to 3 minutes. Exercising for longer duration requires considerable decrease in speed of exercise and ATP consumption as energy is obtained from aerobic metabolism. Thus while 100 m sprint is run at 10.4 m/s, 1000 m race is run at 7.5 m/s and a 42 km marathon at 5.6 m/s. But anaerobic glycolysis requires 17 times more glucose to produce equivalent amount of ATP as aerobic metabolism. Unlike fat cells muscle cells have minimal space to store fuel. This would require a large and compact glucose store with minimum osmotic load and maximum speed of breakdown.

Glycogen structure meets all these demands of compact storage, minimal osmolarity and maximum speed of breakdown.

Each molecule of 42 nm diameter has 55,000 glucose residues and thus exerts very less osmotic pressure. Glycogen equivalent to 400 mM of glucose has concentration of only 0.01 μM, thus reflecting the minimal osmotic pressure created.

Lipid Metabolism

Chapter 6

Q. 1. Differentiate between 'ketone' and 'ketone bodies'.

Ans. Ketone bodies are three different water-soluble molecules that are produced from fatty acids metabolism in liver and are broken down as alternative fuel for energy in other tissues. They include:
- 3-β-hydroxybutyrate
- acetoacetate
- acetone

Even though they are sometimes referred to as ketones, the term 'ketones' should not be used because 3-β-hydroxybutyrate is not a ketone and there are ketones in blood that are not ketone bodies like fructose and pyruvate.

Q. 2. Which produces more ATP: *cis*-Δ^9 C18:1 or *cis*-Δ^6 C18:1?

Ans. *cis* $\Delta 9$ C18:1 – as it has double bond at odd position. Oxidation of unsaturated fatty acid with double bond at even position produces $\Delta 2$-*trans*-4Δ-*cis*-dienoyl CoA during β-oxidation and requires both reductase and isomerase step (Fig. 6.1). So, 1 NADPH is used and one $FADH_2$ is less produced as compared to oxidation of saturated fatty acids. In case of double bond at odd position, $\Delta 3$-*cis*-enoyl CoA is produced during β-oxidation requiring only isomerase step and 1 $FADH_2$ is less produced as compared to oxidation of saturated fatty acid. So *cis*-$\Delta 6$ C18:1 gives lesser amount of ATP.

Q. 3. What is the role of beta oxidation of fatty acids in gluconeogenesis?

Ans. Even though fatty acids and acetyl CoA cannot produce glucose, beta oxidation contributes the process of gluconeogenesis by providing ATP. Further acetyl CoA activates pyruvate carboxylase (regulatory enzyme of gluconeogenesis) and inhibits PDH, thus stimulating gluconeogenesis and inhibiting glycolysis.

Branching and large size allows many phosphorylase molecules to act simultaneously to quickly release large amount of glucose. In fact 20–25 phosphorylase molecules are able to simultaneously bind one glycogen molecule. Glycogen has 2100 non-reducing ends where phosphorylase can possibly act. This high number of non-reducing ends increases the capacity of phosphorylase enzyme to bind to glycogen and has an effect similar to the effect increasing substrate concentration has on enzyme activity. 34.6% of total glucose molecules are directly accessible to phosphorylase enzyme for release. As the phosphorylase is a tetramer of 400 kDa it requires space and excessive branching can cause steric hindrance in binding and continuous activity of the enzyme. Phosphorylase can bind only A chains due to very short tail of B chains. Glycogen has large number of long unbranched A chains in the outermost tier which provide the space and flexibility for phosphorylase action. The large number of long flexible A branches in the outer tier are thus beneficial. Phosphorylase enzyme is present in abundance accounting for 2% of the soluble protein in muscles. Further, a very efficient regulation of glycogen breakdown having an inherent amplification property allows few stimulating signal molecules to quickly activate a very large number of phosphorylase molecules.

The optimized structure of glycogen, large concentration of phosphorylase enzyme and the efficient regulation of glycogen breakdown with inherent amplification ensures maximum speed of glucose-6-phosphate supply to sustain the rapid contraction of white muscle fibres.

Glycogen depletion is the main cause of fatigue in contracting muscles. Any alteration in chain length, order of branching and number of tiers decreases the efficiency and speed of glycogen breakdown. The unique optimized geometry is created by the ratio of synthase and branching enzyme. Thus defects of branching and debranching enzymes have serious clinical implications (glycogen storage diseases).

The ketogenic diet also has been used in glycogenosis type V (McArdle's disease), which is caused by a defect in the muscle-specific isoenzyme of glycogen phosphorylase. Glycogen phosphorylase is necessary to break down glycogen into free glucose for use as an energy source in muscles. When the ketogenic diet was applied to a patient with this disorder (presumably providing an alternative means of energy production), the patient's exercise tolerance improved and there was a trend toward decreased baseline creatine kinase level (indicator of muscle damage).

Q. 16. A 3-month-old male infant had facial dysmorphism, hypotonia, psychomotor retardation and hepatomegaly. He had a brother with same facial features and hypotonia who died of hepatic failure at 4 months of age. Biochemical studies (Tandem Mass Spectrometry – TMS) revealed elevation of blood pipecolic acid and VLCFAs. What is the likely diagnosis?

Ans. Zellweger syndrome. Elevations of VLCFAs are a common feature of peroxisomal diseases as VLCFAs are first metabolized in peroxisomes. The peroxisomal diseases are genetically determined disorders caused either by the failure to form or maintain the peroxisome (Peroxisomal biogenesis disorders – PBD) or by a defect in the function of a single enzyme that is normally located in this organelle. PBD include Zellweger syndrome (ZS), Neonatal adrenoleukodystrophy (NALD), Infantile refsum disease (IRD), and Rhizomelic chondrodysplasia punctata (RCDP). The first 3 disorders are considered to form a clinical continuum, with ZS the most severe, IRD the least severe, and NALD intermediate.

Common lab findings of PBD include:
- Defective oxidation and abnormal accumulation of very long chain fatty acids
- Peroxisomes absent to reduced in number
- Catalase in cytosol
- Deficient synthesis and reduced tissue levels of plasmalogens
- Deficient oxidation of phytanic acid and its age-dependent accumulation
- Defects in certain steps of bile acid formation and accumulation of bile acid intermediates
- Defects in oxidation and accumulation of L-pipecolic acid
- Increased urinary excretion of dicarboxylic acids (derived from omega oxidation of VLCFAs in endoplasmic reticulum).

Newborns with Zellweger syndrome may present with craniofacial abnormalities, profound hypotonia (low muscle tone), seizures, apnea, and an inability to eat, hepatomegaly (enlarged liver), chondrodysplasia punctata (punctate calcification of the cartilage in specific regions of the body), eye abnormalities, and renal cysts. Patients have hypomyelination and psychomotor retardation.

X-linked adrenoleukodystrophy is a single enzyme defect (defect in ABCD1, a membrane transport protein in peroxisomes) of peroxisomes which also has accumulation of VLCFAs. Characteristic lamellar cytoplasmic inclusions can be demonstrated with the electron microscope in adrenocortical cells, testicular Leydig cells, and nervous system macrophages. These are cholesterol esterified with VLCFA. Zona fasciculata of the adrenal cortex at first are distended with lipid and later atrophy. There are 5 relatively distinct phenotypes, 3 of which are present in childhood with symptoms and signs. In all the phenotypes, development is usually normal in the 1st 3–4 years of life.

Also for medium-chain fatty acids:
- Carnitine not required for transport into mitochondria
- Suppress body fat accumulation
- More ketogenic than long chain fatty acids
- Used for dietary therapy of mild to moderate Alzheimer's disease

Medium-chain triglycerides (MCTs) are medium-chain (8 to 12 carbons) fatty acid esters of glycerol. Because of the way that MCFA are digested, they can be absorbed in the stomach, after hydrolysis of MCT by gastric lipase, and can also be solubilized in the aqueous phase of the intestinal contents, where they are absorbed bound to albumin and transported to the liver via the portal vein (longer fatty acids require bile and pancreatic juice for micelle formation and digestion and are absorbed into the lymphatic system as chylomicrons). MCTs do not require bile salts for digestion. Patients that have malnutrition or malabsorption syndromes are treated with MCTs because they do not require bile, pancreatic juice and energy for absorption, utilization, or storage. For these reasons, medium-chain TG has been used as an energy source in syndromes having pancreatic-enzyme deficiency such as cystic fibrosis. Short-chain fatty acids are not utilized until they reach the large intestine, where colonic bacteria use them primarily for energy. Thus, their nutrient value to humans is very low.

Q. 14. Comment on the dietary therapy used for refractory seizures.

Ans. Diet rich in medium chain triglycerides and branched chain amino acids or ketogenic diet is used. Such diet includes 80% fat, 20% combined carbohydrate and protein, by weight. The ketogenic diet results in adaptive changes in brain energy metabolism that increase the energy reserves; ketone bodies are a more efficient fuel than glucose, and the number of mitochondria is increased. This may help the neurons to remain stable in the face of increased energy demand during a seizure, and may confer a neuroprotective effect. Changes in ATP production making neurons more resilient in the face of metabolic demands during seizures; altered brain pH affecting neuronal excitability; direct inhibitory effects of ketone bodies on ion channels; and shifts in amino acid metabolism to favour the synthesis of the inhibitory neurotransmitter GABA are possible mechanisms responsible for anti-seizure effects of ketogenic diet.

Q. 15. What are the various uses of ketogenic diet?

Ans. Ketogenic diet is of therapeutic benefit in –
1. GLUT-1 deficiency
2. PFK deficiency (phosphofructokinase deficiency)
3. PDH deficiency (pyruvate dehydrogenase deficiency)
4. McArdle's disease

The utility of the ketogenic diet in PDH deficiency, PFK deficiency and GLUT-1 deficiency results from its ability to supply acetyl-CoA, increasing the TCA and ATP production. These children respond well to the ketogenic diet, as it is believed to provide an alternative fuel source for their central nervous system. PFK deficiency, GLUT-1 and PDH deficiency impair glycolysis and supply of acetyl CoA for TCA for energy production.

Q. 12. In a newborn screening programme dried filter paper blood spot collected for a neonate was found to have elevated C8 acyl carnitine levels. Testing also revealed decreased free carnitine levels. What is the most likely diagnosis? What will be the clinical manifestations? What will be the biochemical basis of treatment?

Ans. Most likely diagnosis is MCAD deficiency. The child may develop –
- Hypoglycaemia on prolonged fasting
- Fatty liver
- Reduced exercise tolerance
- Sudden infant death
- Dicarboxylic aciduria during fasting

Treatment is mainly avoidance of prolonged fasting.

Disorders of fatty acid metabolism like Medium-chain acyl-CoA dehydrogenase deficiency (MCAD), Very long-chain acyl-CoA dehydrogenase deficiency (VLCAD), Long-chain 3-hydroxy acyl-CoA dehydrogenase deficiency (LCHAD), Trifunctional protein deficiency and Carnitine uptake defect, etc. are recommended for routine mass newborn screening. Clinical manifestations characteristically involve the tissues with a high β-oxidation flux including liver, skeletal, and cardiac muscle. The most common presentation is an acute episode of life-threatening coma and hypoglycemia induced by a period of fasting due to defective hepatic β-oxidation and ketogenesis. Other manifestations include chronic cardiomyopathy and muscle weakness or exercise-induced acute rhabdomyolysis. The fatty acid oxidation defects can be asymptomatic during periods when there is no fasting stress. Acutely presenting disease may be misdiagnosed as Reye syndrome or, if fatal, as sudden unexpected infant death. Fatty acid oxidation disorders are easily overlooked because the only specific clue to the diagnosis may be the finding of inappropriately low concentrations of urinary ketones in an infant who has hypoglycemia. Newborn screening programs using tandem mass spectrometry (MS/MS) detect characteristic acylcarnitines seen in many of these disorders and permit presymptomatic diagnosis.

C8-C10 acyl carnitines are elevated in MCAD as they are not used for β-oxidation and accumulate. Due to defect in β-oxidation ketoacidosis does not occur during fasting phase. Treatment is avoidance of prolonged fasting to avoid hypoglycaemia. This usually requires simply adjusting the diet to ensure that overnight fasting periods are limited to <10–12 hr. Restricting dietary fat or treatment with carnitine is controversial. During fasting stress or at times of acute illness, urinary organic acid profiles by gas chromatography/mass spectrometry show inappropriately low concentrations of ketones and elevated levels of medium-chain dicarboxylic acids (adipic, suberic, and sebacic acids) that are derived from microsomal and peroxisomal omega oxidation of accumulated C8-C10 fatty acids.

Q. 13. Why is coconut oil beneficial for an 8-year-old boy with cystic fibrosis who develops malabsorption?

Ans. Coconut oil contains triglycerides (TG) with medium-chain fatty acids. Cystic fibrosis causes pancreatic malabsorption. Giving medium-chain fatty acid is beneficial as they are absorbed into portal blood directly, and do not require bile and pancreatic juice for digestion and absorption.

of ATP. Thus, production of ketone bodies allows liver to continue beta oxidation of FFA despite limited ATP requirement so as to prevent accumulation of large amount of FFA coming into liver from adipose tissue. Also liver exports ketone bodies as alternative fuel for rest of body to spare glucose for use by brain.

Q. 8. What is the clinical manifestation of in-born error with deficiency of HMG CoA synthase?

Ans. It is manifested by fasting hypoketotic hypoglycaemia and dicarboxylic aciduria. This enzyme is common to pathways of ketone body synthesis and cholesterol synthesis and has 2 iso-enzymes. Mitochondrial isoenzyme of HMG CoA synthase is responsible for ketone body synthesis and made only in liver. It is expressed at high levels in prolonged fasting, while isoenzyme involved in cholesterol synthesis is cytosolic and expressed in low levels in many tissues. Deficiency of the liver mitochondrial enzyme is known and causes fasting hypoketotic hypoglycemia, hepatomegaly and massive dicarboxylic aciduria. The defect is only in liver and cannot be demonstrated in fibroblasts. The occurrence of hypoglycemia and dicarboxylic aciduria shows that defect in ketogenesis can impair beta oxidation as major fate of acetyl-CoA produced by beta oxidation in starved state in liver is ketogenesis. With impaired beta oxidation, gluconeogenesis cannot occur due to shortage of ATP causing hypoglycaemia.

Q. 9. Which ketone bodies can be detected by Rothera's test?

Ans. Rothera's test detects acetone and acetoacetate and not 3-β-hydroxybutyrate, which is the predominant ketone body. It can be modified by addition of hydrogen peroxide to convert 3-β-hydroxybutyrate into acetoacetate.

Q. 10. Out of measurement of ketone bodies in urine or blood, which is the preferred test in a patient of ketoacidosis?

Ans. As there is no fixed renal threshold for KB (varies between individuals) measurement in blood is preferred. Thus different amounts of ketone bodies may be present in urine of different persons having similar amount in blood. Measurement in urine may sometimes completely miss significantly increased levels of ketone bodies in blood.

Q. 11. Why drugs which inhibit fatty acid oxidation are used in treatment of chronic angina?

Ans. Drugs which inhibit fatty acid oxidation are beneficial in treatment of chronic angina because by inhibiting fatty acid oxidation they change the pattern of fuel use by heart. At rest heart uses fatty acids (60%), carb (35%) and amino acids/ketones (5%) for energy. Respiratory quotient for fats is 0.7 and for carbohydrates it is 1.0. Thus fats require more oxygen to burn. By shifting ATP production from fatty acid to carbohydrate oxidation less oxygen is required by heart muscle cells. Ranolazine, a CPT-I inhibitor, shifts ATP production from fatty acid to more oxygen-efficient carbohydrate oxidation. 3-KAT inhibitor, trimetazidine, also inhibits fatty acid oxidation and is used in angina pectoris.

Q. 4. Why is beta oxidation an aerobic process?

Ans. Beta oxidation is an aerobic process and cannot occur in anaerobic condition even though it does not directly use O_2 at any step. This is because it converts NAD into NADH and thus requires steady supply of NAD to continue. A cell has limited amount of NAD. NADH is regenerated back to NAD by electron transport chain, producing ATP in the process. Operation of ETC requires O_2. Thus, in the absence of O_2, NAD cannot be regenerated for beta oxidation to continue.

Q. 5. Which organ can produce ketone bodies and which organs can consume ketone bodies?

Ans. Only liver can produce ketone bodies because HMG CoA lyase enzyme required for their synthesis is present in liver only. However, liver cannot utilize ketone bodies due to absence of succinyl CoA acetoacetate CoA transferase (thiophorase). All other organs including brain can use ketone bodies. In time of need even brain obtains 30% energy from ketone bodies. Thus, ketone bodies are alternative fuel produced by liver for other tissues and organs.

Q. 6. Explain how ketone body synthesis is regulated?

Ans. Ketogenesis is regulated by:

1. Activity of hormone-sensitive lipase and thus FFA levels in blood
2. CAT-1 activity
3. ATP requirement of liver cells
4. Insulin/glucagon ratio.

Ketone bodies are synthesized from fatty acids (under conditions of starvation and insulin deficiency). FFA is supplied to liver from adipose tissue. FFAs are released from adipose tissue by action of hormone-sensitive lipase. Thus, FFA levels in blood are increased by HSL action releasing them from adipose tissue in starved state. These FFAs, once in liver, have to enter mitochondria for oxidation or ketone body synthesis. Entry of FFAs into mitochondria is controlled by carnitine acyl transferase I (CAT I). It is active in time of starvation and inhibited in fed state. Once FFAs enter mitochondria, partition of acetyl CoA between TCA and ketone body synthesis takes place in such a manner that the amount of ATP produced remains constant and meets needs of liver cell. Rest all of acetyl CoA from beta oxidation is shunted to KB synthesis and KBs exported as alternate fuel for tissues. Insulin inhibits ketogenesis by inhibiting hormone-sensitive lipase, and stimulating fatty acid synthesis which produces malonyl CoA – an inhibitor of CAT I. Type 1 DM patients are more susceptible to ketoacidosis as insulin is completely absent. Glucagon and epinephrine increase activity of HSL and β-oxidation enzymes.

Q. 7. How many ATPs are produced from 1 mol of palmitate when 3-β-hydroxybutyrate is end product?

Ans. 21 ATPs are produced from 1 mol of palmitate when 3-β-hydroxybutyrate is end product. This is considerably less than the amount of ATP produced by complete oxidation of palmitate (106 ATPs). Beta oxidation is controlled by the TCA and ETC which supplies back NAD. ETC and oxidative phosphorylation is in turn controlled by supply of ADP or requirement

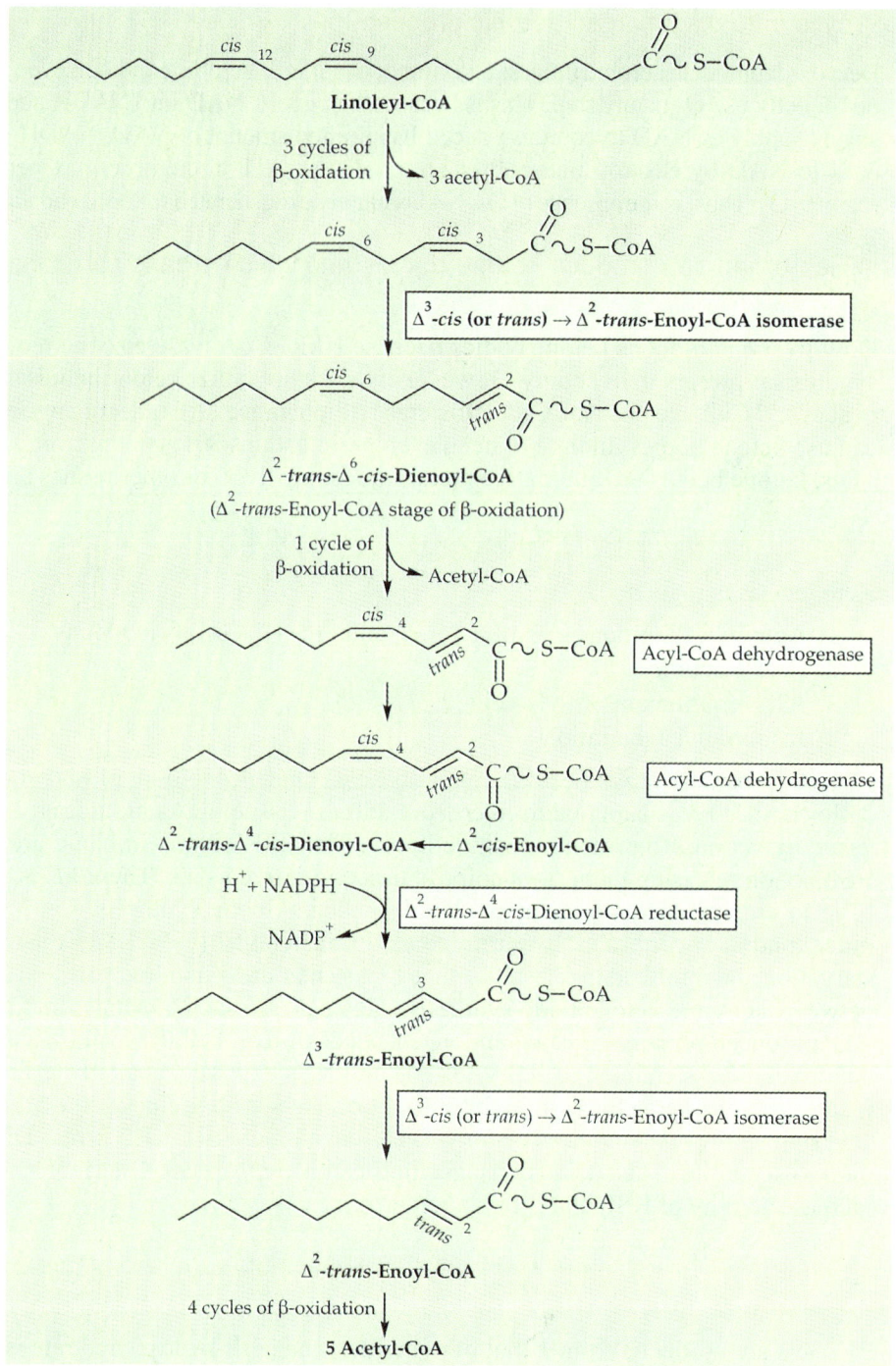

Fig. 6.1. β-oxidation of unsaturated fatty acids. Oxidation of double bond at odd position requires extra step of isomerase besides usual steps of β-oxidation while oxidation of double bond at even position requires extra steps of reductase (consumes 1 ~ ADPH) and isomerase both.

Q. 17. What is the role of lysolecithin in atherosclerosis?

Ans. Lysolecithin or Lysophosphatidylcholine (LPC) forms from partial hydrolysis of phosphatidylcholines, which removes one of the fatty acid groups. The hydrolysis is generally the result of the enzymatic action of phospholipase A2. Lysophosphatidylcholine (LPC) is a bioactive pro-inflammatory lipid generated by pathological activities. LPC is also a major phospholipid component of oxidized low-density lipoprotein (Ox-LDL) and is implicated as a critical factor in the atherogenic activity of oxidised LDL (Ox-LDL). It causes: ROS generation by NADPH oxidase activation, Production of inflammatory cytokines, Chemotaxis of neutrophils and macrophages, Increases adhesion molecules for leukocytes on endothelium, etc. These effects promote atherosclerosis (Fig. 6.2).

LPC can also be formed from action of lecithin cholesterol acyl transferase (LCAT) bound to LDL and HDL in blood. LPCs are present as minor phospholipids in membrane (< 3%) and in blood (8–12%). They are quickly metabolized by lysophospholipases and LPC-acyltransferase.

LPC are neurotoxic as they stimulate phagocytosis of myelin sheath and can alter surface properties of RBCs. Smoking induces phospholipase and increases LPC levels and thus promotes demyelination in patients of multiple sclerosis and also increases ox-LDL and promotes atherosclerosis. Bacteria such as *Legionella pneumoniae* use PLA2 end products (FA and LPC) to cause host cell (macrophage) apoptosis through cytochrome *c* release.

Production of LPC during apoptosis serves as chemotactic signal for macrophage recruitment. LPC acts through G2A and GPR4 (Gi protein coupled receptors) on macrophages and immune cells to cause chemoattraction and macrophage recruitment.

Some food items like processed meat, processed vegetable oils, processed cheese, and bakery products containing egg contain LPC. There is unnaturally high amount of LPC in enzyme processed food. Its presence in vegetable and modified coconut oil has been considered the basis of rinsing mouth with these oils for teeth whitening.

Q. 18. Enumerate the useful compounds synthesized during cholesterol synthesis pathway.

Ans. Useful compounds made by cholesterol synthesis pathway are:
1. Dolichol
2. Side chain of ubiquinone
3. Prenyl and farnesyl groups
4. Side chain of heme A
5. Coenzyme Q

- **Dolichol** – Involved in synthesis of N-linked glycoproteins.
- **Ubiquinone** – Part of electron transport chain (electron carrier in ETC).
- **Prenyl, geranyl and farnesyl groups** – Facilitate attachment of proteins to cell membranes (lipid anchor).
- **Heme A** – Differs from heme B in that a methyl side chain at ring position 8 is oxidized to a formyl group and a hydroxyethylfarnesyl group, an isoprenoid chain, has been attached to the vinyl side chain at ring position 2 of the iron tetrapyrrole heme. Heme A is present in cytochrome *c* oxidase (ETC).
- **CoQ** – Statin-induced rhabdomyolysis is due to the depletion of farnesyl-PP$_i$, which leads to a depletion of CoQ in the electron transport chain of mitochondria, an organelle that is found in great numbers in myocytes.

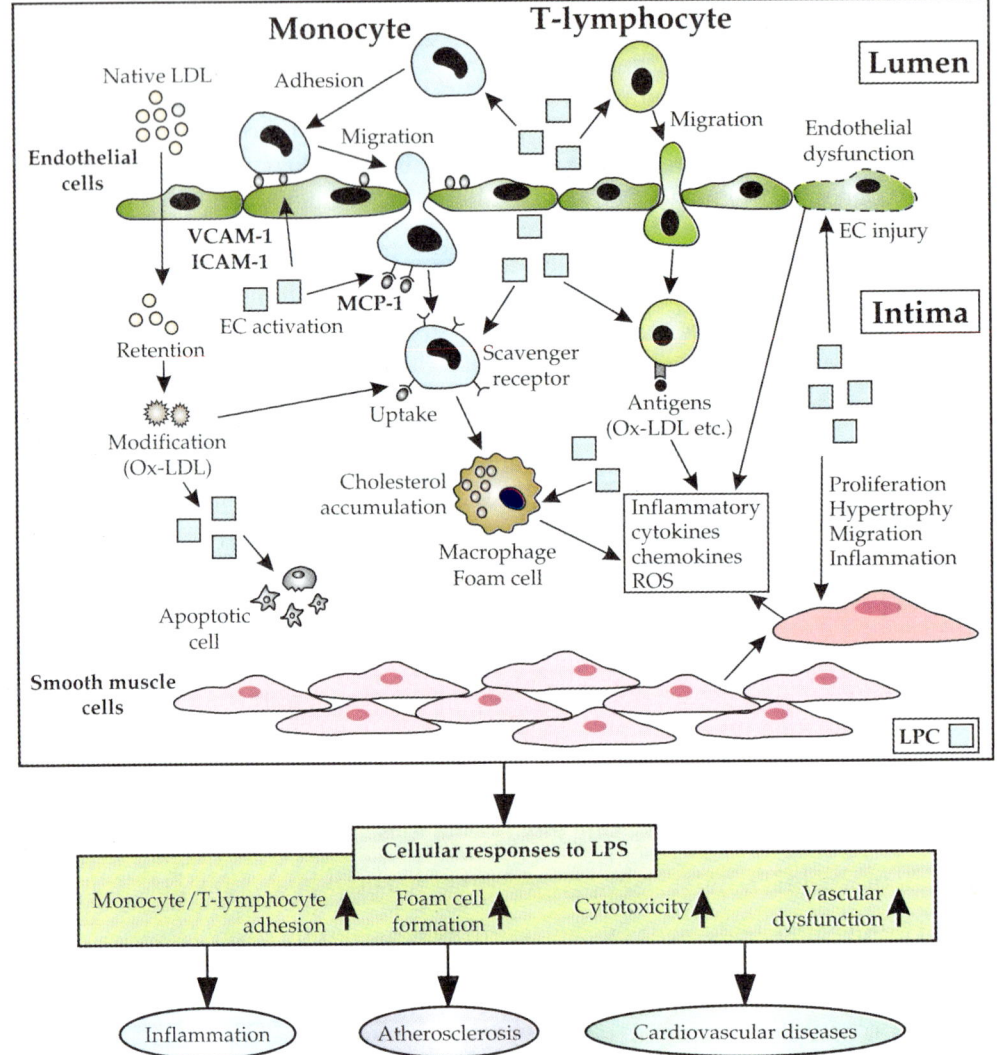

Fig. 6.2. LPC and atherosclerosis.

Q. 19. Why is Butylated hydroxyanisole (BHA)/E320 added to packed food items?

Ans. It is added as a preservative to prevent lipid peroxidation. Peroxidation or auto-oxidation of lipids exposed to oxygen is responsible not only for deterioration of foods (**rancidity**) but also for damage to tissues in vivo, where it may be a cause of cancer, inflammatory diseases, atherosclerosis, and aging. The deleterious effects are considered to be caused by **free radicals** (ROO, RO, OH) produced during peroxide formation from fatty acids containing methylene-interrupted double bonds, i.e., those found in the naturally occurring polyunsaturated fatty acids. Lipid peroxidation is a chain reaction providing a continuous supply of free radicals that initiate further peroxidation and thus has potentially devastating effects (Fig. 6.3). The whole process can be depicted as follows:

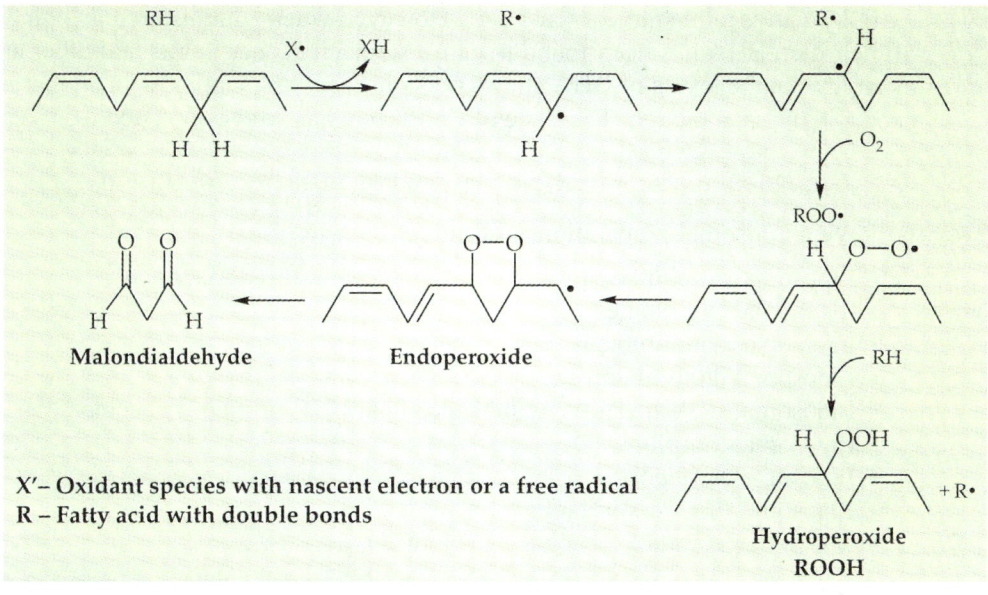

Fig. 6.3. Lipid peroxidation.

1. Initiation
   ROOH + Metal$^{(n)\cdot}$ → ROO$^{\cdot}$ + Metal$^{(n-1)\cdot}$ + H$^{\cdot}$
   X$^{\cdot}$ + RH → R$^{\cdot}$ + XH

2. Propagation
   R$^{\cdot}$ + O$_2$ → ROO$^{\cdot}$
   ROO$^{\cdot}$ + RH → ROOH + R$^{\cdot}$, etc.

3. Termination
   ROO$^{\cdot}$ + ROO$^{\cdot}$ → ROOR + O$_2$
   ROO$^{\cdot}$ + R$^{\cdot}$ → ROOR
   R$^{\cdot}$ + R$^{\cdot}$ → RR

X$^{\cdot}$ – Oxidant species with nascent electron or a free radical
R – Fatty acid with double bonds

Propyl gallate, butylated hydroxyanisole (BHA), and butylated hydroxytoluene (BHT) are antioxidants used as food additives. Naturally occurring antioxidants include vitamin E (tocopherol), which is lipid-soluble, and urate and vitamin C, which are water-soluble. Beta-carotene is an antioxidant at low pO$_2$. Antioxidants fall into two classes: (1) preventive antioxidants, which reduce the rate of chain initiation and (2) chain-breaking antioxidants, which interfere with chain propagation. Preventive antioxidants include catalase and other peroxidases such as glutathione peroxidase that react with ROOH; selenium, which is an essential component of glutathione peroxidase and regulates its activity, and chelators of metal ions such as EDTA (ethylenediaminetetraacetate) and DTPA (diethylenetriaminepenta-acetate). In vivo, the principal chain-breaking antioxidants are superoxide dismutase, which acts in the aqueous phase to trap superoxide free radicals urate, and vitamin E, which acts in the lipid phase to trap ROO radicals.

BHA acts as a free radical scavenger. However, when administered in high doses as part of their diet, BHA has been found to cause stomach cancer in rats and other animals. The usual low intake levels of BHA shows no significant association with an increased risk of cancer in humans though. The State of California, has, however, listed it as a carcinogen.

Q. 20. Give examples of drugs for which liposomes are used for delivery.

Ans. Following liposomal preparations of drugs are in use:
- Liposomal amphotericin B
- Liposomal cytarabine
- Liposomal daunorubicin
- Liposomal doxorubicin
- Liposomal IRIV hepatitis A and Liposomal IRIV influenza vaccine
- Liposomal morphine
- Liposomal verteporfin
- Liposome-PEG doxorubicin
- Micellular estradiol

Liposomes enables hydrophilic drugs to easily cross the cell membrane increasing their movement inside cells. Liposomes when combined with tissue-specific antibodies act as carriers of drugs in the circulation, targeted to specific organs and tissues, e.g., in cancer therapy. They can also be used for gene transfer into vascular cells and as carriers for topical and transdermal delivery of drugs and cosmetics.

Q. 21. What are the various factors regulating fatty acid synthesis?

Ans. Factors regulating fatty acid synthesis include:
1. **Nutritional state** – Synthesis is promoted by fed state and inhibited in starving state.
2. **Type of diet** – Fat or carbohydrate-rich diet promotes synthesis of fats from surplus carbohydrate and storage of fats. While high fat diet inhibits de novo synthesis in body, the excess fats consumed are stored in adipose tissue.
3. **Sucrose feeding** – Sucrose or fructose lead to uncontrolled fatty acid synthesis because metabolism of fructose by fructokinase and aldolase B leads to entry into glycolysis beyond the major regulatory step of phosphofructokinase. This floods glycolysis leading to excess of acetyl CoA which is used for fatty acid synthesis.
4. **PUFA** – Polyunsaturated fatty acids inhibit fatty acid and cholesterol synthesis.

Q. 22. Enumerate the essential fatty acids.

Ans. Essential fatty acids are those which cannot be synthesized in human body. They include linoleic acid and alpha linolenic acid. Arachidonic acid can be synthesized from alpha linolenic acid.

Q. 23. Which unsaturated fatty acids can be synthesized in human body?

Ans. We can synthesize ω_7 or higher unsaturated fatty acids but not ω_6 or ω_3 unsaturated fatty acids because the first double bond is always introduced at $\Delta 9$ or $\Delta 6$ position (ω_7 and ω_{10}

for C16) in a C16 or a higher fatty acid and subsequent double bonds can be introduced at Δ6, Δ5, Δ4 positions (ω_{10}, ω_{11} and ω_{12} for C16) in a C16 or a higher fatty acid (Fig. 6.4). So, double bond can never be introduced between Δ9 and the ω carbon making synthesis of ω_6 or ω_3 series not possible.

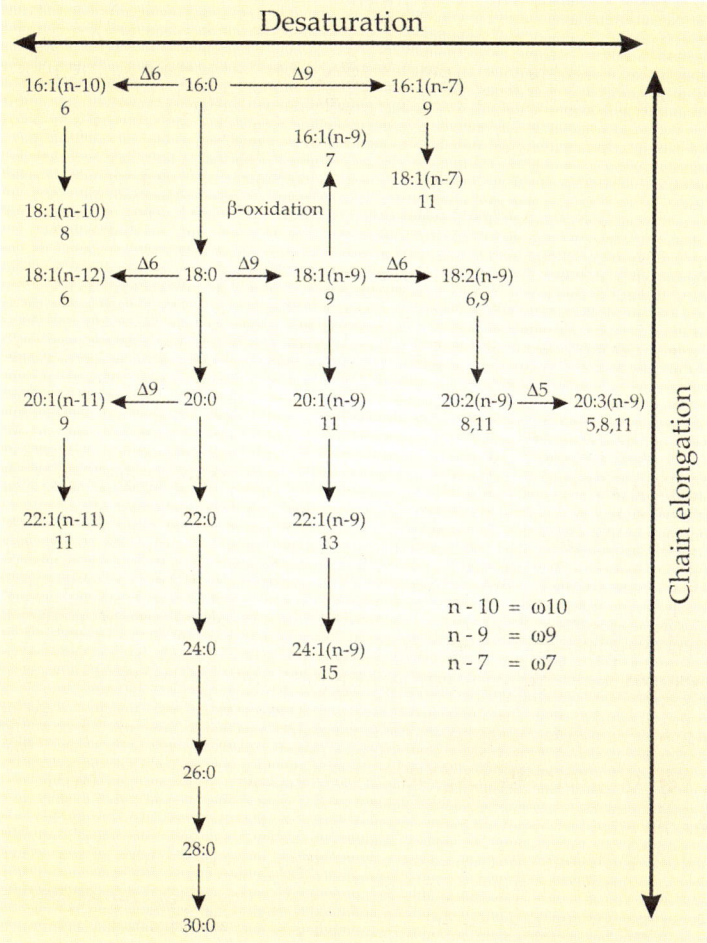

Fig. 6.4. Synthesis of unsaturated fatty acids.

Q. 24. How can diagnosis of essential fatty acid deficiency be confirmed by lab tests?

Ans. In deficiency of EFA, arachidonic acid (20:4 Δ5,8,11,14) synthesis is decreased due to deficiency of alpha linolenate and C20:3 Δ5,8,11 (Meads acid) made from stearate accumulates. Thus triene/tetraene ratio is decreased (to <0.4). This ratio and levels of the essential fatty acids are used for laboratory diagnosis of essential fatty acid deficiency.

Q. 25. Explain giving examples the difference between suicide enzyme and suicide inhibition.

Ans. **Suicide enzyme:** It is an enzyme which catalyzes its own degradation. "Switching off" of prostaglandin activity is partly achieved by a remarkable property of cyclooxygenase—self-catalyzed destruction, i.e., it is a "suicide enzyme".

Suicide inhibition: Also known as suicide inactivation or mechanism-based inhibition, it is a form of irreversible enzyme inhibition that occurs when an enzyme binds a substrate analogue and forms an irreversible complex with it through a covalent bond during the "normal" catalysis reaction. The inhibitor binds to the active site where it is modified by the enzyme to produce a reactive group (e.g. electrophilic α and β unsaturated carbonyl compounds and imines) that reacts irreversibly to form a stable inhibitor-enzyme complex. Some clinical examples of suicide inhibitors include:

- Aspirin, which inhibits cyclooxygenase 1 and 2 enzymes.
- Penicillin, which inhibits DD-transpeptidase from building bacterial cell walls.
- Sulbactam, which prohibits penicillin-resistant strains of bacteria from metabolizing penicillin.
- Allopurinol, which inhibits uric acid production by xanthine oxidase in the treatment of gout.
- AZT (zidovudine) and other chain-terminating nucleoside analogues used to inhibit HIV-1 reverse transcriptase in the treatment of HIV/AIDS.
- Eflornithine, one of the drugs used to treat sleeping sickness, is a suicide inhibitor of ornithine decarboxylase.
- Sarin (nerve gas) is a suicide inhibitor of acetylcholinesterase.
- 5-fluorouracil acts as a suicide inhibitor of thymidylate synthase during the synthesis of thymine from uridine. This reaction is crucial for the proliferation of cells, particularly those that are rapidly proliferating (such as fast-growing cancer tumors). By inhibiting this step, cells die from a thymine-less death because they have no thymine to create more DNA. This is often used in combination with methotrexate, a potent inhibitor of dihydrofolate reductase enzyme.
- Exemestane, a drug used in the treatment of breast cancer, is an inhibitor of the aromatase enzyme.

Q. 26. How is fish oil protective against myocardial infarction (MI)?

Ans. Alpha linolenate forms eicosapentaenoic acid (EPA), which forms PG3 and TX3 series of prostanoids. Linoleic acid forms arachidonic acid which forms PG2 and TX2 series of prostanoids. While PGI3 and PGI2 are equally strong inhibitors of platelet aggregation, TXA3 is weaker aggregator than TXA2. Thus prostanoids formed from alpha linolenate (essential fatty acid) or EPA tilt balance against platelet aggregation and are protective against MI. Fish oil is a good source of eicosapentaenoic acid (EPA) and thus is protective against MI. PG3 and TX3 series prostaglandins also are less inflammatory than PG2 and PG1 series.

Q. 27. Describe the beneficial actions of ω_3 and ω_6 fatty acids.

Ans. ω_3 fatty acids:
- decrease the potent PG2 series prostanoids and have anti-inflammatory action (ω_3 fatty acids produce less inflammatory PG3 series)
- lower TG and cholesterol (inhibit synthesis and increase degradation)
- prevent cancer
- increase insulin sensitivity
- inhibit platelet aggregation

- enhance thermogenesis and lipid metabolism
- benefit skin and brain function.

Primrose oil contains gamma linolenic acid (ω_6) as its active ingredient and has been used for post-menstrual syndrome, fibrofatty breast disease, atopic dermatitis, and eczema.

ω_3 PUFA have a number of effects on lipid and energy metabolism through activation of PPAR-α. They decrease lipogenesis and very low density lipoprotein (VLDL) secretion by suppression of sterol response element binding protein (SREBP-1). ω_3 PUFA increase the activity of lipoprotein lipase, decrease concentrations of apo C-III and potentiate reverse cholesterol transport. ω_3 PUFA induce expression of uncoupling proteins (UCP) and increase density of mitochondria by β-oxidation of FA in muscles. The immunomodulative properties of long chain ω_3 PUFA are related with their ability to suppress the activation of T-lymphocytes. This activation depends on acylated proteins, localized in cell membrane lipid rafts, which leave the raft after increased exposure to long chain ω_3 n-3 PUFA.

Polyunsaturated FA of the ω_6 family are activators of PPAR ($\gamma > \alpha$). Their metabolic effects include affecting cytokine production, increased cholesterol synthesis, increased activity of LDL-receptors resulting from increased mRNA for LDL-receptors, increased activity of cholesterol 7α-hydroxylase (Cyp 7A1) which converts cholesterol to bile acids and decreased conversion of VLDL to LDL. Supplementation with ω_6 PUFA leads to decreased total, LDL- and HDL cholesterol and increased sensitivity of LDL particles to lipoperoxidation. This effect is a result of the "upregulation" of LDL-receptors and the activity of Cyp 7A1. As ligands of PPAR-γ, ω_6 PUFA increase insulin sensitivity and change the distribution of fat and the size of adipocytes.

Q. 28. What is the role of liver X receptors in regulation of cholesterol metabolism?

Ans. LXR form heterodimers with RXR (Retinoid X receptors) and are activated by oxysterols (oxidized cholesterol). Endogenous oxysterols, acting either alone or in concert with membrane cholesterol, participate at multiple steps in the control of cholesterol homeostasis. In response to elevated free cholesterol, enzymatically synthesized oxysterols have feedback effects on multiple pathways to lower the free cholesterol levels in the cell. Oxysterols are ligand for and activate liver X receptors (LXRs) leading to induction of cholesterol efflux and bile acid synthesis and decreased lipoprotein cholesterol uptake and repression of cholesterol synthesizing enzymes. At a transcriptional level, oxysterols and cholesterol inhibit the processing of sterol regulatory element-binding proteins (SREBPs), and transcription factors that are main regulators of cholesterol synthesis and uptake pathways.

Q. 29. How are apo B100 and apo B48 are produced from the same gene?

Ans. By RNA editing as shown in Fig. 6.5.

Q. 30. Which lipoprotein fraction does not move towards charged end in electrophoresis?

Ans. Chylomicrons. On electrophoresis, chylomicrons remain at the origin, LDL migrate into β-globulin region, VLDL migrate into pre-β-globulin region while HDL migrate into α-globulin region. Electrophoretic properties of lipoproteins are based on their charge/size ratio and

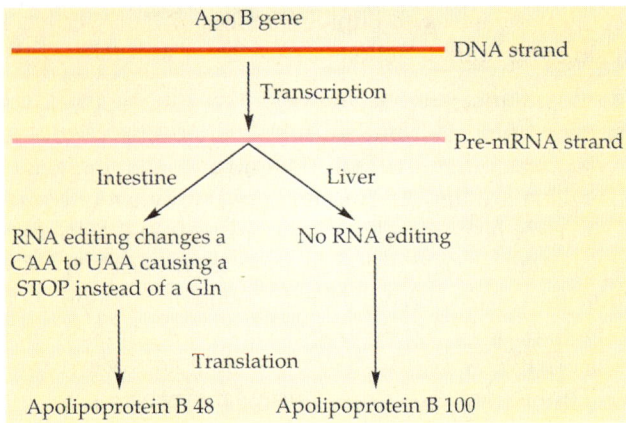

Fig. 6.5. RNA editing for production of Apo B100 and B48.

plasma lipoproteins separated by this technique are classified in relation to comparable migration of serum proteins. As chylomicrons have only 1% protein, the total charge on them is very low, and also as their size is very large they have almost zero mobility on electrophoresis.

Q. 31. How do adipose tissue obtain glycerol-3-phosphate for TG synthesis?

Ans. Glycerol-3-phosphate in adipose tissue is formed from dihydroxyacetone phosphate (from glycolysis) by glycerol-3-phosphate dehydrogenase. Glycerol kinase can catalyze the activation of glycerol to *sn*-glycerol-3-phosphate. But activity of this enzyme is absent or low in muscle and adipose tissue, thus, most of the glycerol-3-phosphate is formed from dihydroxyacetone phosphate by glycerol-3-phosphate dehydrogenase rather than from activation of glycerol to glycerol-3-phosphate.

Q. 32. Which phospholipase is involved in production of prostaglandins?

Ans. PLA2/phospholipase A2. PLA2 cleaves acyl group from sn-2 position of glycerol which has the arachidonic acid or other PUFA from which prostaglandin synthesis occurs. Mellitin present in snake and insect venom activates PLA2 leading to excessive PG synthesis and pain and inflammation at the site of bite.

Q. 33. Which compounds contain ceramide?

Ans. Ceramide is a component of:
1. Sulfatide – sulfogalactosylceramide
2. Gangliosides – formed by addition of glucose, galactose and NANA units to ceramide
3. Shingomylein – formed by addition of phosphatidylcholine to ceramide (Fig. 6.6).

Q. 34. Intravenous imiglucerase or recombinant glucocerebrosidase is used in treatment of which disease?

Ans. Gaucher's disease. Gaucher's disease is characterized by defective lysosomal β-glucocerebrosidase (or β-glucosiadase) which degrades glucocerebroside (glucosylceramide).

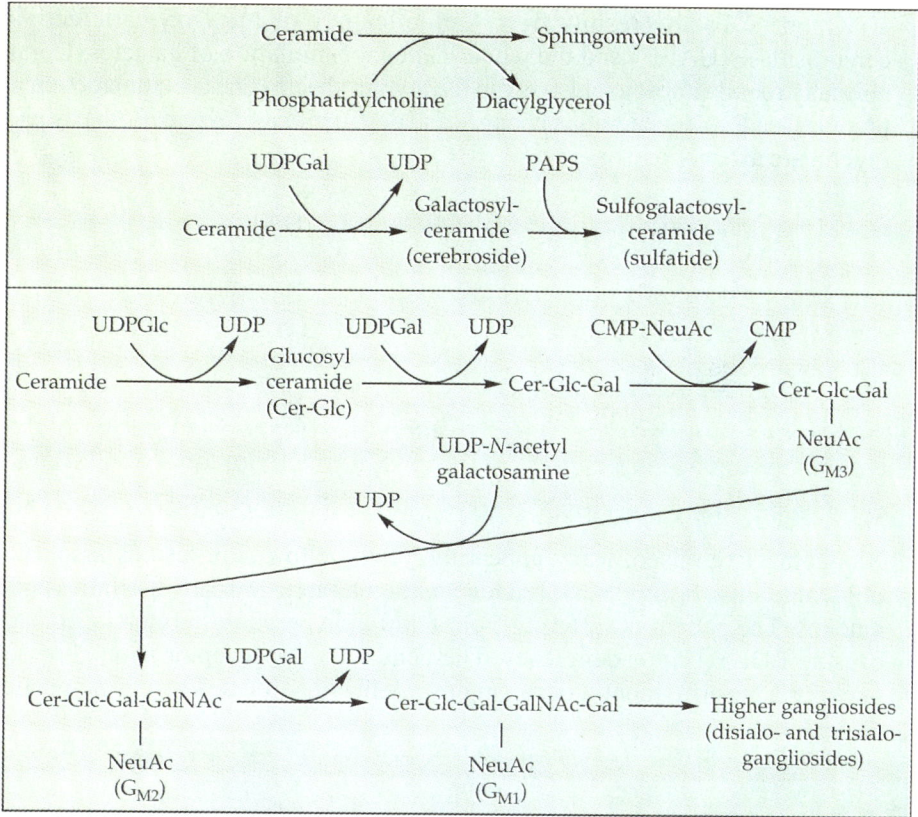

Fig. 6.6. Lipids derived from ceramide.

Glucosylceramide is a cerebroside found mainly in extraneural tissues and occurs in brain in small amounts. Thus, glucosylceramide accumulates mainly in macrophages, WBC, lungs, spleen, liver and marrow causing hepatosplenomegaly, cirrhosis, skeletal abnormalities (Erelmeyer flask in distal femur), and pancytopenia in the most common type I Gaucher's disease. Brain is involved only in the rarer type II and III due to accumulation of glucosylceramide during turnover of complex lipids during brain development and formation of myelin sheath. The pathologic hallmark of Gaucher's disease is the Gaucher cell in the reticuloendothelial system, particularly in the bone marrow. These cells, which are 20–100 μm in diameter, have a characteristic wrinkled paper appearance resulting from the presence of intracytoplasmic substrate inclusions. The cytoplasm of the Gaucher cell reacts strongly positive with the Periodic acid–Schiff stain (PAS stain).

Q. 35. Which lipid storage disease causes severe demyelination?

Ans. Krabbe's disease. Myelin is almost absent in Krabbe's disease. Metachromatic leukodystrophy (MLD) also causes demyelination. Sulfogalactosylceramide (**sulfatide**) is present in high amounts in myelin. It is degraded as:

Sulfatide →[Arylsulfatase (MLD)] Galactocerebroside/Galactosylceramide →[Galactocerebrosidase (Krabbe's disease)] Ceramide

Krabbe's disease results from the deficiency of the enzymatic activity of galactocerebrosidase (GALC) and the white matter accumulation of galactosylceramide, which is normally found almost exclusively in the myelin sheath. The accumulation of un-metabolized products leads to degenerative changes and destruction of myelin. Both peripheral and central myelin are affected.

Q. 36. An 8-year girl was admitted for heart/liver transplant.

History: CHD in family; xanthomas appeared on legs when she was 2 years old; xanthomas appeared on elbows when she was 4 years old; admitted with MI symptoms when she was 7 years old (Total cholesterol = 1240 mg/dl; Triglycerides = 350 mg/dl; Total cholesterol of father = 355 mg/dl; Total cholesterol of mother = 310 mg/dl); 2 weeks after MI she had coronary bypass surgery; past year she had severe angina and second bypass; despite low-fat diet, cholestyramine and lovastatin therapy, total cholesterol = 1000 mg/dl.

What is the likely diagnosis and biochemical explanation for these features?

Ans. Xanthomas are raised, waxy-appearing, often yellow skin lesions associated with hyperlipidemia (Figs. 6.7 and 6.8). Tendon xanthomas are common on achilles and hand extensor tendons. The patient is suffering from familial hypercholesterolemia. It is a genetic defect causing LDL receptor deficiency. The gene for LDL-receptor is on chromosome 19. It is one of the most frequently occurring mendelian disorders. There is no gender difference.

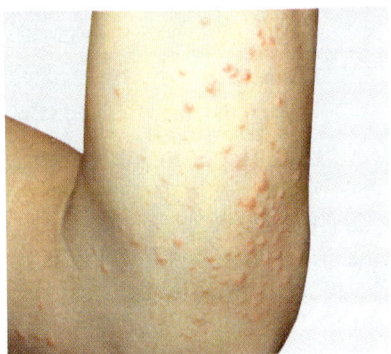

Fig. 6.7. Eruptive xanthomas – generally associated with hypertriglyceridemia.

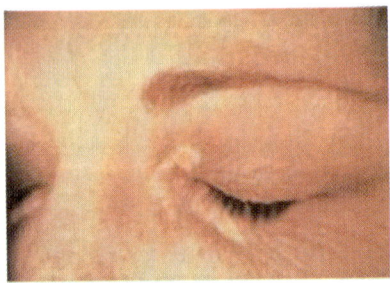

Fig. 6.8. Xanthomas of the eyelid – generally associated with hypercholesterolemia.

Cholesterol balance and transport (Figs. 6.9 and 6.10)

- About 7% of the body's cholesterol circulates in the plasma, mainly as LDL. Liver synthesizes and secretes very-low-density lipoproteins (VLDLs) into the bloodstream. VLDL particles are rich in triglycerides, but they contain lesser amounts of cholesteryl esters.
- When a VLDL particle reaches the capillaries of adipose tissue or muscle, it is cleaved by lipoprotein lipase, extracting most of the triglycerides. The resulting molecule, called intermediate-density lipoprotein (IDL), is reduced in triglyceride content and enriched in cholesteryl esters, and it retains two of the three apoproteins (B-100 and E) present in the parent VLDL particle.
- 50% of newly formed IDL is rapidly taken up by the liver by receptor-mediated transport. The receptor responsible for this recognizes both apo B-100 and apo E. It is called the LDL receptor.
- In the liver cells, IDL is recycled to generate VLDL.
- Remaining IDL undergoes further metabolic processing by lipoprotein lipase that removes most of the remaining triglycerides and apo E, forming cholesterol-rich LDL particles.
- IDL is the immediate and major source of plasma LDL.
- Further, the action of CETP (cholesterol ester transfer protein) transfers cholesterol esters from HDL to IDL and LDL.
- LDL is removed from plasma by two processes: one mediated by an LDL receptor on liver and other tissues and the other by a receptor for oxidized LDL (scavenger receptor B1) on macrophages.
- Many cell types, including fibroblasts, lymphocytes, smooth muscle cells, hepatocytes, and adrenocortical cells, possess high-affinity LDL receptors and clear about 30% of plasma LDL.
- 70% of the plasma LDL is cleared by the liver. Binding of LDL to LDL receptor (clustered in specialized regions of the plasma membrane called coated pits) leads to internalization by invagination (pinocytosis) to form coated vesicles, which fuse with the lysosomes. Here the LDL dissociates from the receptor, which is recycled to the surface.
- In the lysosomes, the LDL molecule is enzymatically degraded; the apoprotein part is hydrolyzed to amino acids, whereas the cholesteryl esters are broken down to free cholesterol. This free cholesterol crosses the lysosomal membrane with help of NPC1 and NPC2 (Neimann Pick type C proteins 1 & 2) to enter the cytoplasm, where it is used for membrane synthesis and as a regulator of cholesterol homeostasis.
- Cholesterol suppresses cholesterol synthesis within the cell by inhibiting the activity of HMG CoA reductase. Cholesterol activates the enzyme acyl-coenzyme A : cholesterol acyltransferase, favouring esterification and storage of excess cholesterol. Cholesterol suppresses the synthesis of LDL receptors, thus protecting the cells from excessive accumulation of cholesterol.

Loss of LDL receptor in familial hypercholesterolemia type IIa

This leads to:
- decreased clearance of LDL from blood;
- decreased hepatic and cellular cholesterol uptake causing increased cholesterol synthesis; and
- increased synthesis of LDL due to decreased hepatic uptake of IDL which is precursor of LDL.

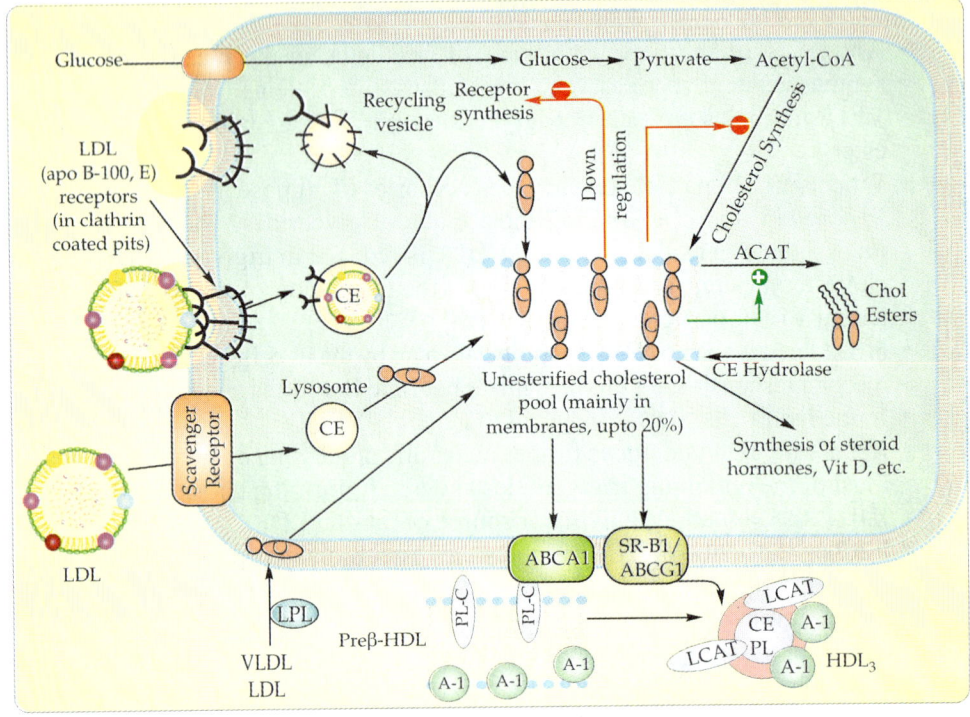

Fig. 6.9. Cholesterol balance in cells.

Longer the LDL stays in blood the more enriched it becomes with cholesterol esters losing triglycerides. When plasma triglycerides exceed a critical threshold of approximately 133 mg/dl, this favours the formation of small, dense LDL from larger, less dense species. The smaller particles are more easily able to penetrate the endothelium. Plasma LDL is transported across the intact endothelium and becomes trapped in the ECM (Extracellular Matrix) of the subendothelial space where it is subjected to oxidative modifications to produce highly oxidized and aggregated LDL, referred to as OxLDL (Oxidized LDL). OxLDLs are believed to be the most atherogenic forms of LDL. Various cellular and biochemical mediators: ROS (Reactive Oxygen Species), the enzymes SMase (Sphingomyelinase), sPLA2 (Secretory Phospholipase-2), other Lipases, and MPO (Myeloperoxidase), initiate and regulate LDL oxidation and aggregation. The various components in OxLDL include Lipid Hydroperoxides, Oxysterols, Lysophosphatidylcholine, and Aldehydes. oxLDL is also better ligand for scavenger receptors than LDL receptors.

Monocytes and macrophages take up oxidized LDL by receptors for chemically altered (e.g., acetylated or oxidized) LDL. These include scavenger receptors A and B1. Normally the amount of LDL transported along this scavenger receptor pathway is less than that mediated by the LDL receptor-dependent mechanisms. In hypercholesterolemia, however, there is a marked increase in the scavenger receptor-mediated traffic of LDL cholesterol into the cells of the mononuclear phagocyte system and possibly the vascular walls. This increase is responsible for the appearance of xanthomas and contributes to the pathogenesis of premature atherosclerosis. LDL oxidation and their harmful effects are inhibited by antioxidants like β-carotene, vitamin E and Paraoxonase-1 (PON1) found in HDL.

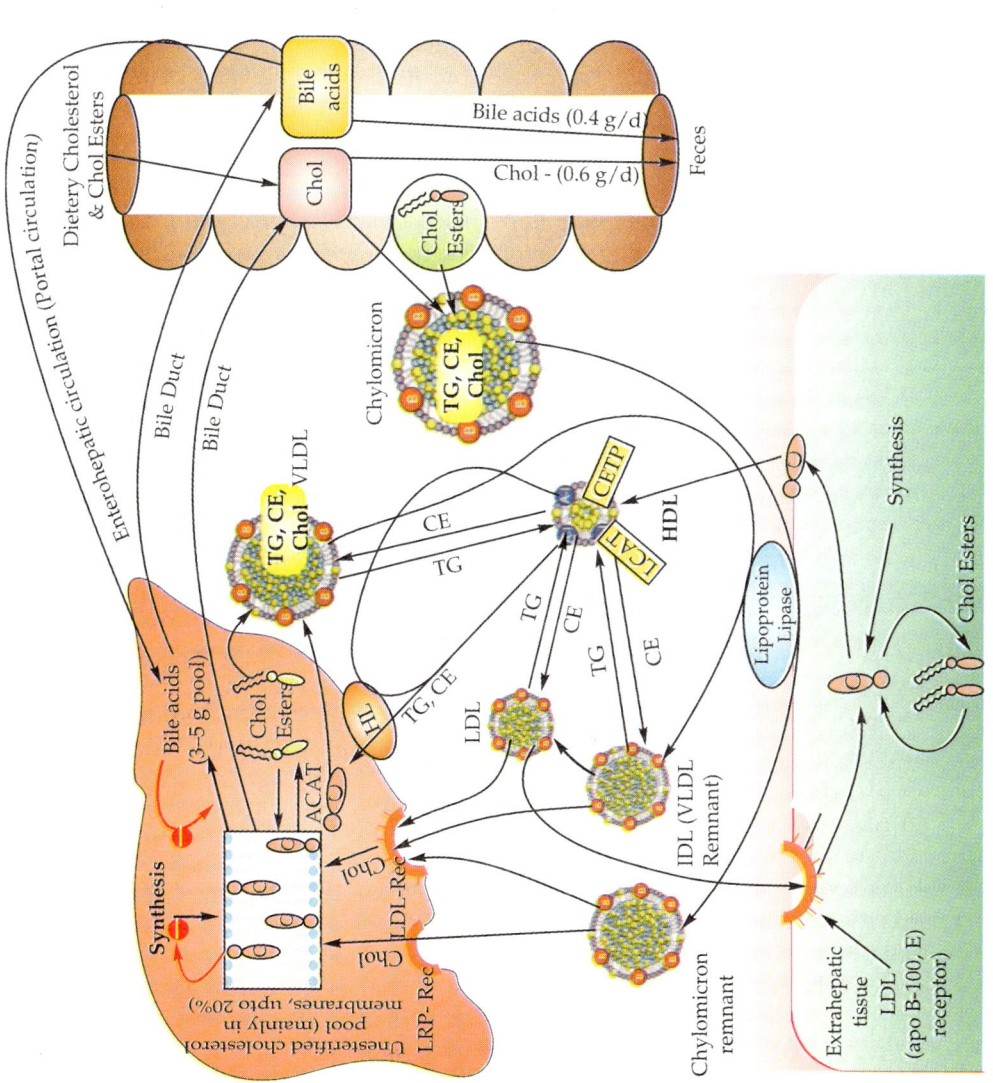

Fig. 6.10. Transport of cholesterol and LDL metabolism.

Familial hypercholesterolemia type IIa

- Heterozygotes (prevalence 1 in 500) have one mutant gene, thus possess only 50% of the normal number of high-affinity LDL receptors. Plasma level of LDL increases approximately two-fold. They have from birth a two-fold to three-fold elevation of plasma cholesterol level, leading to tendinous xanthomas and premature atherosclerosis in adult life.
- Homozygotes (1/1,000,000) having a double dose of the mutant gene, are much more severely affected, and may have five-fold to six-fold elevations in plasma cholesterol levels. These individuals develop skin xanthomas and coronary, cerebral, and peripheral vascular atherosclerosis at an early age. Myocardial infarction may develop before age 20.

More than 900 mutations, including insertions, deletions, and missense and nonsense mutations, involving the LDL receptor gene have been identified. These can be classified into five groups:

1. Class I mutations: Complete failure of synthesis of the receptor protein (null allele).
2. Class II mutations: Encode receptor proteins that accumulate in the endoplasmic reticulum due to misfolding.
3. Class III mutations: Affect the LDL-binding domain of the receptor; the receptor fails to or poorly binds LDL.
4. Class IV mutations: Receptor fails to localize and accumulate in clathrin coated pits, hence the bound LDL is not internalized.
5. Class V mutations: pH-dependent dissociation of receptor and bound LDL fails to occur. Receptors are trapped in the endosome, where they are degraded, and fail to recycle to the cell surface.

Treatment of FH

- Heterozygous FH: Dietary interventions, weight loss and exercise are alone only moderately successful. Cholesterol-lowering drugs in combination with diet will cause up-regulation of LDL-receptors. Most powerful statins at highest dosage will result in ~60% reduction in LDL-C. Other drugs used include Bile Acid Sequestrants (Resins) which prevent reabsorption of bile salts and effect is additive when used with statins.
- Homozygous FH: Diet, exercise, weight loss and drugs are used but have small to no effect on LDL-C as their action is dependent on activity of LDL-receptor. Thus LDL-apheresis is required. Blood is circulated through dextran sulfate cellulose beads which selectively bind to apo B lipoproteins (LDL, VLDL, IDL, LPa) and reduce LDL-C by ~80%. Treatment is used every 2 weeks but is very expensive. Liver transplantation (as ~70% of LDL-receptors in liver) is a long-term solution.

Statins are lower circulating cholesterol levels because statins inhibit HMG-CoA reductase, reducing intracellular synthesis of cholesterol. The reduced cholesterol levels in the cell then upregulate the synthesis of LDL receptors, which remove LDL from circulation, thereby reducing circulating cholesterol levels.

In homozygous familial hypercholesterolemia, both LDL receptor genes are mutated, and the LDL receptors are nonfunctional. Upregulating nonfunctional LDL receptors will not lead to a reduction of LDL in the circulation, so such individuals are resistant to statin action.

Q. 37. Describe briefly the function and consequences of defects in various apolipoproteins and enzymes involved in lipoprotein/lipid transport. Explain with suitable examples the role of LDL and HDL in atherosclerosis. Which is more important – LDL or HDL?

Ans. The defects in various apolipoproteins and enzymes involved in lipoprotein/lipid transport are classified by Fredrickson Classification of Hyperlipoproteinemias (Table 6.1).

Table 6.1. Fredrickson Classification of Hyperlipoproteinemias

Phenotype	I	IIa	IIb	III	IV	V
Lipoprotein, elevated	Chylo-microns	LDL	LDL and VLDL	Chylomicron and VLDL remnants	VLDL	Chylo-microns and VLDL
Triglycerides	↑↑↑	Normal	↑	↑↑	↑↑	↑↑↑
Cholesterol (total)	↑	↑↑↑	↑↑	↑↑	Normal/↑	↑↑
LDL-cholesterol	↓	↑↑↑	↑↑			
HDL-cholesterol	↓↓↓	N/↓	↓	N	↓↓	↓↓↓
Plasma appearance	Lactescent	Clear	Clear	Turbid	Turbid	Lactescent
Xanthomas	Eruptive	Tendon, tuberous	None	Palmar, tubero-eruptive	None	Eruptive
Pancreatitis	+++	0	0	0	0	+++
Coronary atherosclerosis	0	+++	+++	+++	+/–	+/–
Peripheral atherosclerosis	0	+	+	++	+/–	+/–
Molecular defects	LPL and ApoC-II	LDL receptor, ApoB-100, PCSK9, LDLRAP, ABCG5 and ABCG8		ApoE	ApoA-V	ApoA-V and GPIHBP1
Genetic nomenclature	FCS	FH, FDB, ADH, ARH, sitostero-lemia	FCHL	FDBL	FHTG	FHTG

Abbreviations: ADH, autosomal dominant hypercholesterolemia; Apo, apolipoprotein; ARH, autosomal recessive hypercholesterolemia; FCHL, familial combined hyperlipidemia; FCS, familial chylomicronemia syndrome; FDB, familial defective ApoB; FDBL, familial dysbetalipoproteinemia; FH, familial hypercholesterolemia; FHTG, familial hypertriglyceridemia; LPL, lipoprotein lipase; LDLRAP, LDL receptor associated protein; GPIHBP1, glycosylphosphatidylinositol-anchored high density lipoprotein binding protein1; N, normal.

Type I hyperlipoproteinemias

Lipoprotein lipase and Apo CII

- LPL is involved in transport of fatty acids from triglycerides present in chylomicrons, VLDL and IDL into many tissues including adipose tissue. Apo CII is the co-factor required for activity of lipoprotein lipase.
- If there is defect in or deficiency of either of these proteins, lipoprotein lipase cannot work, and the triglyceride in both chylomicrons and VLDL would be unable to be digested. This leads to elevated levels of these particles, and a very high serum triglyceride level. Since VLDL is not being converted to IDL or LDL, cholesterol levels are not elevated.
- Familial chylomicronemia syndrome (Type I hyperlipoproteinemia; Lipoprotein lipase and Apo CII deficiency): Fasting triglyceride levels are almost invariably >1000 mg/dL. Fasting cholesterol levels are also elevated but to a lesser extent.
- These patients can also have elevated plasma levels of VLDL, but chylomicronemia predominates. The fasting plasma is turbid, and if left at 4°C (39.2°F) for a few hours, the chylomicrons float to the top and form a creamy supernatant.
- LPL deficiency has autosomal recessive inheritance and has a frequency of approximately 1 in 1 million in the population. Obligate LPL heterozygotes have normal or mild-to-moderate elevations in plasma triglyceride levels, whereas individuals heterozygous for mutation in apo CII do not have hypertriglyceridemia.
- Apo CII deficiency is also recessive in inheritance pattern and is even less common than LPL deficiency. Familial apolipoprotein CII deficiency is characterized by eruptive xanthomas, hepatosplenomegaly, pancreatitis.
- Both LPL and apo CII deficiency usually present in childhood with recurrent episodes of severe abdominal pain due to acute pancreatitis. On funduscopic examination, the retinal blood vessels are opalescent (lipemia retinalis). Eruptive xanthomas, which are small, yellowish-white papules, often appear in clusters on the back, buttocks, and extensor surfaces of the arms and legs. These typically painless skin lesions may become puritic.
- Hepatosplenomegaly results from the uptake of circulating chylomicrons by reticulo-endothelial cells in the liver and spleen. Some patients with persistent and pronounced chylomicronemia never develop pancreatitis, eruptive xanthomas, or hepatosplenomegaly.
- Premature CHD is not generally a feature of familial chylomicronemia syndromes.

Type IIa hyperlipoproteinemias

LDL-receptor

Discussed in Question 36.

Apo B100

- Structural protein for VLDL, LDL, IDL, Lp(a).
- Ligand for binding to LDL receptor.
- Mutation causes familial defective apo B100 (FDB).
- FDB is caused by mutations in the LDL receptor-binding domain of apo B100, most commonly due to a substitution of glutamine for arginine at position 3500.
- FDB is autosomal dominant.
- Resembles clinically heterozygous familial hypercholesterolemia.

- LDL binds the LDL receptor with reduced affinity, and LDL is removed from the circulation at a reduced rate. Patients with FDB cannot be clinically distinguished from patients with heterozygous FH (familial hypercholesterolemia), although patients with FDB tend to have lower plasma levels of LDL-C than FH heterozygotes.
- Elevated plasma LDL-C levels with normal triglycerides, tendon xanthomas, and an increased incidence of premature atherosclerosis and cardiovascular diseases.

ABCG5

- Phytosterols or plant sterols can diffuse into the intestinal epithelial cells, they are actively transported back into the intestinal lumen by an ABC-cassette (ATP-binding) containing protein, ABCG5 and ABCG8.
- Absorbed phytosterols (<5%) reach liver and are exported by the same proteins in the liver to the bile.
- In the absence of activity of either ABCG5 or ABCG8, the phytosterols are packaged into chylomicrons and are eventually delivered to the liver, where they are packaged into VLDL.
- This condition is called sitosterolemia – an accumulation of plant sterols (phytosterols) in cells and tissues.
- It is rare and autosomal recessive.
- Human cells cannot utilize phytosterols; increased levels interfere with the synthesis of cholesterol and the normal cholesterol recycling.
- Result in severe hypercholesterolemia, tendon xanthomas.
- Patients with this disorder develop premature coronary artery disease.
- High levels of plant sterols in the circulating lipoprotein particles accelerate the deposition of these sterols in the walls of the arteries, promoting atherosclerosis.
- Incorporation of plant sterols into cell membranes results in misshapen red blood cells and megathrombocytes causing episodes of hemolysis.
- The hypercholesterolemia does not respond to HMG-CoA reductase inhibitors, whereas bile acid sequestrants and cholesterol-absorption inhibitors such as ezetimibe, are effective in reducing plasma sterol levels in these patients.

PCSK9 (ADH-PCSK9 or ADH3) - Proprotein convertase subtilisin/kexin type 9 (PCSK9)

- PCSK9 is a secreted protein that binds to the LDL receptor, resulting in its degradation.
- When PCSK9 binds the LDL receptor, the complex is internalized and the receptor is redirected to the lysosome rather than to the cell surface.
- The missense mutations in PCSK9 that cause hypercholesterolemia enhance the activity of PCSK9.
- Autosomal dominant hypercholesterolemia: Rare autosomal dominant disorder.
- Number of hepatic LDL receptors is reduced.
- Patients with ADH-PCSK9 are indistinguishable clinically from patients with FH (familial hypercholesterolemia).

LDLR adaptor protein, LDLRAP

- Involved in LDL receptor-mediated endocytosis in the liver.
- Autosomal recessive hypercholesterolemia (ARH): In the absence of LDLRAP, LDL binds to the LDL receptor but the lipoprotein-receptor complex fails to be internalized.
- Like homozygous FH, it is characterized by hypercholesterolemia, tendon xanthomas, and premature coronary artery disease (CAD).

- The levels of plasma LDL-C tend to be intermediate between the levels present in FH homozygotes and FH heterozygotes, and CAD is not usually symptomatic until at least the third decade.

Type IIb Hyperlipoproteinemias

Familial Combined Hyperlipidemia (FCHL)

- Moderate elevations in plasma levels of triglycerides (VLDL) and cholesterol (LDL) and reduced plasma levels of HDL-C.
- Autosomal dominant with incomplete penetrance and affected family members typically have one of three possible phenotypes: (1) elevated plasma levels of LDL-C, (2) elevated plasma levels of triglycerides due to elevation in VLDL, or (3) elevated plasma levels of both LDL-C and triglyceride.
- Lipoprotein profile can switch among these three phenotypes in the same individual over time and may depend on factors such as diet, exercise, and weight.
- FCHL can manifest in childhood but is usually not fully expressed until adulthood.
- A cluster of other metabolic risk factors are often found in association with this hyperlipidemia, including obesity, glucose intolerance, insulin resistance, and hypertension.
- Always have significantly elevated plasma levels of apo B.
- The levels of apo B are disproportionately high relative to the plasma LDL-C concentration, with the presence of small, dense LDL particles.
- Individuals share the same metabolic defect, which is overproduction of VLDL by the liver.
- Significantly increased risk of premature CHD.

Type III hyperlipoproteinemias

Apo E

- Apolipoprotein E has affinity for the LDL receptor and the LDL receptor-related protein and is important for chylomicron remnant and IDL uptake from the circulation by the liver. The apo E gene is polymorphic in sequence, resulting in the expression of three common isoforms: apo E3, which is the most common; and apo E2 and apo E4, which both differ from apo E3 by a single amino acid.
- Familial dysbetalipoproteinemia (FDBL, Type III hyperlipoproteinemia or familial broad disease): In dysbetalipoproteinemia, a mutation in apolipoprotein E, the patient has the rare E2 form instead of the normal E3 form. With the homozygous E2 form, binding of the particles to their receptors is weak, and the particles circulate longer than normal, contributing to the high cholesterol and triglyceride levels seen in the circulation.
- Approximately 0.5% of the general population are apo E2/E2 homozygotes, but only a small minority of these individuals develop FDBL. About 10% of the individuals who are homozygous for E2 develop this condition, the most common additional precipitating factor being obesity. Others include high-fat diet, diabetes mellitus, hypothyroidism, renal disease, HIV infection, estrogen deficiency, alcohol use, or certain drugs.
- It is characterized by a mixed hyperlipidemia due to the accumulation of remnant lipoprotein particles. Patients with FDBL usually present in adulthood with incidental hyperlipidemia, xanthomas, premature coronary disease, or peripheral vascular disease. The disease seldom presents in women before menopause.

- Two distinctive types of xanthomas, tuberoeruptive and palmar, are seen in FDBL patients. Tuberoeruptive xanthomas begin as clusters of small papules on the elbows, knees, or buttocks and can grow to the size of small grapes. Palmar xanthomas (alternatively called xanthomata striata palmaris) are orange-yellow discolorations of the creases in the palms and wrists.
- Although associated with slightly higher LDL-C levels and increased CHD risk, the apoE4 allele is not associated with FDBL. Patients with apoE4 have an increased incidence of late-onset Alzheimer's disease.

Type IV hyperlipoproteinemias

ApoA-V

- Required for the association of VLDL and chylomicrons with LPL.
- ApoA-V circulates at much lower concentrations than the other major apolipoproteins.
- Individuals harbouring mutations in both ApoA-V alleles can present as adults with chylomicronemia.

Familial hypertriglyceridemia (FHTG)

- FHTG is a relatively common (1 in 500) autosomal dominant disorder.
- Moderately elevated plasma triglycerides accompanied by more modest elevations in cholesterol.
- Increased production of VLDL, impaired catabolism of VLDL, or a combination.
- Some patients with FHTG have a more severe form of hyperlipidemia in which both VLDLs and chylomicrons are elevated (Type V hyperlipidemia), since these two classes of lipoproteins compete for the same lipolytic pathway.
- Increased intake of simple carbohydrates, obesity, insulin resistance, alcohol use, and estrogen treatment, all of which increase VLDL synthesis, can exacerbate this syndrome.
- FHTG appears not to be associated with increased risk of atherosclerosis in many families.

Type V hyperlipoproteinemias

GPIHBP1

- Involved in transport of LPL to endothelial cell after synthesis in adipocytes, myocytes or other cells.
- Homozygosity for mutations that interfere with GPIHBP1 synthesis or folding cause severe hypertriglyceridemia.

Other proteins and disorders

Hepatic lipase (HL)

- HL is a member of the same gene family as LPL and hydrolyzes triglycerides and phospholipids in remnant lipoproteins and HDLs for uptake by liver.
- HL deficiency is a very rare autosomal recessive disorder characterized by elevated plasma levels of cholesterol and triglycerides (mixed hyperlipidemia) due to the accumulation of circulating lipoprotein remnants and either a normal or elevated plasma level of HDL-C.
- Due to the small number of patients with HL deficiency, the association of this genetic defect with atherosclerosis and cardiovascular diseases is not clearly known, but lipid-lowering therapy is recommended.
- This shows that elevation in LDL are more important for pathogenesis of atherosclerosis.

Inherited causes of low levels of apoB-containing lipoproteins

Familial hypobetalipoproteinemia (FHB)
- Low plasma levels of LDL-C (the "β-lipoprotein") with a genetic or inherited basis.
- Mutations in apo B.
- Individuals heterozygous for these mutations usually have LDL-C levels <80 mg/dL and may be protected from atherosclerosis.
- Mutations in both apo B alleles cause homozygous FHB, which resembles abetalipoproteinemia.

PCSK9 deficiency
- Mutations that interfere with the synthesis of PCSK9 result in increased LDL receptor activity and 40% reduction in plasma level of LDL-C.
- Patients are protected from developing CHD again showing significance of LDL for atherosclerosis.

MTTP (Microsomal triglyceride transfer protein)
- Required for synthesis of chylomicrons in intestinal epithelial cells and VLDL in liver cells.
- The patient has abetalipoproteinemia, an absence of apo B-containing proteins in the circulation.
- This leads to low chylomicron and VLDL levels.
- The intestinal cells become laden with lipids obtained from the diet and those which cannot be exported due to the inability to produce chylomicrons.
- Rare autosomal recessive disease.
- Plasma levels of cholesterol and triglyceride are extremely low in this disorder, and chylomicrons, VLDLs, LDLs, and apo B are undetectable in plasma.
- Heterozygotes have normal plasma lipid and apo B levels.
- Abetalipoproteinemia usually presents in early childhood with diarrhea and failure to thrive due to fat malabsorption. Neurologic manifestations: loss of deep-tendon reflexes, decreased distal lower extremity vibratory and proprioceptive sense, dysmetria, ataxia, spastic gait, progressive pigmented retinopathy presenting with decreased night and colour vision, blindness.
- Most clinical manifestations result from defects in the absorption and transport of fat-soluble vitamins E, A and K.

Genetic disorders of HDL metabolism – Low levels of HDL

Apo A1
- Structural protein for HDL activates LCAT.
- Complete genetic deficiency of apo A-I due to deletion of the apo A-I gene results in the complete absence of HDL from the plasma.
- The genes encoding apo A-I, apo CIII, apo A-IV, and apo A-V are clustered together on chromosome 11, and some patients with no apo A-I have genomic deletions that include other genes in the cluster.
- Apo CIII inhibits lipoprotein binding to receptors, apo A-V promotes LPL-mediated triglyceride lipolysis, apo A-IV may be an activator of LCAT and CETP, is mainly made in intestinal epithelial cells and is associated with chylomicrons and HDL.

- In the absence of LCAT activity, free cholesterol levels increase in both HDL and in tissues. The free cholesterol can form deposits in the cornea and in the skin, resulting in corneal opacities and planar xanthomas.
- Premature CHD is a common feature of apo A-I deficiency, especially when additional genes in the complex are also deleted.
- Missense and nonsense mutations in the apo A-I gene have been identified in some patients with low plasma levels of HDL-C (usually 15–30 mg/dL), but these are very rare causes of low HDL-C levels.
- Patients heterozygous for an Arg173Cys substitution in APOAI (so-called apoA-IMilano) have very low plasma levels of HDL due to impaired LCAT activation and rapid catabolism of the mutant apolipoprotein and yet have no increased risk of premature CHD.
- Most other individuals with low plasma HDL-C levels due to missense mutations in apo A-I do not appear to have premature CHD. Thus, low HDL may not be as significant as high LDL for atherosclerosis.
- Some missense mutations in apo A-I and apo A-II promote the formation of amyloid fibrils causing systemic amyloidosis.

ABC1

- It is ATP-binding cassette protein 1 (ABC1), a transporter in cell membranes which is involved in cholesterol efflux from the membrane into the HDL particle (reverse cholesterol transport).
- Mutation causes Tangier disease.
- Tangier disease (ABCA1 deficiency).
- Very rare autosomal co-dominant with extremely low plasma HDL-C levels (<5 mg/dL) and apo A-I (<5 mg/dL).
- Cholesterol accumulates in the reticuloendothelial system causing hepatosplenomegaly and enlarged, grayish-yellow or orange tonsils.
- An intermittent peripheral neuropathy (mononeuritis multiplex) or a sphingomyelia-like neurologic disorder can also be seen in this disorder.
- Increased risk of premature atherosclerotic disease is expected, although the observed association is not as strong.
- Patients with Tangier disease also have low plasma levels of LDL-C, which may attenuate the atherosclerotic risk. This may be because CETP transfers cholesterol esters taken by HDL from HDL to LDL.
- Obligate heterozygotes for ABCA1 mutations have moderately reduced plasma HDL-C levels (15–30 mg/dL) but their risk of premature CHD remains uncertain.
- Thus high LDL which is directly related to pathogenesis of atherosclerosis is a much more important factor for atherosclerosis rather than reduced HDL and reverse cholesterol transport!

LCAT

- Lecithin: Cholesterol acyltransferase (LCAT) activity is associated with HDL-containing apo A-I.
- The enzyme is activated by apo A-I
- LCAT is synthesized in the liver and secreted into the plasma, where it circulates associated with lipoproteins.

- As cholesterol in HDL becomes esterified, it creates a concentration gradient and draws in cholesterol from tissues and other lipoproteins allowing HDL to function in reverse cholesterol transport.
- LCAT deficiency: Very rare autosomal recessive disorder is caused by mutations in LCAT.
- The proportion of free cholesterol in circulating lipoproteins is greatly increased (from 25% to >70% of total plasma cholesterol).
- Lack of normal cholesterol esterification impairs formation of mature HDL particles, resulting in the rapid catabolism of circulating apo A-I.
- Complete deficiency (also called classic LCAT deficiency) and partial deficiency (also called fish-eye disease). Progressive corneal opacification due to the deposition of free cholesterol in the cornea, very low plasma levels of HDL-C (usually <10 mg/dL), and variable hypertriglyceridemia are seen in both.
- Complete LCAT deficiency patients have hemolytic anemia and progressive renal insufficiency that eventually leads to end-stage renal disease (ESRD).
- In partial LCAT deficiency, there are no other known clinical complications.
- Despite the extremely low plasma levels of HDL-C and apoA-I, premature atherosclerosis and cardiovascular diseases is not a consistent feature of either LCAT deficiency or fish-eye disease. Again this proves the higher importance of elevated LDL in these diseases, even though HDL is protective.

Genetic disorders of HDL metabolism – High levels of HDL-C

CETP (Cholesteryl ester transfer protein)

- Associated with HDL, responsible for transfer of cholesteryl ester from HDL to VLDL, IDL, and LDL in exchange for triacylglycerol.
- Thus, much of the cholesteryl ester formed by LCAT finds its way to the liver via VLDL remnants (IDL) or LDL.
- Thus, it relieves product inhibition of the LCAT activity in HDL. The triacylglycerol-enriched HDL2 delivers its cholesterol to the liver in the HDL cycle.
- Familial hyperalphalipoproteinemia: Loss-of-function mutations in both alleles of the gene encoding CETP cause substantially elevated HDL-C levels (usually >150 mg/dL). Seen mainly in Japanese families.
- This increases the cholesteryl ester content of HDL and reduces plasma levels of LDL-C.
- The large, cholesterol-rich HDL particles circulating in these patients are cleared at a reduced rate.
- The relationship of CETP deficiency to atherosclerosis is not clear.
- Heterozygotes for CETP deficiency have only modestly elevated HDL-C levels.
- Based on this information pharmacologic inhibition of CETP is under development as a new therapeutic approach to both raise HDL-C levels and lower LDL-C levels, as a possible way to decreases risk of atherosclerosis.
- Outside Japan increased levels of HDL-C (hyperalphalipoproteinemia) is unlikely to be due to CETP deficiency. Most, but not all, persons with this condition appear to have a reduced risk of CHD and increased longevity. Recent evidence points to mutations in endothelial lipase.

Amino Acid and Heme Metabolism

Chapter 7

Q. 1. What are nutritionally essential and non-essential amino acids?

Ans. Of the 20 amino acids, 9 must be present in the human diet as they cannot be synthesized in the body, and thus are best termed "nutritionally essential". The presence and amount of these 9 amino acids are also used to determine the protein quality. These include Histidine, Isoleucine, Leucine, Lysine, Methionine, Phenylalanine, Threonine, Tryptophan and Valine.

Arginine, cysteine and tyrosine are conditionally essential, i.e. required to be present in diet under certain physiological or pathological conditions like premature infants, liver diseases, etc.

Such distinction has arisen in nature as an evolution due to natural selection. Dependence on an external supply of a given nutrient rather than self-synthesis can be of greater survival value than the ability to biosynthesize it. The distinction in these amino acids is the number of enzymes and amount of ATP or energy required to synthesize each amino acids. These amino acids require significantly larger number of enzymes and have longer biosynthesis pathways than the rest (Table 7.1). Thus, if they are freely available from diet, maintaining extra DNA for all the enzymes and using lot of ATP to synthesize the amino acids is of evolutionary disadvantage. Or if there is a mutation in the pathway and the nutrient is freely available then it has no disadvantage from natural selection view. Thus, this suggests a survival advantage in retaining the ability to manufacture "easy" amino acids while losing the ability to make "difficult" amino acids. The metabolic pathways that form the nutritionally essential amino acids occur in plants and bacteria, but not in humans.

Q. 2. How can nitrogen balance or protein balance be measured?

Ans. Nitrogen balance is a measure of the difference between nitrogen intake (in the form of protein) and nitrogen excretion. During growth and tissue repair, especially after surgery and trauma, the body is in positive nitrogen balance, i.e. intake is greater than loss. In fever,

Table 7.1. Number of enzymes required for the synthesis of amino acids from amphibolic intermediates

Number of enzymes required to synthesize			
Nutritionally essential		*Nutritionally nonessential*	
Arg[1]	7	Ala	1
His	6	Asp	1
Thr	6	Asn	1
Met	5 (4 shared)	Glu	1
Lys	8	Gln	1
Ile	8 (6 shared)	Hyl	1
Val	1 (7 shared)	Hyp	1
Leu	3 (7 shared)	Pro	3
Phe	10	Ser	3
Trp	5 (8 shared)	Gly	1
	59	Cys	2
		Tyr	1
			17

fasting and wasting diseases (cachexia), the loss is greater than intake and the individual is in negative nitrogen balance. As urea is the breakdown product of amino acid nitrogen, the daily nitrogen lost can be calculated from 24-hour urine urea. 24-hour urine urea × 0.467 gives the 24 hour-urine nitrogen (as every 60 g of urea will have 28 g of nitrogen; urea is $CO[NH_2]_2$). To convert grams of protein into nitrogen equivalents, the average weight of an amino acid is taken as 120, of which 16% (average) is due to nitrogen. Thus, amount of nitrogen per g of protein will be 16% of its weight. Or 1 g of nitrogen will be equal to 6.25 g of protein. Thus nitrogen balance is given by:

N_2 balance = (Protein intake per day in g) × 0.16 – [24-hr urine urea nitrogen in g + 4 g]

or Protein balance = Protein intake – [24-h UUN (g) + 4] × 6.25

The fudge factor of 4 is to account for the protein lost in the form of faeces, skin cells and nails.

Q. 3. Describe glycine metabolism and associated clinical implications.

Ans. Glycine is the simplest amino acid with no D/L forms (optical isomers). Average diet contains 3–5 g glycine per day. It is glucogenic. It is an important constituent of proteins, being the every 3rd amino acid in the most abundant protein collagen and is very abundant in elastin also.

Synthesis and catabolism: It can be produced from serine or choline (both the pathways generate one carbon moiety, thus act as input reactions in one carbon metabolism, Figs. 7.1 and 7.2). It is broken down by glycine cleavage complex (also provides one carbon moiety, Fig. 7.3). Even though the inter-conversion of glycine and serine is reversible, the net physiological direction is from serine to glycine. It is glucogenic. Fasting state conversion of glycine to serine is the main source of pyruvate for gluconeogenesis.

Uses: 1 g is daily used for conjugation and detoxification reactions for compounds and drugs like benzoate (converted to hippurate), salicylates (converted to salicyluric acid). Conjugation helps form bile acid glycocholate from cholic acid, and also helps in excretion of accumulated products in certain inborn errors of metabolism (in isovaleric academia isovalerylglycine is excreted, in medium chain acyl CoA dehydrogenase defect phenylpropionylglycine is excreted). Glycine is used for synthesis of glutathione, purines, heme and creatine (Fig. 7.1).

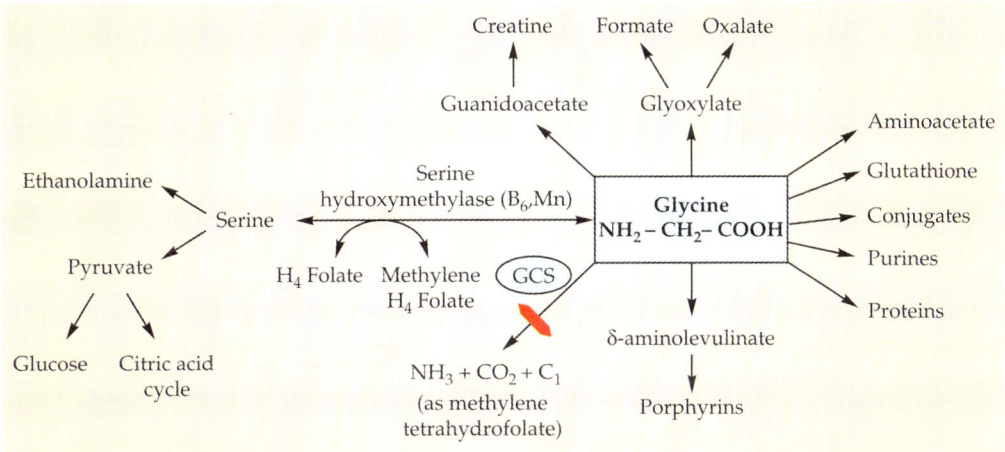

Fig. 7.1. Glycine metabolism (GCS = glycine cleavage system).

Glycine acts as both inhibitory as well as an excitatory neurotransmitter:
- **Inhibitory:** On glycine receptors in brain stem and spinal cord, increases chloride ion permeability like GABA. Strychnine (glycine receptor antagonist and poison) or loss of receptor causes myoclonic jerks.
- **Excitatory:** Glycine is co-agonist at NMDA receptor. It is an allosteric modulator which increases activity and increases frequency of channel opening of NMDA receptor. High levels lead to excitatory events.

Clinical implications

1. **Non-ketotic hyperglycinemia:** Defect in glycine cleavage system: GCS is a 4-protein complex resembling PDH and α-KG dehydrogenase complex (Fig. 7.3). Regulation of GCS activity is increased by glucagon, high protein diet (increases glucagon to insulin ratio), postprandial increase in glucagon, α-agonists – epinephrine and norepinephrine, and vasopressin.

$$\text{Glycine} + H_4 \text{ folate} + NAD^+ \leftrightarrow CO_2 + NH_3 + 5,10\text{-}CH_2\text{-}H_4 \text{ folate} + NADH + H^+$$

Defect in the glycine cleavage system leads to accumulation of large amounts of glycine in all body tissues, including central nervous system. Patient presents in first few days of

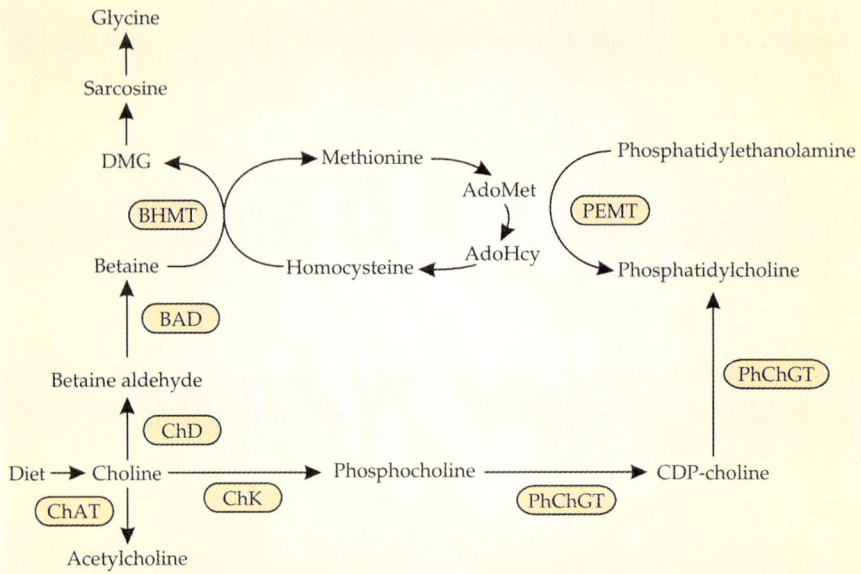

Fig. 7.2. Synthesis of glycine from choline: Choline is oxidized to betaine aldehyde, which is then converted in two steps to betaine. The first step is catalyzed by choline dehydrogenase (ChD), the second step by betaine aldehyde dehydrogenase (BAD). Betaine can be used as a methyl donor in a remethylation reaction from homocysteine to methionine being catalyzed by betaine homocysteine methyltransferase (BHMT). This reaction generates dimethylglycine (DMG). Methionine is the precursor of S-adenosylmethionine, which serves as a methyl donor for numerous physiological reactions resulting in the formation of S-adenosylhomocysteine. ChK = Choline kinase, PhChCT = CTP-phosphocholine cytidyltransferase, PhChGT = Phosphatidylcholine glyceride transferase, ChAT = Choline acetyltransferase, PEMT = Phosphatidylethanolamine-N-methyltransferase.

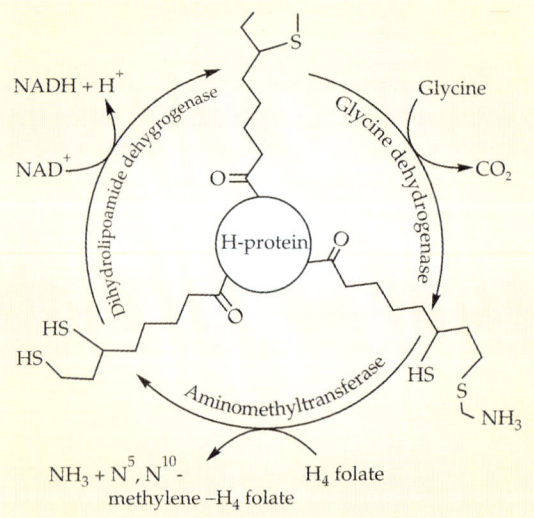

Fig. 7.3. Glycine cleavage system. The glycine cleavage complex consists of three enzymes and an "H-protein" that has covalently attached dihydrolipoate. Enzymes: 1 = glycine dehydrogenase (decarboxylating), 2 = ammonia-forming aminomethyltransferase, 3 = dihydrolipoamide dehydrogenase. The reaction adds one carbon moiety to tetrahydrofolate producing N5,N10-methylenetetrahydrofolate.

life with lethargy, hypotonia, myoclonic jerks, progressing to apnea, and often to death. Those who regain respiration develop intractable seizures and profound mental retardation. There are no other biochemical abnormalities like acidosis or ketosis and anion gap is normal. Plasma, urine, CSF glycine levels are raised and CSF : plasma glycine ratio > 0.08 is diagnostic. Confirmation can be done by assay of glycine cleavage system in liver biopsy, which is often difficult in a critically ill neonate. EEG shows a typical burst suppression pattern (whose most common cause is hyperglycinemia). Transient hyperglycinemia presents similarly but neonate recovers in 2–8 weeks. It is due to immature GCS at birth. Infantile form develops after 6 months of age with mainly seizures and mental retardation.

While suppression of respiration, lethargy and hypotonia are believed be due to action of increased glycine on glycine receptor (inhibitory neurotransmitter), myoclonic jerks, intractable seizures are due to its action as an excitatory neurotransmitter on NMDA receptors. Treatment with strychnine improves respiratory effort and arousal but long-term treatment may worsen seizures and brain damage due activation of NMDA receptors by extra glycine. Treatment with ketamine and dextromethorphan (NMDA antagonists) have led to normalization of myoclonic jerks and EEG. Other treatment includes use of benzoate to increase glycine excretion as hippurate and glycine-serine free diet. Anticonvulsants like phenytoin and phenobarbital, which act by enhancing inhibition by potentiating action of GABA, are not effective; valproate is contraindicated as it is an inhibitor of GCS in liver. Diazepam, carbamazepine, lamotrigine and topiramate are used for controlling seizures.

This disorder shows that even while glycine cleavage system is considered to be reversible and glycine can be converted to serine, the GCS works in the direction of breakdown and serine hydroxymethyl transferase in the direction of glycine formation (serine → glycine) in normal physiology. Defect in GCS cannot be compensated by other reactions using glycine (conversion to serine and oxalate). GCS is the main catabolic pathway.

2. **Benzoate is given for therapy of hyperammonemia** and removes ammonia as glycine by conjugating with it to form hippurate which is lost in urine.

3. **Hyperoxaluria and oxalic acid stones:** Oxalate is a metabolic end product in humans. Urine oxalate comes from diet and endogenous metabolic production, with ~40–50% originating from dietary sources. The upper limit of normal oxalate excretion is generally considered to be 40–50 mg per day. Mild hyperoxaluria (50–80 mg/d) usually is caused by excessive intake of high-oxalate foods such as spinach, nuts, and chocolate. In addition, low-calcium diets promote hyperoxaluria as there is less calcium available to bind oxalate and thus prevent its absorption in the intestine. Oxalic acid cannot be further metabolized in humans and is excreted in the urine as oxalates. Calcium oxalate is relatively insoluble in water and precipitates in tissues (kidneys and joints) if its concentration increases in the body. Diet poor in dairy products (calcium) increases the risk of oxalic acid stone formation by increasing intestinal oxalate absorption.

- **Primary hyperoxaluria type I** (Fig. 7.4): Deficiency of the peroxisomal enzyme alanine-glyoxylate aminotransferase, which is expressed only in the liver peroxisomes and requires pyridoxine (vitamin B_6) as its cofactor. In the absence of this enzyme, glyoxylic acid, which cannot be converted to glycine, is transferred to the cytosol, where it is oxidized to oxalic acid. The majority of patients become symptomatic before 5 years of age. Clinical manifestations are related to renal stones and nephrocalcinosis. A marked increase in urinary

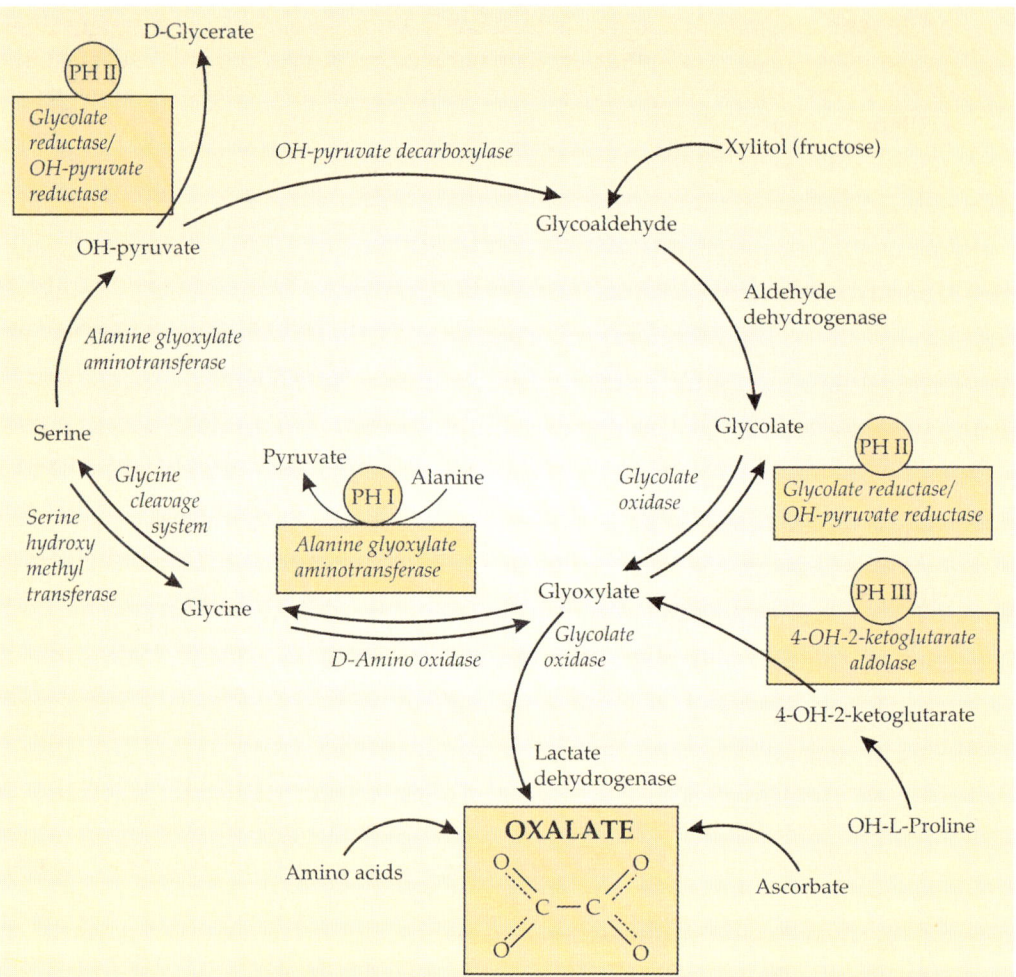

Fig. 7.4. Overview of endogenous oxalate synthesis pathways. PH I–III, primary hyperoxaluria types I–III.

excretion of oxalate (normal excretion 10–50 mg/24 hr) is the most important laboratory finding. The presence of oxalate crystals in urinary sediment is rarely helpful.

- **Primary hyperoxaluria type II (l-glyceric aciduria**, Fig. 7.4): This rare condition is due to a deficiency of D-glycerate dehydrogenase (hydroxypyruvate reductase)/glyoxylate reductase enzyme complex. A deficiency in the activity of this enzyme results in an accumulation of 2 intermediate metabolites, hydroxypyruvate (the ketoacid of serine) and glyoxylic acid. Both these compounds are further metabolized by lactate dehydrogenase (LDH) to L-glyceric acid and oxalic acid, respectively. About 30% of reported patients are from the Saulteaux-Ojibway Indians of Manitoba. Clinical features are similar to type I disorder. Urinary excretion of glycolic acid and glyoxylic acid is not increased. The presence of L-glyceric acid without increased levels of glycolic and glyoxylic acids in urine differentiates this type from type I hyperoxaluria.

- **Secondary hyperoxaluria:** This has been observed in pyridoxine deficiency (cofactor for alanine-glyoxylate aminotransferase), after ingestion of ethylene glycol or high doses of vitamin C, after administration of the anesthetic agent methoxyflurane (which oxidizes directly to oxalic acid), and in patients with inflammatory bowel disease or extensive resection of the bowel, or fat malabsorption (*enteric hyperoxaluria*). With fat malabsorption, calcium in the bowel lumen is bound by fatty acids instead of oxalate, which is left free for absorption in the colon. Acute, fatal hyperoxaluria may develop after ingestion of plants with high oxalic acid content such as sorrel. Precipitation of calcium oxalate in tissues causes hypocalcemia, liver necrosis, renal failure, cardiac arrhythmia, and death. The lethal dose of oxalic acid is estimated to be between 5 and 30 g.

Q. 4. Describe the unique characteristics of branched-chain amino acids metabolism.

Ans. Branched-chain amino acids (BCAA) include valine, leucine and isoleucine. They constitute about 35% of the essential amino acids in muscles and 40% of the essential amino acids required in diet. They are actively metabolized in skeletal muscle and kidney, heart, adipose tissue and brain as an alternative energy source (Fig. 7.5). They yield ketone bodies in liver. Adipose tissue uses the acetyl-CoA produced from their metabolism for lipid synthesis. Leucine promotes insulin release, protein synthesis and inhibits protein degradation. BCAA amino acid infusion can counteract the catabolic state in patients of cirrhosis and chronic renal failure.

Skeletal muscles are the major site of metabolism. In the fed state they are spared by the liver and preferentially taken up by skeletal muscles. In the fasting state they are released by the muscles for use by brain. Pyruvate is produced from muscle glycogen in fasting state, which is then transaminated to alanine for export as part of glucose alanine cycle. Here the BCAAs contribute the amino group. The keto acids formed from BCAA are oxidized for energy production or used to make ketone bodies in liver. The alanine reaching liver is converted back to pyruvate which undergoes gluconeogenesis and amino group is excreted as urea (Fig. 7.6). BCAA metabolism is an excellent source of energy as NADH and $FADH_2$ are formed during their metabolism (Fig. 7.5). They can also be used by brain for energy during starvation. During starvation also they are broken down in muscles to supply amino group to pyruvate for glucose alanine cycle (Fig. 7.6). So, their infusion can help counter the catabolic states in which muscle protein is broken down.

Their metabolism is regulated at the branched-chain keto acid dehydrogenase complex (BCKD complex, similar to pyruvate dehydrogenase and α-KG dehydrogenase complex, Fig. 7.7). Plasma concentrations of BCAA are elevated in starvation, diabetes and obesity. Oxidation is promoted by glucagon and epinephrine and inhibited by insulin. Carnitine and ketone bodies increase oxidation in skeletal muscles while pyruvate inhibits oxidation.

Q. 5. Explain the biochemical basis of maple syrup urine disease and its management.

Ans. Maple syrup urine disease or MSUD is characterized by defect of branched chain α-keto acid dehydrogenase complex (BCKD, Table 7.2) leading to accumulation of the BCAA and corresponding α-keto acids: ketoisocaproate (KIC, from leucine), α-keto-β-methylvalerate (KMV, from isoleucine) and ketoisovalerate (KIV, from valine) (Fig. 7.5). Table 7.3 shows the clinical phenotypes and biochemical features of MSUD.

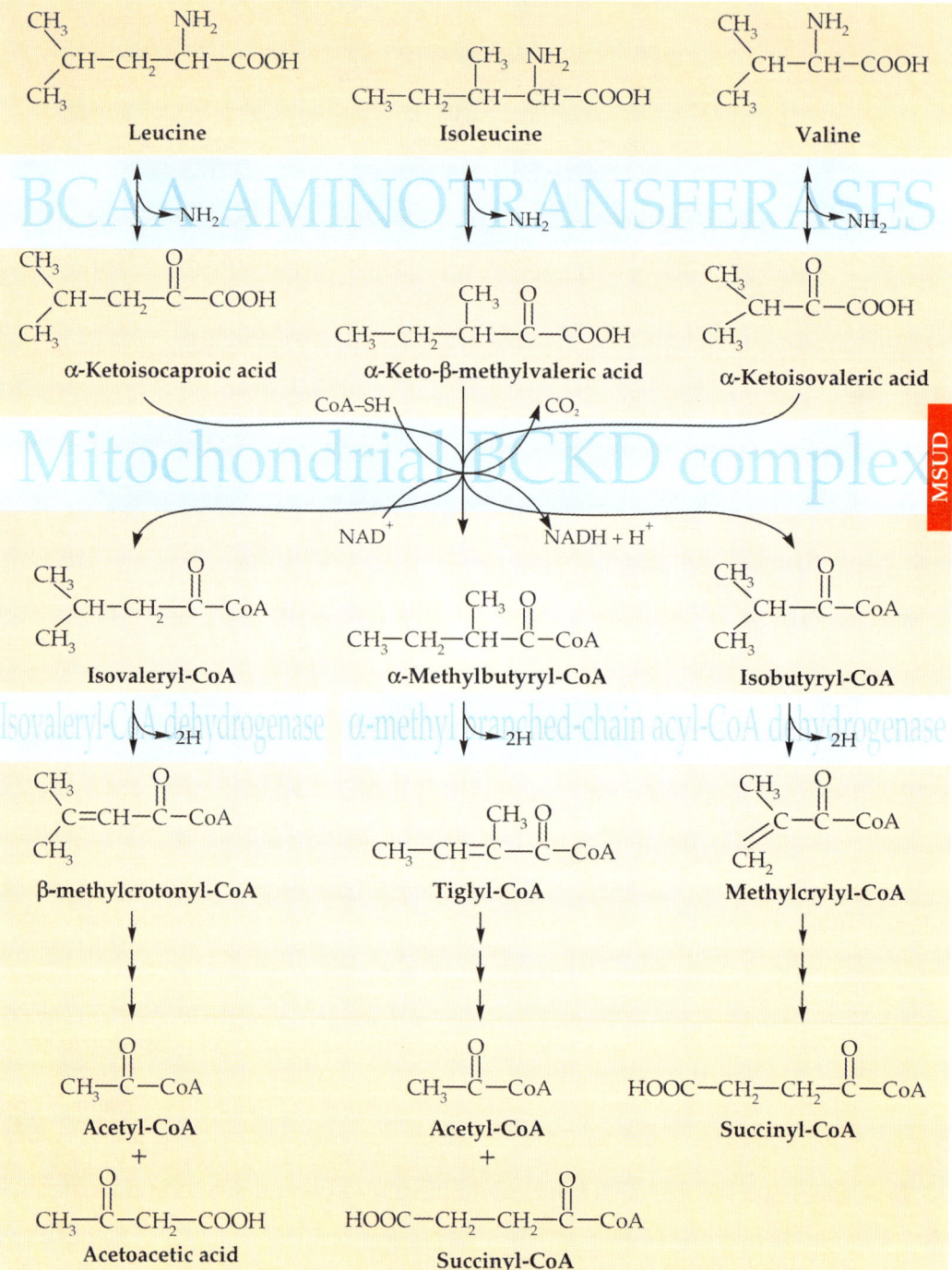

Fig. 7.5. Branched chain amino acid metabolism. 1. BCAA aminotransferases, 2. BCKD complex, 3. Isovaleryl-CoA dehydrogenase, 4. α-methyl branched-chain acyl-CoA dehydrogenase. The NADH and FADH$_2$ produced lead to ATP production in ETC.

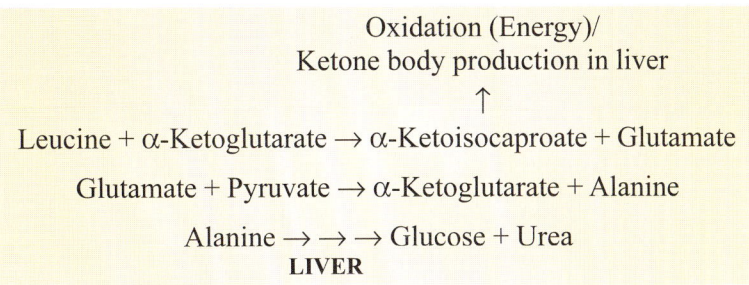

Fig. 7.6. Contribution of BCAA catabolism in muscles to glucose alanine cycle. 25–30% of nitrogen of alanine is derived from BCAA.

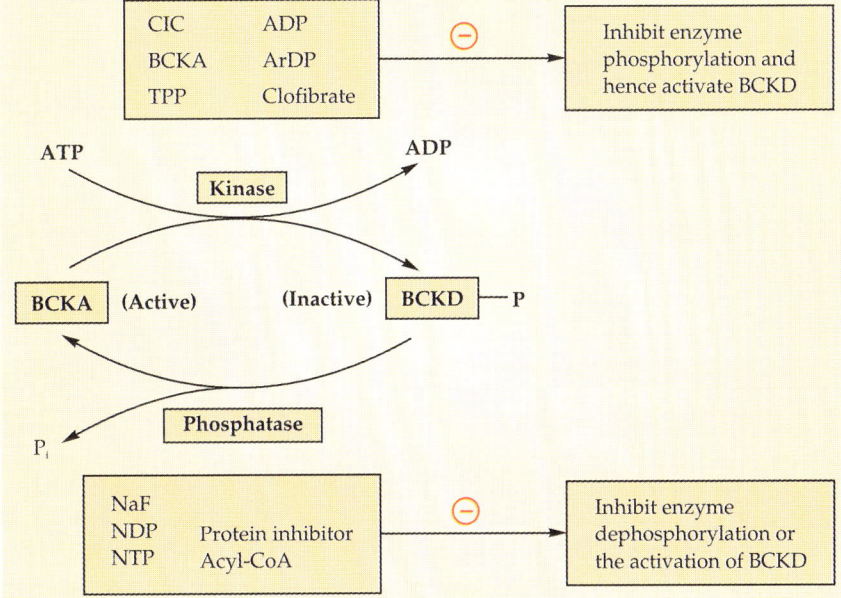

Fig. 7.7. Regulation of branched-chain keto acid dehydrogenase complex. The enzyme is active in dephosphorylated state. CIC = chloroisocaproate, ArDP = arylidenepyruvate, TPP = thymine pyrophosphate, BCKA = branched-chain keto acid, NaF = sodium fluoride, NDP/NTP = nucleoside di/triphosphate.

The brain damage is caused by elevated BCAA and their keto acids. Acute elevation of KIC and leucine can cause brain edema and metabolic encephalopathy.

1. The leucine level may become so elevated as to overwhelm the usual brain mechanisms of water homeostasis and lead to cell swelling.
2. Large neutral amino acids like Leucine, Isoleucine, Valine, Phenylalanine, Tyrosine, Tryptophan, Histidine, Methionine, Threonine are transported across blood-brain barrier by a common sodium independent facilitative transporter LAT1 or SLC7A5. These essential amino acids compete with each other and competitively inhibit transport of others. Thus, maintenance of the physiological ratio of their concentrations is essential.

Table 7.2. Components of BCKA dehydrogenase complex

Component	Molecular mass (daltons)	Prosthetic group (P) and cofactor (C)
BCKA decarboxylase (E1)	1.7×10^5 (α_2, β_2)	TPP (C)
α-Subunit	46,500	Mg^{2+} (C)
β-Subunit	37,200	
Dihydrolipoyl transacylase (E2)	1.1×10^6 (α_{24})	Lipoic acid (P)
Subunit	46,518	
Dihydrolipoyl dehydrogenase (E3)	1.1×10^5	FAD (C)
Subunit	55,000	
BCKA kinase	43,000	Mg^{2+} (C)
Subunit	43,000	
BCKA phosphatase	4.6×10^5	None
Subunit	33,000	

Table 7.3. Clinical phenotypes of maple syrup urine disease

Clinical phenotype	Prominent clinical features	Biochemical features	Decarboxylation activity, % of normal
Classic	Neonatal onset, poor feeding, lethargy, increased/decreased tone, ketoacidosis, and seizures	Markedly increased alloisoleucine, BCAA, and BCKA	0–2
Intermediate	Failure to thrive, often no ketoacidosis, developmental delay	Persistently increased alloisoleucine, BCAA, and BCKA	3–30
Intermittent	Normal early development, episodic ataxia/ketoacidosis precipitated by infection or stress, episodes can be fatal, usually normal intellect	Normal BCAA when asymptomatic	5–20
Thiamine-responsive	Similar to intermediate MSUD	Decreased BCKA and/or BCAA with thiamine therapy	2–40
Lipoamide dehydrogenase (E3) deficiency	Usually no neonatal symptoms, failure to thrive, hypotonia, lactic acidosis, developmental delay, movement disorder, progressive deterioration	Moderately increased BCAA, BCKA; elevated α-ketoglutarate and pyruvate	0–25

The elevated BCAA disturb this balance leading to chronically low uptake of other amino acids in brain cells and high uptake of BCAA. Deficiency of amino acids like tryptophan, tyrosine, phenylalanine effects synthesis of serotonin and catecholamines (epinephrine, norepinephrine and dopamine). Deficiency of methionine affects myelin synthesis. Amino acid deficiency also affects overall protein synthesis in brain cells.

The competitive transport concept is relevant to the pathophysiology of other inborn errors, including phenylketonuria, tyrosinemia, hypermethioninemia, and 5,10-methylenetetrahydrofolate reductase deficiency. In all of these conditions, a pathological pattern of amino acid concentration in blood alters their flow into the nervous system altering neurotransmitter balance and disturbing other biochemical processes.

3. Imbalance in leucine-glutamate cycle: The large concentration of KIC (10–20 fold increase) and its transamination to leucine depletes neuronal glutamate and aspartate (transaminated to α-KG and oxaloacetate to supply amino group to KIC) and neurotransmitters synthesised from them (Fig. 7.8).

4. Depletion of glutamate and aspartate compromises the malate shuttle for transport of NADH into mitochondria effecting ATP production and promoting lactic acidosis due to anaerobic metabolism (Fig. 7.9).

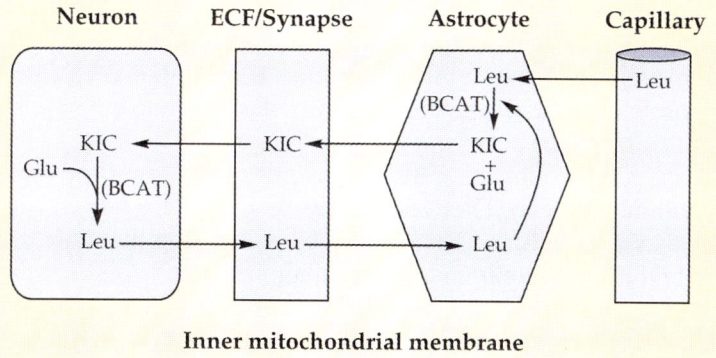

Fig. 7.8. Leucine glutamate cycle in neurons and astrocytes. The extra leucine entering from capillaries depletes Glu in neurons. BCAT = Branched-chain aminotransferase.

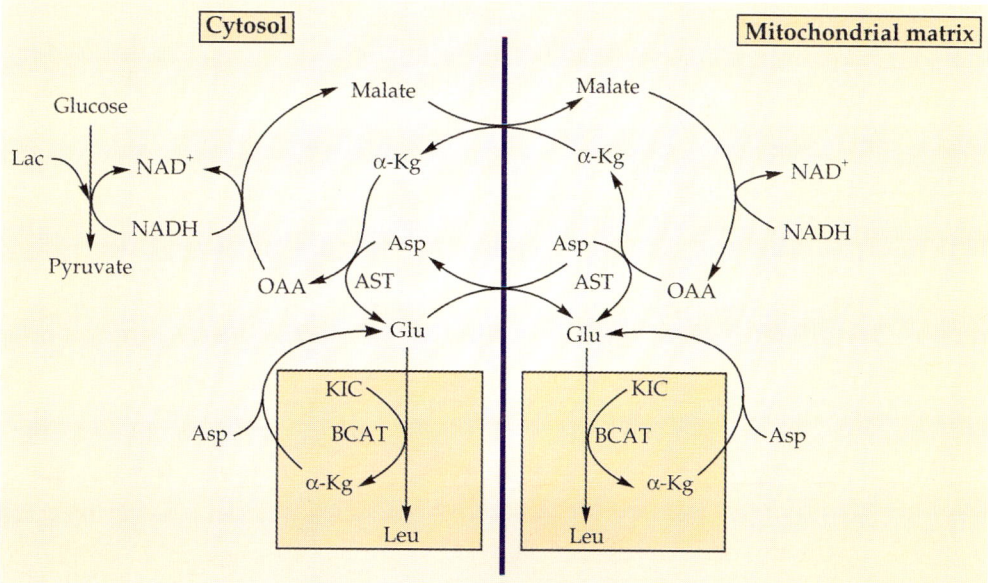

Fig. 7.9. Elevated levels of KIC deplete glutamate and aspartate levels hampering the malate shuttle.

5. In the catabolic muscle increased KIC transaminates to leucine and decreases conversion of pyruvate to alanine (BCAT reaction: KIC + Glu → Leu + α-KG is increased and thus ALT reaction: Glu + Pyruvate → Alanine + α-KG is hampered), disturbing glucose alanine cycle, accounting for the episodes of hypoglycaemia seen.
6. Depletion of glutamate leads to depletion of aspartate, alanine and other amino acids (synthesized from amphibolic intermediates with contribution of NH_3 from glutamate) in brain compromising rate of protein synthesis.

Management

- The dietary composition of amino acids is regulated to optimize the pattern of circulating amino acids for ensuring proper supply of amino acids to nervous tissue, focusing upon brain uptake of each amino acid.
- Conditionally essential amino acids such as glutamine and alanine are fortified to buffer against their depletion by high tissue KIC.
- Based on amino acid monitoring, the dietary prescription is repeatedly adjusted to account for dynamic changes of metabolic homeostasis characteristic of MSUD, especially the frequent catabolic episodes triggered by minor infections.
- BCAA are supplied in just sufficient quantities to support protein synthesis (as they are essential amino acids). Diet completely free from BCAA will lead to their deficiency which is equally harmful. This is done by calculating the growth rate and the associated protein and BCAA requirement to maintain it.
- Essential fatty acids, vitamins, minerals, and micronutrients are given to support normal development and correct existing deficiencies.

Q. 6. How is arginine synthesized in body?

Ans. Arginine is synthesized by coordinated reactions in the intestine and proximal tubules of kidney (Figs. 7.10 and 7.11). In the intestines CPS1 forms carbomoyl phosphate. Ornithine

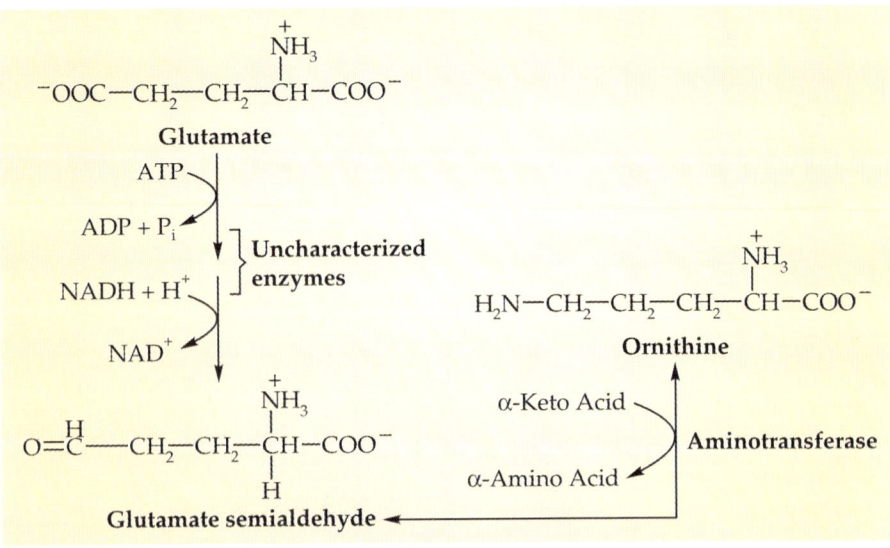

Fig. 7.10. Ornithine synthesis in intestines.

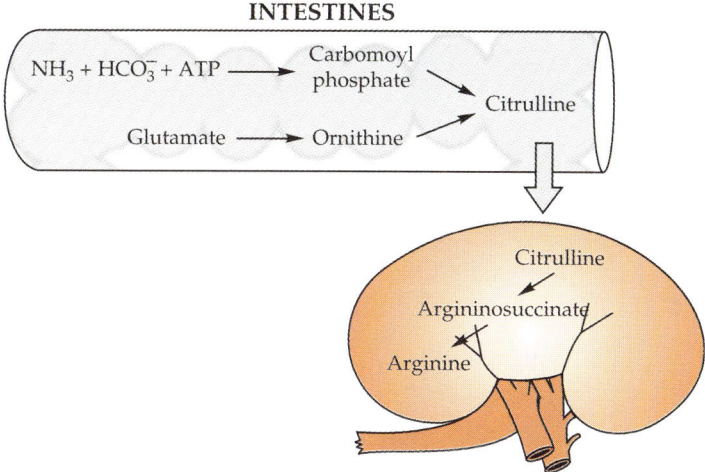

Fig. 7.11. Arginine synthesis: cooperation between intestines and kidney.

is formed from glutamate through glutamic semialdehyde (Fig. 7.10). Ornithine and carbomoyl phosphate form citrulline which then is transported to kidney. These steps also act as sources of ornithine and citrulline in body. In the proximal tubules of kidney citrulline is converted to arginosuccinate and then to arginine as in urea cycle. The proximal tubule cells lack arginase enzyme. Arginine produced is used for synthesis of proteins, creatine, nitric oxide, etc. Urea cycle cannot contribute arginine for export as arginase breaks down the arginine formed in liver.

Q. 7. How is nitrogen transported from tissues for its disposal?

Ans.
- Proteins in the body undergo constant turnover. Under conditions of energy need, proteins are degraded and amino acids used to gain energy and for gluconeogenesis.
- The carbon skeletons of amino acids are used for energy production in liver and muscles. Most important are branched-chain amino acids as their degradation produces large amount of NADH and $FADH_2$.
- The amino group in all these conditions of protein catabolism has to be disposed of. The amino group from most amino acids is channelled by transaminases to glutamine and alanine, the major carriers of nitrogen for disposal in liver. These are produced from α-KG and pyruvate.
- This disposal however is not a solo action of liver but requires co-ordinated action of liver, intestines and kidney. Some glutamine is transported directly to kidney or liver but most is transported to intestines (Fig. 7.12).
- Glutamine is essential for maintenance and proliferation of intestinal cells. Here it is used to maintain the purine and pyrimidine synthesis to support the high rate of division required to maintain the epithelium. It is used for synthesis of citrulline and arginine (in co-ordinated action with kidney) to be supplied to blood. Fate of glutamine in intestines includes citrulline, alanine, ammonia, proline and nucleotide synthesis.
- Glutamine is used in kidneys for synthesis of NH_4^+ (excreted to maintain acid-base balance) and new HCO_3^- generation. This removes the excess hydrogen ions and also conserves HCO_3 which otherwise would be used for urea production in liver. By using glutamine,

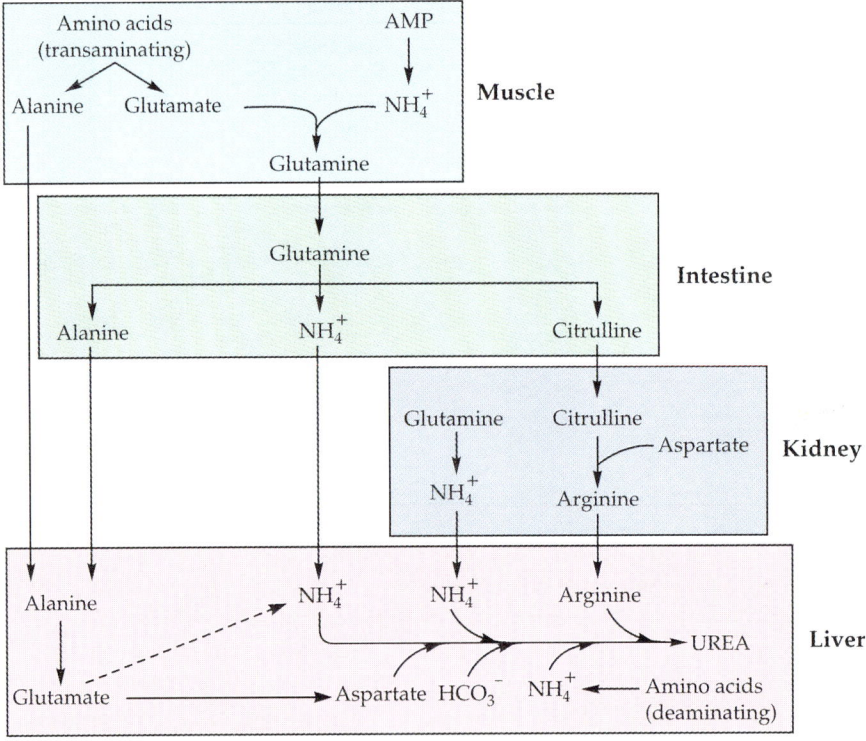

Fig. 7.12. Disposal of amino group during protein catabolism.

kidney decreases glutamine supply to liver and thus decreases HCO_3 consumption in liver for urea production from glutamine. Glutamine requirement and NH_4^+ excretion is increased in metabolic acidosis. Acidosis causes more glutamine to shunt to kidneys by suppressing uptake in liver.
- The alanine from intestines, muscles and other tissues is taken to liver. Here ammonia is released by actions of transaminase and glutamate dehydrogenase and converted to urea by urea cycle.

Q. 8. How many ATPs are required to produce 1 molecule of urea?

Ans. CPS1 reaction converts 2 ATPs to 2 ADPs. Arginosuccinate production converts ATP to AMP and 2 P_i. This is equivalent to 2 ATPs consumed. In the urea bicycle (co-ordinated operation of urea cycle and TCA, Fig. 7.13), fumarate produced by arginosuccinase is converted to oxaloacetate and then aspartate for use in urea cycle. These steps generate 1 NADH equivalent to 2.5 ATPs. It would appear that 1.5 ATPs are thus required. However, about 2/3rds of the oxaloacetate derived from fumarate is metabolized to aspartate and remaining can be used for gluconeogenesis or ATP production. The amount of fumarate used to form energy is approximately equal to that required for urea cycle and gluconeogenesis, so that liver itself gains no net energy. The integration of the urea cycle with gluconeogenesis ensures that the bulk of the NADH required for gluconeogenesis can be provided by the urea bicycle.

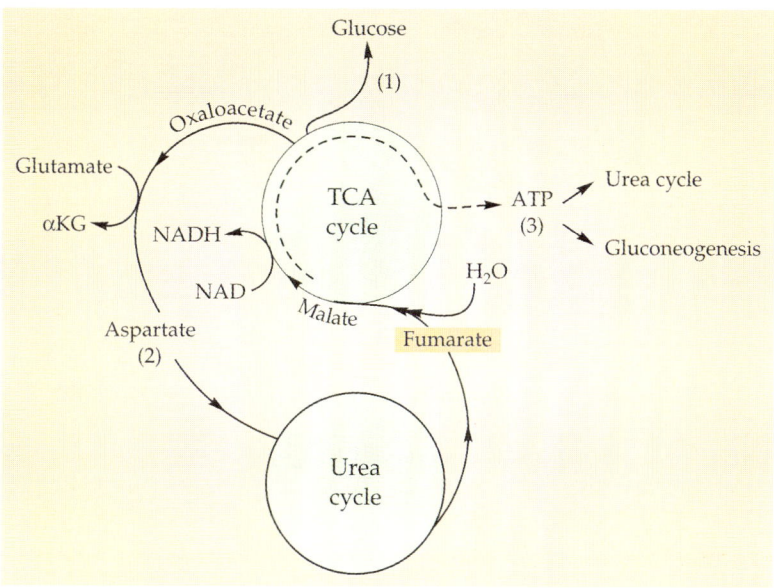

Fig. 7.13. Urea bicycle. OAA = oxaloacetate. Fumarate formed in urea cycle can be used for: (1) gluconeogenesis – OAA can enter gluconeogenesis, (2) OAA is transaminated to aspartate which is used in urea cycle, (3) NADH produced from malate → OAA step generates ATP or the NADH can be used in gluconeogenesis from OAA.

Q. 9. How are amino acids transported across cell membranes?

Ans. There are 'systems' of amino acid transporters. 'Systems' imply that: The functional activity of transporting amino acid appears to be similar in many tissues and that each transporter transports a group of amino acids rather than individual amino acids. These systems have been classified into 5 categories:

1. Neutral amino acids
2. Cationic amino acids and cysteine
3. Anionic amino acids
4. Iminoglycine: Proline, hydroxyproline and glycine
5. Taurine and other beta amino acids.

The known complete list of transporters is summarized in Table 7.4.

The transporters may be sodium-dependent or independent or may use H^+ gradient or gradient of other amino acids. They are responsible for absorption at apical membranes and basolateral membranes of epithelia in GIT and kidney, across cell membranes and blood-brain barrier. A particular amino acid may be transported by multiple transporters. The amino acids transported by a transporter competitively inhibit the transport of each other, e.g. as in MSUD excess BCAA inhibit transport of aromatic amino acids by LAT1 (SLC3A2/SLC7A5). The inhibition can be specific for the transporters or at high concentration may even be non-specific by competing for the Na or proton gradient used by multiple transporters. Mutations in the transporter may selectively alter the affinity for one or more of the substrate amino acids. The transport systems and associated clinical disorders are summarized in Table 7.4.

Table 7.4. Amino acid transporters and associated disorders

SLC	Amino acid substrates	Affinity	Mechanism	Expression	Disorder
SLC38A2	G, P, A, S, C, Q, N, H, M	Medium	S	Ubiquitous	
SLC38A4	G, A, S, C, Q, N, M, AA+	Medium	S	K	
SLC1A4	A, S, C	High	A	K	
SLC1A5	A, S, C, T, Q	High	A	K, I (AM)	
SLC3A2/SLC7A10	G, A, S, C, T	High	A	K	
SLC6A19	AA0	Low	S	K, I (AM)	Hartnup disorder
SLC6A15	P, L, V, I, M	High	S	K	
SLC6A14	AA0, AA+, β-Ala	High	S	I (AM)	
SLC3A1/SLC7A9	R, K, O, cystine	High	A	K, I (AM)	Cystinuria
SLC6A6	Tau, β-Ala	High	S	K (AM, BM)	
SLC6A18	G	NR	NR	K (AM)	Glycinuria
SLC6A20	P, HO-P	Medium	S	K, I (AM)	Iminoglycinuria
SLC3A2/SLC7A5	H, M, L, I, V, F, Y, W	High	A		
SLC3A2/SLC7A8	AA0 except P	Medium	A	K, I (BM)	
SLC43A1	L, I, M, F	Low	U	K	
SLC43A2	L, I, M, F	Low	U		
SLC38A3	Q, N, H	Low	S	K (BM)	
SLC38A5	Q, N, H, S, G	Low	S	K	
SLC36A1	P, G, A GABA, β-Ala	Low	S	K, I (AM)	Iminoglycinuria
SLC36A2	P, G, A	Medium	S	K	
SLC16A10	F, Y, W	Low	U	K, I (BM)	Blue diaper syndrome
SLC1A2	E, D	High	S	K (BM)	
SLC1A1	E, D	High	S	K, I (AM)	Dicarboxylic aminoaciduria
SLC3A2/SLC7A11	E, cystine	High	A	Ub	
SLC7A1	R, K, O, H	Medium	U	Ub	
SLC3A2/SLC7A7	K, R, Q, H, M, L	High	A	K, I (BM)	Lysinuric protein intolerance
SLC3A2/SLC7A6	K, R, Q, H, M, L, A, C	High	A	K, I (BM)	

NR = not reported; A = antiport; AA0 = neutral amino acids; AA+ = cationic amino acids; U = uniport; S = symport; S-AA0 = symport together with neutral amino acids; K = kidney; I = intestine; AM = apical membrane; BM = basolateral membrane; O = ornithine; HO-P = hydroxyproline. Amino acids are given in one-letter codes.

Hartnup syndrome: Occurs due to mutation in SLC6A19 responsible for transport of neutral amino acids. It is characterized by skin rash and cerebellar ataxia. Intestinal absorption of tryptophan is most affected leading to niacin deficiency. Other neutral amino acids can be absorbed to considerable extent and absorption of peptides also compensates for them. Renal excretion of serine, threonine, glutamine, tyrosine, tryptophan and histidine is increased 60–80 times normal and of other neutral amino acids up to 20 times normal. While skin rash can be cured by niacin supplementation, ataxia cannot be, though high protein diet relieves all clinical features. Patients are asymptomatic with high protein diet.

Q. 10. Describe the biochemical basis of clinical features of urea cycle defects.

Ans. Deficiencies of the urea cycle enzymes causing hyperammonemia include:
- Carbamyl phosphate synthetase (CPS, Fig. 7.14 – ①)
- Ornithine transcarbamylase (OTC, Fig. 7.14 – ②)
- Argininosuccinate synthetase (AS, Fig. 7.14 – ③)
- Argininosuccinate lyase (AL, Fig. 7.14 – ④)
- Arginase (Fig. 7.14 – ⑤)
- N-Acetylglutamate synthetase (Fig. 7.14 – ⑦)

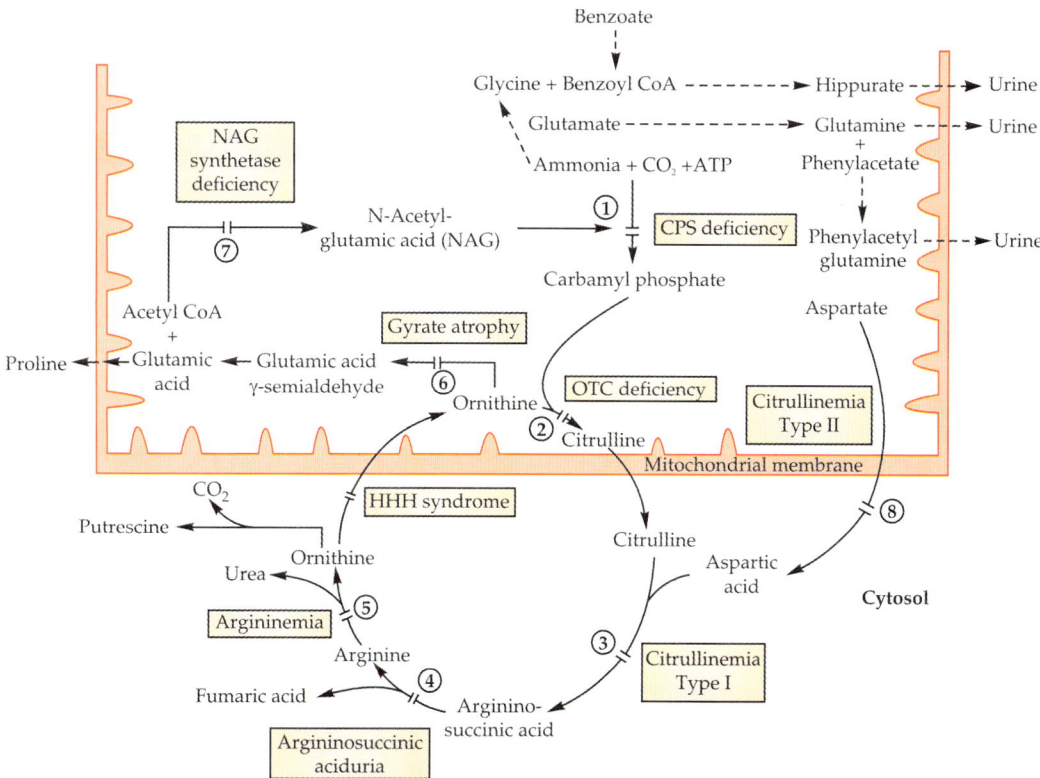

Fig. 7.14. Urea cycle and associated diseases.

Deficiency of urea cycle enzymes leads to
- Hyperammoniemia: accumulation of ammonia and glutamine, the severity and pattern varies with the type of defect
- Arginine becomes essential amino acid (except in arginase deficiency) as synthesis is hampered in intestine and kidney
- Accumulation of intermediates in the cycle before the defective enzyme.

Hyperammonemia

The affected infant is normal at birth but becomes symptomatic within a few days of protein feeding. Refusal to eat, vomiting, tachypnea, and lethargy can quickly progress to a deep coma. Convulsions are common. Physical examination may reveal hepatomegaly in addition to the neurologic signs of deep coma. Hyperammonemia can trigger increased intracranial pressure that may be manifested with bulging fontanel and dilated pupils. In infants and older children acute hyperammonemia is manifested by vomiting and neurologic abnormalities such as ataxia, mental confusion, agitation, irritability, and combativeness. These manifestations may alternate with periods of lethargy and somnolence that may progress to coma.

Biochemical basis:
- Ammonia is metabolised by glutamine synthetase in astrocytes. Hyperammonemia leads to excess glutamine and depletion of glutamate and α-ketoglutarate (Figs. 7.15 and 7.16).
- Depletion of α-ketoglutarate slows TCA and decreases ATP production.
- Decreased glutamate decreases GABA pool (inhibitory neurotransmitter).
- Excess glutamine is exchanged for tryptophan leading to increased serotonin production from tryptophan. Serotonin causes drowsiness (Fig. 7.16).
- Ammonia directly also alters excitatory and inhibitory pathways (neuronal toxin).
- Decreased myoinositol efflux (NH_3 inhibits myoinisitol export from cells) and an increase in glutamine ('osmolytes') leads to cell swelling/edema in astrocytes (Fig. 7.15). Normally efflux of myoinositol from astrocytes helps counteract cell swelling or osmotic stress due to glutamine, etc.
- Increase in astrocyte hydration may be a major pathogenetic event in the development of hepatic encephalopathy.

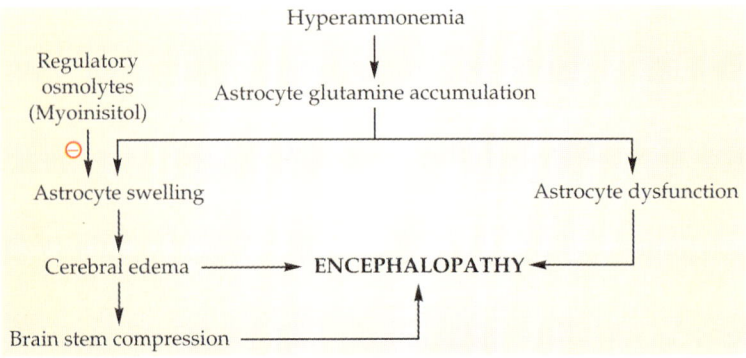

Fig. 7.15. Effects of hyperammonemia on brain.

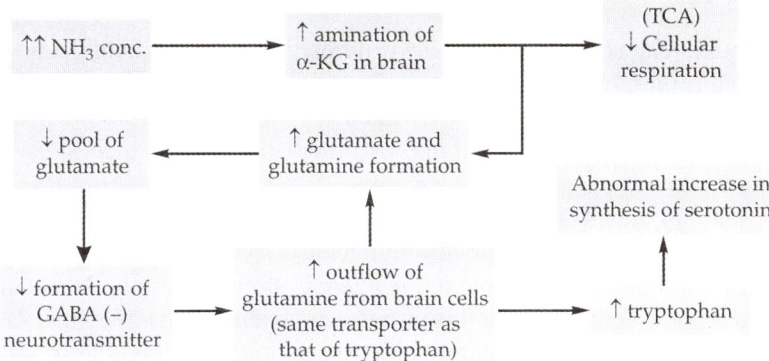

Fig. 7.16. Mechanism of NH$_3$ toxicity.

Arginase deficiency (Fig. 7.14 – ⑤)

The clinical manifestations of this rare condition are quite different from those of other urea cycle enzyme defects. They include progressive spastic diplegia with scissoring of the lower extremities, choreoathetotic movements, and loss of developmental milestones in a previously normal infant. Mental retardation is progressive; seizures are common, but episodes of severe hyperammonemia are not usually seen in this disorder. Treatment includes diet devoid of arginine and benzoate for hyperammonemia.

Gyrate atrophy of retina and choroid (Fig. 7.14 – ⑥)

Ornithine 5-aminotransferase deficiency inhibits ornithine degradation to glutamate (Fig. 7.14). Clinical manifestations are limited to the eyes and include night blindness, myopia, loss of peripheral vision, and posterior subcapsular cataracts. These patients usually have normal intelligence. There is a 10–20-fold increase in plasma levels of ornithine (400–1400 µmol/L). There is no hyperammonemia and no increase in any other amino acids; plasma levels of glutamate, glutamine, lysine, creatine, and creatinine are moderately decreased. Some patients respond partially to high doses of pyridoxine (required by ornithine 5-aminotransferase).

Hyperammonemia-Hyperornithinemia-Homocitrullinemia (HHH) syndrome (Fig. 7.14)

Defect is in the transport system of ornithine from the cytosol into the mitochondria, resulting in accumulation of ornithine in the cytosol and its deficiency in the mitochondria. This causes hyperornithinemia and results in disruption of the urea cycle and hyperammonemia. Homocitrulline occurs from the reaction of mitochondrial carbomyl phosphate with lysine. Ornithine supplementation may produce clinical improvement in some patients.

Q. 11. Explain biochemical basis of management of urea cycle defects.

Ans. Hyperammonemia should be treated promptly and vigorously to avoid permanent neurological defects. The goal of therapy is to lower the concentration of ammonia in the body. This is accomplished in two ways: (1) by removal of ammonia from the body in a form other than urea, and (2) by provision of adequate calories and essential amino acids to minimize the endogenous protein degradation and favour protein synthesis.

Treatment of acute hyperammonemia

- Adequate calories, fluid, and electrolytes are given intravenously. Minimal amounts of protein preferably as a mixture of essential amino acids is given during the 1st 24 hr of therapy. Sodium benzoate, sodium phenylacetate and arginine are given. Peritoneal dialysis or hemodialysis is done if above treatment fails to produce an appreciable decrease in plasma ammonia.
- As soon as the clinical condition of the patient allows, oral feeding with a low-protein formula (0.5–1.0 g/kg/24 hr) through a nasogastric tube is started.
- Use of organic acids to remove nitrogen as adducts with non-essential amino acids: The main organic acids used for this purpose are sodium salts of benzoic acid and phenylacetic acid. Benzoate forms hippuric acid with endogenous glycine in the liver. Each mole of benzoate removes 1 mole of ammonia as glycine. Phenylacetate conjugates with glutamine to form phenylacetylglutamine, which is readily excreted in the urine. One mole of phenyl-acetate removes 2 moles of ammonia as glutamine from the body (Fig. 7.14).
- Arginine administration is effective in the treatment of hyperammonemia that is due to most defects of the urea cycle because it supplies the urea cycle with ornithine and NAG. In patients with citrullinemia, 1 mole of arginine reacts with 1 mole of ammonia (as carbamyl phosphate) to form citrulline. In patients with argininosuccinic acidemia, 2 moles of ammonia (as carbamyl phosphate and aspartate) react with arginine to form argininosuccinic acid. Citrulline and argininosuccinic acid are far less toxic and more readily excreted by the kidneys than ammonia. In patients with CPS or OTC deficiency, arginine administration is indicated because arginine becomes an essential amino acid in these disorders.
- Patients with OTC deficiency benefit from supplementation with citrulline (200 mg/kg/24 hr), which reacts with 1 mole of ammonia (as aspartic acid) to form arginine.
- Administration of arginine or citrulline is contraindicated in patients with arginase deficiency.
- Oral administration of neomycin limits growth of intestinal bacteria that can produce ammonia. Oral lactulose acidifies the intestinal lumen, thereby reducing the diffusion of ammonia across the intestinal epithelium.
- There may be considerable lag between the normalization of ammonia and an improvement in the neurologic status of the patient. Several days may be needed before the infant becomes fully alert.
- Long-term therapy: In general, all patients, regardless of the enzymatic defect, require some degree of protein restriction (1–2 g/kg/24 hr). In patients with defects in the urea cycle, chronic administration of benzoate, phenylacetate, and arginine or citrulline (in patients with OTC deficiency) is effective in maintaining blood ammonia levels within the normal range. Phenylbutyrate may be used in place of phenylacetate, because the patient and the family may not accept the latter owing to its offensive odor.
- Carnitine supplementation is recommended because benzoate and phenylacetate may cause carnitine depletion. Growth parameters, especially head circumference and nutritional indices (blood albumin, prealbumin, pH, electrolytes, amino acids, zinc, selenium), should be monitored.
- Catabolic states (infections, fasting) triggering hyperammonemia should be avoided or treated vigorously.

Q. 12. What are the causes and effects of tetrahydrobiopterin deficiency? Explain the biochemical basis of management.

Ans. Tetrahydrobiopterin is a pteridine which acts as a cofactor of a number of enzymes (Fig. 7.17).

1. Phenylalanine hydroxylase
2. Tyrosine hydroxylase
3. Tryptophan-5-hydroxylase
4. Nitric oxide synthase
5. Glyceryl ether monoxygenase.

It is present in many cells and tissues of the human body. Cells generate BH_4 by two mechanisms.

1. De novo synthesis from GTP (Fig. 7.18)
2. Salvage from pre-existing dihydrobiopterins (Fig. 7.19).

De novo pathway is essential as defects cause life-threatening disorders. Exogenous dihydrobiopterin can be converted to BH_4 by dihydrofolate reductase enzyme (salvage).

Tetrahydrobiopterin deficiency can be caused by mutations in:
- Enzymes involved in de novo synthesis (GTPCH or PTPS, Fig. 7.18)
- Enzymes involved in regeneration of BH_4 (pterin-4-α-carbinolamine dehydratase, PCD or dihydropteridine reductase, DHPR, Fig. 7.20).

It causes:
- Hyperphenylalaninemia
- Deficiency of neurotransmitter precursors: L-dopa and 5-hydroxytryptophan
- Brain nitric oxide synthase may be affected.

Infants with cofactor deficiency are identified during screening programs for phenylketonuria (PKU) because of evidence of hyperphenylalaninemia. However, the clinical manifestations of the BH_4 deficiency differ greatly from classical PKU. Neurologic symptoms of BH_4 deficiency often manifest in the 1st few months of life and include extrapyramidal signs with choreoathetotic or dystonic limb movements, axial and truncal hypotonia, hypokinesia, feeding difficulties, and autonomic problems. Mental retardation, seizures, hypersalivation, and swallowing difficulties are also seen.

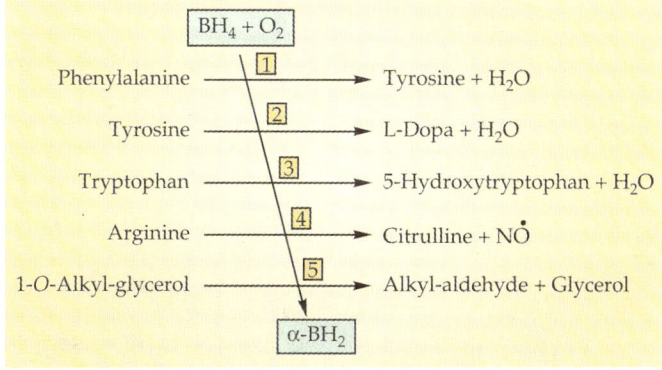

Fig. 7.17. Enzymes requiring tetrahydrobiopterin (BH_4).

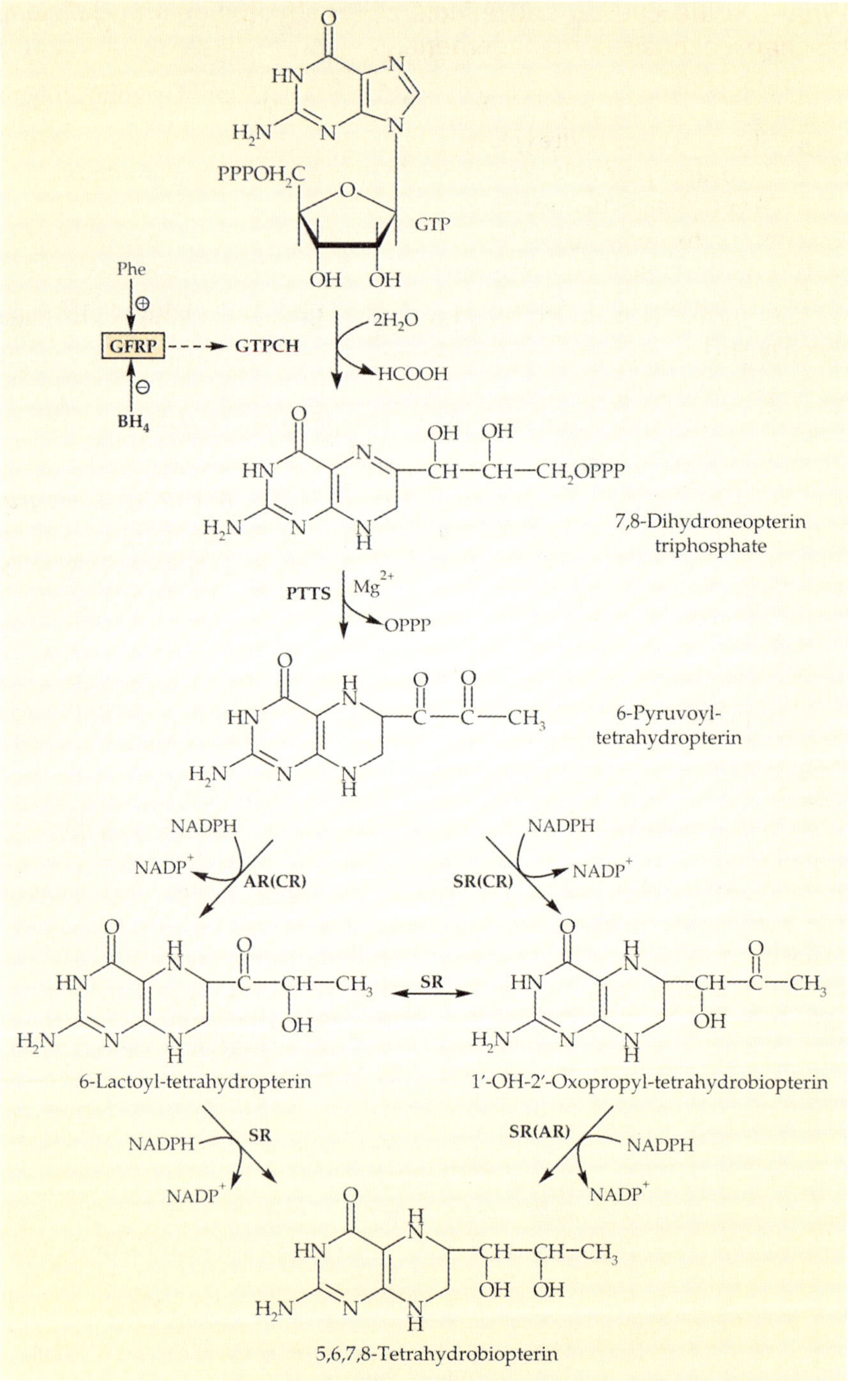

Fig. 7.18. De novo synthesis of BH_4. GTCPH = GTP cyclohydrase I, PTPS= 6-pyruvoyl tetrahydrobiopterin synthase, AR= alsode reductase, SR= sepiapterin reductase, CR= carbonyl reductase, GFRP = GTPCH feedback regulatory protein.

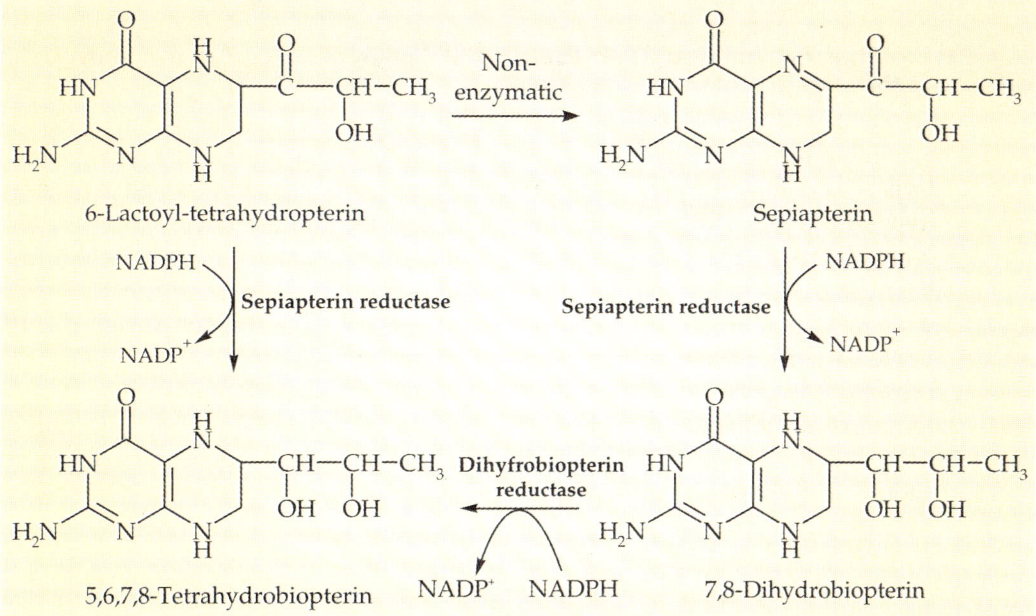

Fig. 7.19. Salvage of BH$_4$. DHPR = dihyfrobiopterin reductase, SR = sepiapterin reductase.

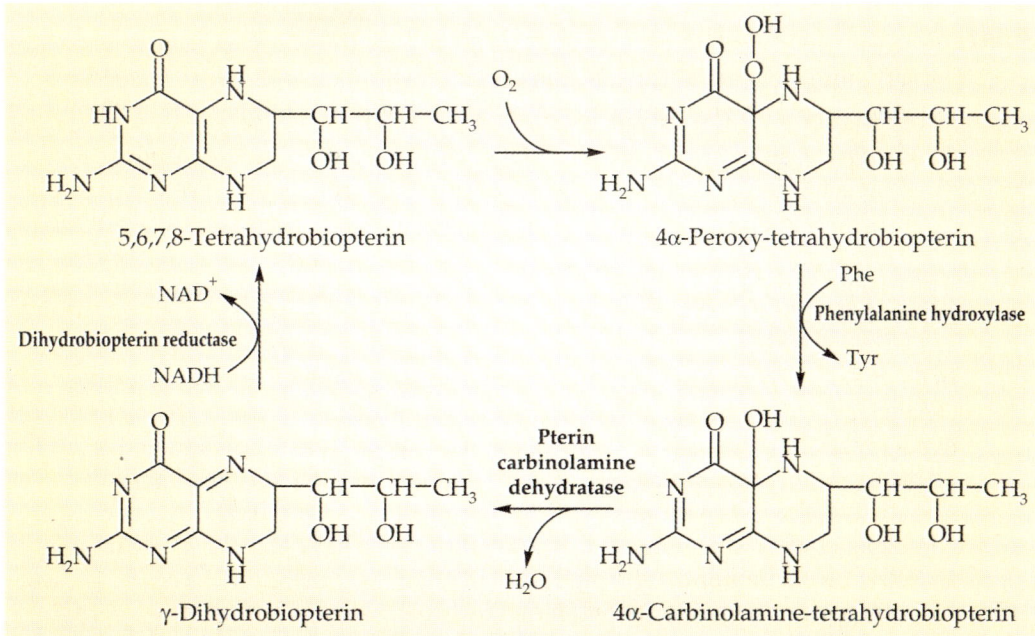

Fig. 7.20. Regeneration of BH$_4$. DHPR = dihyfrobiopterin reductase, PCD = pterin carbinolamine dehydratase, PAH = phenylalanine hydroxylase.

Biochemical basis of therapy

- **Low Phe diet and oral BH4:** The goals of therapy are to correct hyperphenylalaninemia and to restore neurotransmitter deficiencies in the CNS. The control of hyperphenylalaninemia is important in patients with BH4 deficiency, because high levels of phenylalanine competitively interfere with the transport of neurotransmitter precursors (tyrosine, tryptophan) into the brain. Plasma phenylalanine should be maintained as close to normal as possible (<6 mg/dL). Low phenylalanine diet and oral supplementation of BH4 is used.
- **Neurotransmitter replacement:** Lifelong supplementation with neurotransmitter precursors such as L-dopa and 5-hydroxytryptophan is necessary in most of these patients even when treatment with BH4 normalizes plasma levels of phenylalanine as BH4 does not readily enter the brain. Supplementation with folinic acid (co-factor of DHPR) is also recommended in patients with dihydropteridine reductase deficiency.
- **Drug precautions:** Drugs such as trimethoprim sulfamethoxazole, methotrexate, and other antileukemic agents, are known to inhibit dihydropteridine reductase enzyme activity and should be used with great caution.
- **Monitoring:** Hyperprolactinemia occurs in patients with BH4 deficiency and may be due to hypothalamic dopamine deficiency. Measurement of serum prolactin levels provides a convenient method for monitoring adequacy of neurotransmitter replacement in affected patients.

Q. 13. What are the biological functions of heme degradation products – carbon monoxide and bilirubin/biliverdin?

Ans. Carbon monoxide and biliverdin are not merely the passive waste products of heme degradation but serve important biological functions. Free heme, which is toxic, is degraded via cleavage of its tetrapyrrolole ring by heme oxygenase (HO). Two major forms of HO exist:

1. HO-1 is an inducible enzyme that occurs in many tissues but is most abundant in the spleen where it is activated by heme emerging from degraded red blood cells. HO-1 is rapidly induced by diverse cytotoxic stimuli and is regarded as one of the heat shock proteins.
2. HO-2 is constitutive and most concentrated in brain and testes.

Functions of CO

In the brain and peripheral nervous system carbon monoxide, formed when the heme ring is cleaved, appears to be a neurotransmitter. Its synthesis is regulated by neuronal activity, as depolarization of neurons leads to calcium entry with calcium-calmodulin binding to and activating HO-2. CO structurally resembles nitric oxide (NO) and also acts via cGMP on smooth muscles as a vasodilator. It has a protective effect in stroke patients. CO can act complementary or antagonistic to NO. While NO can have protective (in low concentration) as well as deleterious effects (in high concentration, by generation of reactive nitrogen species) CO generated in body has mainly protective role.

Functions of bilirubin/biliverdin

Biliverdin generated from cleavage of tetrapyrrolole ring of heme by HO accumulates very little in most tissues being rapidly reduced to bilirubin by the high tissue densities of biliverdin reductase (BVR). Because bilirubin is toxic and insoluble, it must be glucuronidated before excretion in the bile. The glucuronidation pathway is poorly developed in most newborns leading to accumulation of bilirubin whose yellow colour conveys the physiologic jaundice of many babies. Substantial elevations of bilirubin lead to its deposition in the brain with kernicteric damage. Because biliverdin is more water-soluble than bilirubin, hence more readily excreted, the physiologic rationale for the existence of the BVR pathway has been unclear.

Bilirubin is a potent antioxidant. However, tissue concentrations of bilirubin, about 20–50 nM, are much too low to cope with the 1000 times higher (mM) levels of reactive oxygen species that most cells encounter. By contrast, GSH, a well-accepted physiologic cytoprotectant antioxidant, occurs in levels of 5–10 mM in most tissues. Despite tissue levels that are thousands of times lower than glutathione GSH, bilirubin is effective because of the biosynthetic cycle wherein it is generated from biliverdin by biliverdin reductase (BVR). When bilirubin acts as an antioxidant, it is oxidized to biliverdin, which is immediately reduced by BVR to bilirubin. Thus, as little as 10 nM bilirubin protects against 10,000 higherfold concentrations of hydrogen peroxide H_2O_2. The antioxidant actions of bilirubin are dramatically amplified by BVR in a biliverdin–bilirubin cycle. The reducing power for BVR comes from NADPH.

Bilirubin protects against lipid peroxidation of cell membranes and other lipids while GSH largely protects water-soluble proteins. Knockout mice with targeted deletion of HO-2 have reduced bilirubin levels and are more susceptible to neurotoxic damage, seizures, stroke damage, and traumatic brain injury. The complementary functions of bilirubin and GSH are physiologically relevant, as depletion of bilirubin by HO-2 or BVR deletion selectively enhances lipid peroxidation, while depletion of GSH selectively increases water-soluble protein oxidation. Depletion of BVR or GSH leads to cell death due to oxidant damage.

While very high levels of bilirubin are neurotoxic, but mildly elevated levels of bilirubin can be beneficial. Elevated serum levels of bilirubin are associated with diminished risk of coronary artery disease. Gilbert syndrome is a common genetic condition involving impairment of bilirubin conjugation leading to mildly elevated serum bilirubin levels. The prevalence of ischemic heart disease in individuals with Gilbert syndrome is 2%, about one-sixth that of general population.

Other functions of bilirubin/biliverdin

- Bilirubin can inhibit oxidant-associated neutrophil chemotaxis.
- BVR can act as a serine/threonine-tyrosine kinase and as a transcription factor.
- Bilirubin inhibits expression of inducible nitric oxide synthase (iNOS).

Nucleotide Metabolism

Chapter 8

Q. 1. Why pyrimidines and purines are called 'Bases'?

Ans. Purine and pyrimidines are heterocyclic rings made of carbon and nitrogen. In the free form in solution they are moderately basic in nature and hence called 'bases'. Electron delocalization among atoms in the ring (aromatic nature) gives most of the bonds partial double bond character. This makes the rings near planar, hydrophobic and relatively insoluble in water at the near-neutral pH of cells. In the 3-dimensional structure of DNA two or more bases are positioned with planes of their rings parallel (like a stack of coins). This stacking

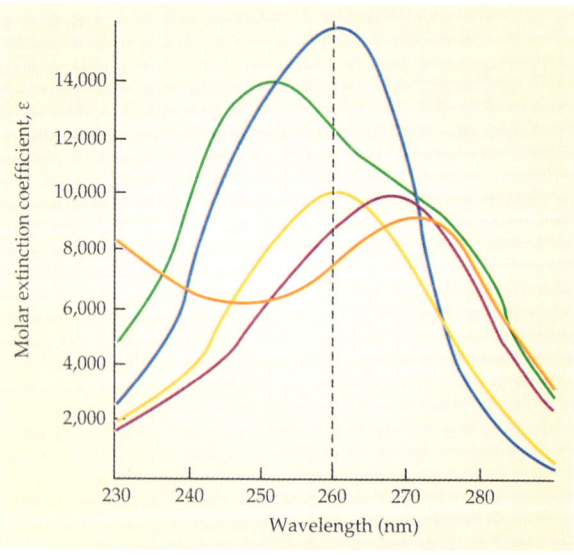

Fig. 8.1. Different purine and pyrimidine bases absorb light maximally around 260 nm.

is due to mainly hydrophobic interaction (minimizing contact with water) and also due to van der Waals and dipole-dipole interaction. This stacking is most important in maintaining the 3D structure of nucleic acids. Their aromatic nature and electron delocalization also makes them strongly absorb UV light of 260 nm, a property used to measure concentration of nucleic acids using Lambert–Beer law and spectrophotometry (Fig. 8.1).

Q. 2. **What is the fate of nucleic acids and nucleotides consumed in diet?**

Ans. 2′(3′)-GMP and 5′-GMP → Guanosine → Guanine → Xanthine → Uric acid

2′(3′)-AMP and 5′-AMP → Adenosine → Inosine → Hypoxanthine → Xanthine
$$\downarrow$$
Uric acid

RNA is digested in the small intestine via the action of the pancreatic ribonuclease to the nucleotides. Nucleotides are then hydrolyzed to the nucleosides – adenosine, guanosine, cytidine and uridine – via the action of the enzymes, alkaline phosphatase and nucleotidase, present in intestinal brush border. Adenosine is deaminated to ionosine. Most of the nucleoside and base are absorbed via both facilitated diffusion and sodium-dependent carrier-mediated processes.

In the enterocyte ionosine and guanine are converted to hypoxanthine and xanthine and ultimately to uric acid by xanthine oxidase. Uric acid is absorbed into blood and excreted in urine. Pyrimidine bases are also catabolised to beta-alanine (further catabolised to acetyl CoA and urea) and β-aminoisobutyrate or salvaged and used by the enterocytes or other tissues. Dietary uridine can be salvaged and used by the body and it is used in the treatment of UMP synthase defect (hereditary oroticaciduria). Purines hypoxanthine and guanine can also be salvaged by HPRT but under normal conditions most are degraded (Fig. 8.2).

Nucleosides and bases that are not catabolized in the enterocytes are transported via the portal circulation to the liver, where they are also catabolized. A small percentage of ingested bases and nucleosides reach the systemic circulation and is transported to various tissues of the body. Even under normal conditions, a small percentage (from 2% to 5%) of dietary bases and nucleosides is incorporated into nucleic acids, especially in the small intestine, liver and skeletal muscle. This occurs via the salvage pathways of purine nucleotide and pyrimidine nucleotide synthesis.

During conditions of metabolic stress, including trauma, rapid growth and limited food supply, there is apparently greater conversion of dietary bases into tissue nucleotides and nucleic acids. Xanthine oxidase in the enterocytes is downregulated and salvage is increased.

DNA is digested in the small intestine via the action of the pancreatic enzyme deoxyribonuclease to deoxynucleotides; these, in turn, are hydrolyzed to deoxynucleosides and finally to the pyrimidine bases cytosine and thymine and the purine bases adenine and guanine. The deoxynucleosides and bases are absorbed by the enterocytes and processed as described above for the nucleosides.

Human milk contains relatively high amounts of nucleotides accounting for 0.15% of total nitrogen. Artificial infant feed formulas are regularly supplemented with nucleotides. They have been shown to have number of beneficial effects like:

1. Growth and maturation of intestinal epithelium
2. Decreased incidence of diarrhoea

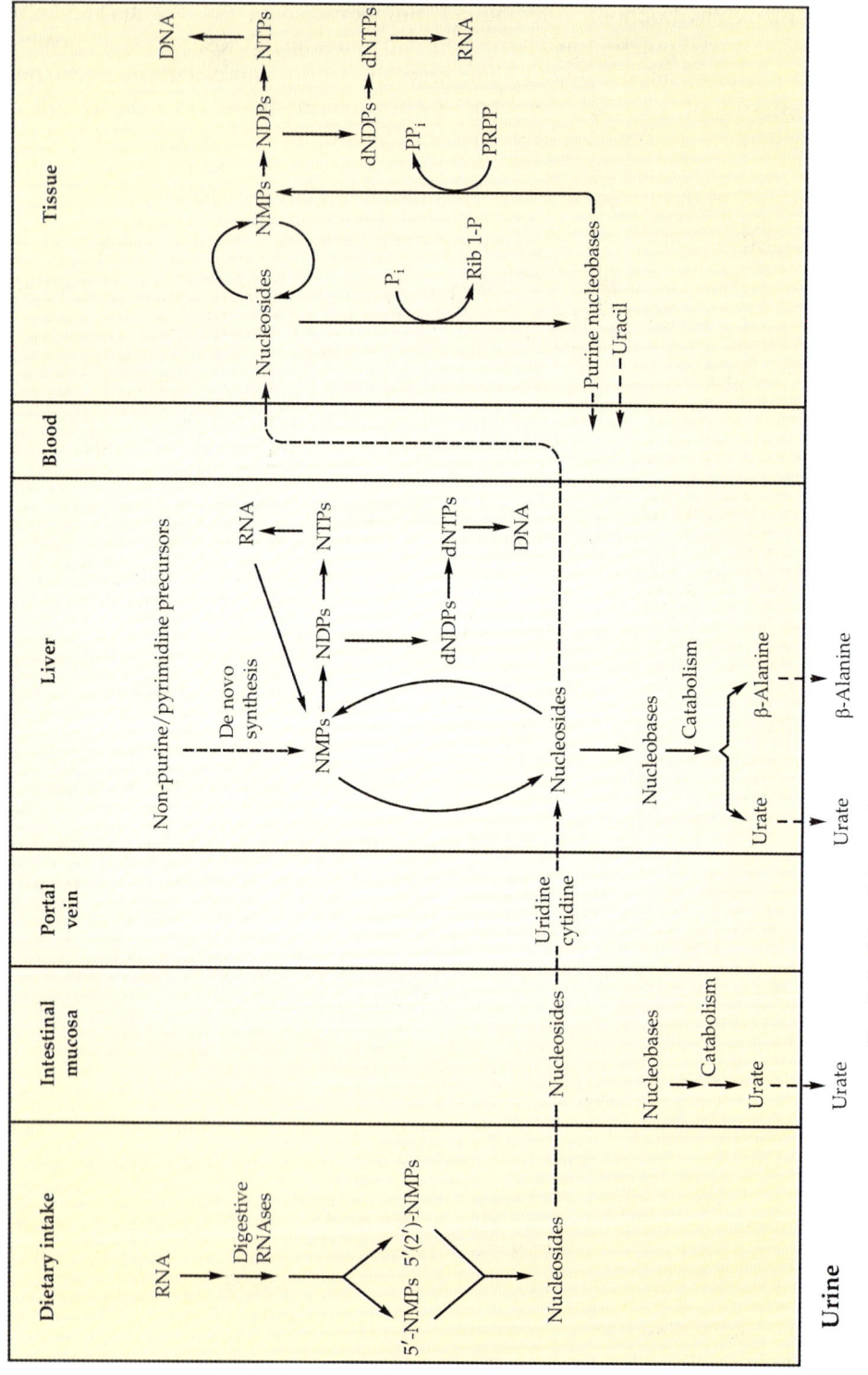

Fig. 8.2. Fate of dietary bases and nucleosides derived from RNA in food.

3. Promotion of growth of bifidobacter and lactobacilli (good commensals) in GIT
4. Boosting of immune function, improved response to sepsis, lymphocyte proliferation, increased antibody production, better response to vaccination (WBC rely on salvage pathway for supply of nucleotides)
5. Increased synthesis of omega 3 & 6 PUFA with C18 or higher
6. Beneficial for regenerating liver.

Q. 3. What are the different biological functions of nucleotides?

Ans.
1. Energy metabolism – energy currency of cell – ATP.
2. Monomeric units of DNA and RNA.
3. Precursor function – GTP is used for mRNA capping and synthesis of tetrahydrobiopterin.
4. Component of coenzymes – NAD, NADP, FMN, FAD and coenzyme A.
5. Activated metabolic intermediates – UDP-glucose, CDP-choline, SAM (methylation reactions), PAPS (activated sulphur).
6. Allosteric regulators of many enzymes – ATP, AMP, dATP, CTP.
7. Physiological mediator – adenosine (coronary blood flow), ADP (platelet aggregation), cAMP and cGMP (second messengers).
8. Nucleotide cycle in muscles.

Q. 4. What is salvage pathway and what is its importance?

Ans. **Purine salvage pathway**

De novo synthesis of purines requires 6 ATPs for each purine nucleotide formed. The pathways of nucleotide interconversion, base and nucleoside salvage allow efficient reutilization of preformed purines. Reutilization of purine bases from cell turnover allows for more economical functioning of purine metabolism. A portion of purine bases and nucleosides derived from food is also taken up from gut into bloodstream and incorporated into utilizable purines in liver by salvage enzymes. Liver exports purine bases for use by other tissues especially those lacking de novo synthetic pathway like RBC, WBC and brain. These tissues are dependent on salvage pathway for purine nucleotide production. Therefore, absence of salvage would result in inability to recycle purines produced through intracellular metabolism as well as purines derived from extracellular sources. It is also important because free purines are somewhat toxic, and the liver, which synthesizes most nucleotides, releases the compounds as either free bases or free nucleotides.

Enzymes and reactions involved are:
- HPRT (Hypoxanthine-guanine phosphoribosyltransferase)
  PRPP + hypoxanthine/guanine → IMP/GMP + PP_i
- APRT (Adenine phosphoribosyltransferase)
  PRPP + adenine → AMP + PP_i
- Adenosine kinase
  Adenosine + ATP → AMP + ADP

Pyrimidine salvage

De novo synthesis requires 5 ATP for each UMP, while reutilization of uridine from cell turnover or dietary sources costs only 1 ATP for making UMP. Enzymes and reactions involved in pyrimidine salvage are:

- Pyrimidine phosphoribosyltransferase

    PRPP + orotate/uracil/thymine → OMP/UMP/TMP + PP_i

- Thymidine phosphorylase

    Thymidine + phosphate ↔ thymine + deoxyribose 1-phosphate

- Uridine phosphorylase

    Uridine + phosphate ↔ uracil + ribose 1-phosphate

- Thymidine kinase

    ATP + thymidine ↔ ADP + TMP

- Uridine monophosphokinase

    ATP + uridine ↔ ADP + UMP

    ATP + cytidine ↔ ADP + CMP

- Deoxycytidine kinase

    NTP + deoxycytidine ↔ NDP + dCMP

Most of the normal pyrimidine requirement can be met from the de novo synthesis but under conditions of increased requirement like in cancer cells, salvage pathway is 100 to 300 times more active. During treatment of hereditary orotic aciduria (defect of UMP synthase, defective de novo synthetic pathway) exogenous uridine is given in food which is converted to UMP by salvage pathway.

Q. 5. Which reactions use PRPP and how its levels are regulated?

Ans. Reactions and pathways requiring PRPP are:

1. De novo synthesis of purines:

    PRPP + glutamine → 5-phosphoribosylamine + glutamate + PP_i

2. Salvage of purines:

    PRPP + hypoxanthine/guanine → IMP/GMP + PP_i

    PRPP + adenine → AMP + PP_i

3. De novo synthesis of pyrimidines:

    PRPP + orotate → OMP + PP_i

4. Salvage of pyrimidine bases:

    PRPP + uracil → UMP + PP_i

5. NAD synthesis:

    PRPP + nicotinate → nicotinate mononucleotide + PP_i

    PRPP + nicotinamide → nicotinamide mononucleotide + PP_i

    PRPP + quinolate → nicotinate mononucleotide + PP_i

Synthesis of PRPP is regulated in a complex manner by:
1. Allosteric feedback inhibition by end products of all the pathways using PRPP
2. Response to mitogens (substances which increase cell division/proliferation)
3. Change in divalent ion concentration
4. Multiple PRPS (phosphoribosyl-pyrophosphate synthetase or PRP synthetase) isoforms with different kinetic properties exist in different tissues. PRPS1 is constitutively expressed while PRPS2 expression is stimulated by mitogens or transformation.

Superactivity or increased activity of PRPS is a known genetic cause of gout. Defects include: impaired response to allosteric regulators, overabundance of PRPS1 or increased affinity for ribose-5-phosphate. It is an X-linked trait presenting as two clinical phenotypes:
1. Severe childhood onset gout and neurological impairment in homozygous males and gout during pregnancy in the heterozygous female carriers.
2. Early adult onset gout in males but no neurological defects.

Q. 6. What is tumor lysis syndrome?

Ans. Tumor lysis syndrome represents a group of metabolic consequences that result from cancer treatment. When cancer patients with bulky, rapidly proliferating, treatment-responsive tumors undergo chemotherapy or radiotherapy large number of cancer cells are killed in a short period of time. Tumor lysis syndrome is typically associated with acute leukemias and high-grade non-Hodgkin lymphomas, such as Burkitt lymphoma, other hematologic malignancies and with solid tumors such as hepatoblastoma and stage IV neuroblastoma.

When large numbers of neoplastic cells are killed rapidly, release of intracellular ions and metabolic byproducts occurs into the systemic circulation. The released DNA, RNA and cellular nucleotides are ultimately degraded to uric acid. This can lead to hyperuricemia. Breakdown of large number of cells also leads to hyperphosphatemia, hyperkalemia and hypocalcemia. Hyperkalemia and hyperphosphatemia result directly from rapid cell lysis. Hypocalcemia is a consequence of acute hyperphosphatemia with subsequent precipitation of calcium phosphate in soft tissues.

Clinically, there is rapid development of hyperuricemia, hyperkalemia, hyper-phosphatemia, hypocalcemia, and acute renal failure. Rapid release of intracellular contents into the circulation can overwhelm renal excretion and cellular buffering mechanisms, leading to many metabolic derangements. Clinically significant tumor lysis syndrome can occur spontaneously, but occurs most often 48–72 hours after initiation of cancer treatment. Hyperkalemia is often the earliest laboratory manifestation.

Complications
- Acute renal failure: There is oliguria (urine output < 400 mL daily), leading to volume overload and complications liken hypertension and pulmonary edema. High blood urea levels due to increased protein catabolism and renal failure can result in pericarditis, platelet dysfunction, and defective cellular immunity. Renal dysfunction can be severe enough to require dialysis. With prompt treatment, it is usually reversible.

Causes
- Uric acid nephropathy is the major cause of acute renal failure. It develops due to mechanical obstruction in the renal tubules by uric acid crystals. Uric acid precipitation is enhanced by high acidity (pKa of uric acid is 5.6) and high concentration in the renal tubular fluid. Renal medullary hemoconcentration and decreased tubular flow rate also contribute to crystallization.
- Acute nephrocalcinosis from calcium phosphate crystal precipitation. This develops in the setting of hyperphosphatemia and is exacerbated by overzealous iatrogenic alkalinization, because calcium phosphate, unlike uric acid, becomes less soluble at an alkaline pH.
- Precipitation of xanthine (even less soluble than uric acid), or other purine metabolites whose excretion is increased by use of allopurinol.

- Cardiac arrhythmia: Hyperkalemia can lead to electrocardiographic changes and life-threatening cardiac arrhythmia, including asystole. Severe potassium elevation can cause electrocardiographic alterations such as peaked T waves, flattened P waves, prolonged PR interval, widened QRS complexes, deep S wave, and sine waves. Hypocalcemia can lead to QT interval lengthening, which predisposes patients to ventricular arrhythmia.
- Seizures due to hyperkalemia and hypocalcemia.
- Iatrogenic complications like pulmonary edema: Occur due to overly vigorous hydration or metabolic alkalosis from excess exogenous administration of bicarbonate.
- Metabolic acidosis: Occurs due to acute renal failure and the liberation of large amounts of endogenous intracellular acids from cellular catabolism. It causes a decrease in serum bicarbonate concentration and a high anion gap acidosis. It can worsen the already existing electrolyte imbalances – intracellular uptake of potassium is inhibited, uric acid solubility is decreased, and extracellular shift of phosphate is promoted. Calcium phosphate solubility, however, improves in acidic conditions.
- Hypocalcemia can be severe enough to cause tetany, sudden mental incapacity, parkinsonian (extrapyramidal) movement disorders, papilledema, seizures and myopathy.

Treatment
Proper fluid management, alkalinization of the urine, correction of acidosis, and treatment of infections are the main supportive therapy. Drugs are used to correct metabolic disturbances. Use of these medications should be started before the start of chemotherapy; the goal is to achieve optimal metabolic stability.

Allopurinol, a xanthine oxidase inhibitor, reduces the conversion of nucleic acid by-products to uric acid, preventing urate nephropathy and subsequent oliguric renal failure. Rasburicase (urate oxidase made by recombinant DNA technologgy), which controls hyperuricemia by converting uric acid to water-soluble allantoin can also be used.

Q. 7. Describe regulation of purine synthesis and its clinical implications.

Ans. Purine synthesis is regulated at the following reactions:
1. The reaction catalysed by glutamine PRPP amidotransferase is the committed as well the major regulated step. It is also rate limiting step of purine synthesis. IMP, GMP and AMP are negative allosteric effectors and PRPP is a positive allosteric effector. AMP has

synergistic inhibition with IMP/GMP. The dependence of rate of reaction of this enzyme on glutamine and PRPP concentration is shown in Fig. 8.3. It has hyperbolic kinetics with respect to glutamine and sigmoidal with respect to PRPP (positive effector).

The cellular concentration of glutamine varies little and is close to K_m of the enzyme. However, anticancer drug asparaginase decreases glutamine concentration and thus decreases purine de novo synthesis.

The normal cellular concentration of PRPP varies widely and is 10 to 100 times less than the K_m. Thus, increased PRPP availability in Von Gierke's disease and PRPS superactivity thus can greatly increase the rate of purine de novo synthesis (due to sigmoidal kinetics for PRPP) despite feedback inhibition by products leading to increased purine turnover and gout.

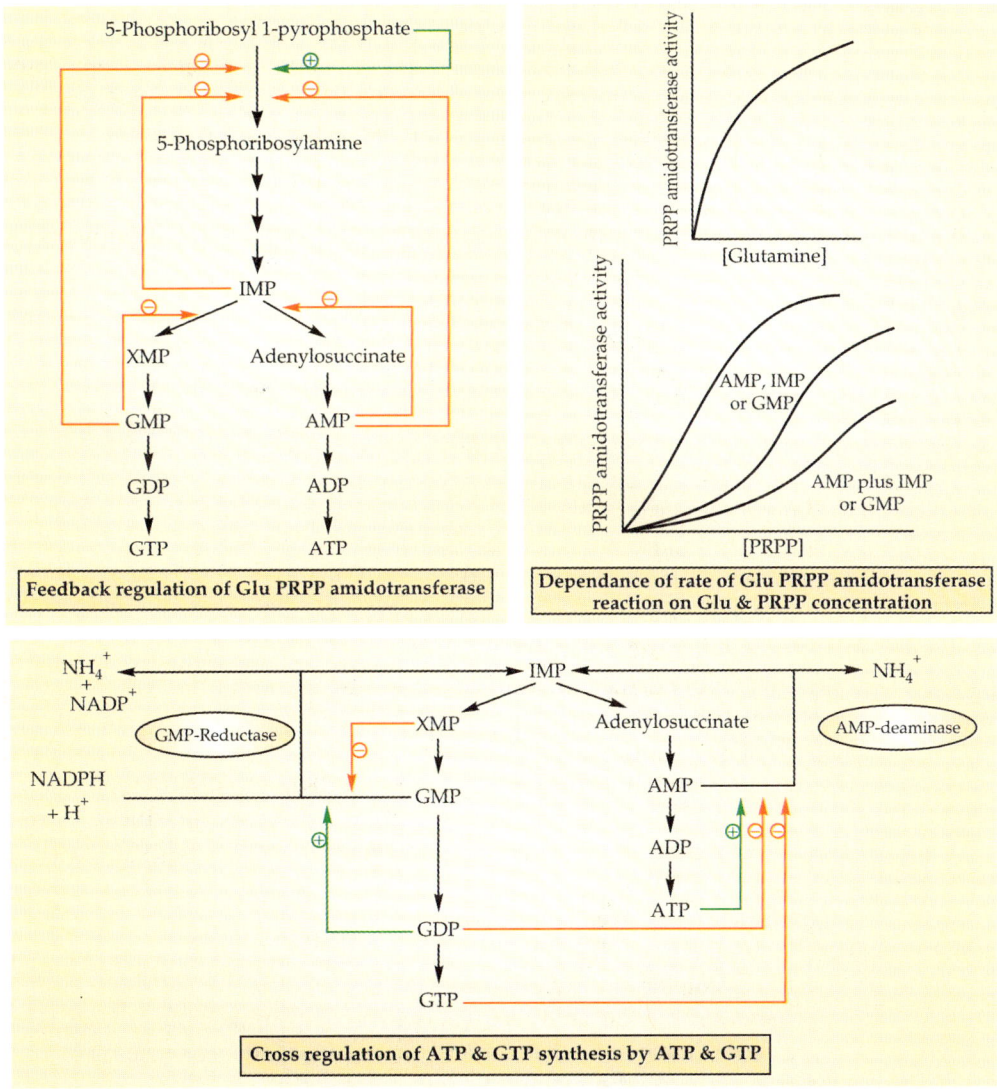

Fig. 8.3. Regulation of purine synthesis.

2. AMP and GMP feedback inhibit their formation from IMP. Further, ATP is required for GMP synthesis and GTP for AMP synthesis. Further, GMP can be converted back to IMP and this step is inhibited by XMP and stimulated by GTP. Similarly, AMP can be converted back to IMP and this step is inhibited by GDP/GTP and stimulated by ATP (Fig. 8.3). These maintain a constant ratio of adenine and guanine nucleotides in the cell with total adenine nucleotides being 4–6 times total guanine nucleotides. The enzyme IMPDH is involved in GMP synthesis and has two isoenzymes. First being constitutively active and the other is induced at time of cell growth and proliferation. IMPDH-II is amplified in tumors and rapidly proliferating tissues and IMPDH inhibitors (e.g. mizoribine, mycophenolic acid and ribavirin) are now widely used in immunosuppressive and antiviral chemotherapy.
3. ADP and GDP feedback inhibit PRPP synthetase, however, not completely as PRPP is also required in other pathways. This is not the major regulatory step. Thus, increased ribose-5-phosphate availability in Von Gierke's disease increases PRPP synthesis which greatly increases purine de novo synthesis despite feedback inhibition of PRPPS by ADP and GDP.

Q. 8. Classify the different causes of hyperuricemia and explain the underlying biochemical basis.

Ans. Hyperuricemia is defined as a plasma (or serum) urate concentration > 7.0 mg/dL in men and 6.8 mg/dL in women. Clinical manifestations can be:
- Asymptomatic
- Gout
- Gouty nephropathy with urate deposition in parenchyma
- Acute intratubular deposition of urate crystals
- Urate nephrolithiasis
- Lesch-Nyhan syndrome
- Pregnancy-induced hypertension
- Hyperuricemia and metabolic syndrome.

Causes can be classified into:
1. **Essential hyperuricemia:** Polygenic – cause uncertain in 99% cases but involves combination of metabolic overproduction, decreased renal excretion and increased dietary intake of purines.
2. **Gout occurring in in-born errors of metabolism** is due to overproduction of PRPP (HGPRT deficiency, glucose-6-phosphatase deficiency and PRPP synthetase overactivity) or increased ATP turnover (glucogen storage diseases III, V, VII and fructose-1-phosphate aldolase deficiency).
3. **Secondary or acquired** can be due to:
   (i) Overproduction which can be due to:
   - Excess dietary intake of purines
   - Increased nucleic acid turnover (cancer, leukemia, radiotherapy, chemotherapy, trauma, hemolysis, rhabdomyolysis, exercise, Paget's disease)
   - Excessive ATP metabolism – Exercise, alcohol, tissue hypoxia, myocardial infarction, smoke inhalation, acute respiratory failure and tissue hypoxia

- Obesity – Metabolic syndrome
- Pregnancy-induced hypertension (tissue hypoxia, excessive ATP metabolism).

(ii) Decreased renal excretion which can be due to:
- Renal insufficiency
- Diabetes insipidus
- Hypertension, pregnancy-induced hypertension
- Acidosis – Lactic acidosis, diabetic ketoacidosis, starvation ketosis
- Hyperparathyroidism
- Hypothyroidism
- Alcohol
- Drugs – Salicylates, diuretics, ethambutol, pyrazinamide, nicotinic acid.

During hypoxia or ischemia ATP degradation to uric acid is increased. Both these conditions limit ATP regeneration from both ADP and AMP and hence enhance ATP consumption. The myokinase reaction converts 2 ADPs into ATP and AMP to salvage some ATP from ADP under such conditions (ADP + ADP → ATP + AMP). Normally most of the AMP formed can be used for ATP synthesis by production of ADP first by the reversal of same myokinase reaction when sufficient ATP is available (AMP + ATP → 2ADPs, under condition of adequate oxygen and fuel supply). However, in tissue hypoxia or ischemia the increased amount of AMP is not recycled back to ATP, but the excessive AMP formed enters the purine nucleotide degradation pathway, leading to uric acid synthesis.

Q. 9. Discuss renal handling of uric acid and its clinical implications.

Ans. Until recently, a four-component model has been used to describe the renal handling of urate/uric acid:

1. Glomerular filtration
2. Tubular reabsorption
3. Secretion
4. Postsecretory reabsorption

Although these processes have been considered sequential, it is now apparent that they are carried out in parallel by specific organic anion transporters. The combined activities of URAT1 (uric acid transporter), other OATs (organic anion transporter), and sodium anion-dependent transporter result in 8–12% of the filtered urate being excreted as uric acid (Fig. 8.4).

URAT1 and OAT4 cause reabsorption of uric acid from apical (brush border) side in exchange for monocarboxylate and dicarboxylate organic anions. This reabsorbed uric acid moves to blood on basolateral side with the help of OAT and hUAT. The mono- and dicarboxylates enter back the cells through SLC5 and SLC13. The sodium-coupled mono-carboxyl transporters SMCT1 and 2 (SLC5A8, SLC5A12) in the brush border of the proximal tubular cells mediate sodium-dependent loading of these cells with monocarboxylates. A similar transporter, SLC13A3, mediates sodium-dependent influx of dicarboxylates into the epithelial cell from the basolateral membrane. Some of these carboxylates are well known to cause hyperuricemia. They include pyrazinoate (from pyrazinamide treatment), nicotinate (from niacin therapy), and the organic acids lactate, hydroxybutyrate, and acetoacetate. These

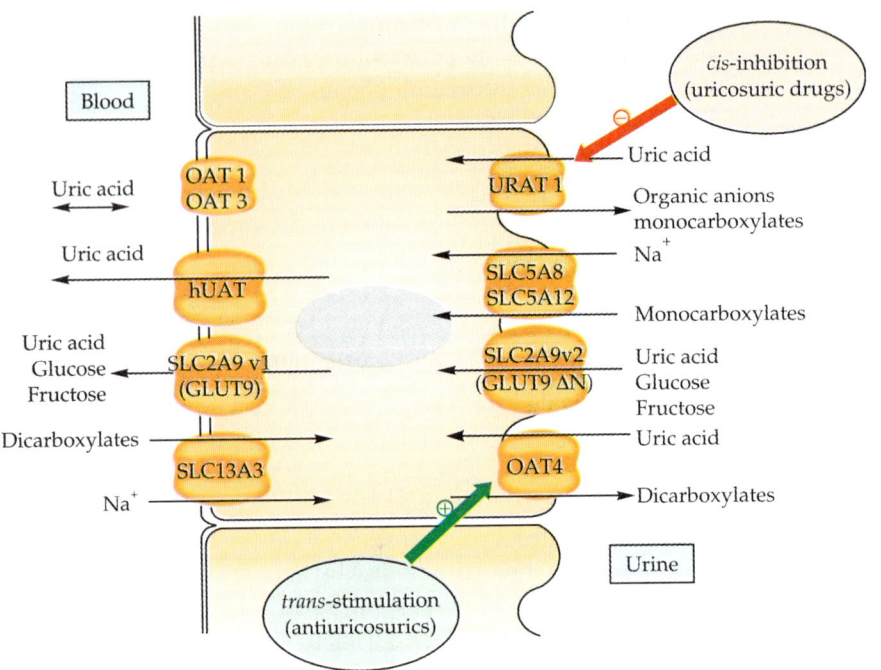

Fig. 8.4. Renal handling of uric acid. OAT = organic acid transporter, hUAT = human uric acid transporter, SLC = sodium dependent co-transporter.

mono- and divalent anions become substrates for URAT1 and organic anion transporter (OAT4), respectively, and are exchanged for uric acid from the proximal tubule. Increased blood levels of these anions result in their increased glomerular filtration and greater reabsorption by proximal tubular cells. The increased intraepithelial cell concentrations lead to increased uric acid reabsorption by promoting URAT1- and OAT4-dependent anion exchange. This is known as trans-stimulation of uric acid reabsorption. Low doses of salicylates also promote hyperuricemia by this mechanism. Uricosuric drugs like probenecid which decrease uric acid reabsorption act by inhibiting URAT 1 (*cis*-inhibition).

Sodium loading of proximal tubular cells also provokes urate retention by reducing extracellular fluid volume and increasing angiotensin II, insulin, and parathyroid hormone release. Glucose transporter 9 (GLUT9, SLC2A9) mediates co-reabsorption of uric acid along with glucose and fructose at the apical membrane as well as their transport to blood through the basolateral membrane. GLUT 9 polymorphisms may play an important role in susceptibility to gout. Thus increased blood sugar and high fructose consumption increases blood uric acid levels.

Q. 10. What is the role of alcohol in gout?

Ans. Ingestion of ethanol can lead to formation of lactic acid, which inhibits secretion of uric acid in renal tubules. In addition, ethanol appears to promote hepatic breakdown of ATP, leading to increased production of purines from which uric acid is formed. Also, the solubility of monosodium urate is markedly diminished as the pH in tissues drops, a situation favored by increased production of lactic acid. The high purine content in some alcoholic beverages such as beer may also be a factor.

Q. 11. Why is hypouricemic therapy not given during attacks of acute gout?

Ans. Acute attack of gout is treated with anti-inflammatory drugs such as nonsteroidal anti-inflammatory drugs (NSAIDs), colchicine, or glucocorticoids. Hypouricemic therapy is not given because acute fluctuations or decrease in serum uric acid levels can also precipitate acute gout as shown in Fig. 8.5.

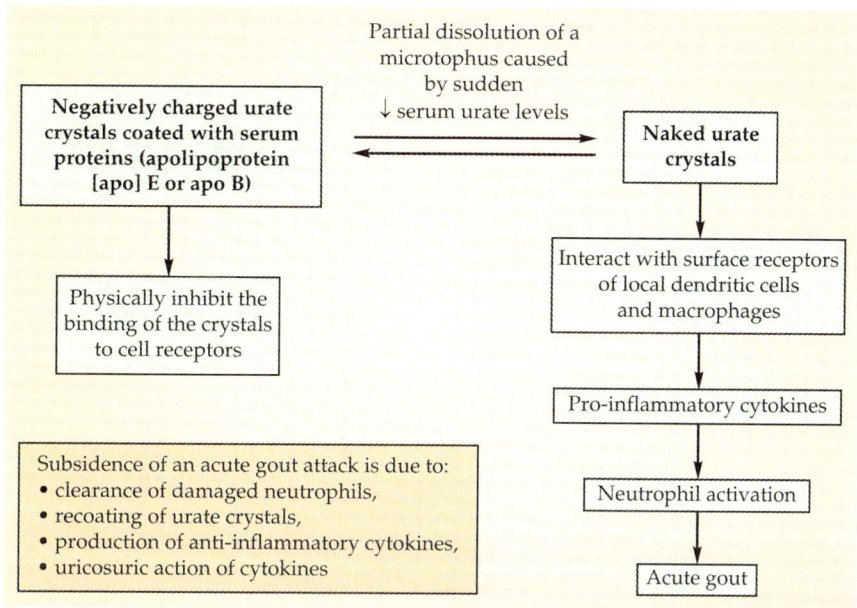

Fig. 8.5. Pathophysiology of gout.

Hypouricosemic therapy includes uricosuric drug like probenecid, xanthine oxidase inhibitor allopurinol, recombinant urate oxidase Rabsuricase and Febuxostat. Febuxostat is a non-purine selective inhibitor of xanthine oxidase. It works by non-competitively blocking the molybdenum pterin centre which is the active site on xanthine oxidase. These are used in chronic gout after inflammation has been controlled.

Q. 12. What is the difference in action of allopurinol in gout and Lesch-Nyhan syndrome (HGPRT deficiency)?

Ans. Allopurinol inhibits xanthine oxidase enzyme reducing uric acid production. This spares hypoxanthine and xanthine which can be salvaged by HGPRT to IMP and XMP. This consumes PRPP (positive regulator of de novo pathway) and generates nucleotides which feedback inhibit de novo synthesis. Thus, allopurinol decreases uric acid production as well as reduces de novo synthesis. However, Lesch-Nyhan syndrome patients have a marked reduction in HGPRT activity which blocks salvage and spares PRPP. This excess PRPP overrides the feedback regulation of de novo synthesis greatly increasing the rate of de novo synthesis. Allopurinol is not able to decrease the rate of de novo synthesis in these patients due to lack of salvage pathway. Further, urinary excretion of xanthine and hypoxanthine increases and these purine bases may form stones despite allopurinol treatment.

Q. 13. What is the physiological significance of β-alanine and β-aminoisobutyric acid (BAIBA)?

Ans. *β-Alanine*

β-Alanine is produced in our body by the degradation of pyrimidines, valine and carnosine. It is a component of the naturally occurring peptides carnosine and anserine and also of pantothenic acid (vitamin B_5), which itself is a component of coenzyme A. Under normal conditions, β-alanine is metabolized into acetic acid.

Carnosine is a dipeptide, formed from the amino acids histidine and β-alanine. It is found in large amounts in the brain and muscle. It has anti-oxidant properties as well as accounts for about 10% of the muscle's ability to buffer the acidity (H^+ ions) produced by high intensity exercise.

β-Alanine is the rate-limiting precursor of carnosine, i.e. carnosine levels are limited by the amount of available β-alanine, and not histidine. Supplementation with β-alanine has been shown to increase the concentration of carnosine in muscles, decrease fatigue in athletes and increase total muscular work done. Supplementing with carnosine is not as effective since carnosine, when taken orally, is broken down during digestion to its components, histidine and β-alanine. This results in only about 40% of the total dose being available as β-alanine. Supplementation with 5–6 g/d β-alanine can increase muscle carnosine content by ~60% after 4 weeks and ~80% after 10 weeks of supplementation. Increasing muscle carnosine levels may offer an alternative to bicarbonate/citrate loading for high-intensity exercise. It offers an additional strategy since muscle carnosine is an intracellular buffer, while bicarbonate/citrate loading provides extracellular buffering.

There is emerging evidence to support the use of β-alanine by athletes undertaking athletic events that are limited by the lowering of pH (build-up of H^+ ion) in the muscle in association with high-intensity exercises like:

- Sustained competitive events lasting 1–7 minutes (e.g. rowing, swimming, track cycling, middle distance running)
- Repeated bouts of high-intensity work (sprints, lifts) which cause an exercise-limiting increase in H^+ ions over time. This includes:
  – Interval training and resistance training
  – Team and racquet sports.

In these situations, β-alanine supplementation leads to increased muscle buffering capacity against H^+ ions. It also reduces the damage associated with high levels of muscle acidity. Antioxidant property of carnosine may also contribute. A rapid rise in blood β-alanine levels is associated with side-effects of paraesthesia (tingling sensation in the skin) which may be uncomfortable in some individuals.

3-Aminoisobutyric acid (or β-aminoisobutyric acid, 'BAIBA')

It is formed by the catabolism of thymine. It has recently been postulated to play a role in cell metabolism, how body burns fat and regulates insulin, triglycerides, and total cholesterol.

The transcriptional coactivator-peroxisome proliferator-activated receptor gamma coactivator-1α (PGC-1α) regulates metabolic genes in skeletal muscle and contributes to the response of muscle to exercise. During exercise, the increase of PGC-1α protein triggers the secretion of BAIBA from exercising muscles to blood (Fig. 8.6). BAIBA increases the

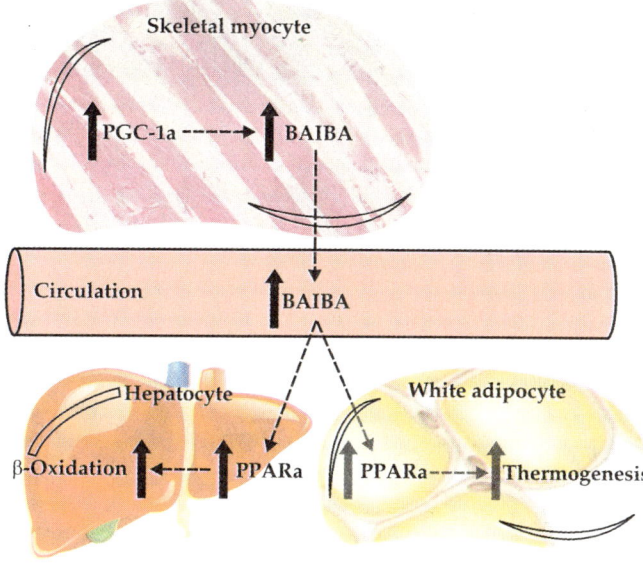

Fig. 8.6. Secretion and action of 3-aminoisobutyric acid (or β-aminoisobutyric acid, 'BAIBA').

expression of brown adipocyte-specific genes in white adipocytes, increases β-oxidation in hepatocytes through a PPARα-mediated mechanism, induces a brown adipose-like phenotype in human pluripotent stem cells, and improves glucose homeostasis. When BAIBA reaches the white fat tissue, it activates the expression of thermogenic genes via PPARα receptors, resulting in a browning of white fat cells. It increase of the basal metabolism of the target cells. Plasma BAIBA concentrations are increased with exercise and inversely associated with metabolic risk factors. BAIBA may thus contribute to exercise-induced protection from metabolic diseases. Thus β-aminoisobutyric acid (BAIBA) may act as a small molecule myokine!

Q. 14. What is the difference between xanthine oxidase and xanthine dehydrogenase?

Ans. Xanthine oxidoreductases (XOR) was isolated in its xanthine oxidase (XO) form (which uses oxygen as the electron acceptor) from cow's milk, whereas it has been purified in its xanthine dehydrogenase (XDH) form (which uses NAD^+ as the electron acceptor). Both enzymes, XO and XDH, are interconvertible products of the same gene. The enzyme originally exists in its XDH form but is readily converted to XO either irreversibly by proteolysis or reversibly by oxidation of Cys residues to form disulfide groups. The process of reversible or irreversible conversion of XDH to the XO form generates reactive oxygen species (i.e., H_2O_2 and O_2^-). The main product of the reversible conversion of XDH to its XO form is O_2^-, and that of XO to its XDH form is H_2O_2. Both processes have role in many physiologic and pathologic mechanisms such as reduction of cytochrome c, defence against infectious pathogens, or in the pathology of post ischemia-reperfusion injury.

Nutrition, Vitamins and Minerals

Chapter 9

Q. 1. What is thermic effect of food?

Ans. Thermic effect of food is the amount of energy expenditure above the resting metabolic rate due to the cost of processing food for use and storage. It is the energy used in digestion, absorption and distribution of nutrients. It is also called the specific dynamic action of food (SDA) or dietary-induced thermogenesis (DIT). It depends on the quantity and quality of food consumed. The type, size, composition, and temperature of the meal, as well as body size, body composition, and several environmental factors (e.g., ambient temperature and gas concentration) can each significantly impact the magnitude and duration of the SDA response.

It has 3 contributing components (Fig. 9.1):

1. Preabsorptive: Involve the energetic costs of meal heating, gut peristalsis, enzyme secretion, protein catabolism, acid secretion, intestinal remodelling, blood pH regulation.
2. Absorptive: Involve energetic costs related to intestinal absorption and nutrient transport across cell membranes.
3. Postabsorptive: Involve costs of protein synthesis, ketogenesis, amino acid deamination and/or oxidation, glycogen production, renal excretion, and general costs of growth.

It accounts for 6–17% of energy budget in humans. SDA for different macronutrients are:

Carbohydrates	5–15% of the energy consumed
Protein	20–35%
Fats	5–15%

Foods referred to as Negative Energy/Calorie Foods are called so as their specific dynamic action is more than the energy they can provide themselves! For example,

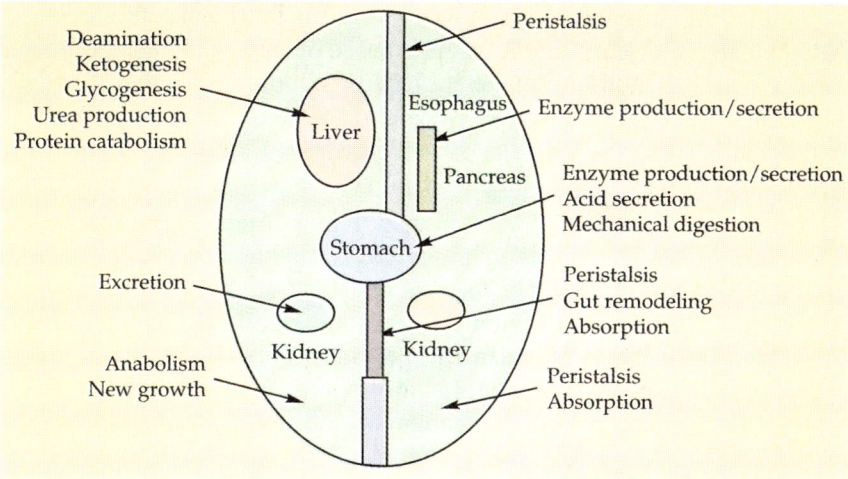

Fig. 9.1. Components of SDA.

- Vegetables: Asparagus, Bean sprouts, Beets, Broccoli, Cabbage, Carrots, Cauliflower, Celery, Chicory/Radicchio, Cucumbers, Endives, Green beans, Jicama, Kale, Leeks, Lettuce, Radishes, Spinach, Squash, Tomatoes, Turnips, Zucchini.
- Fruits: Apples, Blueberries, Cantaloupe, Cranberries, Grapefruits, Honeydew, Lemons/Limes, Mangoes, Oranges, Papaya, Peaches, Pineapple, Raspberries, Strawberries, Tangerines, Watermelon.
- Spices and fresh or dried herbs: Anise, Cayenne, Chili peppers, Cinnamon, Cloves, Coriander/Cilantro, Cumin, Dill, Fennel seeds, Flax seeds, Garden cress, Garlic, Ginger, Parsley, Onion, Mustard seeds, Watercress.

Q. 2. How are nutritional recommendations on quantities of different nutrients to be consumed daily made?

Ans. Too much, as well as too little, intake of a nutrient can have adverse effects or alter the health benefits conferred by another nutrient. Therefore, recommendations regarding nutrient intakes have been developed. These quantitative estimates of nutrient intakes are collectively referred to as the *dietary reference intakes* (DRIs). DRIs include the estimated average requirement (EAR) for nutrients, the recommended daily allowance (RDA), the adequate intake (AI), and the tolerable upper level (UL).

EAR: The EAR is the amount of a nutrient estimated to be adequate for half of the healthy individuals of a specific age and sex. The EAR is not an effective estimate of nutrient adequacy in individuals because it is a median requirement for a group; 50% of individuals in a group fall below the requirement and 50% fall above it. Thus, a person with a usual intake at the EAR has a 50% risk of an inadequate intake.

RDA: The RDA is the average daily dietary intake level that meets the nutrient requirements of nearly all healthy persons of a specific sex, age, life stage, or physiologic condition (such as pregnancy or lactation). The RDA is the nutrient-intake goal for planning diets of individuals. The RDA is defined statistically as two standard deviations (SD) above the EAR to ensure that the needs of any given individual are met.

AI: If it is not possible to set an RDA for some nutrients that do not have an established EAR, then, in this circumstance, the AI is based on observed, or experimentally determined, approximations of nutrient intakes in healthy people. AIs rather than RDAs are used for infants up to age 1 year, as well as for calcium, chromium, vitamin D, fluoride, manganese, pantothenic acid, biotin, and choline for persons of all ages. Vitamin D and calcium are currently being re-evaluated, and more precise values may be available in the near future.

UL: Excessive nutrient intake can disturb body functions and cause acute, progressive, or permanent disabilities. The tolerable UL is the highest level of chronic nutrient intake (usually daily) that is unlikely to pose a risk of adverse health effects for most of the population. Nutrients in commonly eaten foods rarely exceed the UL. However, highly fortified foods and dietary supplements provide more concentrated amounts of nutrients per serving and, thus, pose a potential risk of toxicity. Nutrient supplements are labelled with supplement facts that express the amount of nutrient in absolute units or as the per cent of the daily value (DV) provided per recommended serving size. Total nutrient consumption, including foods, supplements, and over-the-counter medications, such as antacids, should not exceed RDA levels.

Q. 3. What is FIGLU test? What are the functions of folate in body and why daily intake is required if it is a coenzyme? Which other tests are used to detect folate deficiency?

Ans. FIGLU test is a test to diagnose folate deficiency. Tetrahydrofolate is required for conversion of N-formiminoglutamate (FIGLU) to glutamate in histidine metabolism (Fig. 9.2). After a histidine load (oral intake of 15 or 20 g of histidine), patients excrete more N-formimino-glutamate in the urine. Normally, people only excrete less than 30 µg/mL or 0.1 to 18 mg/day. If there is a deficiency of active folate, the excreted amounts are increased (up to 2 g/day). However, this test is rarely carried out these days.

Folate deficiency is associated with megaloblastic anaemia, higher incidence of neural tube defects (folate deficiency in first 12 weeks of pregnancy), homocystinemia and homocystinuria (associated with increased risk of cardiovascular and peripheral vascular disease) and malignancies in persons with some polymorphism of folate processing enzymes.

Folate is required for formate activation, purine synthesis, pyrimidine (thymidine) synthesis, serine glycine interconversion, homocysteine to methionine conversion, and in histidine metabolism (FIGLU to glutamate conversion). Even though folate being a coenzyme recycled in the body, a small amount is not recycled but degraded during the thymidylate synthesis reaction. 60-90 µg of folate is excreted in bile daily and this along with the sloughed intestinal mucosal cells leads to daily folate loss from body. Thus folate needs to be taken daily in diet.

Fig. 9.3 summarises the time course of appearance of biochemical, haematological and clinical defects due to folate deficiency. Folate deficiency can be diagnosed by the tests listed in Table 9.1. Even though homocysteine levels are a sensitive marker for folate deficiency, they are not specific or confirmatory as homocysteine elevation can be caused by deficiency of vitamin B_{12} and B_6, chronic kidney disease, alcohol intake, hypothyroidism, drugs like OCP, steroids, cyclosporine and some inborn errors of metabolism.

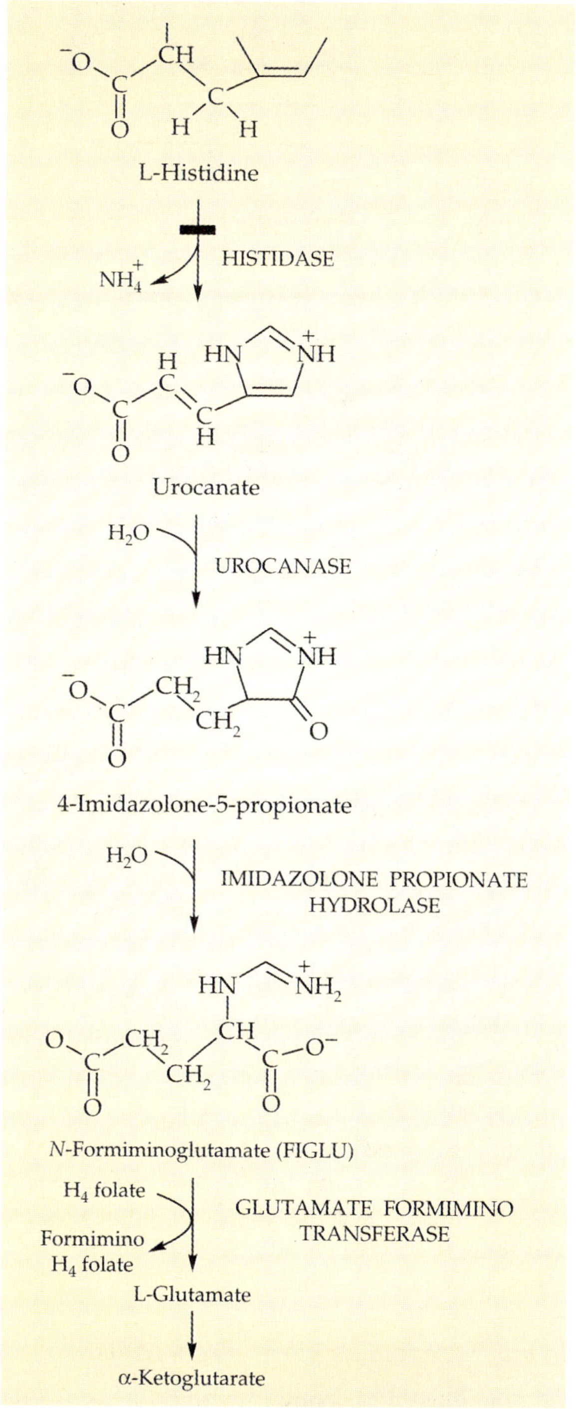

Fig. 9.2. Histidine metabolism – H_4 folate is required for action of glutamate formiminotransferase enzyme which converts FIGLU to glutamate.

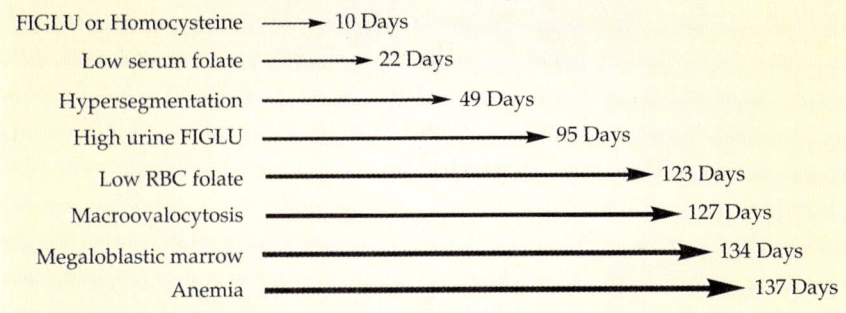

Fig. 9.3. Biochemical and clinical consequences of folate deficiency and their time course of appearance.

Table 9.1. Folic acid deficiency tests

Test/Marker	Deficiency indication
Homocysteine, urine	> 25 mg/mg creatinine
Homocysteine, plasma	> 15 nmol/mL
Serum folate	< 3 ng/ml
FIGLU	> 50 mg/day following 5–25 gm His
Erythrocyte folate	< 160 ng/ml
Leukocyte folate	< 500 ng/ml

RBC and leukocyte folate levels are good tests of general folate status and not affected by daily dietary fluctuations and small amount of hemolysis but are decreased only in later stages of deficiency. They can be falsely high with blood transfusion and high reticulocyte count. Serum folate levels are more affected by short-term fluctuations in diet and thus may be normal even in folate deficiency status. Thus patient must be fasting before test and intake of supplements and multivitamins avoided. Further hemolysis must be avoided and sample transported in dark as folate is light sensitive. Measurement of plasma folate records the fluctuations of the folate supply ingested with food somewhat better while erythrocyte folate levels are a good indicator of the tissue concentration or the long-term supply. Folate trap due to B_{12} deficiency will lead to high serum folate while RBC folate will be low and there is a functional deficiency of folate in cells.

The deoxyuridine-suppression test is another test used earlier for diagnosing folate deficiency. It consists in assessing the capacity of leucocytes or bone marrow cells to incorporate 3[H]-thymidine into the DNA after a supply of the co-factor (folic acid or vitamin B_{12}). It is a very sensitive and specific test to establish folate deficiency, which, however, these days, is not used much anymore.

Q. 4. What is folate trap? Explain its biochemical basis.

Ans. Folate trap is a functional deficiency of active forms of folate in cells with folate being trapped in the inactive form due to vitamin B_{12} deficiency. The mechanisms responsible for it are:

1. Folate is present in food as polyglutamate forms of DHF/THF. After absorption into the intestinal epithelial cells all is converted to monoglutamate form by conjugase enzyme which requires zinc. Most of the dietary folate undergoes reduction and methylation within the intestinal mucosa and what enters the portal blood stream is mostly 5-methyl-tetrahydrofolate. This 5-methyl THF entering the blood is the transported bound to albumin. Small amounts of other one-carbon substituted folates also circulate (about 10% to 15% of plasma folate is 10-formyltetrahydrofolate) and are also available for tissue uptake. The cells uptake the 5-methyltetrahydrofolate. This form is used only by the reaction methionine synthase. This reaction requires B_{12} as co-factor. This is the only way in which methyltetrahydrofolate can be demethylated to yield free tetrahydrofolate in tissues (Fig. 9.4). Methionine synthase thus provides the link between the physiological functions of folate and vitamin B_{12}. This reaction generates THF which is converted to polyglutamate forms by polyglutamate synthase enzyme. This enzyme uses only THF and not 5-methyl THF. All other reactions need folate as polyglutamate form to function as co-enzyme. In B_{12} deficiency 5-methyl THF is not converted to THF and then to polyglutamated forms required for other reactions like thymidylate synthase, etc. The 5-methyl THF is not used and lost from cells and excreted in urine. Thus even as plasma folate is raised there is a deficiency of the functionally active folate inside cells. Impairment of methionine synthase activity, for example, in vitamin B_{12} deficiency, will result in the accumulation of methyl-tetrahydrofolate. This can neither be utilized for any other one-carbon transfer reactions nor demethylated to provide free tetrahydrofolate. As a result of this, vitamin B_{12} deficiency is frequently accompanied by biochemical evidence of functional folate deficiency, including impaired metabolism of histidine (excretion of formiminoglutamate) and impaired thymidylate synthetase activity, although plasma concentrations of methyltetra-hydrofolate are normal or elevated.
2. Further, in the reactions that can interconvert various forms of folate the reduction of N5N10-methylene-tetrahydrofolate to methyltetrahydrofolate by MTHFR is irreversible (Fig. 9.4). This further leads to trapping of folate as 5-methyl THF. SAM is an inhibitor of this reaction. However, in B_{12} deficiency methionine and SAM are decreased and inhibition of this reaction is relieved exacerbating the trapping of folate as 5-methyl THF.
3. The activity of 10-formyltetrahydrofolate dehydrogenase, which catalyzes the oxidation of 10-formyltetrahydrofolate to CO_2 and tetrahydrofolate, is reduced at times of low methionine availability as a means of conserving valuable one-carbon fragments. Therefore, there is no sink for one-carbon substituted tetrahydrofolate, and increasing amounts of folate are trapped as methyltetrahydrofolate that cannot be used because of the lack of vitamin B_{12}.

Q. 5. Excessive intake of vitamin D can cause toxicity but excessive exposure to sunlight does not, why?

Ans. 7-dehydrocholesterol is synthesized by the sebaceous glands and secreted onto the surface of skin from where it is absorbed and maximum concentration is in stratum spinosum and basale of skin epithelium. It is reversibly isomerized to previtamin D by UV light (UV-B light: 290–320 nm, maximum by 296.5 nm). Previtamin D converts to calciferol by slow thermal isomerization (Fig. 9.5). Removal of the product aids the isomerization reaction in

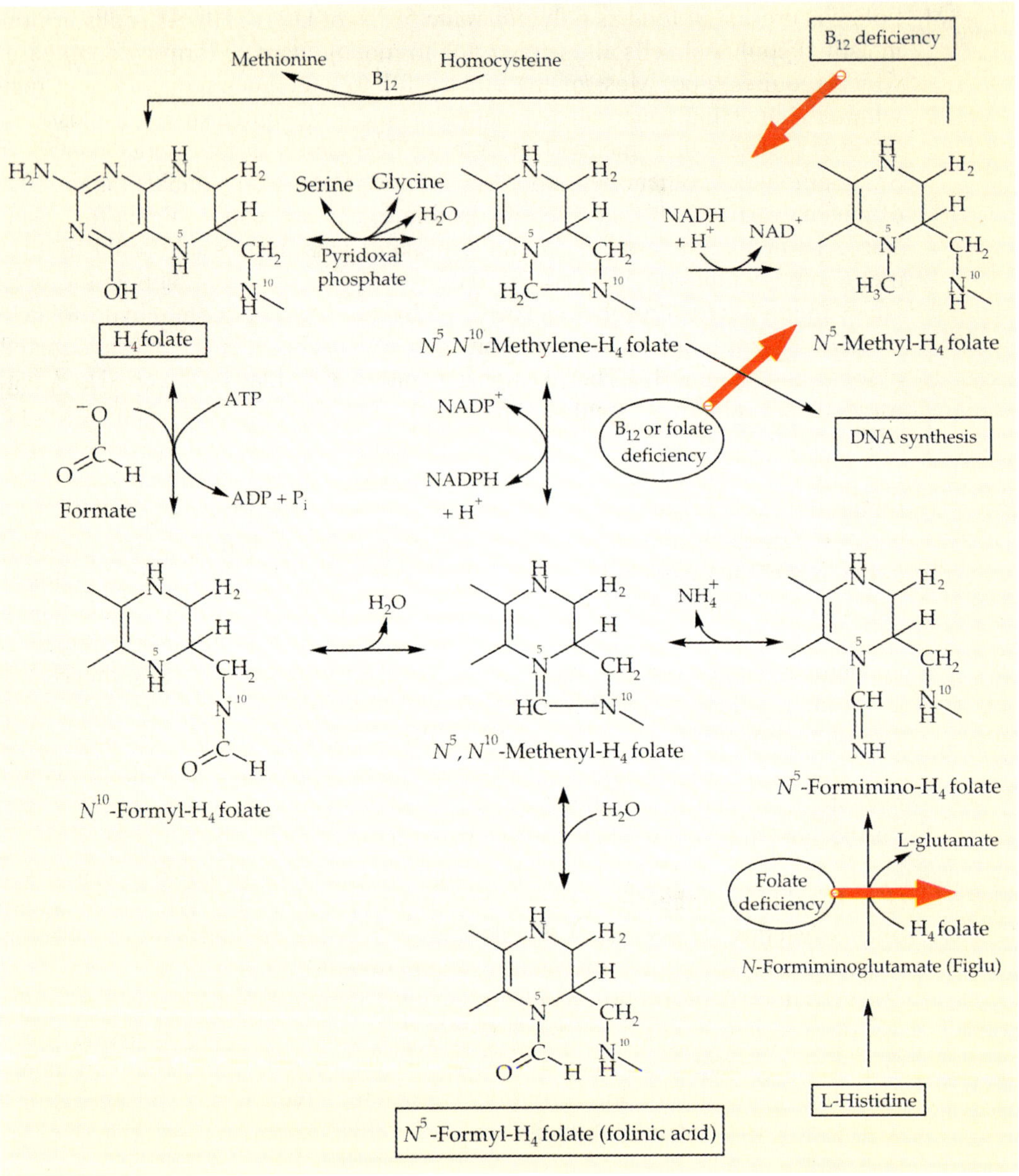

Fig. 9.4. Folate metabolism and folate trap.

the cells. Formation of vitamin D does not require direct exposure to sunlight as UV-B can penetrate light clothing also and it can penetrate clouds also. It is also unaffected by skin pigmentation.

Excessive oral diet vitamin D intake can lead to toxicity at levels greater than 400 nmol/L. However, with excessive exposure to sunlight levels never cross more than 200 nmol/L. This is because:

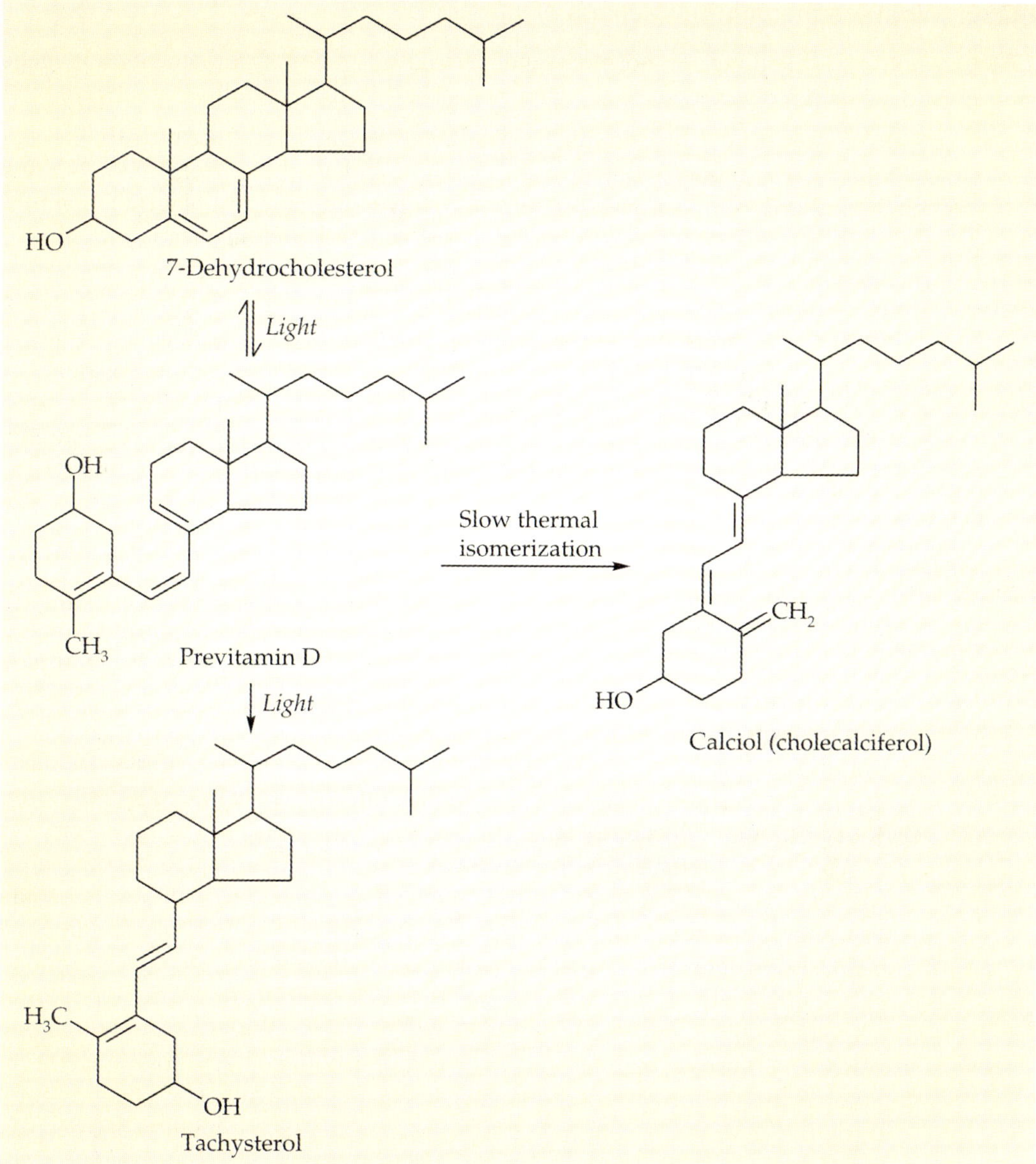

Fig. 9.5. Synthesis of cholecalciferol from 7-dehydrocholesterol in skin.

1. Isomerization step by light is reversible (Fig. 9.5).
2. Thermal isomerization to calciferol is very slow. *In vitro*, at 37°C, 50% conversion occurs in 4 days and at equilibrium, 83% is converted. *In vivo* removal of calciferol drives the reaction to right.
3. Light also converts previtamin D to inactive forms like lumisterol and tachysterol.

So, with increased exposure to light as formation of previtamin D increases its breakdown also increases. Formation of calciferol in body is not regulated by any feedback or other regulation.

Q. 6. What are the different actions of vitamin D?

Ans. Vitamin D functions as a hormone and has multiple actions mediated by both genome level and cell surface receptors. Both calcitriol and 24-hydroxycalcidiol are active biologically.

- **Nuclear receptor** is a zinc finger protein and forms heterodimers with RXR (retinoid X receptor). It is found in osteoblasts, intestine, kidney, beta islet, liver, PTH gland, skin, thymus, uterus, monocytes/macrophages, active lymphocytes, placenta, mammary glands and pituitary. Their expression is increased by PTH and calcitriol. Vitamin D regulates expression of > 50 genes, either increasing or decreasing their expression, e.g. 1-α-hydroxylase, 24-hydroxylase, calbindin, osteocalcin, osteopontin, collagen, etc.
- **Cell surface G-protein coupled receptor** found in intestines, keratinocytes and osteoblasts, etc. They act through phospholipase-C, diacylglycerol, ionositol triphosphate, protein kinase C, and MAP kinases. They mediate actions like inhibition of proliferation and induction of differentiation, maturation of chondrocytes, arachidonic acid release and increase production of prostaglandins like PGE1 and PGE2, regulation of calcium transporters and ion channels.

Actions of vitamin D

1. The primary function of vitamin D is to maintain plasma calcium levels.
2. **Intestines:** Increases absorption of calcium and phosphorus in intestines. There is a rapid increase in calcium uptake mediated by rapid recruitment of calcium transporters to cell membrane, and a slow increase mediated by increased expression of calcium binding protein calbindin.
3. **Kidney:** Increase in renal reabsorption of calcium in distal tubule (transcellular absorption through increased expression of calbindin), thus decrease in loss of calcium in urine.
4. **Bone:** Vitamin D receptors are present only on osteoblasts. The immediate response of osteoblasts is increased osteoblastic resorption of calcium to blood, and decreased synthesis of collagen and ALP. Osteoblastic resorption of minerals occurs without resorption of bone matrix. Osteoblasts also show a rapid increase in calcium uptake in response to calcitriol. Osteoclasts are stimulated indirectly. Osteoblasts produce RANKL and other growth factors for osteoclast which lead to osteoclastic resorption (minerals and matrix both).

    However, over 24–48 hours there is increase in collagen, ALP, osteocalcin, bone matrix protein, osteonectin, osteopontin and osteoprotegrin synthesis. This promotes mineralization of new bone or replacement of absorbed bone and inhibition of osteoclast activity.

    Calcitriol stimulation of osteoblast resorptive activity also causes the synthesis and release of a variety of growth factors from the osteoblasts. These accumulate in the bone and act as delayed activators of osteoblast proliferation and activation. The combined effect of the delayed autocrine activators of osteoblast proliferation and the delayed induction of collagen, osteocalcin, and alkaline phosphatase synthesis is thus to promote the formation and mineralization of new bone matrix to replace that resorbed. Non-genomic actions on bone include activation of voltage-gated calcium channels, increase phospholipid turnover and potentiation of PTH action.
5. **Secretion of insulin, PTH and thyroid hormones:** Occurs secondary to increase in intracellular calcium ion concentration due to up-regulation of calbindin expression.

6. **Protective against metabolic syndrome X:** It increases insulin release and inhibits adipocyte development.
7. **Immune system:** Differentiation and maturation of monocytes (thus Vit. D has been used in treatment of leukemia), terminal differentiation of keratinocytes (used in treatment of psoriasis), regulation of T cell activity. Calcitriol promotes the differentiation of monocyte precursor cells to form monocytes and macrophages, and enhances monocyte function.
8. **Hair growth**.
9. **Decreased response to TSH in thyroid gland:** Genomic (decreases G proteins) and non-genomic (decreases responsiveness to cAMP).
10. **Effects on cancer tissue:** Low concentrations stimulate growth while high concentrations inhibit growth.

24-hydroxycalcidiol, previously considered biologically inactive, is also active. In hypocalcaemic vitamin D deficiency rickets, administration of both 24-hydroxycalcidiol and calcitriol reverts the PTH gland hypertrophy rather than administration of calcitriol only. It also has role in maturation of chondrocytes and intramembranous ossification of bone.

Q. 7. What is glycemic index and glycemic load?

Ans. Glycemic index is a relative measure which ranks food items in terms of the rapidity with which they can raise blood glucose levels as compared to pure glucose taken orally.

The glycemic index of a food is measured as the area under the two-hour blood glucose response curve (area under curve) following a 12-hour fast and ingestion of a food with a certain quantity of available carbohydrate (usually tested with 50 g, Fig. 9.6). The AUC of the test food is divided by the area under curve (AUC) of the standard (glucose) and multiplied by 100 to obtain the GI. The average GI value is calculated from data collected in 10 human subjects. Both the standard and test food must contain an equal amount of available carbohydrate. The current methods use glucose as the reference food, giving it a glycemic index value of 100 by definition.

Foods with carbohydrates that break down quickly during digestion and release glucose rapidly into the bloodstream tend to have a high GI; foods with carbohydrates that break

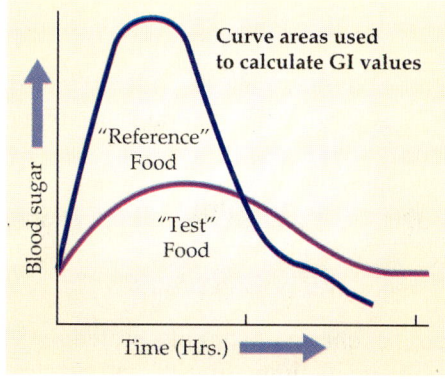

Fig. 9.6. Curve areas from glucose tolerance test used to calculate GI values.

down more slowly, releasing glucose more gradually into the bloodstream, tend to have a low GI. Thus complex carbohydrates have low glycemic index and refined foods have high glycemic index.

A low-GI food will release glucose more slowly and steadily, which leads to more suitable postprandial (after meal) blood glucose readings and lesser insulin release and requirement thus being very beneficial for diabetics.

GI provides a measure of how quickly blood sugar levels rise after eating a particular type of food but does no tell about the total carbohydrate consumed per serving of any food, which is measured by the glycemic load.

Glycemic load is based on the glycemic index (GI), and is defined as the percentage of available carbohydrate in the food times the food's GI for a 100 g serving of the food. GL is usually calculated as the glycemic index (GI) multiplied by the weight of the available carbohydrate in the food for that particular amount of food.

Glycemic load estimates the impact of carbohydrate consumption using the glycemic index while taking into account the amount of carbohydrate that is consumed. Thus it is a GI-weighted measure of carbohydrate content. Lesser the glycemic load, lesser is the rise in blood glucose and insulin release and lesser the amount of carbohydrate consumption as well. **It is equal to the amount of glucose added to the blood in the next 2 hours after consumption of a particular food.** Thus, it takes into account both the absolute carbohydrate content as well as the speed with which that food can raise the blood glucose levels. Fig. 9.7 shows the classification of glycemic index and load values into low, moderate and high.

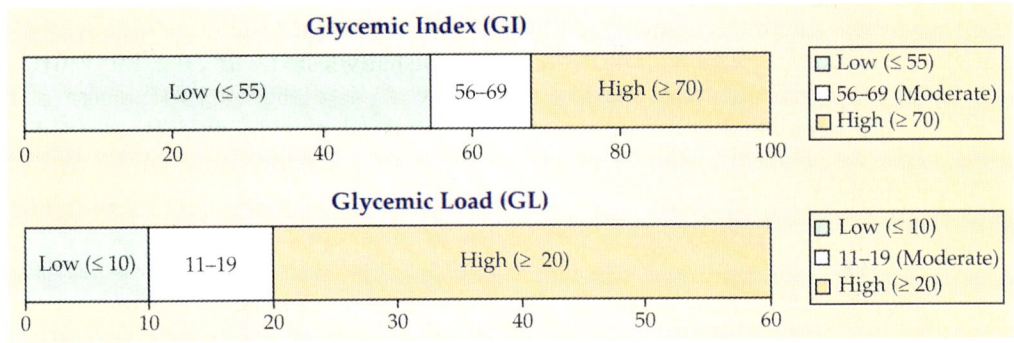

Fig. 9.7. Classification of glycemic index and glycemic load values.

Take watermelon as an example for calculating glycemic load. Its glycemic index is pretty high, about 72. A serving of 120 grams has 6 grams of available carbohydrate, so its glycemic load is pretty low (72/100) × 6 = 4.32 for 120 g or 3.6 for 100 g. It is a way of saying that 100 g of watermelon will provide only 3.6 g of glucose in blood in the 2 hours after it is consumed. Low GI and GL foods are beneficial in DM and obesity.

Q. 8. What is protein quality and how is protein quality assessed?

Ans. Protein quality describes characteristics of a protein in relation to its ability to achieve defined metabolic actions like maintaining muscle and bone protein mass, satisfying demands for biosynthetic pathways, and special needs for growth, pregnancy, or lactation.

A number of methods for evaluating the quality of food proteins have been used over the years. Older methodologies include rat bioassays such as biological value (BV), net protein utilisation (NPU), and protein efficiency ratio (PER).

Biological value is measured using nitrogen balance techniques to determine the amount of absorbed nitrogen that is retained in the body for repair and maintenance.

$$BV = \frac{\text{Retained N}}{\text{Absorbed N}} \times 100$$

Net protein utilisation is based on a combination of biologic value and the food protein's digestibility.

$$NPU = \frac{\text{Retained N}}{\text{N-application (N given in diet)}} \times 100$$

Protein efficiency ratio (PER) is based on the weight gain of a growing rat divided by its intake of a particular food protein during the test period.

The practical difficulties, poor sensitivity and differences between humans and animals associated with these nitrogen balance method has led to the adoption of the protein digestibility-corrected amino acid score (PDCAAS) approach to measure protein quality.

Complete proteins are those food proteins that contain all nine indispensable or essential amino acids in concentrations sufficient to meet effectively the requirements of humans.

Protein digestibility-corrected amino acid score, or PDCAAS is a more accurate method for evaluating the quality of food proteins or their completeness. It is based on a food protein's amino acid content, its true digestibility, and its ability to supply indispensable amino acids in amounts adequate to meet the amino acid requirements of a 2- to 5-year old child, the age group used as the standard.

$$AAS = \frac{\text{\% amino acid in test protein}}{\text{\% corresponding amino acid requirement}}$$

The amino acid content used as the standard should reflect the amounts of the various essential amino acids needed to carry out the tasks of growth, repair, and maintenance of living tissues in humans. The FAO/WHO Expert Consultation, for example, uses the amino acid requirements of a 2- to 5-year-old child as the standard. This age group has the most demanding amino acid requirements of any group except infants.

The PDCAAS is based on a food protein's completeness—
1. Amino acid content of essential amino acids,
2. Digestibility, and
3. Ability to supply essential amino acids in the amounts adequate to meet human needs.

The highest PDCAAS value that any protein can achieve is 1.0. This score means that after digestion of the food protein, it provides per unit of protein 100% or more of the indispensable amino acids required by the two- to five-year-old child.

A score above 1.0 is rounded down to 1.0. Any amino acids in excess of those required to build and repair tissue would not be used for protein synthesis, but would be catabolised and eliminated from the body or stored as fat.

The following steps are necessary to calculate the PDCAAS of a food protein:

1. The food protein must be analysed for its nitrogen content.
2. Protein content is calculated by multiplying the nitrogen content by 6.25.
3. The food protein is analysed to determine its essential amino acid content.
4. The uncorrected amino acid score is calculated by dividing the milligrams of a particular essential amino acid in one gram of the test protein by the milligrams of the essential amino acids in one gram of the reference protein which is the amino acid requirement pattern for the 2- to 5-year-old child.
5. The true digestibility of food protein needs to be determined. The traditional method for determining true digestibility is based on the nitrogen balance obtained from rat feeding trials.

$$\text{True digestibility} = \frac{\text{N uptake} - (\text{N in faeces} - \text{Endogenous N in faeces})}{\text{N uptake}} \times 100$$

This method has been recommended by the FAO/WHO Expert Consultation Group for human digestibility model studies as well.

Amino acids in a food are not necessarily entirely available. The protein degradation as well as the absorption can be incomplete. With animal proteins the digestion and absorption rate lies over 90%, with vegetable proteins it is around 60–70% only. This is because of unfavourable conformations for action of proteases, bound factors (metals, lipids, nucleic acids, cellulose or other polysaccharides), antinutritional factors such as trypsin or chymotrypsin inhibitors, and size and surface area of the protein particle. Digestibility can be improved by heat treatment i.e. cooking (denaturation) and fine grinding to increase particle surface area.

6. The PDCAAS is calculated by multiplying the lowest uncorrected amino acid score (of all the essential amino acids) by the food protein's digestibility. PDCAAS = AAS × True digestibility.

Evaluating protein quality on the basis of content of essential amino acid is logical as even if one essential amino acid is deficient (called limiting amino acid of a food) it will halt the protein synthesis midway when its chance comes to be added to the growing polypeptide during translation. Neither will be the complete protein synthesized and also the partially synthesized peptide will be degraded and ATP used to make it wasted. This will lead to negative nitrogen balance.

Table 9.2 shows the calculation of PDCAAS for isolated soy protein, the most concentrated type of soy protein ingredient. Take a look at histidine, for example. Isolated soy protein has 26 milligrams of histidine per gram of protein. The digestibility factor of 97% means that out of 26 milligrams of histidine reaching the intestinal tract, 25.2 milligrams are absorbed. A two- to five-year-old child requires 19 milligrams of histidine per gram of protein, giving isolated soy protein a PDCAAS of 1.3 for this amino acid. This means that isolated soy protein provides 130% of the histidine required by the reference pattern, which reflects the requirements of a two- to five-year-old child. The PDCAAS for a food protein is equal to the lowest score for a single indispensable amino acid (or amino acid pair). In this case, methionine and cysteine have a PDCAAS of 1.0, which becomes the score for the entire protein. Had all of the individual amino acid scores exceeded 1.0, the PDCAAS would still have been rounded down to 1.0, the highest PDCAAS possible.

Table 9.2. Calculation of protein digestibility – Corrected amino acid score of soy protein

Indispensable amino acid	Isolated soy protein (mg/g protein)	Digestibility (AA × 97%) (mg/g protein)	Reference pattern (mg/g protein)	PDCAAS
Histidine	26	25.2	19	1.3
Isoleucine	49	47.5	28	1.7
Leucine	82	79.5	66	1.2
Lysine	63	61.1	58	1.1
Methionine and Cysteine#	26	25.2	25	1.0
Phenylalanine and Tyrosine##	90	87.3	63	1.4
Threonine	38	36.9	34	1.1
Tryptophan	13	12.6	11	1.1
Valine	50	48.5	35	1.4
				PDCAAS = 1.0

AA = Amino acids; PDCAAS = Protein digestibility-corrected amino acid score.
 # Methionine is a precursor of cysteine.
 ## Phenylalanine is a precursor of tyrosine.

Adoption of the PDCAAS to evaluate protein quality has shown that some soy proteins are also complete proteins; that is, they provide all the essential amino acids in sufficient quantity to meet the needs of humans. The PDCAAS of some soy protein products is equal to milk protein and egg white. PDCAAS of some common proteins are shown in Fig. 9.8.

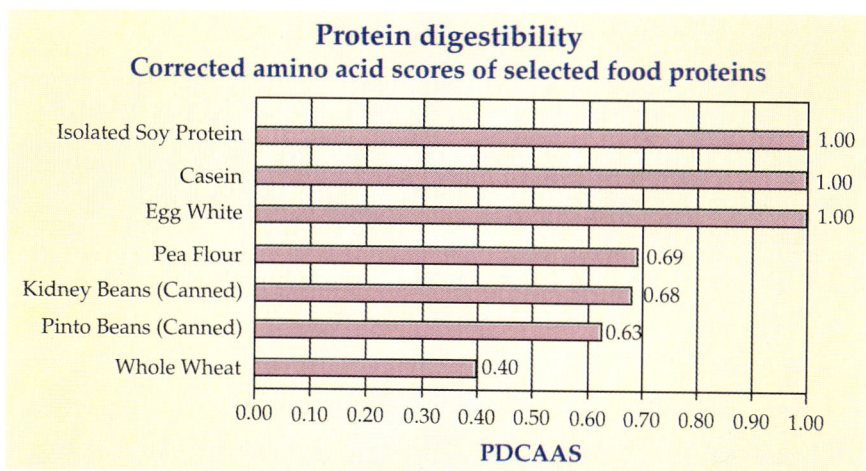

Fig. 9.8. PDCAAS of some common food proteins.

Q. 9. What is the pharmacological application of niacin and its biochemical basis?

Ans. Niacin (nicotinic acid) in pharmacological doses (1.4–4 g/day) is used to lower LDL cholesterol and triglyceride and increase HDL cholesterol levels.

Decrease in LDL cholesterol level is due to direct non-competitive inhibition by niacin of liver diacylglycerol acyltransferase-2, a key enzyme in triglyceride synthesis. The decrease in hepatic triglyceride synthesis results in degradation of intracellular apo B and decreased secretion of VLDL.

Increase in HDL appears to be due to an effect of niacin on a hepatic apo AI receptor; this leads to decrease in the hepatic removal of HDL from blood.

Such pharmacological doses of niacin can have toxicity like flushing of skin, hyper-uricemia, macular oedema, macular cysts, glucose intolerance and elevation of liver enzymes. Flushing can be avoided with preparations which release niacin slowly in intestines, but monitoring liver enzymes is required. Prostaglandin-mediated flushing due to binding of niacin to a G protein-coupled receptor has been observed at daily doses as low as 50 mg of niacin.

Q. 10. Enumerate nutritional/dietary factors related to risk of metabolic syndrome and cardiovascular diseases.

Ans.

Factor	Biochemical basis
B_{12}, folic acid and B_6	Decrease homocysteine levels, deficiency elevates homocysteine
Vitamin D	Inhibits adipocyte development and increases insulin release
Choline	Source of one carbon moiety in one carbon metabolism, helps decrease homocysteine. Decreases SAH and increases SAM. Decreases nitric oxide and increases GSH
Dietary fibre	Decreases lipid absorption, improves glycemic index of diet
ω-3 PUFA, eicosapentaenoic acid (EPA) + docosahexaenoic acid (DHA) + alpha linolenic acid	Decrease cholesterol, platelet aggregation and inflammation, improve insulin resistance and membrane fluidity
Low glycemic index/load foods	Decrease insulin release, beneficial for metabolic syndrome
Salt restriction (< 4 g/day)	Improves hypertension
Limiting saturated fatty acid (SFA) intake to < 7% and trans fatty acid (tFA) intake to < 1% of total energy intake	Trans fat: insulin resistance, decrease membrane fluidity
Plant sterols	Decrease cholesterol absorption competitively in GIT
Antioxidants, flavinoids	Decrease free radical-mediated damage of lipids, proteins and DNA; decrease inflammation

Q. 11. What are goitrogenic factors? How selenium deficiency affects thyroid function?

Ans. Goitrogens are variety of naturally occurring agents in food or environment exposure to which has been identified to cause goitre. Goitrogens are usually active only if iodine supply is limited and/or goitrogen intake is of long duration. Many of these have only been tested in animals and/or have been shown to possess antithyroid effects *in vitro*. These compounds belong to the following chemical groups:

- Sulfurated organics (like thiocyanate, isothiocyanate, goitrin and disulphides)
- Perchlorate and pertechnate
- Flavonoids (polyphenols)
- Polyhydroxyphenols and phenol derivatives
- Pyridines, phthalate esters and metabolites,
- Polychlorinated (PCB) and polybrominated (PBB) biphenyls
- Organochlorines (like DDT)
- Polycyclic aromatic hydrocarbons (PAH)
- Inorganic iodine (in excess)
- Lithium

Goitrogens can be classified into agents acting directly on the thyroid gland and those causing goitre by indirect action.

Directly-acting agents are subdivided as:

- Those inhibiting transport of iodide into the thyroid by inhibiting the sodium iodine symporter (like thiocyanate, isothiocyanate, perchlorate, pertechnate).
- Those acting on the intrathyroidal oxidation and organic binding process of iodide and/or the coupling reaction (like phenolic compounds, some phthalate derivatives, disulfides and goitrin).
- Those interfering with proteolysis, dehalogenation and hormone release (like iodide and lithium).

Indirect goitrogens increase the rate of thyroid hormone metabolism (like 2,4-dinitrophenol, PCBs and PBBs). Soybean, an important protein source in many third world countries, interrupts the enterohepatic cycle of thyroid hormone and may cause goitre when iodine intake is limited.

Firm evidence for goitrogenic action in humans has only been shown for a few compounds: thiocyanate, goitrin, resorcinol, dinitrophenol, PBBs and its oxides, excess iodine and high doses of lithium. Deficiencies of iron and vitamin A may also have a goitrogenic effect in areas of iodine deficiency. Dietary goitrogens are summarized in Table 9.3.

Selenium deficiency

- Has profound effects on thyroid hormone metabolism and possibly also on the thyroid gland itself.
- The function of type I deiodinase (a selenoprotein) is impaired. Type I deiodinase plays a major role in T4 deiodination in peripheral tissues.
- It has been shown that when, in an area of combined iodine and selenium deficiency, only selenium is supplemented, serum T4 decreases. This effect is explained by restoration of type I deiodinase activity leading to normalization of T4 deiodination while T4 synthesis remains impaired because of continued iodine deficiency.

Table 9.3. Dietary goitrogens

Goitrogen	Mechanism
Foods	
Cassava, lima beans, linseed, sorghum, sweet potato	Contain cyanogenic glucosides; they are metabolized to thiocyanates that compete with iodine for thyroidal uptake
Cruciferous vegetables: cabbage, kale, cauliflower, broccoli, turnips, rapeseed	Contains glucosinolates; metabolites compete with iodine for thyroidal uptake
Soy, millet	Flavonoids impair thyroid peroxidase activity
Nutrients	
Selenium deficiency	Accumulated peroxides may damage the thyroid, and deiodinase deficiency impairs thyroid hormone synthesis
Iron deficiency	Reduces heme-dependent thyroperoxidase activity in the thyroid and may blunt the efficacy of iodine prophylaxis
Vitamin A deficiency	Increases TSH stimulation and goitre through decreased vitamin A-mediated suppression of the pituitary TSHβ gene

- Reduction of the selenium-containing enzyme glutathione peroxidase. Glutathione peroxidase detoxifies H_2O_2 which is abundantly present in the thyroid gland as a substrate for the thyroperoxidase that catalyzes iodide oxidation and binding to thyroglobulin, and the oxidative coupling of iodotyrosines into iodothyronines. Reduced detoxification of H_2O_2 may lead to thyroid cell death. Elevated H_2O_2 levels in thyrocytes may be more toxic under situations of increased TSH stimulation such as is present in areas with severe iodine deficiency.

Q. 12. **What are the different consequences of Iodine deficiency and their biochemical basis?**

Ans. Iodine is an essential component of the thyroid hormones which are essential for mammalian life. The recommended daily allowance is given in Table 9.4. In order for the thyroid gland to synthesize adequate amounts of thyroxin (T4), approximately 52 µg of iodide must be taken up daily by the thyroid gland. Severe iodine deficiency develops when iodide intake is

Table 9.4. Recommendations for iodine intake (µg/day) by age or population group

Age or population group[a]	Iodine intake (µg/day)
Infants 0–12 months[b]	110–130
Children 1–8 years	90
Children 9–13 years	120
Adults ≥ 14 years	150
Pregnancy	250
Lactation	250

a = Recommended daily allowance; b = Adequate intake.

chronically <20 µg/day. In India, out of 321 districts surveyed 260 districts are endemic i.e. where the prevalence of Iodine Deficiency Disorders (IDDs) is more than 10%.

Iodine deficiency disorders (IDD)

The term IDD refers to all the ill-effects of iodine deficiency in a population that can be prevented by ensuring that the population has an adequate intake of iodine (Table 9.5). Brain damage and irreversible mental retardation are the most important disorders induced by iodine deficiency. Inadequate iodine intake leads to inadequate thyroid hormone production, and all the consequences of iodine deficiency stem from the associated hypothyroidism.

Table 9.5. Spectrum of iodine deficiency disorders (IDD)

Fetus	• Miscarriage • Stillbirths • Congenital anomalies • Increased perinatal morbidity and mortality • Endemic cretinism
Neonate	• Neonatal goitre • Neonatal hypothyroidism • Endemic mental retardation • Increased susceptibility of the thyroid gland to nuclear radiation
Child and adolescent	• Goitre • (Subclinical) hypothyroidism • Impaired mental function • Retarded physical development • Increased susceptibility of the thyroid gland to nuclear radiation
Adult	• Goitre with its complications • Hypothyroidism • Impaired mental function • Spontaneous hyperthyroidism in the elderly • Iodine-induced hyperthyroidism • Increased susceptibility of the thyroid gland to nuclear radiation

Diffuse and nodular goitre

- Goitre is the most obvious manifestation of iodine deficiency. Low iodine intake leads to reduced thyroxin (T4) and triiodothyronine (T3) production, which results in increased thyrotropin (TSH) secretion in an attempt to restore T4 and T3 production to normal. TSH also stimulates thyroid growth; thus, goitre occurs as part of the compensatory response to iodine deficiency.
- Development of goitre – Biochemical basis:
  – The first functional consequence of iodine deficiency is an increase in the uptake of iodide by the thyroid mediated via a transmembrane protein, the sodium iodide symporter (NIS).
  – Both the sensitivity of the thyroid to TSH and the TSH level itself increase with decreased iodide supply.

- For adequate adjustment of iodine supply to the thyroid, iodide trapping must fulfil two conditions.
    - First, it must reduce the amount of iodide excreted in the urine to a level corresponding to the level of iodine intake in order to preserve the pre-existing iodine stores.
    - Second, it must ensure the accumulation in the thyroid of definite amounts of iodide per day, estimated at least 100 µg/day in adolescents and adults.
- The increase in the iodide clearance/uptake by the thyroid despite the decrease in the serum concentration of iodide maintains a normal absolute uptake of iodide by the thyroid and an organic iodine content of the thyroid which remains within the limits of normal (i.e., 10–20 mg) as long as the iodine intake remains above a threshold of about 50 µg/day.
- Below this critical level of iodine intake, despite a further increase of thyroid iodide clearance, the absolute uptake of iodide diminishes and the iodine content of the thyroid decreases with functional consequences resulting in the development of a goitre (explained below as maladaptation of thyroid).
- Thyroid hyperplasia induced by iodine deficiency is associated with an altered pattern of thyroid hormone synthesis: the abnormal configuration of the poorly iodinated thyroglobulin in the thyroid colloid is accompanied by an increase in poorly iodinated compounds, monoiodotyrosine (MIT) and T3, and a decrease in diiodotyrosine (DIT) and T4. The increase of the MIT/DIT and T3/T4 ratios is closely related to the degree of iodine depletion of the gland.
- The T3/T4 ratio in the serum may be elevated in conditions of iodine deficiency because:
    - thyroidal secretion of T4 and T3 is in the proportion in which they exist within the gland; and
    - preferential secretion of T3 or increased peripheral conversion of T4 to T3.

    The shift to increased T3 secretion plays an important role in the adaptation to iodine deficiency because T3 possesses about 4 times the metabolic potency of T4 but requires only 75 % as much iodine for synthesis.
- Thus efficient adaptation to iodine deficiency is possible even in the absence of goitre or with minimal gland enlargement due to the above described mechanisms.
- Large colloid goitres in endemic iodine deficiency represents maladaptation:
    - In large goitres, the major part of the gland is occupied by extremely distended vesicles filled with colloid with a flattened epithelium.
    - The mechanism responsible for the development of colloid goitre appears to be TSH hyperstimulation.
    - It is the consequence of an imbalance between thyroglobulin synthesis and hydrolysis.
    - In these conditions, iodide is diluted while thyroglobulin is in excess, resulting in a lesser degree of iodization of thyroglobulin and, consequently, in a decrease in iodothyronine synthesis and secretion.
    - Hydrolysis of large amounts of poorly iodinated thyroglobulin results in the leak of iodide from thyroid gland and enhanced urinary loss of iodide, further aggravating the state of iodine deficiency.

    Therefore, large colloid goitres in endemic iodine deficiency represent maladaptation instead of adaptation to iodine deficiency because they may produce a vicious cycle of iodine loss and defective thyroid hormones synthesis.

- The goitre is initially diffuse but eventually becomes nodular because the cells in some thyroid follicles proliferate more than others. Therefore, in regions of iodine deficiency, children and adolescents generally have diffuse goitres, while adults who lived in conditions of long-standing iodine deficiency have nodular goitre.
- Iodine deficiency favouring thyroid follicular cell replication also increases the chance of mutations in the TSH-receptor gene that may lead to constitutive activation of the receptor and TSH-independent growth and function. With continued growth of one or more TSH-independent nodules, hyperthyroidism may occur if iodine deficiency is not extremely severe. Hyperthyroidism is more likely to develop if iodine intake is supplemented.

Endemic goitre

Endemic goitre is characterized by enlargement of the thyroid gland in a significantly large fraction of a population group, and is generally considered to be due to insufficient iodine in the daily diet. Endemic goitre exists in a population when >5% of 6–12-year-old children have enlarged thyroid glands.

Hypothyroidism

- Hypothyroidism due to very low iodine intake.
- Adults have the typical clinical manifestations of hypothyroidism and usually a goitre. There is reduced mental function due to cerebral hypothyroidism and high degree of apathy. There is detrimental effect on their initiative and decision-making.
- Fetus and neonate: Fig. 9.9 shows the time course of the development of the brain and of thyroid function in the human fetus and neonate.
    - Brain growth is characterized by two periods of maximal growth velocity:
        * The first one occurs during the first and second trimesters between 8 to 20 weeks of gestation. This phase corresponds to neuronal multiplication, migration and organization.
        * The second phase takes place from the third trimester onwards up to the second and third years postnatally. It corresponds to glial cell multiplication, migration and myelinization.
    - The first phase occurs before fetal thyroid has reached its functional capacity.
    - During the first phase, the supply of thyroid hormones to the growing fetus is almost exclusively of maternal origin while during the second phase, the supply of thyroid hormones to the fetus is essentially of fetal origin.
    - Nuclear T3 receptors and the amount of T3 bound to these receptors increases six- to ten-fold between 10 and 16 weeks.
    - Onset of secretion of T4 by the fetal thyroid occurs at the 24th week of gestation. The transfer of maternal thyroid hormones decreases but persists during later gestation. Up to 30% of serum T4 in cord blood at birth may be of maternal origin.
- Developing fetus or infant: Untreated maternal hypothyroidism due to severe iodine deficiency causes permanent mental retardation, which, in its most severe form, is known as cretinism.

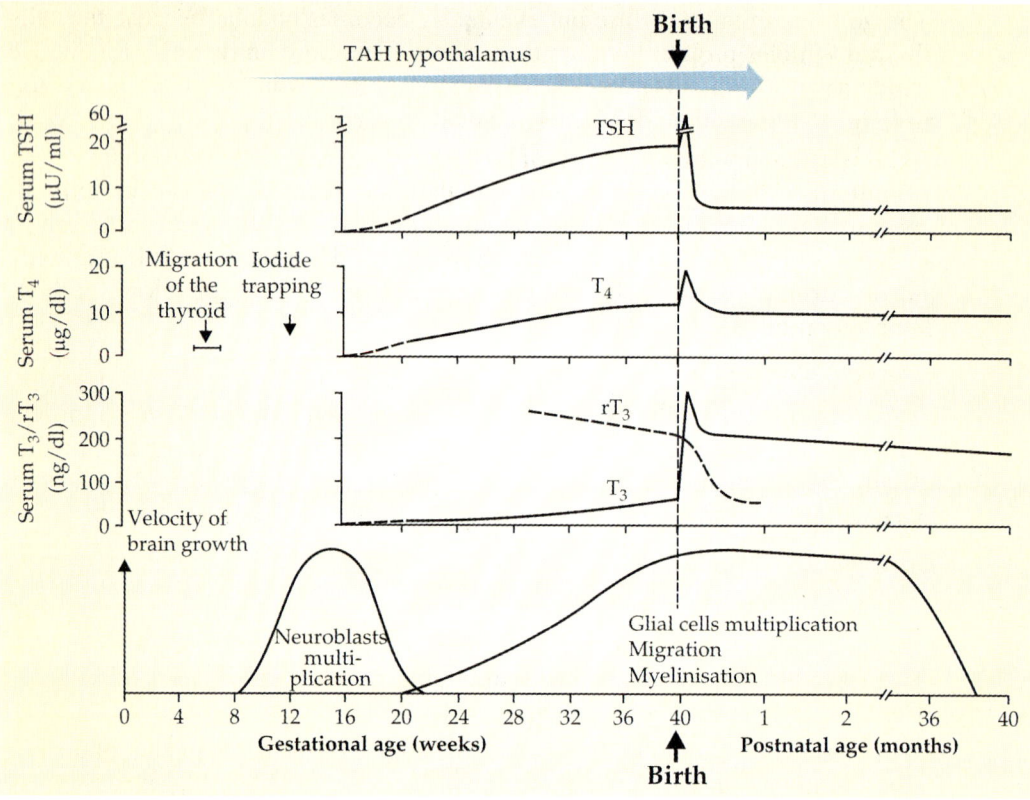

Fig. 9.9. Ontogenesis of thyroid function and regulation in humans during fetal and early postnatal life in relation to the velocity of brain growth.

- In addition to mental retardation, cretinism is accompanied by other neurologic and somatic defects. This has led to cretinism being subdivided into neurologic and myxedematous types:
  - Neurological cretinism
    * Characterized by mental retardation, deaf mutism, gait disturbances, and spasticity, but not hypothyroidism.
    * It is thought to result from hypothyroidism in the mother during early pregnancy, but a euthyroid state postnatally.
    * The neuropathological basis of the clinical picture includes under-development of the cochlea for deafness; maldevelopment of the cerebral neocortex for mental retardation; and maldevelopment of the corpus striatum (especially putamen and globus pallidus) for the motor disorder.
    * The cerebellum, hypothalamus, visual system, and hippocampus are relatively spared.
    * Iodine deficiency has an early effect on neuroblast multiplication. Brain weight is reduced.
  - Myxedematous cretinism
    * Characterized by mental retardation, short stature, and hypothyroidism.
    * It is thought to result from iodine deficiency and thyroid injury predominantly late in pregnancy and continuing after birth.

- Has a less severe degree of mental retardation than the neurological cretin, but has all the features of extremely severe hypothyroidism present since early life: severe growth retardation, incomplete maturation of the facial features including the naso-orbital configuration, atrophy of the mandibles, puffy features, myxedematous, thickened and dry skin, dry and decreased hair, eyelashes and eyebrows and much delayed sexual maturation.
- Goitre is usually absent and the thyroid is often not palpable, suggesting thyroid atrophy.
- Three additional factors besides iodine deficiency, acting alone or in combination, have been proposed for explaining the thyroid atrophy characteristic of the myxedematous type of cretinism: Thiocyanate overload, Selenium deficiency, Immunological mechanisms.

Neonatal and infant mortality

- Severe iodine deficiency increases neonatal and infant mortality, an effect that can be reduced by up to 50% with correction of severe iodine deficiency. The mechanism of this benefit is not known, but multiple factors are probably involved.
- Hypothyroid or retarded infants may suffer more birth trauma and be more prone to infectious diseases and nutritional deficiencies typical of the poor rural communities in which iodine deficiency is prominent.

Increased susceptibility of the thyroid gland to radiation and radioiodine

- Thyroidal uptake of radioiodine reaches its maximum value in the earliest years of life and then decline progressively into adult life.
- The thyroidal iodine turnover rate is much higher in young infants (25–30 times higher) than in adults and decreased progressively with age. This is also the reason for the greatly increased susceptibility of the neonate and fetus to iodine deficiency.
- Iodine deficiency leads to increased uptake of radioiodine.

Subclinical neurological defects

- Minor neuropsychological defects have been described in children born to mothers exposed to mild to moderate iodine deficiency during pregnancy.
- An increased auditory threshold may be another clinical manifestation of iodine deficiency.

Intellectual disability

- Iodine deficiency also appears to have adverse effects on growth and development in the postnatal period.
- Children and adolescents in regions of iodine deficiency are at risk for some degree of intellectual disability and have an average loss of 13.5 intelligence quotient (IQ) points.
- Intellectual disability resulting from the effects of iodine deficiency on the central nervous system during fetal development is not reversible.
- The additional impairment caused by continuing postnatal hypothyroidism and/or iodine deficiency may improve with appropriate thyroid hormone replacement and/or iodine supplementation.

Socioeconomic effects

People in iodine-deficient communities are typically less educable and less economically productive. Correction of the deficiency has resulted in dramatic improvement in school performance, agricultural output, and per capita income.

Assessment of iodine status

Four methods are generally recommended for assessment of iodine nutrition in populations: urinary iodine concentration (UI), the goitre rate, serum thyroid stimulating hormone (TSH), and serum thyroglobulin (Tg). These indicators are complementary, in that UI (Table 9.6) is a sensitive indicator of recent iodine intake (days) and Tg shows an intermediate response (weeks to months), whereas changes in the goitre rate reflect long-term iodine nutrition (months to years). Approximately 90 percent or more of ingested iodine eventually appears in the urine. A median average daily iodine intake of 150 µg corresponds to a median urinary iodine concentration of 100 µg/L.

Table 9.6. Criteria for assessing iodine nutrition based on median urinary iodine concentrations in school-age children

Median urinary iodine (µg/L)	Iodine intake	Iodine nutrition
< 20	Insufficient	Severe iodine deficiency
20–49	Insufficient	Moderate iodine deficiency
50–99	Insufficient	Mild iodine deficiency
100–199	Adequate	Optimal
200–299	More than adequate	Risk of iodine-induced hyperthyroidism
≥ 300	Excessive	Risk of adverse health consequences (iodine-induced hyperthyroidism, autoimmune thyroid disease)

Q. 13. What are the different consequences of iodine excess and their biochemical basis?

Ans. Iodine excess, including overcorrection of a previous state of iodine deficiency, can also impair thyroid function. Both low and high iodine intake are associated with an increased risk of thyroid disorders. Healthy adults can tolerate up to 600–1100 µg iodine/day without any side effects (Table 9.7). However, this upper limit is much lower in a population which has been exposed to iodine deficiency for a prolonged period in the past.

Table 9.7. Tolerable upper intake level for iodine (µg/day)

Age group	Tolerable upper intake level for iodine (µg/day)
1–3 years	200
4–6 years	250
7–10 years	300
11–14 years	450
15–17 years	500
Adults	600
Pregnant women > 19 years	600

Consequent risks of excess iodine intake

Iodide goitre and iodine-induced hypothyroidism
- Thyroid enlargement and goitre, subclinical hypothyroidism.
- The mechanisms are iodine enhancement of thyroid autoimmunity and reversible inhibition of thyroid function (especially sodium iodine symporter) by excess iodine (the Wolff-Chaikoff effect) in susceptible subjects.
- Increased thyroid volume in children due to iodine excess has been observed when the median urinary iodine is > 500 µg/L.

Iodine-induced hyperthyroidism (IIH)
- Main complication of iodine prophylaxis.
- IIH following iodine fortification of salt cannot be entirely avoided even when fortification provides only physiological amounts of iodine.
- Iodine deficiency increases thyrocyte proliferation and mutation rates which, in turn, trigger the development of multifocal autonomous growth with scattered cell clones harbouring activating mutations of the TSH receptors. Only some nodules keep their capacity to store iodine, become autonomous and cause hyperthyroidism which is promoted by iodine fortification. Thus, IIH can be considered one of the iodine deficiency disorders, and it may be largely unavoidable in the early phase of iodine repletion in iodine deficient populations, particularly in those with moderate to severe iodine deficiency.
- Increased iodine intake in patients with Graves' disease may exacerbate hyperthyroidism.

Iodine-induced thyroiditis
- Aggravation or the induction of autoimmune thyroiditis by iodine supplementation.
- Mechanisms involved are:
  - triggering of thyroid autoimmune reactivity by increasing the immunogenicity of thyroglobulin; and
  - damage to the thyroid and cell injury by free radicals.

Thyroid cancer
- Chronic overstimulation of the thyroid (cell proliferation and thus increased rate of mutations) by TSH can produce thyroid neoplasms especially in the autonomous thyroid nodules (constitutive activation of TSH receptor due to mutation).
- Iodine supplementation is accompanied by a change in the epidemiological pattern of thyroid cancer with an increased prevalence of occult papillary cancer discovered at autopsy.
- It appears the prognosis of thyroid cancer is significantly improved following iodine supplementation due to a shift towards differentiated forms of thyroid cancer that are diagnosed at earlier stages.

Excessive iodine ingestion during pregnancy may also have adverse effects on fetal thyroid function. Sudden exposure to excess serum iodide inhibits organification of iodide, thereby diminishing hormone biosynthesis (the Wolff-Chaikoff effect). The fetal thyroid gland is particularly susceptible to the inhibitory effects of excess iodine during the third trimester, which can result in a prolonged inhibition of thyroid hormone synthesis, an increase in thyrotropin (TSH), and fetal goitre.

The benefits of correcting iodine deficiency far outweigh its risks and hence food fortification and salt iodization is recommended especially in endemic areas. Iodine-induced hyperthyroidism and other adverse effects can be majorly avoided by adequate and sustained quality assurance and monitoring of iodine supplementation which should also confirm adequate iodine intake.

Chapter 10

Genetics

Q. 1. What is DNA tautomerization and what is its significance?

Ans. Isomers that differ in the position of atoms, and the bonds between them are tautomers. Tautomeric forms are in equilibrium. Many tautomers are formed by migration of a hydrogen atom, accompanied by a switch of a single bond and neighbouring double bond. In cyclic structures, H– atoms can move from one atom to another or from one ring to another, so they cannot be assigned a fixed location. This movement is called tautomeric shift.

In DNA, H– atoms usually prefer specific atomic location in purine and pyrimidine bases (Fig. 10.1).
- Keto (C=O), Enol (C–OH)
- Amino (NH_2), Imino (=NH)

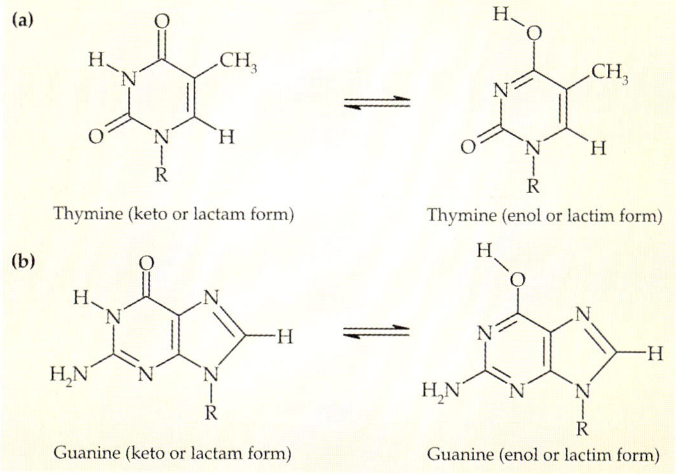

(a) Thymine (keto or lactam form) ⇌ Thymine (enol or lactim form)

(b) Guanine (keto or lactam form) ⇌ Guanine (enol or lactim form)

Fig. 10.1. Tautomers of thymine and guanine.

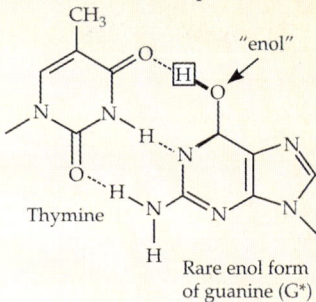

Fig. 10.2. Effect of tautomerization on base pairing.

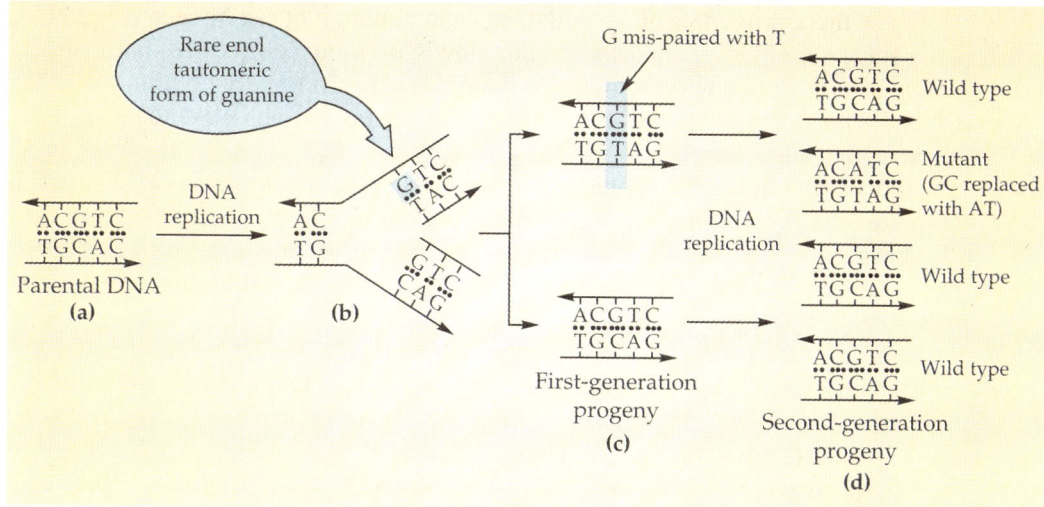

Fig. 10.3. Mutation due to tautomerization.

Normally, the N– atoms attached to C, G and A are in the amino form (–NH_2). The O– atom in G and T are in keto form (=O). A pairs with T and G with C in DNA. Due to tautomerism A can pair with C and G with T as shown in Fig. 10.2. When such DNA replicates it leads to change in sequence or mutation. It causes transitions or replacement of purine with purine (A instead of G or vice versa) or replacement of pyrimidine with pyrimidine (C instead of T or vice versa) (Fig. 10.3).

Q. 2. What is DNA damage and mutation? What are differences between them?

Ans. Damages are physical abnormalities in the DNA, e.g. single- and double-strand breaks, 8-hydroxydeoxyguanosine residues, and polycyclic aromatic hydrocarbon adducts. Mutation is a permanent change in the base sequence of the DNA. DNA damage and mutation are fundamentally different.

- DNA damages can be recognized by enzymes, and, thus, they can be correctly repaired if redundant information, such as the undamaged sequence in the complementary DNA strand or in a homologous chromosome, is available for copying.
- If a cell retains DNA damage, transcription of a gene can be prevented, and, thus, translation into a protein will also be blocked. Replication may also be blocked and/or the cell may die.
- A mutation cannot be recognized by enzymes once the base change is present in both DNA strands, and, thus, a mutation cannot be repaired.
- At the cellular level, mutations can cause alterations in protein function and regulation.
- Mutations are replicated when the cell replicates.
- In a population of cells, mutant cells will increase or decrease in frequency according to the effects of the mutation on the ability of the cell to survive and reproduce.
- Although distinctly different from each other, DNA damages and mutations are related because DNA damages often cause errors of DNA synthesis during replication or repair; these errors are a major source of mutations.

Given these properties of DNA damage and mutation, it can be seen that DNA damages are a special problem in non-dividing or slowly dividing cells, where unrepaired damages will tend to accumulate over time. On the other hand, in rapidly dividing cells, unrepaired DNA damages that do not kill the cell by blocking replication will tend to cause replication errors and thus mutation.

Human genome has 2 copies of 23 chromosomes. Totally there are 6×10^9 bp. Each chromosome contains a single DNA molecule ranging from 34 million bp in the smallest chromosome to 263 million bp in the largest. During a single cycle of cell replication or replication of the entire DNA of a cell, only 1 error/10^9 bp is introduced or only 6 errors or mutations occur in the whole genome of a cell.

Cells need to ensure that:
- DNA replication is very accurate to prevent heritable mutations.
- All parts of the genome/DNA are replicated only once during each cell cycle to avoid chromosomal abnormalities and imbalance.
- Integrity of DNA is maintained as DNA is continuously subject to attack and damage by chemical and physical agents.

Q. 3. Describe the different types of DNA damages and their causes.

Ans. DNA damage, due to environmental factors and normal metabolic processes inside the cell, occurs at a rate of 1,000 to 1,000,000 molecular lesions per cell per day. While this constitutes only 0.000165% of the human genome's approximately 6 billion bases (3 billion base pairs), unrepaired lesions in critical genes (such as tumor suppressor genes) can impede a cell's ability to carry out its function and increase the risk of tumor formation.

Sources and types of damage

Endogenous

Naturally occurring DNA damages arise more than 60,000 times per day per mammalian cell and include:
- Replication errors – if uncorrected by repair pathways lead to mutations.
  - Mismatch or mispairing due to tautomerism or due to ionization of bases – leads to base substitutions.
  - Deletion or extra insertion of bases – leads to frame shifts. These occur due to slipping of newly synthesized strand during replication or recombination (crossing over) and usually occurs at repetitive sequences.
- Attack by free radicals generated during metabolism: 10,000/cell/day.
  - Reactive oxygen species (O_2^*, H_2O_2, OH^* from aerobic metabolism in mitochondria, Haber-Weiss reaction, Fenton reaction) – oxidation of bases [e.g. 8-oxo-7,8-dihydro-guanine (oxoG), 2,800 oxoG/cell/day], thymine glycol, 8-hydroxyguanine, etc. (Fig. 10.4). oxoG mispairs with A, thus after replication G is replaced by T causing mutation. Thymine glycol blocks replication.
  - Oxidative deamination, abasic sites and generation of DNA strand interruptions.
  - Reactive nitrogen species – Nitrous acid converts amine groups on A and C to diazo groups, altering their hydrogen bonding patterns which leads to incorrect base pairing during replication.
  - Lipid peroxidation products – Malondialdehyde-deoxyguanine adduct.

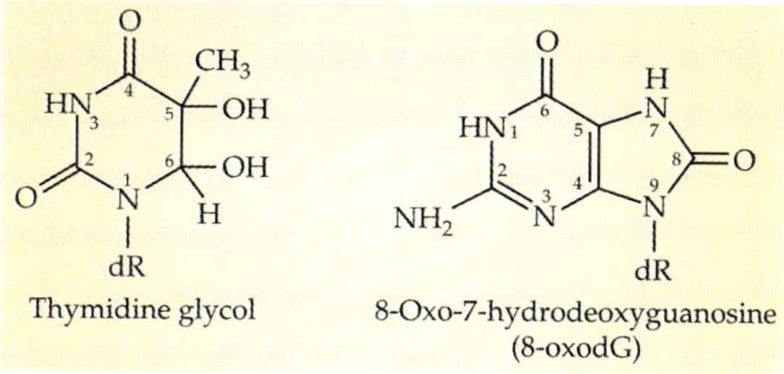

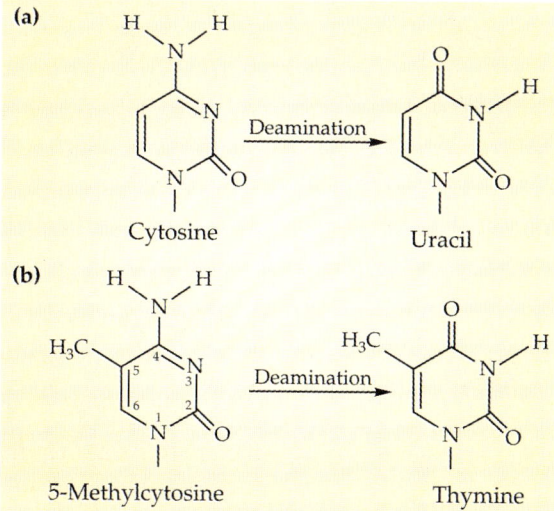

Fig. 10.4. Examples of damaged bases in DNA.

- Methylation – Formation of 7-methylguanine, 1-methyladenine, 6-O-methylguanine (O6-methylguanines – 3,000/cell/day).
- Spontaneous hydrolysis – Hydrolysis of bases, such as deamination, depurination, and depyrimidination.
  - Deamination – Deamination of C to U (190/cell/day).
  - Hydrolysis changes a normal base to an atypical base containing a keto group in place of the original amine group. Examples include C → U and A → HX (hypoxanthine), which can be corrected by DNA repair mechanisms; and 5MeC (5-methylcytosine) → T, which is less likely to be detected as a mutation because thymine is a normal DNA base (Fig. 10.5).
  - Depurination (10,000/cell/day) (Fig. 10.6).
  - Depyrimidination (600/cell/day).

Fig. 10.5. Spontaneous deamination of cytosine → uracil and 5-methyl cytosine → thymine.

Exogenous

- Ultraviolet radiation from the sun [UV 200–400 nm]
  - UV-A (400–315 nm) light creates free radicals which cause damage to DNA like single-strand breaks (indirect damage).

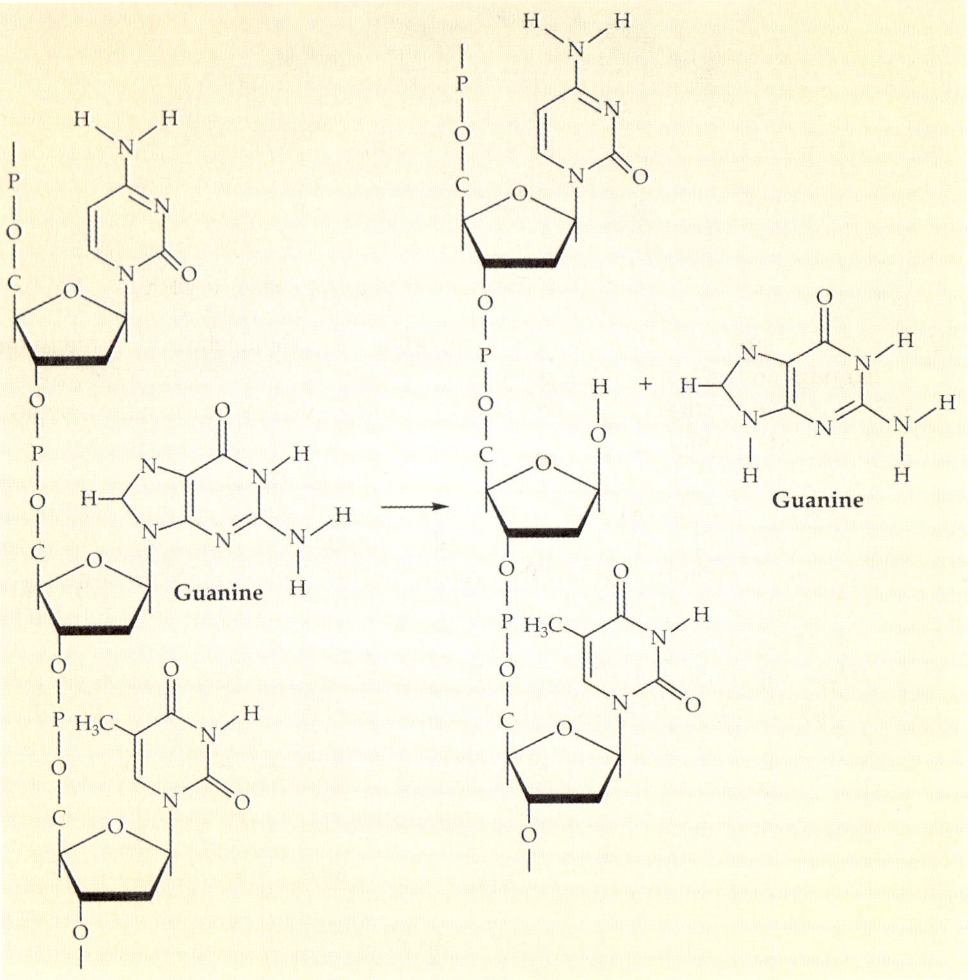

Fig. 10.6. Depurination of DNA.

- UV-B (315–280), UV-C (280–100 nm) light can produce direct damage:
  * Pyrimidine dimers (TT dimers, TC/CT dimers, CC dimers) (Fig. 10.7).
  * Cyclobutane Pyrimidine Dimers (CPDs).
  * UV-generated endonuclease-sensitive sites (ESS).

When DNA polymerase comes along to replicate a strand of DNA with an unrepaired pyrimidine dimer, it reads a CC dimer as AA and not the original CC. This causes the DNA replication mechanism to add a TT on the growing strand (mutation). This mutation can result in cancerous growths (skin cancers), and is known as a "classical C-T mutation". This cancer connection is one reason for concern about ozone depletion and the ozone hole. Individuals with an inherited defect in one of the proteins necessary for nucleotide excision repair (which repairs pyrimidine dimers) suffer from a condition called xeroderma pigmentosum that is characterized by extreme sun-sensitivity and by a high incidence of skin cancers.

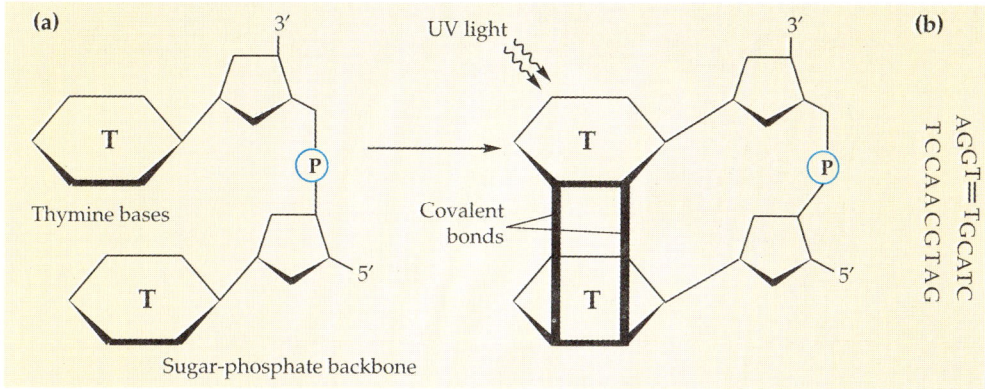

Fig. 10.7. TT dimer generated due to UV light.

- Other radiation frequencies, including X-rays, gamma rays and cosmic rays: These are ionizing radiation which damage DNA by producing single- or double-strand breaks as well as by generating free radicals. Deletion of DNA segments is the predominant form of radiation damage in cells that survive irradiation. It is caused by misrepair of double-strand breaks.
  - Double-strand breaks – 10/cell/day
  - Single-strand breaks – 55,000/cell/day
- Human-made mutagenic chemicals/industrial chemicals – vinyl chloride, hydrogen peroxide, ethylene oxide and environmental chemicals such as polycyclic aromatic hydrocarbons (PAH). Most of these form DNA adducts, increase oxidative damage and lead to mutations and cancers.
  - PAH like benzo[*a*]pyrene is found in tobacco smoke, coal tar, in automobile exhaust fumes (especially from diesel engines), in all smoke resulting from the combustion of organic material (including cigarette smoke), and in charbroiled/barbecued food. Associated with lung and colon cancer.
  - Benzo[*a*]pyrene is a procarcinogen and activated to active carcinogen as shown in Fig. 10.8. The dihydroepoxide product intercalates in DNA, covalently bonding to the nucleophilic guanine nucleobases at the N2 position forming "bulky adducts" (i.e., benzo[*a*]pyrene diol epoxide-dG adduct) (Fig. 10.9). This distorts structure of DNA and during replication G (guanine) to T (thymidine) transversions occur. It may specifically target the tumor suppressor gene p53, leading to cancer.
  - Ethylene oxide used in industries produces N7-(2-hydroxyethyl)guanine (7-HEG) adducts, alkylation at N7 of guanine with subsequent production of abasic sites by spontaneous or enzymatic depurination and promotes base substitutions, frameshift mutations or large deletions.
- Certain plant toxins:
  - Exposure to aristolochic acid (AA), a component of *Aristolochia* plants used in herbal remedies, is associated with chronic kidney disease and urothelial carcinomas of the upper urinary tract. Following metabolic activation, AA reacts with dA and dG residues in DNA to form aristolactam (AL)-DNA adducts.
  - Aflatoxin – Aflatoxin metabolites can intercalate into DNA and alkylate the bases through its epoxide moiety. Mutations in p53 gene leads to liver cancer.

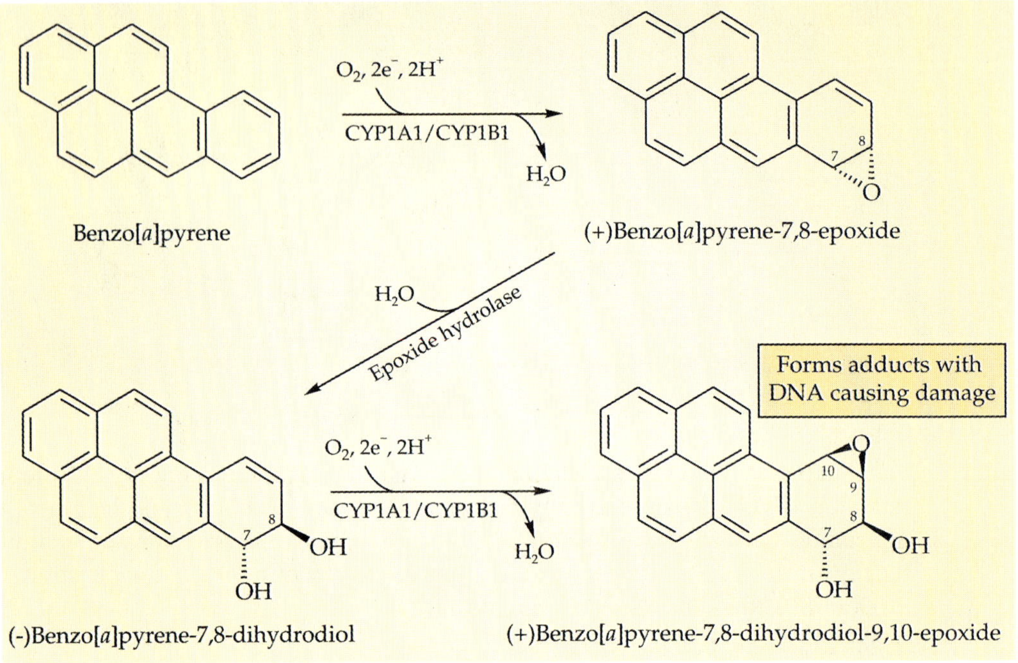

Fig. 10.8. Activation of procarcinogen benzo(a)pyrene to active carcinogen.

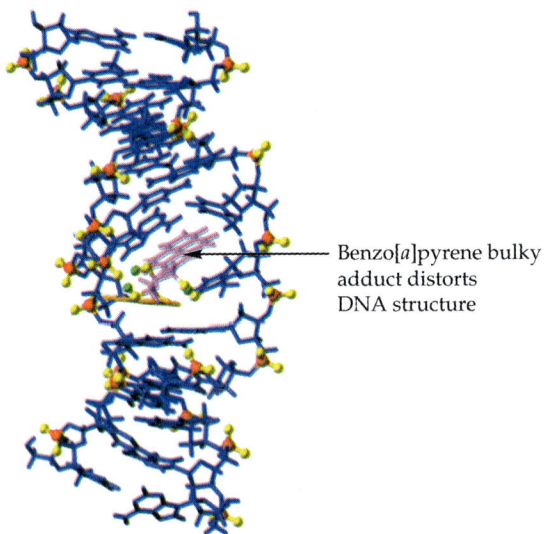

Fig. 10.9. Bulky adduct formed by benzo(a)pyrene.

- Hydrolysis or thermal disruption – Thermal disruption at elevated temperature increases the rate of depurination (loss of purine bases from the DNA backbone) and single-strand breaks.
- Free radical damage – Exogenous compounds can also increase generation of free radicals.

Cells have many repair mechanisms to counter these damages and prevent them from becoming mutations. Thus there is a constant fight between these damaging agents and cellular DNA repair mechanisms and at any particular time many DNA damages can be detected in a cell (Table 10.1). These numbers vary with age, cell and organ type.

Table 10.1. Steady-state amounts of DNA damages

Lesions	Number per cell
Abasic sites	30,000
N7-(2-hydroxyethyl)guanine (7HEG)	3,000
8-hydroxyguanine	2,400
7-(2-oxoethyl)guanine	1,500
Formaldehyde adducts	960
Acrolein-deoxyguanine	120
Malondialdehyde-deoxyguanine	60

Q. 4. What are the consequences of DNA damage/mutations?

Ans.
- Apoptosis
- Ageing
- Cancer
- Diseases – heritable and acquired
- Evolution

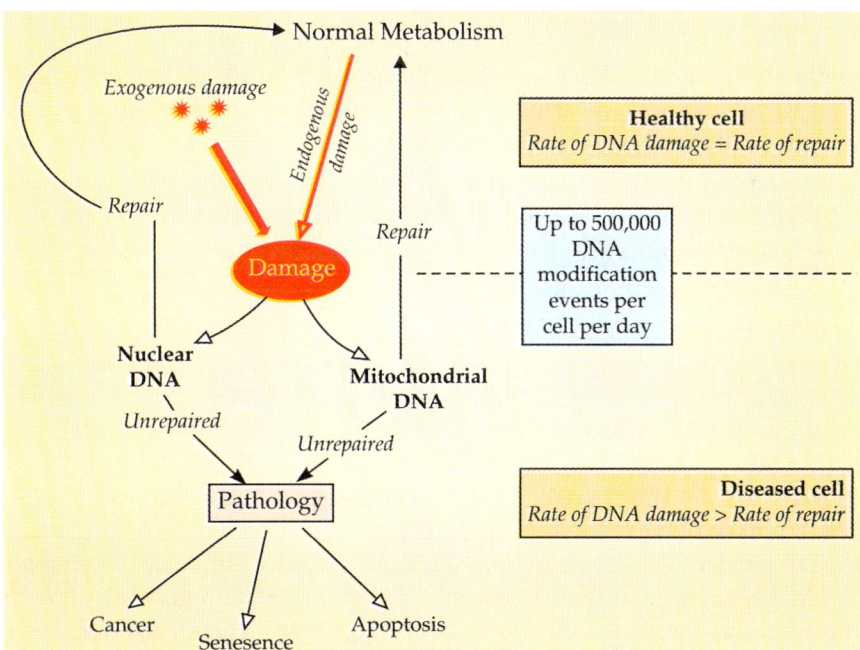

Fig. 10.10. Consequences of DNA damage and mutation.

Apoptosis

- DNA damage can be detected and repaired before next cell replication. If it cannot be repaired the cell is destined to undergo apoptosis or programmed cell death (mediated by p53 and Rb genes).
- Undetected damage and mutations can alter the normal gene function. Many mutations may be silent i.e. not have any impact on protein synthesis and function. However, other mutations alter cell function and lead to pathological consequences.
- DNA damages are a special problem in non-dividing or slowly dividing cells, where unrepaired damages will tend to accumulate over time. The accumulation of unrepaired DNA damage is more prevalent in certain types of cells, particularly in non-replicating or slowly replicating cells, such as cells in the brain, skeletal and cardiac muscle.
- On the other hand, in rapidly dividing cells, unrepaired DNA damages that do not kill the cell by blocking replication will tend to cause replication errors and thus mutation. The great majority of mutations that are not neutral in their effect are deleterious to a cell's survival. Thus, in a population of cells comprising a tissue with replicating cells, mutant cells will tend to be lost or die out.
- However, infrequent mutations that provide a survival advantage will tend to clonally expand at the expense of neighboring cells in the tissue. This advantage to the cell is disadvantageous to the whole organism, and such mutant cells can give rise to cancer. Thus, DNA damages in frequently dividing cells, because they give rise to mutations, are a prominent cause of cancer.
- In contrast, DNA damages in infrequently dividing cells are a prominent cause of ageing.

Ageing

Slow accumulation of unrepaired DNA damage and mutations in infrequently dividing cells gradually cause loss of critical functions and decreased cell functionality, e.g.

- Reduction in both renal blood flow and glomerular filtration rate, and impairment in the ability to concentrate urine and to conserve sodium and water with age.
- Loss of long-lived stem cells, decreased healing capacity.
- Increased oxidative damage, decreased protein synthesis.
- Decreased muscle strength and stamina.
- Decreased memory, cognitive power, vision, hearing loss, etc.

With age the markers of DNA damage have been found to increase and evidence also comes from the genetic diseases which hamper DNA repair (defects in DNA repair) which are associated with premature ageing, e.g. Werner's syndrome (mean lifespan 47 years), Hutchinson–Gilford progeria syndrome (mean lifespan 13 years), and Cockayne syndrome (mean lifespan 13 years). Werner's syndrome is due to an inherited defect in an enzyme (a helicase and exonuclease) that acts in base excision repair of DNA. Hutchinson–Gilford progeria syndrome is due to a defect in Lamin A protein which forms a scaffolding within the cell nucleus to organize chromatin and is needed for repair of double-strand breaks in DNA. Cockayne syndrome is due to a defect in a protein necessary for the repair process, transcription-coupled nucleotide excision repair, which can remove damages, particularly oxidative DNA damages, that block transcription. In addition to these three conditions, several other human syndromes, that also have defective DNA repair, show several features of premature ageing. These include ataxia telangiectasia, Nijmegen breakage syndrome, some subgroups of xeroderma pigmentosum, trichothiodystrophy, Fanconi anemia, Bloom's syndrome and Rothmund–Thomson syndrome.

Cancer

Inactivating/loss of function mutations in tumor suppressor genes greatly increase the likelihood of tumor formation. Tumor suppressor genes are involved in keeping a check on cell cycle/cell growth and replication. They also are involved in DNA repair. Defects in DNA repair lead to significant increase in mutations in many genes, including other tumor suppressor genes and oncogenes accelerating the process of cancer development. Oncogenes are usually growth factors or their receptors. Gain of function mutation in these cause unregulated activation of cell replication and growth stimulating pathways, development of new blood vessels, telomerase activation, etc. This leads to uncontrolled cell multiplication and growth or, in other words, cancer.

Diseases

New mutations in gametes may lead to fetal death in any trimester (most common in 1st trimester). If not lethal they are transferred to progeny leading to genetic or heritable diseases like sickle cell anaemia, phenylketonuria, Down's syndrome, etc.

Mutations in somatic cells in a multicellular organism and humans lead to ageing and cancer. Mutations in tissue like hemopoietic stem cells can cause both excessive replication (neoplasia) or failure of tissue repair (aplasia, e.g. aplastic anemia).

Evolution

Just like mutations can increase cell survival, inherited mutations (in gametes) can confer increased survival advantage to the organism. Natural selection leads to their increased survival and over the time evolution. Mutations produce variability, some of which may confer advantage in a changed environment and thus become adaptation and lead to evolution.

Q. 5. What is photoreactivation?

Ans. Photoreactivation is a specific mechanism for repair of cyclobutane pyrimidine dimers produced by UV radiation (Fig. 10.11).

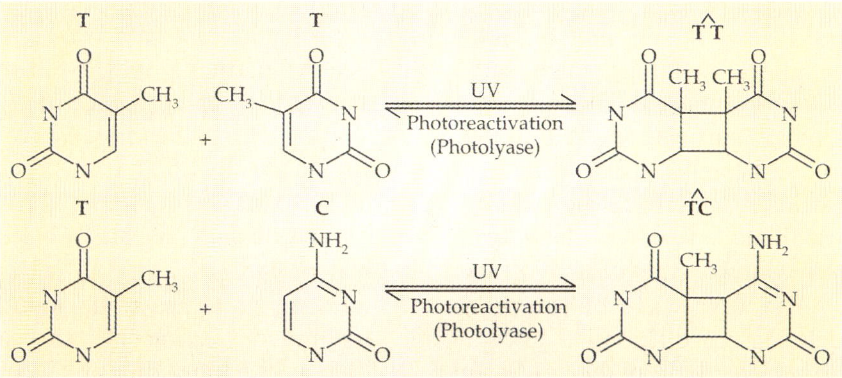

Fig. 10.11. Photoreactivation.

This mechanism requires visible light, preferentially from the violet/blue end of the spectrum, and an enzyme photolyase.

Photolyase is a phylogenetically old enzyme, which is present and functional in many species in the bacteria, fungi, plants and animals. Photolyase is particularly important in repairing UV-induced damage in plants. However, it is no longer working in humans and other placental mammals who instead rely on the less efficient nucleotide excision repair mechanism.

Photolyases bind complementary DNA strands and break certain types of pyrimidine dimers that arise when a pair of thymine or cytosine bases on the same strand of DNA become covalently linked due to action of UV light. These dimers result in a 'bulge' of the DNA structure and photolyases have a high affinity for these lesions and reversibly bind and convert them back to the original bases.

Photolyases are flavoproteins and contain two light-harvesting cofactors. All photolyases contain the two electron-reduced FADH and either the pterin methenyltetrahydrofolate (MTHF) in folate photolyases or the deazaflavin 8-hydroxy-7,8-didemethyl-5-deazariboflavin (8-HDF) in deazaflavin photolyases. Some sunscreens include photolyase in their ingredients, claiming a reparative action on UV-damaged skin.

Q. 6. Why combination therapy is required in HIV treatment?

Ans. HIV (Human immunodeficiency virus) infection causes AIDS. The virus has two strands of RNA as its genome. A key event in the viral life cycle is the synthesis of copy of DNA of the viral genome by reverse transcriptase (Fig. 10.12). Unlike DNA polymerase reverse transcriptase does not carry out proofreading. This leads to very high rates of mutations (hypermutation) in the viral genome. Combined with a very high replicative rate, a very large number of mutants are present in a single patient. Molecular analyses of HIV isolates reveal varying levels of sequence diversity over all regions of the viral genome. For example, the degree of difference in the coding sequences of the viral envelope protein ranges from a few percent to 50%. The mutations may be of disadvantage or advantage to the virus. The virus particles with deleterious mutations in critical regions quickly die out and are compensated by the extremely high proliferation rate in the virus population.

But the rapid mutations in the surface proteins allow the virus particles to evade the immune system as the antibodies synthesized by the body against the surface proteins become useless against the mutated proteins. Their selection pressure allows the virus to adapt. Similarly, mutations which confer resistance to a particular drug by changing the structure of reverse transcriptase or protease are of benefit in the presence of the particular drug. Quickly particles resistant to the drug become predominant as sensitive strains are killed and resistant ones survive and keep multiplying at a very high rate. This is like accelerated evolution. To prevent any single drug from developing resistance quickly multiple drugs are used simultaneously as it is very unlikely that a particular viral particle will develop mutations that confer resistance to all of them simultaneously.

HIV can evolve by several means, including simple base substitution, insertions and deletions, recombination, and gain and loss of glycosylation sites. HIV sequence diversity arises directly from the limited fidelity of the reverse transcriptase. The balance of immune pressure and functional constraints on proteins influence the regional level of variation within

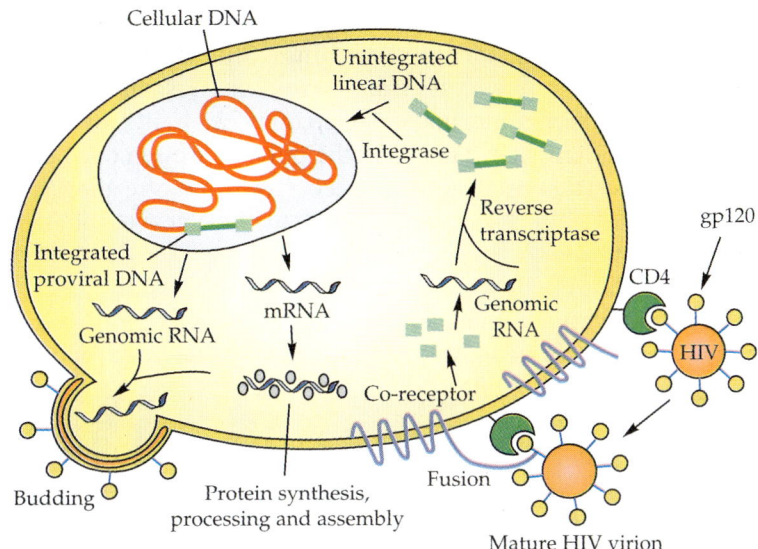

Fig. 10.12. Life cycle of HIV virus.

proteins. For example, envelope, which is exposed on the surface of the virion and is under immune selective pressure from both antibodies and cytolytic T lymphocytes, is extremely variable, with clusters of mutations in hypervariable domains.

Q. 7. What is proofreading by DNA polymerase and how does it occur?

Ans. Proofreading simply means the process of checking or revising the sequence of nucleotides added during replication so as to find any mismatch/error and correct it. It is like reading each word gain as it is typed or written before going to next word to check for spelling errors and correct it there and then only. DNA polymerase has the capability to simultaneously check the previous few nucleotides added for any mismatch and halt if there is any error and to correct it.

The bacterial polymerase III has a high processivity of adding around 50,000 bases at a stretch at very high speed (10^5 bases per minute) before dissociating from template strand. The eukaryotic polymerase δ replicates the entire available template with the help of sliding clamp (PCNA) at a speed of 5,000 bases per minute. Thus, DNA polymerase does not pass over the newly synthesized strand or added bases again once it moves forward. Proofreading is actually achieved by having both 5′ to 3′ polymerase and 3′ to 5′ exonuclease activity. As long as there is no mispairing in previous 8–10 bases added, the new strand is bound to template neatly and the last nucleotide is a poor substrate for exonuclease activity but good substrate for polymerase activity allowing replication to continue at high speed.

If a wrong base is added then it disturbs the hydrogen bonding between the two strands producing a physical bulge. This makes it a poor substrate for polymerase activity and good one for exonuclease activity. The polymerase is then unable to add the next base and pauses. The pause allows the new strand to separate a little from the template and reposition into the exonuclease site of DNA polymerase. Then the enzyme cleaves the wrongly added last base and sometimes a few more bases along with it and then again resumes polymerase activity as the deformity is corrected (Fig. 10.13).

Without proofreading the error rate is $1/10^4$ to $1/10^6$ which is unacceptable. Proofreading improves accuracy by a hundred million times. Still, despite the vastly improved accuracy due to proofreading, replication errors can occur (mispairing due to tautomerism, etc.). Sometimes due to thermal fluctuations there may be slight movement in between the bases of new strand and template. Then also the polymerase removes the correct base also and adds it again. This is the cost of achieving accuracy by proofreading (having 3′–5′ exonuclease activity). A mutated polymerase very sensitive to movements or physical disturbance between new and template strand or having stronger exonuclease activity will be more accurate (better proofreading) but will remove more correct bases also, and hence becomes slower and energetically very wasteful. The rare errors left after proofreading can be corrected by repair mechanisms and errors still remaining (mutations) are fodder for evolution!

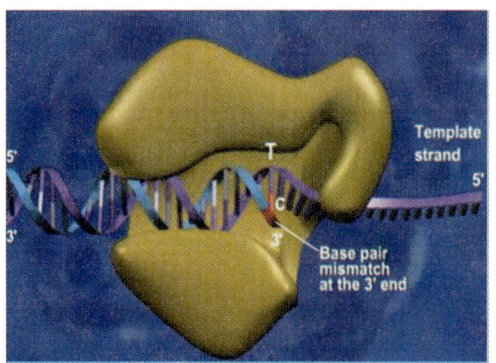 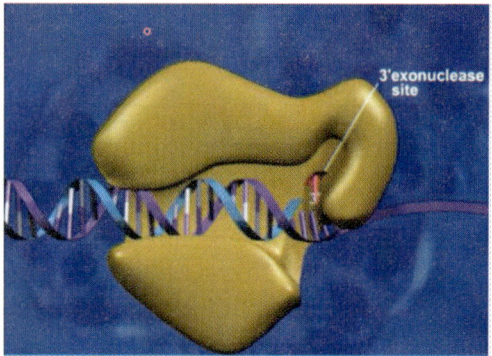

Fig. 10.13. Mechanism of proofreading. Mismatched base inhibits polymerase activity and leads to physical repositioning of base to the 3′ exonuclease site.

Q. 8. Why primer is required for DNA replication?

Ans. RNA polymerase can synthesize RNA without any primer but DNA polymerases require a RNA primer to initiate synthesis. The most likely explanation lies in relation to proofreading activity of DNA polymerase. The ability to discriminate between properly and incorrectly incorporated bases is hampered when the growing chain is very short (< 8 nucleotides) as the overall strength of base pairing between a short chain and template is weak. Thus DNA polymerases have evolved to start from a RNA primer which is eventually replaced by DNA later during replication. This prevents replication errors in the first few bases which would otherwise be missed due to lack of proofreading. Proofreading can easily occur during gap filling when RNA primers are removed and replaced by DNA.

Q. 9. What is end replication problem?

Ans. As the replication bubble reaches the end of the chromosome or the telomere the synthesis of the leading strand on the 3′ to 5′ template is completed continuously without any problems. But on the 5′ to 3′ template strand where synthesis occurs by formation of Okazaki fragments there occurs a problem called the end replication problem. As shown in Fig. 10.14 synthesis of the last primer at the 3′ end leaves a few bases where the primase sits (step 2). Further when the primer is removed (step 4) the total remaining gap cannot be filled as there is no

CHROMOSOME SHORTENING DURING NORMAL DNA REPLICATION

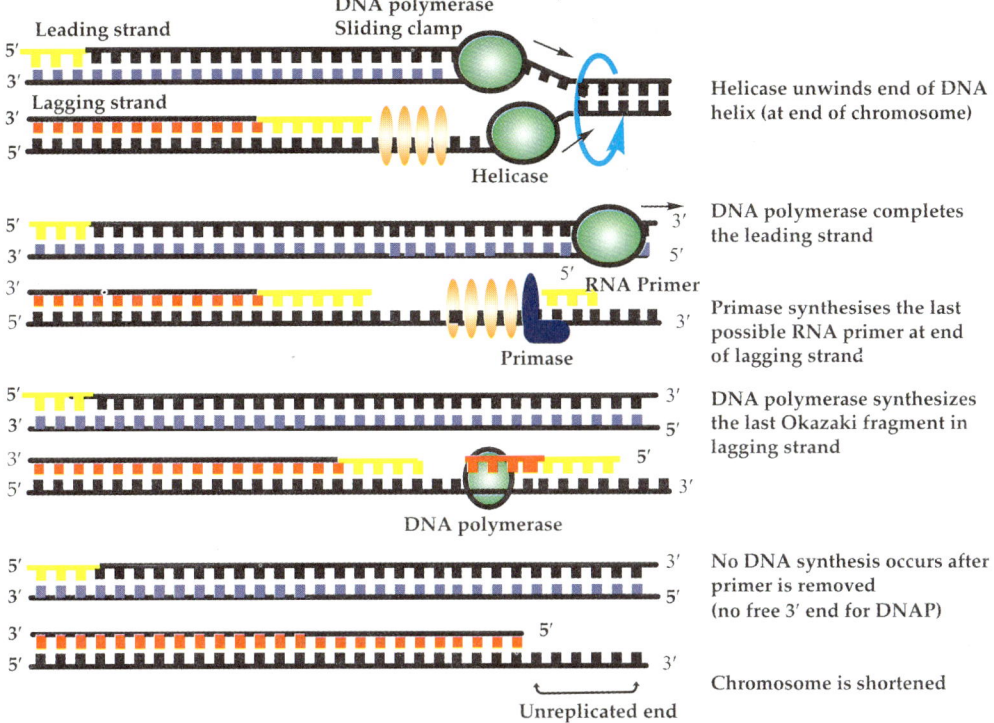

Fig. 10.14. End replication problem.

DNA template to make new primer. Thus one of the daughter strands (lagging strand on 5′ to 3′ parent strand) remains shorter. This shortening would repeat each time cell replication occurs leading to chromosomal shortening until it reaches some critical gene (after a finite number of cell replications) when it will hamper cellular function leading to apoptosis. This leads to ageing or senescence of the cell population. Without preventing this shortening cell lines cannot be maintained for many generations (Fig. 10.15).

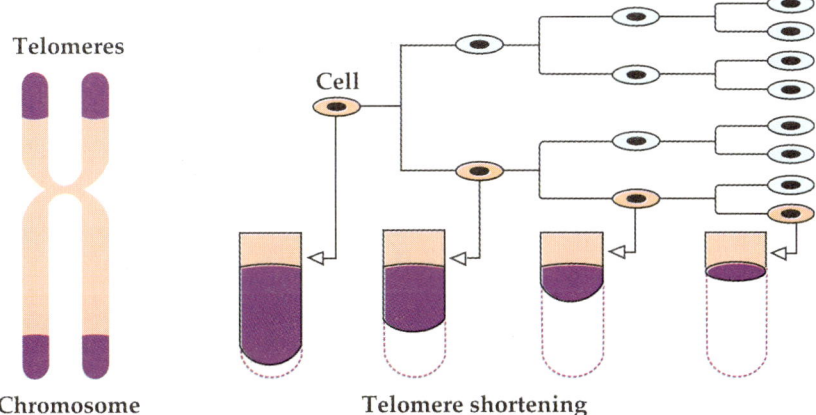

Fig. 10.15. Telomere shortening.

To overcome this problem and also to protect the ends of DNA from exonuclease digestion the linear ends of the eukaryotic chromosomes have specialized structures called telomeres (Fig. 10.16) at the end of the chromosomes. The ends in humans contain repeat of TTAGGG (5' to 3') for multiple times extending upto 1000 base pairs (Fig. 10.17). Further, the end is modified into a circular T loop to prevent exonuclease digestion. These repeats ensure that the critical genes are not shortened till many cell replications (Figs. 10.17 and 10.18).

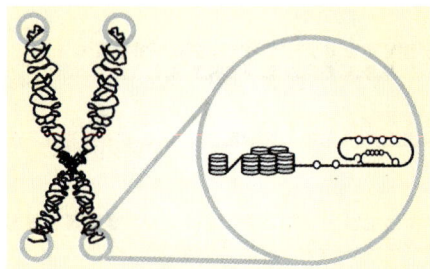

Fig. 10.16. The structure of telomeres.

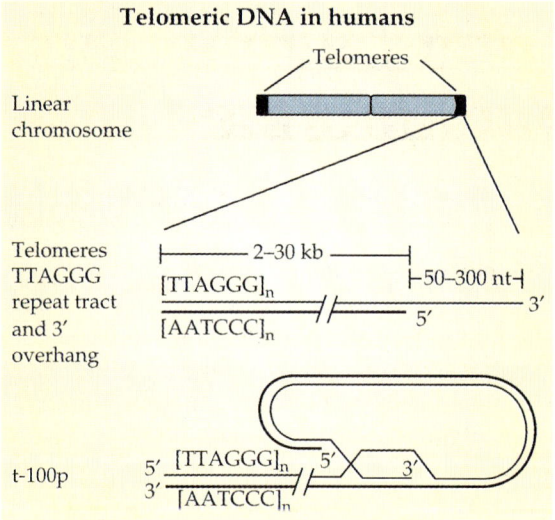

Fig. 10.17. TTAGGG repeats in telomeres and the T loop.

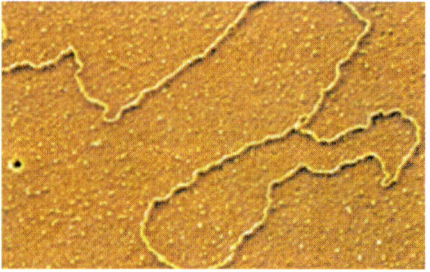

Fig. 10.18. T loop at the end of a chromosome. It prevents exonuclease digestion.

Further, the provision of enzyme telomerase is there to prevent shortening in rapidly dividing cells, stem cells and in cancer cells. This enzyme has reverse transcriptase activity and contains an in-built RNA template (CCCAAUCCC) complementary to the telomeric repeat. This enzyme binds to the 5′ to 3′ parent template strand and extends it using the in-built RNA template. It moves down the DNA to add additional TTAGGG repeats. Then, on the extended parent strand primase makes new primer and DNA polymerase extends it to complete the lagging daughter strand. A unpaired hang of TTAGGG is still left on the parent strand. This prevents DNA shortening (Fig. 10.19). After this the T loop is resynthesized to complete the telomeric end.

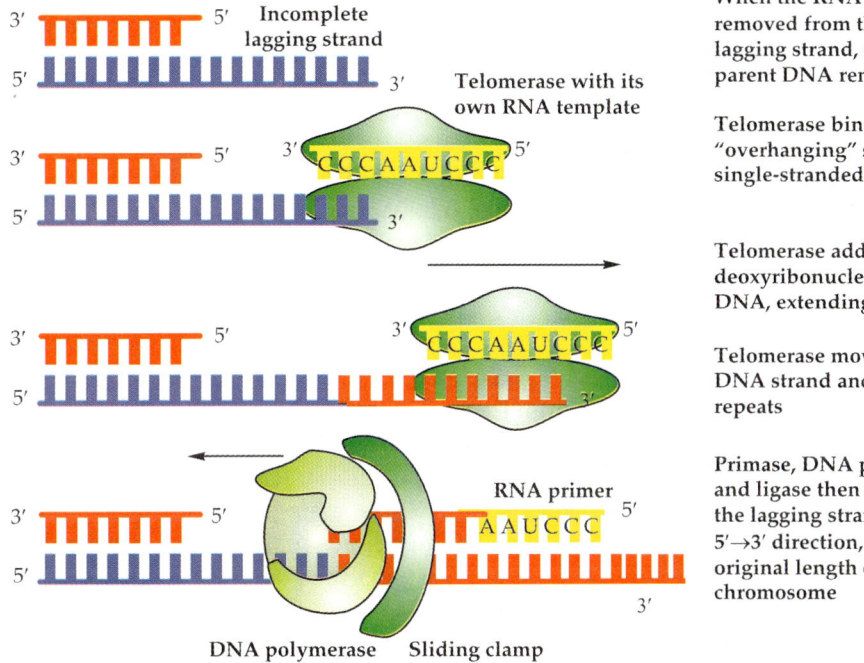

Fig. 10.19. Action of telomerase.

Q. 10. What are the similarities and differences between eukaryotes and prokaryotes in DNA replication?

Ans. Cell division in eukaryotes is carried out in the context of the cell cycle. Unlike prokaryotes, which can double under optimal conditions in as little as 20 min, the eukaryotic cell cycle takes some 18 to 24 hours.

Similarities between prokaryotic and eukaryotic replication
- Both are bi-directional processes.
- DNA polymerases work 5′ to 3′.
- Leading and lagging strands (Okazaki fragments).
- Primers are required.
- Topoisomerases are required to remove supercoiling.

Unique problems faced by eukaryotes that are not faced by prokaryotes

- Linear chromosomes with ends unlike circular chromosome in prokaryotes.
- Much more genetic material – the typical animal cell has 50 times more DNA than the average bacterium (*E. coli* has 4.6 million base pairs, humans have 3000 million base pairs or 650 times as much!!).
- Much more packaging – the nucleosomes (DNA wound around histones) and all the scaffolds and higher order packing. Dissociation of nucleosome is required for replication and limits the rate of DNA replication.
- DNA polymerases that are found in eukaryotes work much slower. At the rate they work it would take 30 days to copy the human genome if it was left to 2 replication forks! The average *E. coli* replication fork works around the chromosome at a staggering 10^5 bases per minute. Eukaryotic enzymes can only manage somewhere between 500 and 5000 bases per minute.

To overcome these problems, eukaryotes have:

- **Multiple initiation sites:** There are multiple initiation sites scattered some 30 to 300 kilobases apart. Mammalian cells have ~20,000 initiation sites. Prokaryotic genomes have only one initiation site (origin of replication) and a circular genome, thus replication starts once, proceeds bidirectionally and is terminated at the opposite end of circular genome when both replication forks meet. In eukaryotes the multiple origin sites and replication bubbles mean that mechanisms are required to prevent reinitiation and ensure that entire genome is replicated during one S phase of cell cycle.
- **Differences in Okazaki fragments:** Each origin of replication begins with the binding of a large protein complex – the Origin Recognition Complex (ORC). Following it the mini-chromosome maintenance protein (MCM) with helicase activity binds and catalyses strand separation to form replication bubble. Then SSBs or single-strand binding proteins keep the strands separate. Then the primase/pol α complex makes the 10 nucleotide primer of RNA and then switches to dNTPs, elongating the primer by 15–30 nucleotides after which pol α takes over. pol β works continuously on leading strand while on lagging strand Okazaki fragments of 130–200 bp are formed. Prokaryotic Okazaki fragments are 10 times longer. Eukaryotic size of 200 bp is due to the fact that dissociation of one nucleosome frees about 200 bp of DNA only.
- **Prevention of reinitiation:** The ORC and MCM complexes accumulate during G1 phase of the cell cycle. Their assembly can occur only in presence of 'licensing factors' – CDC6 (cell division cycle protein 6) and Cdt1 (chromatin licensing and cell division factor 1). The initiation complex is now described as licensed to begin replication. After initiation CDC6 and MCM are phosphorylated by cyclin-dependent and other kinases. The protein geminin binds and inactivates Cdt1 preventing premature reinitiation during single cell cycle. For that origin to be reused new CDC6 and licensing factors are required which are available only in next G1 phase. Thus in the G1 phase all origins are licensed and initiated only once. Replication occurs in the following S phase. After G1 phase the MCM are no longer available.
- The whole genome is not simultaneously replicated. It appears that clusters of 20 to 80 sites are initiated together. Forks extend from both sides of each initiation site and move in opposite directions until they fuse with an approaching fork from an adjacent site. New clusters are activated throughout S phase of the cell cycle and it takes several hours to copy the whole genome.

- Different regions of genome are replicated at different times in the S phase. Actively transcribed regions replicate early and heterochromatin (condensed chromatin, not actively transcribed) replicates late in S phase.
- **Different enzymes** (Table 10.2): The enzymes used by eukaryotes are different. There are many, named pol α, pol γ, pol δ1 and pol ε. Not only do they have different enzymes but eukaryotic cells have more copies of these enzymes than do prokaryotes. One typical animal cell has between 20,000 and 60,000 molecules of pol α whereas a regular bacterium, *E. coli*, has 10 to 20 molecules of DNA pol III.
- The ends of chromosomes are protected by repeated sequence and T loops. They may get progressively shortened leading to senescence or are maintained by telomerase in rapidly dividing cells, stem cells and cancer cells.
- Once the DNA has replicated in eukaryotes it must be packaged. This happens rapidly after replication. The cell must synthesise the required histones as replication proceeds (it doesn't have enough stored histones to do the packing).

Table 10.2. Enzymes and proteins involved in replication in prokaryotes and eukaryotes

Protein	Prokaryotic/ Eukaryotic	Activity/Role
DNA Polymerase I	Prokaryotic	5' to 3' polymerase, 3' to 5' exonuclease, 5' to 3' exonuclease
DNA Polymerase III	Prokaryotic	5' to 3' polymerase, 3' to 5' exonuclease, proofreading
DNA Polymerase α	Eukaryotic	5' to 3' polymerase, complexes with primase then begins DNA synthesis from RNA primers, low processivity (~100 nt), no exonuclease activity
DNA Polymerase δ	Eukaryotic	5' to 3' polymerase, 3' to 5' exonuclease (proof reading), high processivity when complexed with PCNA, replicates entire leading strand
DNA Polymerase ε	Eukaryotic	5' to 3' polymerase, high processivity, probable regulatory role
DNA Polymerase γ	Eukaryotic	Mitochondrial DNA polymerase (5' to 3')
Primase	Both	RNA polymerase (5' to 3') makes primers
DNA helicase	Both	Untwists DNA
Single-stranded binding protein (SSBP)	Both	Coats DNA to prevent strands re-annealing
Topoisomerases (Type I and Type II)	Both	Relieves stress of supercoiling (type I) and introduces negative supercoiling (type II)
DNA gyrase	Prokaryotic	Type II topoisomerase
DNA ligase	Both	Seals breaks in the DNA backbone between 3' OH and 5' PO_4 requires energy source
Initiator proteins	Both	Bind at the origin of replication
Telomerase	Eukaryotic	Reverse transcriptase activity (5' to 3') using an endogenous RNA template
pols β, η, ι, κ and ζ	Eukaryotic	Repair enzymes

Q. 11. A 3-year-old male child presented with brownish-black pigmentation on the sun exposed part of the body like face, hands and neck at the age of 2 years. Dry skin was also evident. He also complained of burning sensation on exposure to sunlight. There were no other findings. What is the probable diagnosis? How can it be confirmed and managed?

Ans. The child is suffering from a form of xeroderma pigmentosum, a disorder in which thymine dimers (created by exposure to UV light) cannot be appropriately repaired in DNA. Xeroderma pigmentosum is a rare disorder transmitted in an autosomal recessive manner. It is characterized by photosensitivity, pigmentary changes, premature skin aging, and malignant tumor development. Some subjects also have progressive neurological degeneration. These manifestations are due to a cellular hypersensitivity to ultraviolet (UV) radiation resulting from a defect in nucleotide excision repair (NER).

Besides thymine dimers produced by UV light, damage due to cisplatin (anticancer drug), benzopyrene and aflatoxin (bulky adducts) are also repaired by this mechanism. Recognition of the damage leads to removal of a short single-stranded DNA segment that contains the lesion. The undamaged single-stranded DNA remains and DNA polymerase uses it as a template to synthesize a short complementary sequence. Final ligation to complete NER and form a double-stranded DNA is carried out by DNA ligase.

Two types of NER exist: global genome (GG-NER) and transcription coupled (TC-NER). Seven xeroderma pigmentosum repair genes, XPA through XP, are involved. These genes play key roles in GG-NER and TC-NER. The two sub-pathways differ in how they recognize DNA damage but they share the same process for lesion incision, repair, and ligation (Fig. 10.20).

Damage recognition

Global genomic NER is not dependent on transcription and repairs both actively transcribed and other regions. This pathway employs several "damage sensing" proteins including the DNA-damage binding (DDB) and XPC-Rad23B complexes that constantly scan the genome and recognize helix distortions. XPA is also involved. Upon identification and binding of a damaged site, subsequent repair proteins are then recruited to the damaged DNA to verify presence of DNA damage, excise the damaged DNA surrounding the lesion and then fill in the repair patch.

NER repairs the transcribed strands of transcriptionally active genes faster than it repairs nontranscribed strands and transcriptionally silent DNA. For this TC-NER is initiated when RNA polymerase stalls/halts at a lesion in DNA – the blocked RNA polymerase serves as a damage recognition signal. Then CS proteins CSA and CSB bind the DNA damage site.

Common pathway

- TFIIH and XPG are then first recruited to the site of DNA damage (XPG stabilizes TFIIH). The TFIIH subunits of XPD and XPB act as a helicase and ATPase respectively – they help unwind DNA and generate a junction between the double-stranded and single-stranded DNA around the transcription bubble. In addition to stabilizing TFIIH, XPG also has endonuclease activity; it cuts DNA damage on the 3′ side while the XPF-ERCC1 heterodimeric protein cuts on the 5′ side. The dual incision leads to the removal of a ssDNA with a single strand gap of 25~30 nucleotides (Fig. 10.20).

- Replication protein A (RPA) and XPA are the last two proteins associated with the main NER repair complex. These two proteins are present prior to TFIIH binding since they are involved with verifying DNA damage. They may also protect single-stranded DNA. After verification, the 5' side incision is made and DNA repair begins before the 3' side incision. This helps reduce exposed single-stranded DNA during the repair process.
- Replication factor C (RFC) loads the Proliferating Cell Nuclear Antigen (PCNA) onto the DNA strand. This allows DNA polymerases implicated in repair (δ, ε and/or κ) to copy the undamaged strand via translocation. DNA ligase I and Flap endonuclease 1 or the Ligase-III-XRCC1 complex seal the nicks to complete NER.

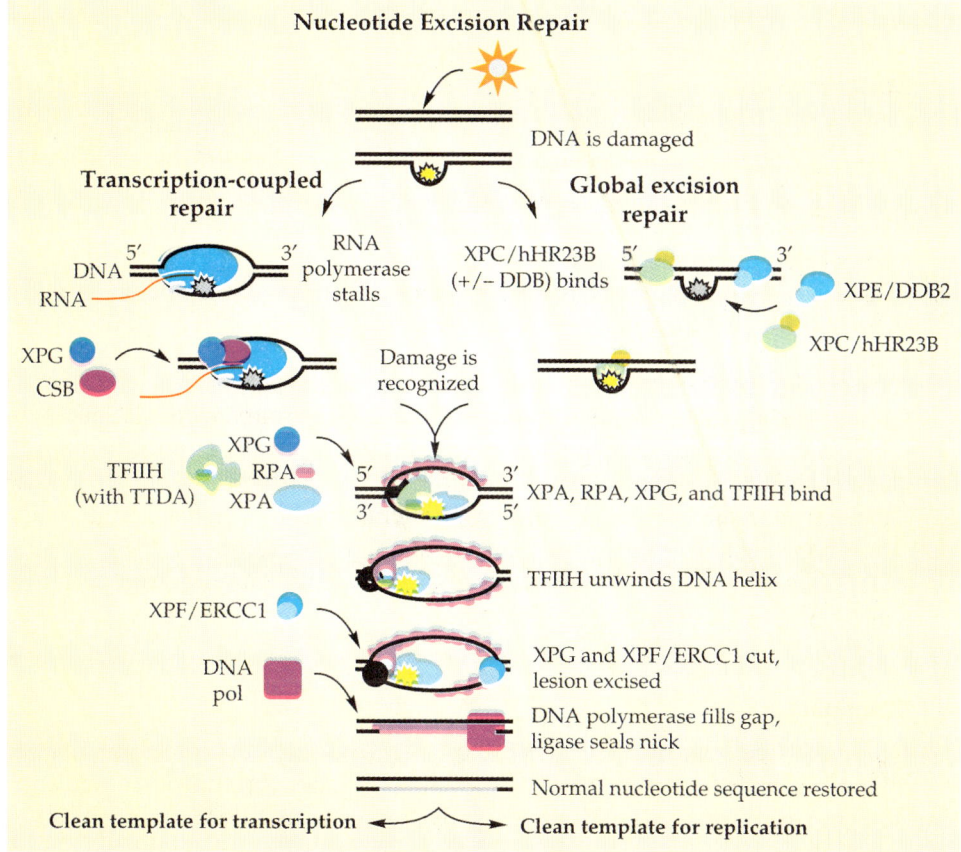

Fig. 10.20. Nucleotide excision repair.

Defects in any of XPA to XPG or XPV (XP variant) causes xeroderma pigmentosum (7 complementation groups).

Features

Skin

- The skin is healthy at birth. The first stage appears after age of 6 months. This stage is characterized by diffuse erythema, scaling, and freckle-like areas of increased pigmentation

over light-exposed areas, appearing initially on the face (photosensitivity to 290–320 nm). With progression of the disease, the skin changes appear on the lower legs, the neck, and even the trunk in extreme cases. While these features tend to diminish during the winter months with decreased sun exposure, as time passes, these findings become permanent.
- The second stage is characterized by poikiloderma. Poikiloderma consists of skin atrophy, telangiectasias, and mottled hyperpigmentation and hypopigmentation, giving rise to an appearance similar to that of chronic radiodermatitis.
- The third stage is heralded by the appearance of numerous malignancies, including squamous cell carcinomas, malignant melanoma, basal cell carcinoma, and fibrosarcoma. These malignancies may occur as early as age 4–5 years and are more prevalent in sun-exposed areas.

Ocular problems
- Occur in nearly 80% of individuals with xeroderma pigmentosum.
- They include photophobia, conjunctivitis, eyelid solar lentigines, malignant melanoma, ectropion, symblepharon with ulceration, repeated conjunctival inflammation, infections, and scarring.
- Vascular pterygia, fibrovascular pannus of the cornea, and epitheliomas of the lids, the conjunctivae, and the cornea can occur.
- Squamous cell carcinoma, basal cell carcinoma, sebaceous cell carcinoma, and fibrosarcoma can also involve the eyes.

Neurologic problems
- Seen in nearly 20% of patients, more commonly in groups with XPA and XPD mutations.
- Microcephaly, spasticity, hyporeflexia or areflexia, ataxia, chorea, motor neuron signs or segmental demyelination, sensorineural deafness, supranuclear ophthalmoplegia, and mental retardation. The neurologic problems might overshadow the cutaneous manifestations in some patients with xeroderma pigmentosum.
- De Sanctis-Cacchione syndrome refers to the combination of xeroderma pigmentosum and neurologic abnormalities (including mental retardation and cerebellar ataxia), hypogonadism, and dwarfism.

Diagnosis
- Studies of cellular hypersensitivity to UV radiation and chromosomal breakage studies: In the cellular hypersensitivity to UV radiation and chromosomal breakage studies, the xeroderma pigmentosum fibroblasts are stressed with different doses of UV radiation and chromosomal breakage is evaluated in at least 100–200 cells. Prenatal diagnosis of xeroderma pigmentosum can be accomplished using similar chromosomal breakage studies on amniocytes from at-risk fetuses.
- Complementation studies: The xeroderma pigmentosum complementation groups can be determined using cell-fusion techniques followed by assessment of DNA repair.
- Gene sequencing: Gene sequencing to identify the specific gene complementation group.

Management
- Protection from sunlight by physical and chemical sunscreens and protective clothing. Patients are also sensitive to tobacco smoke (benzopyrene, etc.) and need to be protected.

- Oral retinoids have been shown to decrease the incidence of skin cancer in patients with xeroderma pigmentosum.
- Chemical therapy with 5-fluorouracil for actinic keratosis.
- Surgery for malignancies.
- A new approach to photoprotection is to repair DNA damage after UV exposure. This can be accomplished by delivery of a DNA repair enzyme into the skin by means of specially engineered liposomes. T4 endonuclease V has been shown to repair cyclobutane pyrimidine dimers resulting from DNA damage.
- Gene therapy (using adeno- and retroviruses) for xeroderma pigmentosum is still in a theoretical and experimental stage.

Mutations in TC-NER machinery are responsible for multiple genetic disorders including:

- Trichothiodystrophy (TTD): In some individuals – photosensitivity, ichthyosis, mental/physical retardation.
- Cockayne syndrome (CS): Photosensitivity, mental retardation, progeria-like features, microcephaly, mutations occur in CSA or CSB.

Membrane and Transport

Chapter 11

Q. 1. What are the different types of lipids present in membranes and their significance?

Ans. Membranes contain three major types of lipids: Glycerophospholipids, Cholesterol and Shingolipids. All these lipids are amphiphatic and, besides forming the structural bilayer of the membrane, they also serve specific active functions. Membranes of different tissues and different cell organelles have different proportion of these lipids but the composition of each type of membrane is constant and unique. This suggests a relationship between specific function of these membranes and lipids contained in them (Fig. 11.1).

Different lipids have different shapes and their distribution affects the membrane shape, fluidity, vesicle and endosome formation and fusion. The shape of a membrane lipid depends on the relative size of its polar head group and non-polar tails. When the head group and lipid backbone have similar cross-sectional areas, the molecule has a cylindrical shape (phosphatidylcholine (PC) and phosphatidylserine (PS)). Lipids with a small head group like phosphatidylethanolamine (PE) are cone-shaped. By contrast, when the hydrophobic part occupies a relatively smaller surface area, the molecule has the shape of an inverted cone (lysophosphatidylcholine (LPC) and, to some extent, sphingomyelin). This 'lipid polymorphism' has a physiological role in the generation of curvature as during vesicle budding, and membrane fusion. Cholesterol and sphingomyelin are also important for stabilizing membranes during fusion, and phosphatidylethanolamine greatly stimulates membrane fusion (Fig. 11.2).

Arachidonic acid and other PUFA are released by phospholipase A2 for synthesis of eicosanoids. Membrane lipids are also involved in correct folding of transmembrane proteins and are called lipidochaperones.

1. Glycerophospholipids
These include:

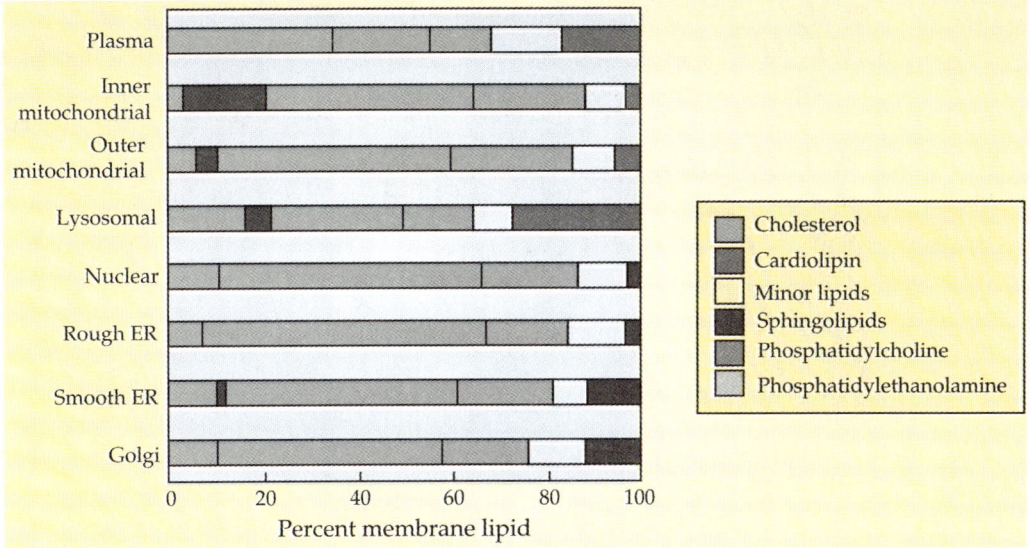

Fig. 11.1. Distribution of different lipids in different membrane types.

Phosphatidylcholine or lecithin

Phosphatidylcholine is a major constituent of cell membranes and pulmonary surfactant, and is more commonly found in the exoplasmic or outer leaflet of a cell membrane. Surfactant is a mixture of lipids, proteins, and glycoproteins, lecithin and sphingomyelin being two of them. Lecithin makes the surfactant mixture more effective. L/S ratio in amniotic fluid is measured to assess the maturity of fetal lungs. An L/S ratio of 2 or more indicates fetal lung maturity and a relatively low risk of infant respiratory distress syndrome, and an L/S ratio of less than 1.5 is associated with a high risk of infant respiratory distress syndrome.

Phosphatidylcholine is transported between membranes within the cell by phosphatidylcholine transfer protein (PCTP). Phosphatidylcholine also plays a role in membrane-mediated cell signalling and PCTP activation of other enzymes. PCTP has role in hepatobiliary lipid homeostasis, reverse cholesterol transport, and high density lipoprotein metabolism. Phosphatidylcholine is necessary for activity of β-hydroxybutyrate dehydrogenase.

Phosphatidylethanolamine or cephalin

Phosphatidylethanolamines are found in all living cells, composing 25% of all phospholipids. They are found particularly in nervous tissue such as the white matter of brain, nerves, neural tissue, and in spinal cord, where they make up to 45% of all phospholipids.

Phosphatidylcholine, phosphatidylserine and phosphatidylinositol provide for hydrated or charged membrane surfaces, allowing water and/or ions to bind to their polar head groups. In contrast, surfaces rich in phosphatidylethanolamine are hydrophobic, poorly hydrated and promote surface-to-surface interactions without direct protein binding. This is necessary

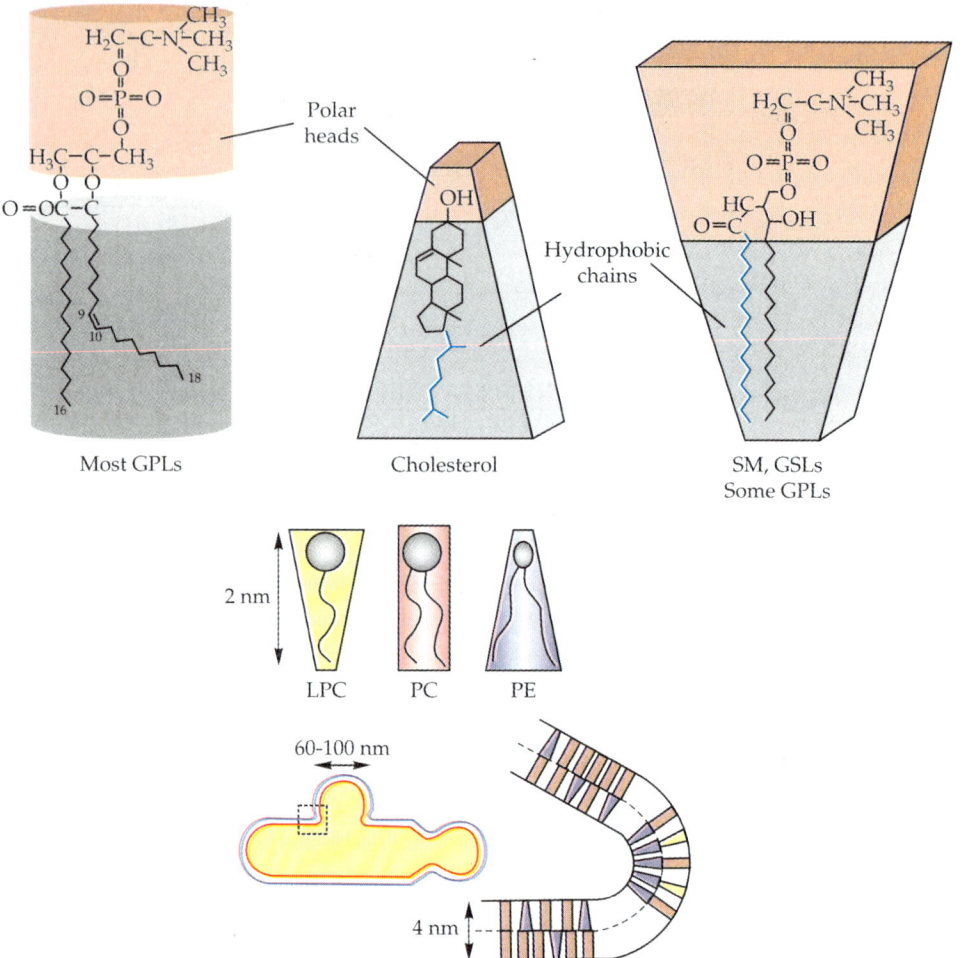

Fig. 11.2. Shapes of different lipids in membrane and their role in membrane curvature.

for membrane fusion. PEs play a role in membrane fusion and in disassembly of the contractile ring during cytokinesis in cell division.

It is also essential for activity of Ca^{2+}-ATPase in muscle sarcoplasmic reticulum.

Phosphatidylserine

Phosphatidylserine (PS), like PE, is usually kept on the inner leaflet. Increase in intracellular Ca^{2+} during coagulation in platelets and during apoptosis activates phospholipid scramblase which moves PS and PE to outer leaflet of cell membrane. PS provides an anionic surface for activation of factor X and binding of factors Xa and Va to form active prothrombinase leading to prothrombin activation. PE also promotes this binding. PS is recognized by macrophages by specific receptors and leads to phagocytosis of apoptotic cells. Annexin V dye binds to PS and is used to identify apoptotic cells in histological slides. Rare genetic defect in PS translocation to outer leaflet possibly due to defective scramblase leads to Scott syndrome, a rare congenital bleeding disorder.

Phosphatidylglycerol phosphoglyceride or cardiolipin (a symmetric molecule)

It is present mainly in inner mitochondrial membrane (upto 25%) and about 4% in mitochondrial outer membrane. It is essential for activity of ADP/ATP exchanger in inner mitochondrial membrane. It is also a component in 3-dimensional structure of mitochondrial complex III, complex IV and the ADP-ATP carrier. It also anchors two kinases, mitochondrial creatine kinase and nucleoside diphosphate kinase, to the inner and possibly the outer mitochondrial membranes where they come in contact.

Cardiolipin has been implicated in the process of apoptosis (programmed cell death) in animal cells through its interactions with a variety of death-inducing proteins, including cytochrome c. Cytochrome c is believed to act as a peroxidase, which reacts quite specifically with cardiolipin but not with other more abundant phospholipids, causing oxidation and then hydrolysis. The consequence is that the cytochrome c is released into the intermembrane space, while the oxidized cardiolipin is translocated to the outer mitochondrial membrane and participates in the formation of the mitochondrial permeability transition pore that facilitates egress of pro-apoptopic factors from mitochondria into the cytosol where they trigger apoptosis. During this process, cardiolipin is also involved in the anchoring, translocation, and embedding of caspase, a key protein in the process of apoptosis, in the mitochondrial membrane, and thereby causes further release of apoptotic factors into the cytosol.

Mutations in the tafazzin gene (TAZ, also called G4.5) lead to Barth syndrome. The tafazzin gene encodes for an acyltransferase involved in complex lipid metabolism. Mutation leads to abnormalities in structure of cardiolipin. The characteristics of this multi-system disorder include: cardiomyopathy, exercise intolerance, neutropenia, underdeveloped skeletal musculature and muscle weakness, growth delay, and 3-methylglutaconic aciduria.

Phosphatidylinositol

Phosphatidylinositol-4,5-bisphosphate is a source of second messengers like IP_3 and DAG. Phosphatidylinositol-3-phosphate and phosphatidylinositol-3,5-bisphosphate are involved in control of membrane traffic in endosomes.

Glycophosphatidylinositol (GPI) is involved in anchoring many proteins like acetylcholine esterase, carbonic anhydrase, lipoprotein lipase, etc. to membranes. It is also involved in activation of ion channels – phosphatidylinositol-4,5-bisphosphate is involved in opening of Na^+ channels during release of growth hormone by GHRH.

Phosphatidylinositol-4,5-bisphosphate and PI triphosphate also serve as docking phospholipids that bind specific domains that promote the recruitment of proteins to the plasma membrane and subsequent activation of signalling cascades. Examples of proteins activated by PI(3,4,5)P3 are AKT, PDPK1, Btk1.

Glycerol ether phospholipids – ethanolamine plasmalogen and choline plasmalogen

Plasmalogens are found in numerous human tissues, with particular enrichment in the nervous, immune, and cardiovascular system. In human heart tissue, nearly 30–40% of choline glycerophospholipids are plasmalogens. Almost 30% of the glycerophospholipids in the adult human brain and up to 70% of myelin sheath ethanolamine glycerophospholipids are plasmalogens. Plasmalogens can protect mammalian cells against the damaging effects of reactive oxygen species. Also, they have been implicated as being signalling molecules and modulators of membrane dynamics.

Plasmalogen deficiencies due to peroxisome biogenesis disorders lead to the development of rhizomelic chondrodysplasia punctata (RCDP). Individuals with severe plasmalogen deficiencies frequently show abnormal neurological development, skeletal malformation, impaired respiration, and cataracts.

2. Sphingolipids

Sphingolipids are believed to protect the cell surface against harmful environmental factors by forming a mechanically stable and chemically resistant outer leaflet of the plasma membrane lipid bilayer. Sphingolipids are virtually absent from mitochondria and the ER, but constitute a 20–35% of plasma membrane lipids.

Sphingomyelins

These are involved in formation of myelin (myelin sphingomyelins have mainly longer chain FA like C24) and lipid rafts.

Glycosphingolipids – glucocerebrosides, galactocerebrosides, phrenosine, sulfatides

Galactosylceramides are present in all nervous tissues, and compose up to 2% dry weight of grey matter and 12% of white matter. They are major constituents of oligodendrocytes. Galactocerebrosides and sulfatides mainly have fatty acids with C22-26. Myelin – galactocerebrosides and sphingomyelin form myelin sheath responsible for saltatory conduction and electrical insulation in neurons.

Glucosylceramide is found at low levels in animal cells such as the spleen, erythrocytes, and nervous tissues, especially neurons. Glucosylceramide is a major constituent of skin lipids, where it is essential for lamellar body formation in the stratum corneum and to maintain the water permeability barrier of the skin.

Galactocerebrosides are used as cellular binding sites by a wide variety of pathogens, including viruses, bacteria, fungi and parasites. GalCer is recognized by HIV-1, prions and also of *Borrelia burgdorferi* (the causative agent of Lyme disease).

Gangliosides

These are also predominantly found in CNS. Gangliosides are involved in cell-cell recognition and binding of hormones and bacterial toxins like cholera toxin (GM1), tetanus toxin, and certain viruses like influenza virus.

Q. 2. Describe the role and functions of cholesterol in plasma membranes.

Ans. The planar/flat sterol ring and the hydrophobic tail orient cholesterol within the membrane core, while the 3-β-hydroxyl group (polar head) allows cholesterol to contribute to the surface properties of the bilayer. Pure glycerophospholipids exist in a fluid liquid crystalline phase (Lc) at 37°C and a solid gel-like crystalline phase (Lβ) at lower temperature. The mid point of this temperature range is called T_m. Addition of cholesterol inhibits the organization of lipids into the Lβ phase at lower temperatures (increasing fluidity at low temperatures), but favour a less fluid and more ordered structure than the Lc phase at body temperature (decreasing fluidity) (Fig. 11.3). The planar structure of cholesterol allows it to reduce the freedom of movement of phospholipid acyl chains or reduce their rotation and coiling, thus rigidifying the membrane at body temperature, which can have a dramatic impact upon membrane function. This phenomenon is referred to as a 'condensing effect'.

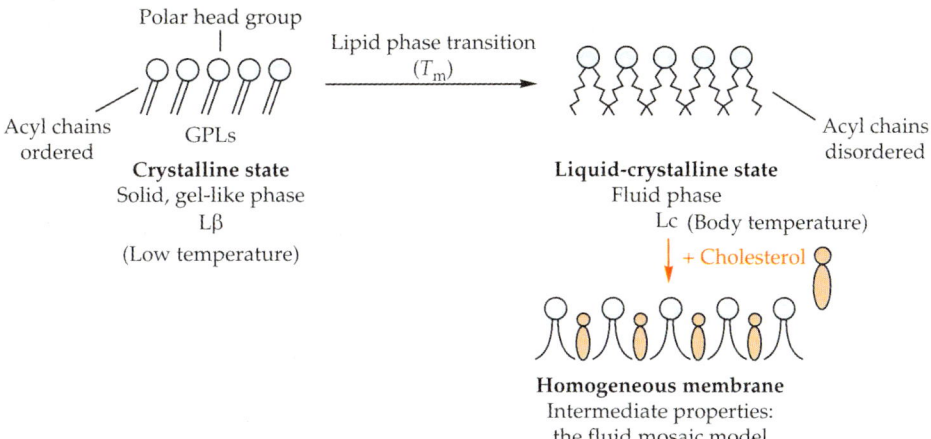

Fig. 11.3. Orientation of cholesterol in membrane and its role in physical properties of membrane.

Thus, cholesterol functions as a buffer, preventing lower temperatures from inhibiting fluidity and preventing higher temperatures from increasing fluidity too much. It does not change transition temperature of a membrane, but increases the temperature-range of the transition. Cholesterol stiffens membranes above the transition temperature and keeps them fluid below the transition temperature (Fig. 11.4).

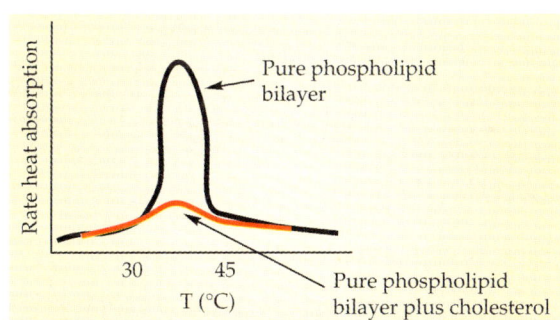

Fig. 11.4. Effect of cholesterol on temperature range of transition and transition temperature of membrane.

Further, the geranyl, prenyl and farnesyl groups produced during cholesterol synthesis are important for anchoring proteins to membranes. Ubiquinone and Heme A (a component of cytochrome) are also derived from isoprenoid units and are important in the inner mitochondrial membrane electron transport chain.

Cholesterol molecules in membrane are associated with Na/K ATPase and Band 3 anion transporter and essential for their activity by specific interaction. Cholesterol also serves other functions, such as organizing clusters of transmembrane proteins into lipid rafts, which are very important for signal transduction, neurotransmission and receptor function. Cholesterol, phosphatidylserine and sphingomyelin are important for exocytosis and membrane fusion. The importance of the contribution of cholesterol to membrane properties is reflected in its ubiquitous distribution and its necessity for normal cell growth and function.

Most of the cellular cholesterol is present in the plasma membranes. Free cholesterol in membrane is maintained in a narrow range. Cholesterol is derived from de novo synthesis or from uptake from LDL. Excess free cholesterol is stored in the form of droplets in cytoplasm. When membrane-free cholesterol exceeds a threshold it is transported to endoplasmic reticulum where ACAT esterifies it or it is removed to HDL by reverse cholesterol transport.

Decreased cholesterol in membrane alters lipid rafts and these alterations play critical role in the pathophysiology of multiple CNS disorders, including Smith-Lemli-Opitz syndrome, Huntington, and Alzheimer's disease.

High levels of membrane cholesterol, often secondary to high levels of serum cholesterol, exert deleterious effects on cells. RBCs cannot synthesize cholesterol and cholesterol content of their membranes depends on the plasma cholesterol. When it increases, their membrane cholesterol increases by 25–65% leading to reduced fluidity of membrane and decreased flexibility and a spiny shape (cholesterol reduces fluidity at body temperature). These RBCs are destroyed prematurely in the spleen leading to 'spur' cell anaemia. Hypercholesterolemia also leads to decreased membrane fluidity making them more sensitive to thrombin and other stimuli promoting aggregation.

In hypercholesterolemia, the membrane cholesterol contents of erythrocytes, platelets, leukocytes, smooth muscle cells and endothelial cells have been shown to increase. This increase causes the enhanced production of oxygen-free radicals as cholesterol undergoes oxidation, giving rise to a variety of epoxides and alcohols involved in atherosclerosis. Increased membrane cholesterol increases activity of many ion channels including Ca^{2+} channels and decreases activity of active transporters with ATPase activity by decreasing membrane fluidity. In hypercholesterolemia the increased membrane cholesterol content leads to increased calcium entry into vascular smooth muscle cells and promotes calcium-dependent atherogenetic cell processes, such as migration, proliferation, and stimulus-secretion coupling.

Gram-positive bacteria like *Streptococcus* produce cholesterol-dependent cytolysins (CDC) which can lyse cells and induce apoptosis.

Q. 3. How are proteins held in the plasma membrane?

Ans. Membrane proteins are of two types: integral and peripheral (Fig. 11.5). Integral proteins are embedded in the membrane and have a transmembrane domain which contains sequences rich in hydrophobic amino acids which come in contact with the hydrophobic membrane

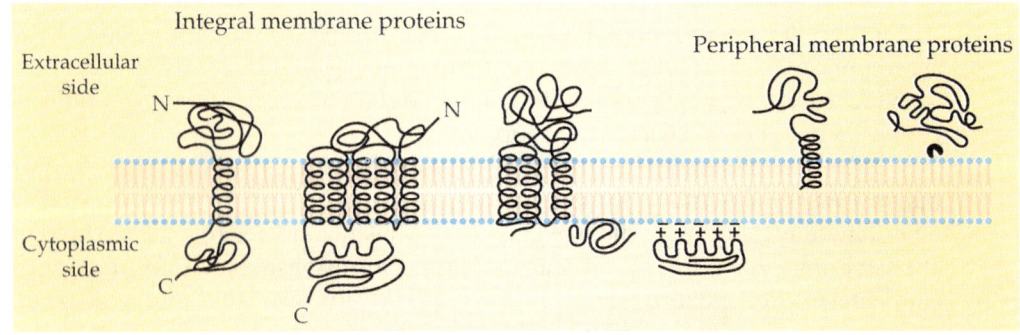

Fig. 11.5. Integral and peripheral membrane proteins.

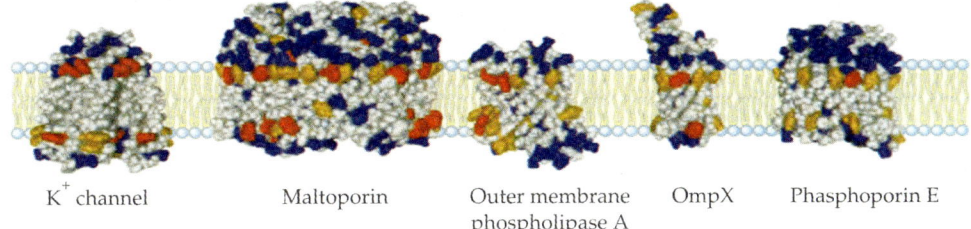

K⁺ channel   Maltoporin   Outer membrane   OmpX   Phasphoporin E
                            phospholipase A

Fig. 11.6. Distribution of Tyr and Trp in integral membrane proteins (Red & Orange spheres).

core. A remarkable feature of many transmembrane proteins is the presence of Tyr and Trp residues (Fig. 11.6) at the interface between lipid and water. The planar aromatic side chains of these residues apparently serve as membrane interface anchors, able to interact simultaneously with the central lipid phase and the aqueous phases on either side of the membrane.

Peripheral proteins are on the surface of membranes and can be easily removed without disrupting the membranes. Some are associated transiently with membrane with cyclic attachment and detachment. This controls their activity and they are involved in signal transduction.

Peripheral proteins may be attached by:

1. Binding to an integral protein, e.g. ankyrin binding to anion channel in RBC.
2. Electrostatic interaction: Negatively charged phospholipids interact with positively charged regions of proteins.
3. Insertion of short hydrophobic sequence of amino acids into the membrane as an anchor.
4. Non-covalent binding to inositol-3-phosphate head group of phosphatidylinositol of membrane by specific protein domains.
5. Lipid anchors: Covalently linked lipid is inserted into the membrane (Table 11.1 and Figs. 11.7 and 11.8). These may be:
   - GPI anchor – Glycosylphosphatidylinositol anchor – the carboxy terminal of protein is bound to ethanolamine which is linked to a chain of glycan (made of mannose and glucosamine) which is covalently bound to phosphatidylinositol whose acyl chain is inserted in the membrane.
   - Myristoyl anchor: Myristic acid is linked by amide linkage to N-terminal glycine of the protein.
   - Thioester or hydroxyester anchor: Myristic acid, palmitic acid, stearic acid or oleic acid are linked to –SH or –OH group of cysteine, serine or threonine.
   - Thioether linked anchor: Isoprenoid lipids like farnesyl, geranylgeranyl or dolichol are linked to cysteine of protein. Such proteins are called prenylated proteins. Such proteins are usually found on the cytoplasmic side of membrane.

Defects in the GPI anchor synthesis occur in the rare acquired diseases such as paroxysmal nocturnal hemoglobinuria (PNH) and congenital diseases such as hyperphosphatasia with mental retardation syndrome (HPMRS). In PNH a somatic defect in blood stem cells in the pathway required for GPI synthesis, results in faulty GPI linkage of decay-accelerating factor (DAF) and CD59 in red blood cells. The most common cause of PNH are somatic mutations in the X-chromosomal gene PIGA. This gene encodes a protein required for synthesis of N-acetylglucosaminyl phosphatidylinositol (GlcNAc-PI), the first intermediate in the biosynthetic pathway of GPI anchor. CD59 is an inhibitor of membrane attack complex

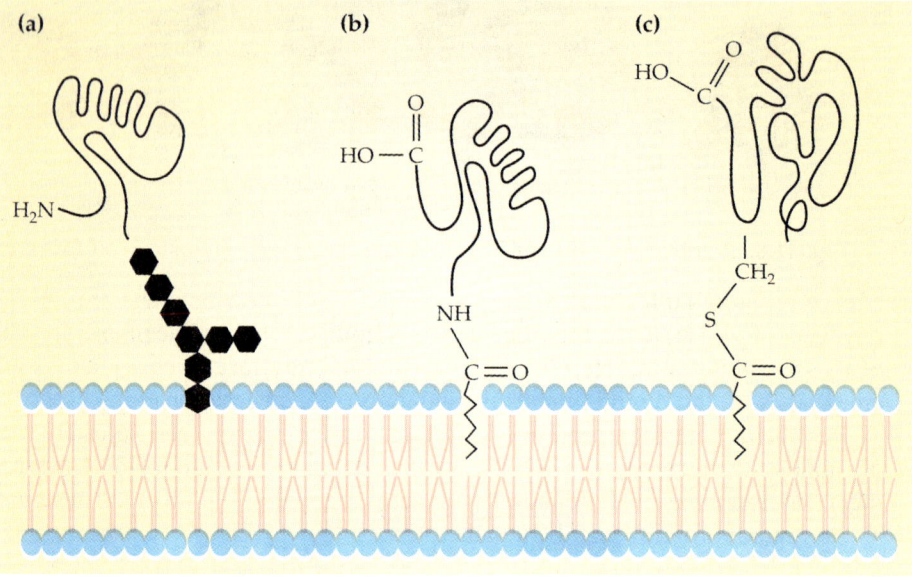

Fig. 11.7. Types of lipid anchors for attachment of membrane proteins. (a) Glycosylphosphatidylinositol (GPI) anchor; (b) Myristoyl anchor; and (c) Thioester anchor.

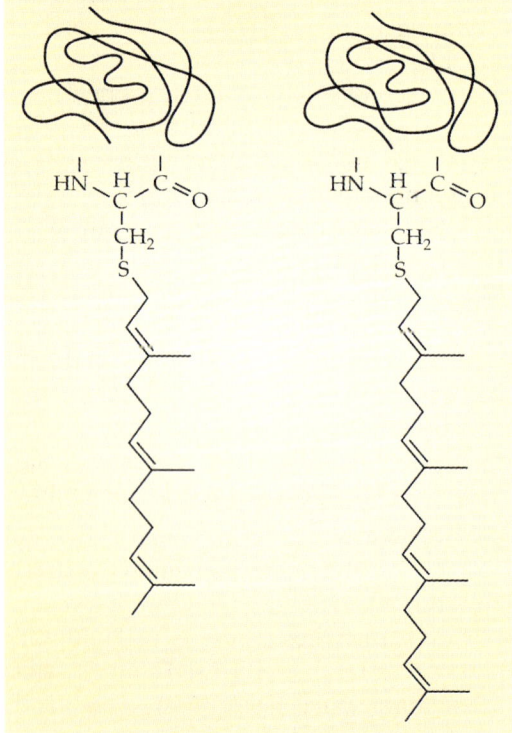

Fig. 11.8. Lipid anchors – Isoprenoid anchors – Farnesyl anchor and geranylgeranyl anchor.

Table 11.1. Different types of lipid anchors

Type of anchor	Lipid involved in attachment	Attachment	Examples
Phosphatidylinositol (GPI)	Phosphatidylinositol	Glycan (ethanolamine, phosphate, mannose and glucosamine)	Acetylcholine esterase, alkaline phosphodiesterase, carbonic anhydrase, cell-cell adhesion molecules, cell surface hydrolases, lipoprotein lipase, scrapie prion protein, surface antigens
Myristoyl	Myristic acid (C_{14})	Amide linkage at N-terminal glycine	β-adrenergic receptor, c-CAMP protein kinase, insulin receptor, α-subunit of G protein
Thioester and hydroxyester	Myristic acid (C_{14}), palmitic acid (C_{16}), stearic acid (C_{18}), oleic acid (C_{18})	—SH or —OH of cysteine, serine, threonine	G protein-coupled receptors, transferrin receptor
Thioether-linked	Isoprenoid lipid: farnesyl (C_{15}), geranylgeranyl (C_{20}), dolichol	Cysteine	Many GTP-binding proteins, nuclear lamins, protein kinases, protein phosphatases

of complement system. Without DAF and CD59 proteins linked to the cell surface, the complement system can lyse the cell, and high numbers of RBCs are destroyed, leading to hemoglobinuria.

Q. 4. What is asymmetric distribution of lipids? How is it maintained and what is its significance?

Ans. Different types of lipids are asymmetrically distributed in the inner and outer leaflet of the bilayer of membranes (Fig. 11.9). While sphingomyelin and phosphatidylcholine predominate in outer leaflet, phosphatidylserine and phosphatidylethanolamine are found mainly in the inner leaflet. Phosphatidylinositols are primarily located on the inner leaflet. The asymmetry is established during the biosynthesis of plasma membrane on the endoplasmic reticulum. Uncatalyzed transverse movement of lipids (flip-flop) is very slow (Fig. 11.10). Asymmetry is maintained by lipid transporters which catalyse unidirectional movement of specific lipids from one leaflet to other against the concentration gradient. ATP-dependent aminophospholipid translocase or flippases transport phosphatidylserine and ethanolamine from extra-cytoplasmic to cytoplasmic side (Fig. 11.11).

Scramblases are ATP-independent and Ca stimulated transporters which facilitate bidirectional mixing of phospholipids and thus randomizing the phospholipids. Their action increases PE and PS content of the outer leaflet. This is important during coagulation cascade in platelets where exposure of PE and PS promote prothrombinase activation and in apoptotic cells where PS on outer surface is recognized by receptors on macrophages which then phagocytose the apoptotic cells.

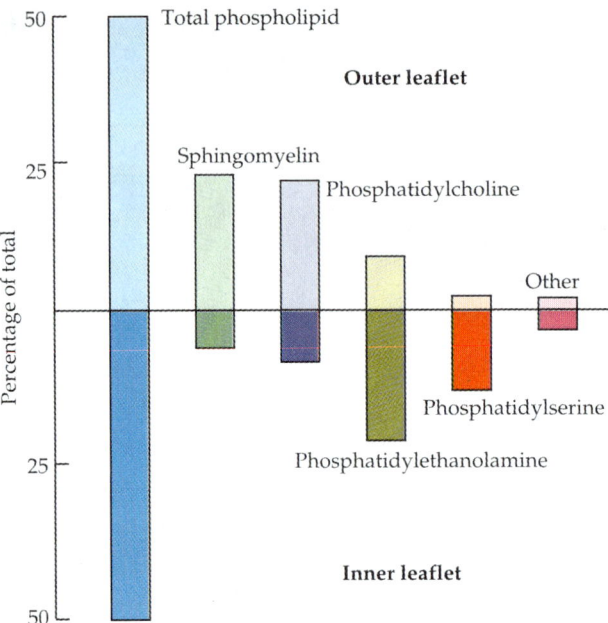

Fig. 11.9. Asymmetric distribution of lipids in the two leaflets of a membrane.

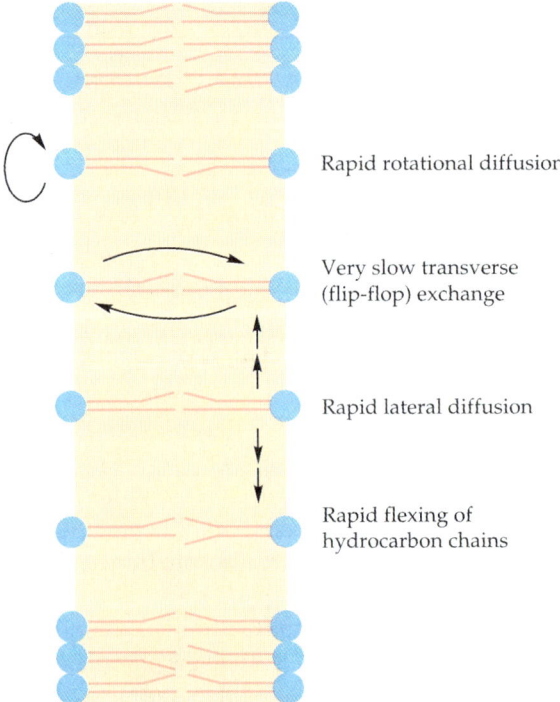

Fig. 11.10. Movements of lipid molecules in membrane. While rotational movement and lateral diffusion occur freely, transverse movement between leaflets is restricted.

Membrane and Transport

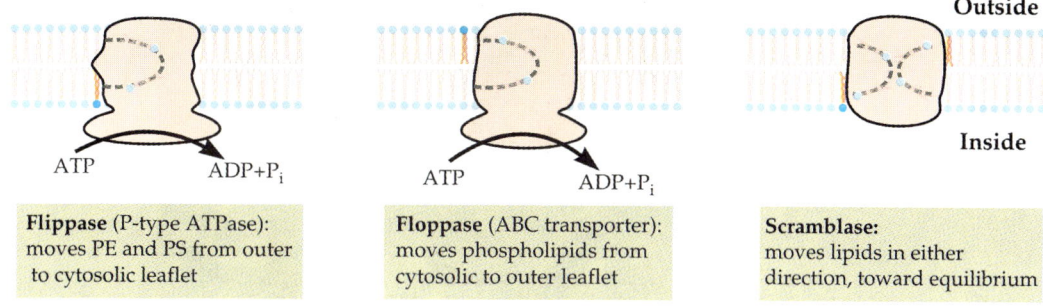

Fig. 11.11. Enzyme-dependent movement of lipids between the two leaflets of a membrane.

Q. 5. What are lipid rafts and caveolae and what is their significance?

Ans. Lipids and proteins are distributed in a heterogenous rather than homogenous fashion in the membranes. Lipid rafts are small (10–200 nm), heterogenous, highly dynamic, sterol- and sphingolipid-enriched microdomains of membranes that compartmentalize cellular processes. Their organized bilayer structure (lipid and protein composition) is different from surrounding membrane (Fig. 11.12).

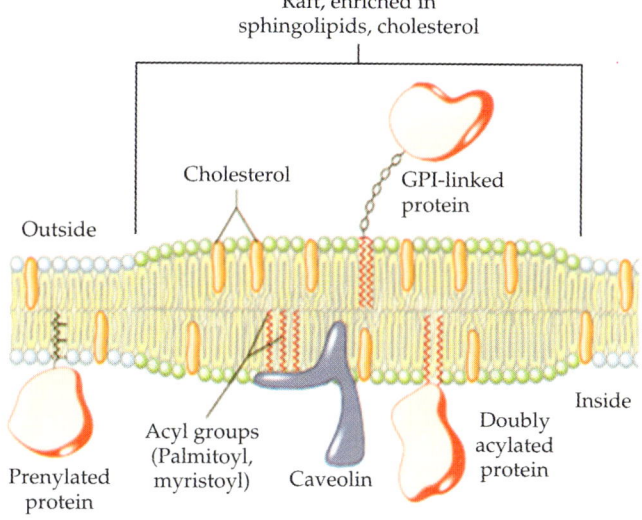

Fig. 11.12. Lipid raft.

Structure
- Cholesterol and sphingolipid-enriched membrane microdomains or platforms.
- Cholesterol levels double and sphingomyelin levels elevated by 50%.
- Concentrate and segregate proteins within the plane of the bilayer to facilitate their coordinated activity.
- More ordered and tightly packed than surrounding bilayer (Fig. 11.13): Outer leaflets of rafts have higher concentration of ceramides and glycosphingolipids which usually contain longer chain fatty acid. This leads to increased membrane thickness. Inner leaflet of rafts have more saturated acyl chains allowing more compact packing than surrounding membrane.

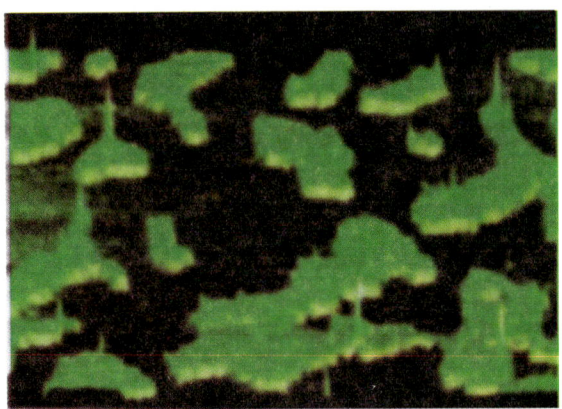

Fig. 11.13. Lipid rafts are like thick floating ice shelves (less fluid) in the more fluid sea of membrane.

- Float freely in liquid crystalline lipid bilayer (Fig. 11.13).
- True resident proteins: GPI-anchored proteins – prion protein (PrPc), caveolin and flotillin – are found mainly in the rafts than in surrounding membrane and thus are called 'true resident proteins'.
- Sequestered proteins: signalling proteins like G-protein, non-receptor tyrosine kinases.
- Sequestered proteins may be attached to cytoskeletal/adhesion proteins like actin, myosin, vinculin, cofilin, cadherin and ezrin.
- Rafts are of two types:
  - Caveolae: small, flask-shaped invaginations of the plasma membrane enriched in caveolin.
  - Planar lipid rafts: found in neurons and enriched in flotillin.
- Caveolin and flotillin recruit signalling proteins.

Formation

- Cholesterol is the dynamic "glue" that holds the raft together (Fig. 11.14).
- Due to the rigid nature of the sterol group, cholesterol partitions preferentially into the lipid rafts where acyl chains of the lipids tend to be more rigid and in a less fluid state (Fig. 11.14).
- Fig. 11.15 shows the inverted cone-like shape of sphingomyelin and the cone-like shape of cholesterol based on the area of space occupied by the hydrophobic and hydrophilic regions. Cholesterol has the ability to pack in between the lipids in rafts, serving as a molecular spacer and filling any voids between associated sphingolipids.

Functions

- Organizing centres – assembly of signalling molecules.
- Signalling can be promoted or dampened (Fig. 11.16).
- Signalling molecules may be maintained in inactive state in different rafts and may become activated when the rafts cluster together.
- Small rafts can act as concentrating platforms after ligand binding activates receptors. If receptor activation takes place in a lipid raft, the signalling complex is protected from non-raft enzymes such as membrane phosphatases. Overall, raft binding recruits proteins to a new micro-environment so that the phosphorylation state can be modified by local

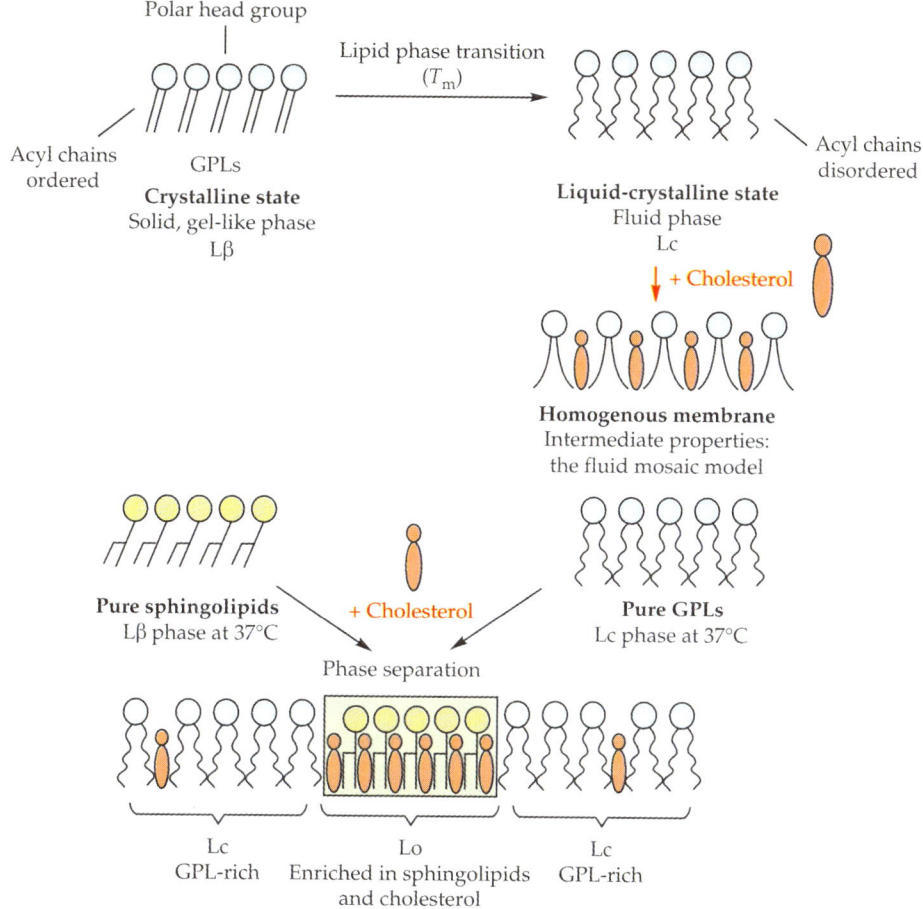

Fig. 11.14. How cholesterol helps in raft formation. It favours the phase separation of membrane lipids forming the Lo phase of rafts. Sphingolipids and cholesterol are responsible for raft formation in the glycerophosphate lipid membranes.

kinases and phosphatases to give downstream signalling. Lipid rafts have been found to be involved in many signal transduction processes, such as immunoglobulin E signalling, T cell antigen receptor signalling, B cell antigen receptor signalling, EGF receptor signalling, insulin receptor signalling, etc.
- Affects membrane fluidity.
- Involved in trafficking of membrane proteins.
- Regulation of neurotransmission and receptor trafficking.

Rafts and diseases
- HIV virus: Budding may occur from lipid rafts.
- Influenza virus: Has raft-associated glycoproteins in envelope.
- Alzheimer's disease: Rafts are platforms for production of β-amyloid (neurotoxic protein).
- Prion disorder: Normal prion protein (PrPc) is converted to abnormal proteins (PrPsc) in lipid rafts (GPI anchor required).

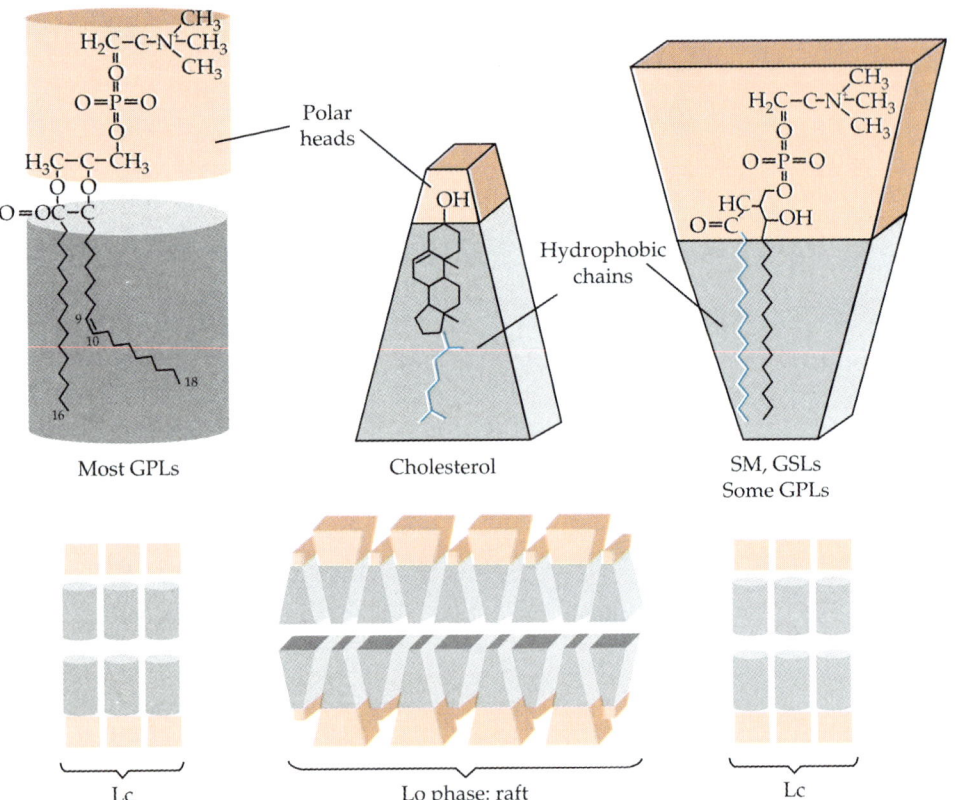

Fig. 11.15. Lipid organisation in raft microdomains: A simplified model based on the shape of membrane lipids. GPL – glycerophospholipid, SM – Sphingomyelin, GSL – Glycerosphingolipid.

- In the nervous tissue various molecular complexes are assembled in lipid rafts, thus mediating a diversity of downstream cellular events such as neurotransmitter processing and release, cell division, cell adhesion, and neuronal outgrowth. Neurotrophin receptors are embedded in lipid rafts and BDNF, NGF and GDNF signalling depends on the normal functioning of lipid rafts. The neurotrophin system is also capable of regulating the lipid and cholesterol content of the rafts themselves. Lipid rafts are likely to play a critical role in the pathophysiology of multiple CNS disorders, including Smith-Lemli-Opitz syndrome, Huntington, Alzheimer's, and Niemann–Pick Type C diseases.

Caveolae (Fig. 11.16)

- Caveolin is an integral membrane protein with two globular domains connected by a hairpin-shaped hydrophobic domain, which binds the protein to the cytoplasmic leaflet of the plasma membrane (Fig. 11.17).
- Three palmitoyl groups attached to the carboxyl-terminal globular domain further anchor it to the membrane.
- Caveolin binds cholesterol in the membrane, and the presence of caveolin forces the associated lipid bilayer to curve inwards, forming caveolae ("little caves") in the surface of the cell (Fig. 11.17).

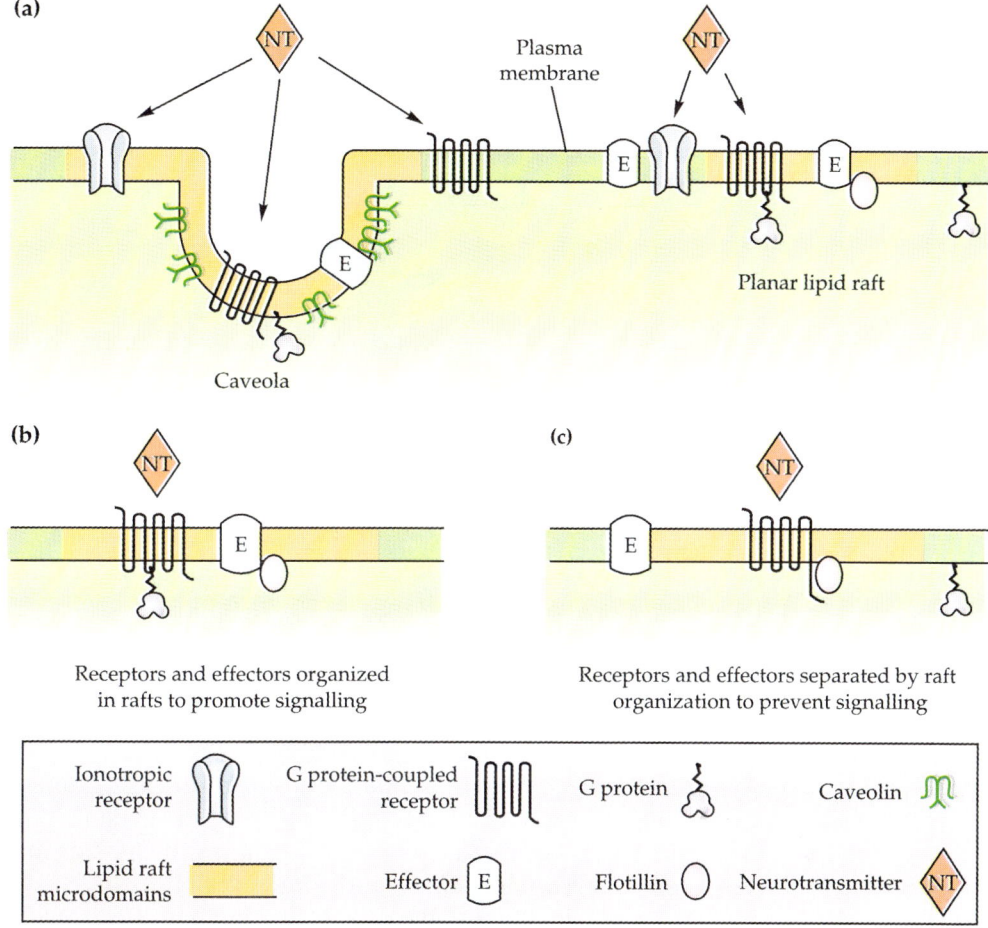

Fig. 11.16. (a) Caveolae and planar lipid rafts. (b) Enhancement and dampening of receptor signalling by rafts.

- Caveolae are unusual rafts. They involve both leaflets of the bilayer – the cytoplasmic leaflet, from which the caveolin globular domains project, and the exoplasmic leaflet, a typical sphingolipid/cholesterol raft with associated GPI-anchored proteins.
- Caveolae are implicated in a variety of cellular functions, including membrane trafficking within cells and the transduction of external signals into cellular responses.
- The receptors for insulin and other growth factors, as well as certain GTP-binding proteins and protein kinases associated with transmembrane signalling, appear to be localized in rafts and caveolae.
- Effective insulin signalling in the adipocyte depends on localization of insulin receptor and GLUT-4 to caveolae as well as on a direct functional interaction between caveolin-1 and the insulin receptor. Increased GM3 gangliosides accumulate in caveolae which weakens insulin receptor caveolin interaction and causes loss of insulin receptors from caveolae. This has been found to occur in insulin resistance and insulin resistance is now being considered a membrane microdomain disorder.

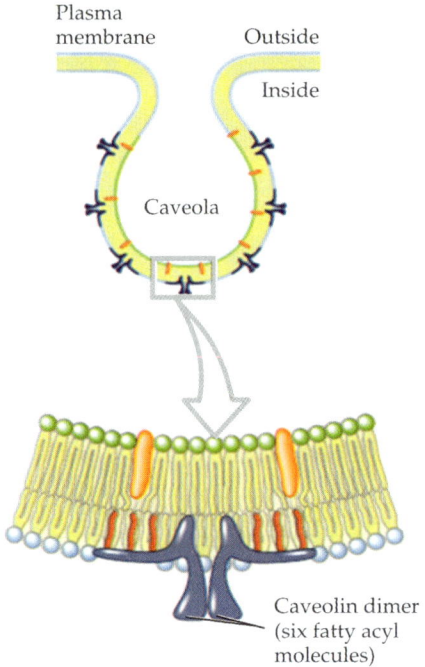

Fig. 11.17. Caveolin.

Q. 6. What are the factors which affect membrane fluidity?

Ans. The term "fluidity" reflects the tightness of packing of acyl parts of the membrane phospholipid molecules. The membrane is fluid but also fairly rigid and can burst if penetrated or if a cell takes in too much water. The mosaic nature of the plasma membrane allows a very fine needle to easily penetrate it without causing it to burst and allows it to self-seal when the needle is extracted. Individual lipids and proteins can rapidly move across the surface. Fluidity depends on:

- The mosaic characteristic of the membrane helps the plasma membrane remain fluid. The integral proteins and lipids exist in the membrane as separate but loosely-attached molecules.
- Temperature: Decreasing temperature decreases the fluidity.
- Saturation of acyl groups: In their saturated form, the fatty acids in phospholipid tails are relatively straight. A *cis* double bond results in a bend of approximately 30 degrees in the string of carbons. This leads to kinks in the hydrocarbon chain preventing tight packing and increasing fluidity. Many organisms (fish are one example) are capable of adapting to cold environments by changing the proportion of unsaturated fatty acids in their membranes in response to the lowering of the temperature (Fig. 11.18).
- Chain length of the acyl groups: Shorter the length more the fluidity.
- Cholesterol content: It lies alongside the phospholipids in the membrane and tends to dampen the effects of temperature on the membrane. Thus, cholesterol functions as a buffer, preventing lower temperatures from inhibiting fluidity and preventing higher temperatures from increasing fluidity too much. Cholesterol extends the range of temperature in which the membrane is appropriately fluid and, consequently, functional.

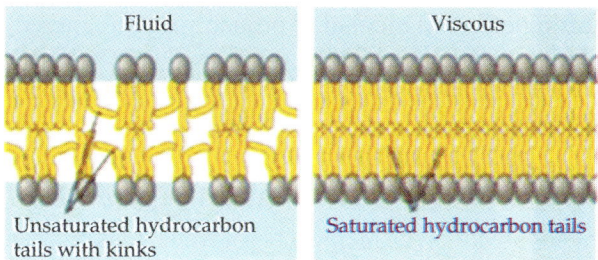

Fig. 11.18. Effect of unsaturated fatty acids on membrane fluidity.

- Calcium ion: It decreases fluidity because of its interaction with negatively charged head groups of phospholipids, reducing repulsion between the polar head groups and increasing the packing of lipid molecules.
- Asymmetric distribution of phospholipids and sphingolipids in the two leaflets leads to a difference in the fluidity of the two leaflets.

The composition of fatty acyl chains of phospholipids can be altered by changes in diet, cellular Ca^{2+}, free radicals and lipid peroxidation leading to change in membrane fluidity. Anaesthetic agents increase fluidity. Changes in fluidity occur in hypercholesterolemia, hypertension, diabetes, obesity, alcoholism, schizophrenia, LCAT deficiency and Alzheimer's disease. Replacement of *cis*-unsaturated fatty acids with *trans*-unsaturated fat decreases fluidity as they are shaped more like saturated fatty acids (Fig. 11.19). Presence of PUFA increases fluidity. Individuals with abetalipoproteinemia have increase in sphingomyelin content and decrease in phosphatidylcholine content in membranes leading to decreased fluidity.

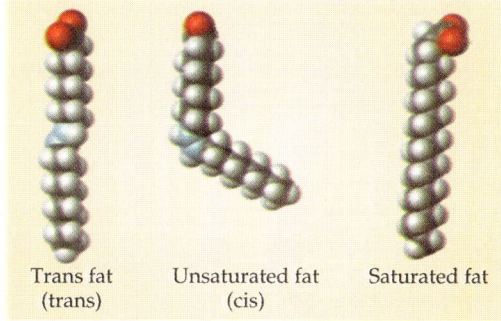

Fig. 11.19. Shapes of *trans*-unsaturated, *cis*-unsaturated and saturated fatty acids.

Effects of alterations in fluidity

- Fluidity influences considerably the molecular mobility and thus the sensitivity and reactivity of membrane bound transporters, receptors and enzyme systems. Membrane fluidity can control the activity of membrane-bound receptors, enzymes and functions such as phagocytosis, cell growth and death.
- In spur cell anaemia due to hypercholesterolemia RBC, membrane cholesterol content is increased leading to increased stiffness of RBC membrane and hence increased destruction in spleen and a spiny shape of RBCs. Hypercholesterolemia similarly decreases membrane fluidity of platelets and makes them more sensitive to aggregation.

- The intoxicating effect of alcohol is probably due to altered fluidity, altering membrane receptors, and ion channel in CNS.
- PUFA may improve insulin sensitivity by increasing membrane fluidity besides their actions through peroxisome proliferation activation receptors.

Q. 7. How are transport proteins classified?

Ans. Transport proteins are involved in transport of water, ions, nutrients, metabolic waste products and macromolecules across membranes.

Classification

Type	Subtype	Human examples
1. Pores and channels	A. α-helical channels	Ryanodine-inositol-1,4,5-triphosphate receptor Ca^{2+} channel; cellular sensors responding to smell, taste, touch, pain, osmolarity; voltage-gated ion channels; epithelial Na channel, glutamate-gated ion channel of neurotransmitter receptors; gap-junction-forming connexion; urea transporter; nuclear pores
	B. β-strand porins	Mitochondrial porin in outer mitochondrial membrane
	C. Pore forming toxins	Defensins, complement C9, perforins, Anthrax toxin
	D. Non-ribosomally synthesized toxins	Gramicidin A
2. Electrochemical potential driven transporters	A. Transporters or carriers (uni-, syn- and antiporters)	Amino acid transporters, GLUT, anion exchange protein, Na/H exchanger, ADP/ATP exchanger, phosphate/H symporter, etc.
	B. Non-ribosomally synthesized transporters	Valinomycin, nigericin
3. Primary active transporters	A. P-P bond hydrolysis driven transporters	ATP-binding-cassette proteins; ATPases: P type – Na/K ATPase, F type – F0F1 ATP synthase, V type – vacuolar VoV1 ATPase (acidification of lysosomes)
	B. Decarboxylation driven transporters	
	C. Methyl driven transporters	
	D. Oxidoreduction driven transporters	Proton-translocating NADH dehydrogenase
	E. Light driven transporters	
4. Group translocators	A. Phosphotransferases	
5. Transmembrane electron carriers	A. Two electron carriers	
	B. One electron carrier	Phagocyte NADPH oxidase

Q. 8. What are the similarities between transporters and enzymes?

Ans. Just like enzymes work by lowering the activation energy, membrane proteins lower the activation energy for transport of polar compounds and ions by providing an alternative path through the bilayer for specific solutes (Fig. 11.20). Proteins that bring about this facilitated diffusion, or passive transport, are not enzymes in the usual sense; their "substrates" are moved from one compartment to another, but are not chemically altered (Fig. 11.21). Like enzymes, transporters bind their substrates with stereochemical specificity through multiple weak, noncovalent interactions. They follow saturation kinetics characterized by V_{max} and K_m like that of enzymes. Just like enzymes they have high degree of specificity and stereospecificity for substrates.

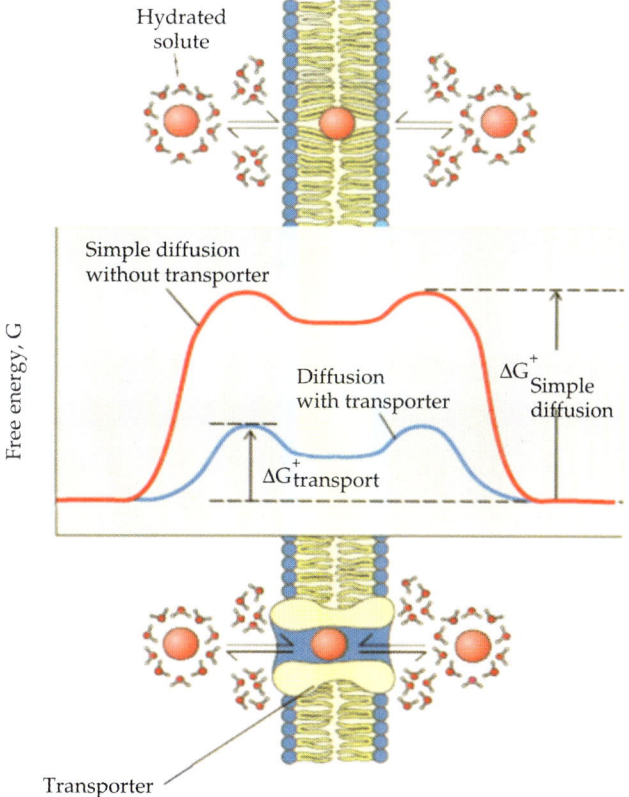

Fig. 11.20. Polar molecules cannot cross the hydrophobic part of membrane. This is because removal of hydration shell requires energy. Transporters, by providing an alternate pathway, decrease this activation energy required. Energy is released again when hydration shell of polar molecule is reformed (b).

Q. 9. What are pore-forming toxins and ionophores?

Ans. Pore-forming toxins are peptides and proteins made by few mammalian tissues and bacteria. They are secreted by cells and form transmembrane pores in membranes of other cells. These pores allow flow of electrolytes and small solutes through the membrane leading to toxic effect.

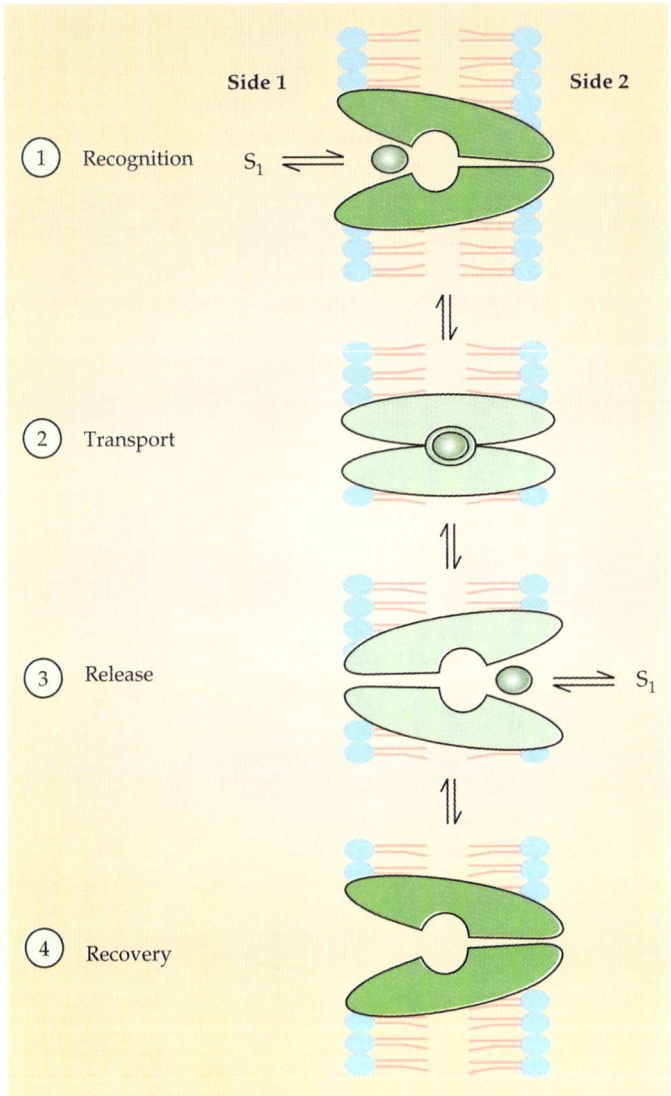

Fig. 11.21. Transporter proteins act just like enzymes.

Human pore-forming proteins
- Defensins: Defensin is produced by epithelial cells and hematopoietic cells, have broad-spectrum anti-bacterial activity and important in innate immunity. It is also present in tears, breast milk and saliva.
- Membrane attack complex of complement system: C9 functions by punching holes in the membrane of pathogenic Gram-negative bacteria. Deficiency of C9, or other components of the MAC, results in an increased susceptibility to diseases caused by Gram-negative bacteria such as meningococcal meningitis. Deficiency of the MAC inhibitor CD59 results in an overactivity of complement and paroxysmal nocturnal hemoglobinuria.

- Perforins: Perforin is released by cytotoxic T cells and lyses virally infected and cancer cells. In addition perforin permits delivery of cytotoxic proteases called granzymes that cause cell death. Perforin deficiency results in the fatal disorder familial hemophagocytic lymphohistiocytosis (FHL or HLH). This disease is characterised by an overactivation of lymphocytes which results in cytokine-mediated organ damage.

Bacterial toxins

- α-pore-forming toxin: Cytolysin of *E. coli*.
- β-pore-forming toxin: Hemolysin, Panton-Valentine leukocidin.
- Binary toxin: Anthrax toxin.
- Cholesterol-dependent cytolysin of *Streptococcus*.
- Small pore-forming toxin: Gramicidin A.

Binary toxins, such as Anthrax lethal and edema toxins, *C. perfringens* Iota toxin and *C. difficile* cyto-lethal toxins consist of two components (hence binary) – An enzymatic component A, and a membrane-altering component B. The B component facilitates the entry of the enzymatic 'payload' into the target cell by forming homooligomeric pores. The A component then enters the cytosol and inhibits normal cell functions by one of the following means:

- Mono-ADP-ribosylation of G-actin: ADP-ribosylation is a common enzymatic method used by various bacterial toxins from various species. These toxins (including *C. perfringens* Iota toxin and *C. botulinum* C2 toxin) attach a ribosyl-ADP moiety to surface arginine residue 177 of G-actin. This prevents G-actin assembling to form F-actin, and thus, the cytoskeleton breaks down, resulting in cell death.
- Proteolysis of mitogen-activated protein kinase kinases (MAPKK): The A component of Anthrax toxin lethal toxin is zinc-metalloprotease, which shows specificity for a conserved family of mitogen-activated protein kinases. The loss of these proteins results in a break down of cell signalling, which, in turn, renders the cell insensitive to outside stimuli – therefore no immune response is triggered.
- Increasing intracellular levels of cAMP: Anthrax toxin (Edema toxin) triggers a calcium ion influx into the target cell. This subsequently elevates intracellular cAMP levels.

Ionophores

These are non-ribosomally derived channels which include:

- Chemical compounds (mobile ion carriers) that bind to a particular ion, shielding its charge from the surrounding environment, and thus facilitating its crossing of the hydrophobic interior of the lipid membrane (Fig. 11.22).
- Channel formers that introduce a hydrophilic pore into the membrane, allowing ions to pass through while avoiding contact with the membrane's hydrophobic interior.

Uses

Experimental tool in studies of ion translocation in biological membranes and for manipulation of ionic composition of cells. Gramicidin is used as antibiotic. For example, of ionophores:

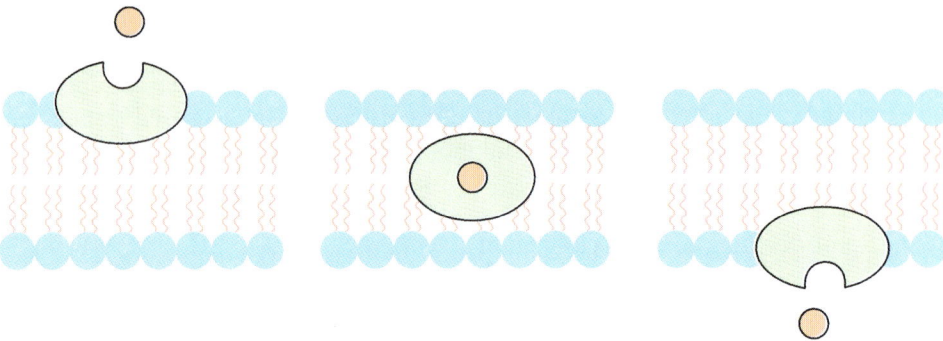

Fig. 11.22. Action of Ionophores.

- A23187 (Ca^{2+})
- Enniatin (ammonium)
- Gramicidin A (H^+, Na^+, K^+)
- Ionomycin (Ca^{2+})
- Monensin (Na^+, H^+)
- Nigericin (K^+, H^+, Pb^{2+})
- Nystatin
- Salinomycin (K^+)
- Valinomycin (potassium ionophore I)

Q. 10. What are ABC transporters and describe their clinical significance.

Ans. ABC transporters are transmembrane proteins that utilize the energy of adenosine triphosphate (ATP) to carry out certain biological processes including translocation of various substrates across membranes and non-transport-related processes such as translation of RNA and DNA repair. In humans they transport a wide variety of substrates across extra- and intracellular membranes, including metabolic products, lipids (phospholipids, long chain fatty acyl CoA, bile salts, cholesterol) and sterols, peptides, toxic organic molecules, and chemotherapeutic drugs.

Proteins are classified as ABC transporters based on the sequence and organization of their ATP-binding cassette (ABC) domain(s). They have a modular structure with a six-transmembrane-segment domain, and a cytosolic ATP binding domain (or cassette). Individual members function as channels or transporters. ATP binding induces a conformational change in transmembrane domain, but ATP hydrolysis does not lead to phosphorylation of the transporter. Although, most eukaryotic ABC transporters are effluxers, some are not directly involved in transporting substrates. In the cystic fibrosis transmembrane regulator (CFTR) and in the sulfonylurea receptor (SUR), ATP hydrolysis is associated with the regulation of opening and closing of ion channels carried by the ABC protein itself or other proteins. ABC transporters have been shown to exist within the placenta, indicating they could play a protective role for the developing fetus against various drugs (xenobiotics) and harmful substances in maternal circulation.

There are 48 known ABC transporters present in humans, which are classified into seven families by the Human Genome Organization (Table 11.2).

Membrane and Transport

Table 11.2. Different ABC transporters present in human tissues

Family	Function	Disease due to mutations
ABCA	Responsible for the transportation of cholesterol and lipids, among other things	Tangier disease (ABCA1, phospholipid); Juvenile macular degeneration, Retinitis pigmentosa (ABCA5/ABCR, phosphatidyl-ethanolamine)
ABCB	Some are located in the blood–brain barrier, liver, mitochondria and transports peptides and bile	Sideroblastic anemia with ataxia (ABCB7, iron); Progressive familial intrahepatic cholestasis (ABCB11/BSEP, bile salts); Cholestasis of pregnancy (ABCB4/PGY3, long chain phosphatidylcholine); Ankylosing spondylitis, insulin-dependent DM, celiac disease (ABCB2 and 3/TAP1 and 2, peptide transporter)
ABCC	Used in ion transport, cell-surface receptors, toxin secretion. Includes the CFTR protein, which causes cystic fibrosis when deficient	Multi-drug resistance (ABCC1/MRP1, drugs); Dubin–Johnson syndrome (ABCC2/MRP2, bilirubin glucoronides); Cystic fibrosis (CF) and congenital bilateral aplasia of the vas deferens (CBAVD) (ABCC7/CFTR, chloride channel)
ABCD	All are used in peroxisomes	Adrenoleukodystrophy (ABCD1/ALD)
ABCE/ ABCF	These are not actually transporters but merely ATP-binding domains that were derived from the ABC family, but without the transmembrane domains. These proteins mainly regulate protein synthesis or expression	
ABCG	Transports lipids, diverse drug substrates, bile, cholesterol, and other steroids	Sitosterolemia (ABCG5)

P Glycoprotein (MDR1) or ATP-binding cassette sub-family B member 1 (ABCB1)/CD243

P-gp is extensively distributed and expressed in the intestinal epithelium where it pumps xenobiotics (such as toxins or drugs) back into the intestinal lumen, in liver cells where it pumps them into bile ducts, in the cells of the proximal tubular of the kidney where it pumps them into urine-conducting ducts, and in the capillary endothelial cells comprising the blood–brain barrier and blood–testis barrier, where it pumps them back into the capillaries. Some cancer cells also express large amounts of P-gp, which renders these cancers multi-drug resistant. It is responsible for multiple drug resistance (MDR) against a variety of structurally unrelated drugs.

P-gp transports various substrates across the cell membrane including:
- Drugs such as colchicine, tacrolimus and quinidine
- Chemotherapeutic agents such as etoposide, doxorubicin, and vinblastine
- Lipids

- Steroids
- Xenobiotics
- Peptides
- Bilirubin
- Cardiac glycosides like digoxin
- Immunosuppressive agents
- Glucocorticoids like dexamethasone
- HIV-type 1 antiretroviral therapy agents like protease inhibitors and non-nucleoside reverse transcriptase inhibitors.

Its ability to transport the above substrates accounts for the many roles of P-gp including:

- Regulating the distribution and bioavailability of drugs.
- Increased intestinal expression of P-glycoprotein can reduce the absorption of drugs that are substrates for P-glycoprotein. Thus, there is a reduced bioavailability, and therapeutic plasma concentrations are not attained. On the other hand, supratherapeutic plasma concentrations and drug toxicity may result because of decreased P-glycoprotein expression.
- Active cellular transport of antineoplastics resulting in multidrug resistance to these drugs.
- The removal of toxic metabolites and xenobiotics from cells into urine, bile, and the intestinal lumen.
- The transport of compounds out of the brain across the blood–brain barrier.
- Digoxin uptake.
- Prevention of ivermectin and loperamide entry into the central nervous system.
- The migration of dendritic cells.
- Protection of hematopoietic stem cells from toxins.

ABCB1 or MDR1 P-glycoprotein is also involved in other biological processes for which lipid transport is the main function. It mediates the secretion of the steroid aldosterone by the adrenals, and its inhibition blocks the migration of dendritic immune cells, possibly related to the outward transport of the lipid platelet activating factor (PAF). It has also been reported that ABCB1 mediates transport of cortisol and dexamethasone. MDR1 can also transport cholesterol, short-chain and long-chain analogs of phosphatidylcholine (PC), phosphatidylethanolamine (PE), phosphatidylserine (PS), sphingomyelin (SM), and glucosylceramide (GlcCer).

Integration of Metabolism and Endocrinology

Chapter 12

Q. 1. How is eating behaviour regulated in humans?

Ans. Body weight is regulated by both endocrine and neural components that influence the balance between energy intake and expenditure. This complex regulatory system is necessary because even small imbalances between energy intake and expenditure will ultimately have large effects on body weight. For example, even a 0.3% positive imbalance over 30 years would result in a 9-kg weight gain. Alterations in stable weight by forced overfeeding or food deprivation induce physiologic changes that resist these disturbances. With weight loss, appetite increases and energy expenditure falls and with overfeeding, appetite falls and energy expenditure increases. However, the compensatory mechanism for overfeeding frequently fails, permitting obesity to develop when food is abundant and physical activity is limited. This may be of survival advantage in evolution, allowing storage of food reserves for times with limited availability of food.

Eating behaviour and satiety control

Eating behaviour and satiety are important because overeating or consumption of excess calories than required is the most important significant cause of obesity world over. Appetite and weight are regulated by multiple hormones secreted by different tissues. It involves a complex neuroendocrine system of hormones produced in the stomach, small intestines, pancreas, adipose tissue, and central nervous system. Mechanisms of satiety are responsible for regulating the termination of feeding at a given meal and the interval between meals.

As shown in Figs. 12.1 and 12.2, ventromedial hypothalamus (VMH) and ventrolateral hypothalamus (VLH) control the appetite.

- Ventromedial hypothalamus (VMH) acts as satiety centre to inhibit appetite. Damage to VMH causes excessive feeding till body weight is set at a new higher point when food consumption stabilizes to maintain the obese weight.

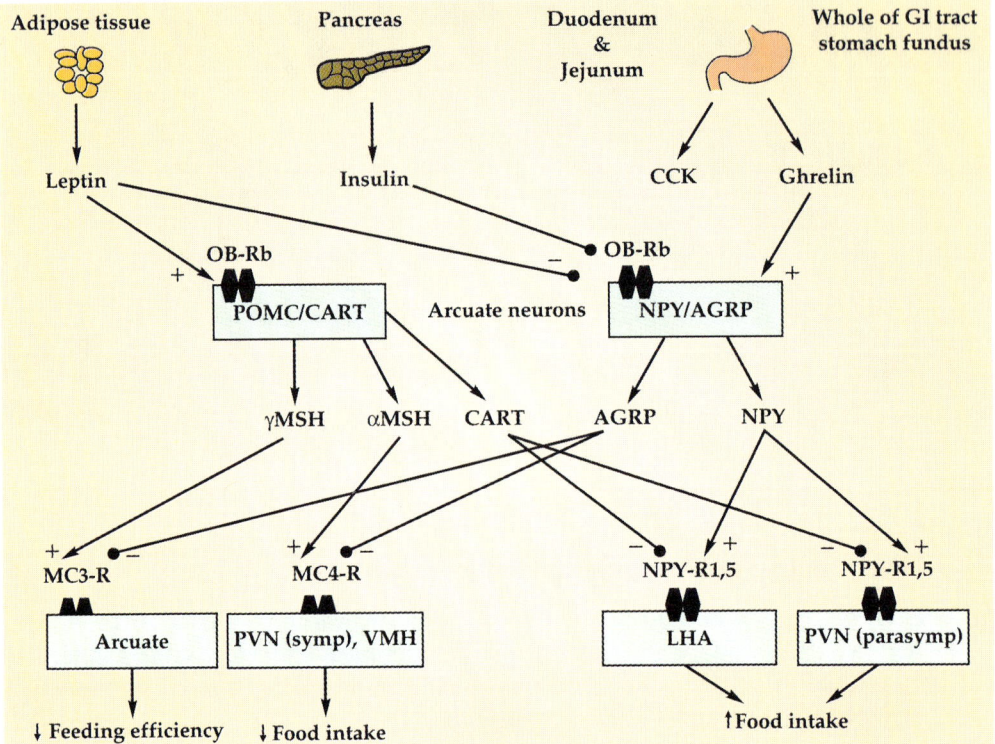

Fig. 12.1. Neurochemistry of hypothalamic satiety network (POMC, CART, PVN, VMH, LHA). OB-Rb = Leptin receptor, POMC = Propiomelanocortin, CART = Cocaine and amphetamine regulated transcript, NPY = Neuropeptide Y, AGRP = Agouti-related protein, MSH = Melanocyte stimulated hormone, PVN = Periventricular nucleus, VMH = Ventromedial hypothalamus, LHA = Lateral hypothalamus, MC3/4-R = Melanocortin receptor, NPY-R = Neuropeptide Y receptor, CCK = Cholecystokinin.

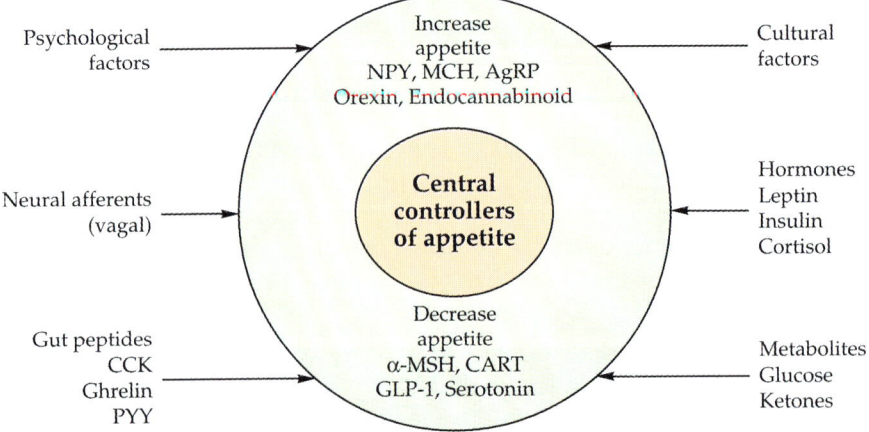

Fig. 12.2. Central control of appetite. GLP-1 = Glucagon-like peptide 1, PYY = Peptide YY (tyrosine tyrosine).

- Ventrolateral hypothalamus (VLH) acts as the feeding centre to stimulate appetite. VLH lesions lead to decreased feeding leading to weight loss and finally stabilization of decreased feeding levels to maintain the new lower body weight set-point.

The activity of these two centres is regulated by output from the arcuate nucleus. Arcuate nucleus is responsible for maintenance of body weight, body temperature, blood pressure, and other vital functions. Arcuate nucleus has two subsets of neurons (Fig. 12.1):

1. NPY/AgRP-producing neurons – release mainly NPY (neuropeptide Y) and AgRP. They activate feeding centre (NPY) and inhibit satiety centre (AgRP).
2. Melanocortin producing neurons – release mainly MSH and CART. They activate satiety centre (MSH) and inhibit feeding centre (CART).

Several neurotransmitters are involved in hypothalamic regulation of feeding and body mass. These can be classified based on their behavioral effects into anabolic/orexigenic peptides that promote feeding and increase of body mass or as catabolic/anorexigenic peptides which act opposite (Fig. 12.2).

- Anabolic/orexigenic peptides: Include neuropeptide Y (NPY), agouti-related protein (AGRP), melanin-concentrating hormone (MCH), orexin, and galanin. NPY is the key feeding-promoting neuropeptide and NPY-receptor subtype 5 is the key site of action. NPY increases in the arcuate nucleus within 6 hours of food deprivation. AGRP is an antagonist for the anorexigenic/catabolic peptides as it blocks the action of α- and γ-MSH on MC3 and MC4 receptors.
- Catabolic/anorexigenic peptides include α-MSH, cocaine- and amphetamine-regulated transcript (CART), glucagon-like peptides 1 and 2 (GLP-1, GLP-2) and prolactin-releasing peptide (PrlRP). Their levels fall with food deprivation and rise with forced overfeeding. Corticotropin-releasing factor (CRF) increases in the paraventricular nucleus (PVN) and pro-opiomelanocortin (POMC) increases in the arcuate nucleus with overfeeding. The main anorexigenic signals are α-MSH and γ-MSH acting at the MC4 and MC3 receptors, respectively. CART is an antagonist of the orexigenic/anabolic peptide NPY.

Many hormones and neural signals act as inputs on neurons within the arcuate nucleus region of the hypothalamus to regulate appetite and energy balance:

- *Neural signals:* Mediated by vagus nerve. Information from stretch receptors in the stomach wall and sensors in the portal blood vessels for cholecystokinin (CCK), glucose, osmolality and pH is conveyed to the brain by vagus to limit meal size. Vagal afferents synapse in the nucleus of the solitary tract and the area postrema. These sites send projections to the paraventricular nucleus to inhibit feeding.
- *Vagus and insulin:* Message from the vagus to the pancreas mediates the cephalic phase of insulin release. The sight and smell of food initiates activity in limbic cortex that in turn activates the central autonomic network. Outflow to the dorsal motor nucleus of the vagus and finally to the pancreas results in the first surge of insulin in the blood that accompanies a meal. Two additional increases in plasma insulin later occur as food enters the gut (the gastrointestinal phase) and then as nutrients enter the intestines (the substrate phase). These stimuli also result in satiety as insulin not only promotes energy storage but also acts as a humoral signal back to the brain for satiety.

- *Humoral signals:* Insulin, leptin, glucose, and CCK. Insulin, leptin and glucose gain access to the CNS at the circumventricular organs of the median eminence and the area postrema and act on specific receptors in neurons of the nuclear cell groups adjoining these areas. Insulin and leptin act as the mediators of satiety signals related to the caloric content of a meal and also act in relation to maintenance of a body weight set point. CCK exerts its main effects on satiety in the periphery by an action on the vagus to potentiate the responses to glucose, pH, and osmolality in the portal blood. Metabolites, including glucose, can influence appetite, as seen by the effect of hypoglycemia to induce hunger; however, glucose is not normally a major regulator of appetite.

Hormones that regulate eating behaviour can be divided into short-term regulators that determine individual meals and long-term regulators that act to stabilize the levels of body fat deposits.

Short-term regulators – Ghrelin and Cholecystokinin (Fig. 12.1)

- Ghrelin is an appetite-stimulating peptide hormone produced in the stomach. Production of ghrelin is maximal when the stomach is empty, but ghrelin levels fall quickly once food is consumed. Cholecystokinin, a peptide hormone, is released from the GIT during eating. Cholecystokinin signals satiety (the sense of fullness) and tends to curtail further eating. Together, ghrelin and cholecystokinin constitute a meal-to-meal control system that regulates the onset and end of eating behaviour. The activity of this control system is also modulated by the long-term regulators (insulin and leptin).

Long-term regulators of eating behaviour – Insulin and Leptin

- Both inhibit eating and promote energy expenditure. They inhibit release of NPY and AgRP in arcuate nucleus neurons. Leptin stimulates release of MSH and CART from melanocortin producing neurons in arcuate nucleus (Fig. 12.1).
- Insulin is released from the β-cells of the pancreas when blood glucose levels rise. It stimulates glucose uptake from the blood into muscle and fat tissues. Insulin stimulates fat cells to make leptin.
- Leptin (from the Greek word *lepto*, meaning "thin") is a 146–amino acid protein produced principally in adipocytes (fat cells). Leptin has a tertiary structure similar to that of cytokines. As fat deposits accumulate in adipocytes, more and more leptin is produced in these cells and released into the blood. Leptin levels in the blood communicate the status of triacylglycerol levels in the adipocytes to the central nervous system so that appropriate changes in appetite take place. If leptin levels are low (starvation), appetite increases; if leptin levels are high (overfeeding), appetite is suppressed. Leptin also regulates fat metabolism in adipocytes, inhibiting fatty acid biosynthesis and stimulating fat metabolism. Leptin induces synthesis of the enzymes in the fatty acid oxidation pathway and increases expression of uncoupling protein 2 (UCP2), a mitochondrial protein that uncouples oxidation from phosphorylation so that the energy of oxidation is lost as heat (thermogenesis). Functional leptin receptors are also essential for pituitary function, growth hormone secretion, and normal puberty. When body fat stores decline, the circulating levels of leptin and insulin also decline.

Intermediate regulation of eating behaviour
- Accomplished by the gut hormone PYY3-36. PYY3-36 is produced in endocrine cells found in distal regions of the small intestine, areas that receive ingested food some time after a meal is eaten. PYY3-36 inhibits eating for many hours after a meal by acting on the NPY/AgRP-producing neurons in the arcuate nucleus.

Role of AMPK
AMPK (AMP activated kinase) mediates many of the hypothalamic responses to all these hormones: The actions of leptin, ghrelin, and NPY converge at AMPK. Leptin inhibits AMPK activity in the arcuate nucleus neurons through melanocortin-4 receptor producing anorexic affect, while ghrelin and NPY activate hypothalamic AMPK, which stimulates food intake and leads, over time, to increased body weight. The effects of AMPK in the hypothalamus that lead to alterations in eating behaviour may be mediated through changes in malonyl-CoA levels. Low [malonyl-CoA] in hypothalamic neurons is associated with increased food intake, and elevated malonyl-CoA levels are associated with suppression of eating. The inhibition of acetyl-CoA carboxylase (and thus, malonyl-CoA synthesis) as a result of phosphorylation by AMPK plays an important part in the regulation of our eating behaviour in hypothalamic neurons.

Defects in these controls are common and also these systems are biased in favour of overeating, which may confer survival advantage in times when food is unavailable.

Control of energy expenditure
Energy expenditure includes the following components:
1. Resting or basal metabolic rate.
2. The energy cost of metabolizing and storing food – specific dynamic action.
3. The thermic effect of exercise.
4. Adaptive thermogenesis.

- Basal metabolic rate accounts for around 70% of daily energy expenditure, whereas active physical activity contributes 5–10%. Thus, a significant component of daily energy consumption is fixed.
- Adaptive thermogenesis varies in response to long-term caloric intake, rising with increased intake. Adaptive thermogenesis occurs in brown adipose tissue (BAT), which plays an important role in energy metabolism in many mammals. In contrast to white adipose tissue, which is used to store energy in the form of lipids, BAT expends stored energy as heat. A mitochondrial uncoupling protein (UCP-1) in BAT dissipates the hydrogen ion gradient in the oxidative respiration chain and releases energy as heat. Leptin and thyroid hormones act in the CNS (hypothalamus) to stimulate the sympathetic supply to BAT which increases the metabolic activity of BAT. Thus, leptin and thyroid hormones increase activity of BAT through a central action.
- Increased weight produces extra leptin which acts to inhibit feeding and increase energy expenditure.
- Weight loss decreases leptin and also peripheral conversion of T_4 to active T_3 to reduce basal metabolic rate.

Disorders of feeding and satiety

- **Obesity** is excess of adipose tissue in an amount that creates a health risk (20% or greater above the ideal body weight). Excess intake of calories is the major contributor to obesity. Basal metabolic rate in a 70-kg man is about 1500 calories/day, so anything above this in a sedentary, healthy individual will result in weight gain. Another mechanism besides excess caloric intake that may contribute to obesity is the lipoprotein lipase hypothesis in which an excess of adipose tissue lipoprotein lipase preferentially stores lipid calories as adipose tissue.
- **Frohlich's syndrome** is characterized by obesity, hypogonadotropic hypogonadism and other variable features including diabetes insipidus, visual impairment and mental retardation. It is thought to result due to a hypothalamic lesion.
- **Anorexia nervosa** is a disorder almost exclusively seen in young, white women of middle-class background, with a prevalence of as high as 1 per 100 being reported. Subclinical prevalence may be as high as 5 percent. Patients observed to be below about 80% of ideal body weight are suspect when no other medical (psychological) causes can be identified. A disordered attitude toward eating, food or weight that overrides hunger, ritualized exercise, amenorrhea, bradycardia, hypotension, and hypothermia complete the usual clinical picture. Patients with anorexia are vulnerable to sudden death from ventricular tachyarrhythmias. There is no specific treatment as yet because the underlying mechanisms are not defined. However, recent studies have shown that a significant number of these patients and those with bulimia have plasma antibodies against pituitary and hypothalamic melanotropes and/or corticotropes suggesting an underlying autoimmune disorder.
- **Bulimia** is often considered a disorder related to anorexia nervosa. The disorder is characterized by the episodic ingestion of large amounts of food in a compulsive fashion ("ox-hunger") coupled with the awareness that the eating pattern is abnormal, that it cannot be stopped, and depression at completion of the act. There is usually a morbid fear of becoming fat, although body weight is usually in the normal range. Induced vomiting that eventually becomes reflexive usually follows episodes of binge eating. Patients frequently have additional behavioral/psychiatric abnormalities.

Q. 2. Describe the changes in metabolism in starve–feed cycle and with different phases of glucose homeostasis.

Ans. Starve–feed cycle

Allows a variable fuel and nitrogen intake to meet variable metabolic and anabolic needs. Feeding refers to intake of meals (variable fuel input), after which fuel is stored (as glycogen and triacylglycerol) to meet metabolic needs during fasting. Fuel from meals or storage ensures that levels of ATP can be always maintained. Humans can consume food at a rate far greater than the basal caloric requirement, this allow them to survive between meals. However, an almost unlimited capacity to consume food is matched by a similar capacity to store excess fat and carbohydrate (after conversion) as triacylglycerol.

Phases of starve–feed cycle

Phase I: Well-fed state (3-4 hours after meal) (Fig. 12.3)

Meal supplies energy requirement.

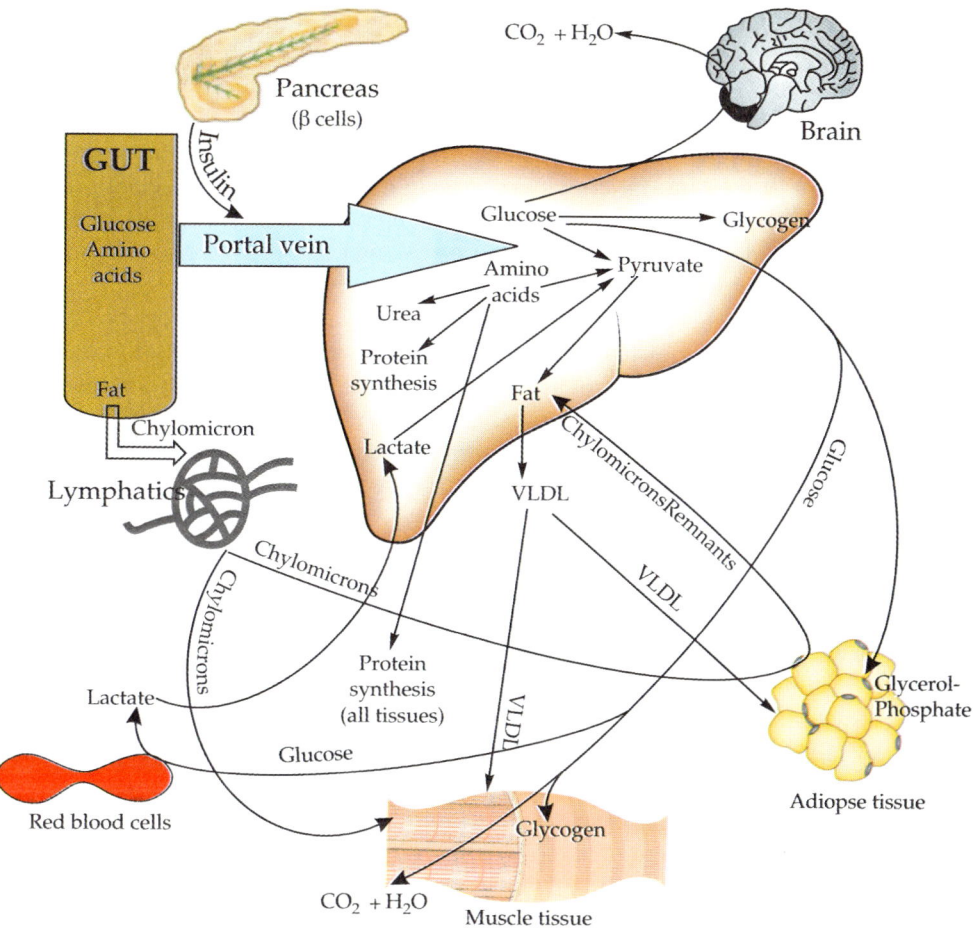

Fig. 12.3. The fed state.

- Glucose passes from intestinal epithelial cells to portal blood to liver – converted to glycogen for storage, used in HMP pathway to produce NADPH for synthetic reactions and to acetyl-CoA by glycolysis. The acetyl-CoA can be used in TCA for ATP production and can be converted to fatty acid and then triglycerides for export as VLDL. Most of the dietary glucose passes through liver to reach other organs including brain, red cells, renal medulla and adipose tissue. While brain, adrenal medulla and RBC are exclusively dependent on glucose for ATP, adipocytes use it to produce glycerol. Muscles use blood glucose to replenish glycogen or for aerobic exercise.

- In this state liver uses glucose and gluconeogenesis is at its minimum possible level. Thus, Cori's cycle is not working in this phase.

- Chylomicrons (made from absorbed triacylglycerols and lipids) are secreted by intestinal cells into lymphatics, which empty into thoracic duct and then to subclavian vein and circulate to rest of the body tissues. The TG from chylomicrons and VLDL is taken up by

tissues to get FFA for energy production and by adipocyte for storage with the help of lipoprotein lipase (LPL). LPL is present on endothelial cells of most capillaries (except brain) and breaks TG from chylomicrons and VLDL into FFA and glycerol. FFA is taken up by the fat or other cells, while glycerol is released into blood. Adipose cells re-esterify the FFA with glycerol-3-phosphate derived from glycolysis to produce and store TG. Because of the high fat content of human diet most TG of fat cells originates from diet rather than from de novo TG synthesis in liver (supplied to fat cells from liver by VLDL).
- Lactate produced by tissues is taken up by liver and oxidized to CO_2 or converted to TG (lactate → pyruvate → acetyl CoA → FFA → TG).
- Some amino acids absorbed are used by intestinal cells for energy production (Fig. 12.6), but most are transported into portal blood. Liver uses some amino acids but most pass through to be distributed to all tissues for protein synthesis. This is especially important for essential amino acids. Liver can catabolize amino acids, but the K_m values of enzymes involved are high, implying that amino acids have to be present in high concentration before significant catabolism can occur. The low K_m values of tRNA charging enzymes ensure that protein synthesis can occur at lower concentrations too. Excess amino acids are oxidized to CO_2 and urea with production of ATP but in the fed state the carbon skeletons are mainly used for lipogenesis in liver.
- The major hormone active in this state is insulin. High glucose levels in portal blood stimulates insulin secretion from pancreatic β cells. This insulin first reaches and acts on liver and then is circulated all over the body.
- Insulin acts in liver to promote – glycogen synthesis, fatty acid and triglyceride synthesis, VLDL production and export, and protein synthesis. It inhibits glycogen breakdown, ketone body synthesis and gluconeogenesis.
- In muscle it promotes glucose and amino acid entry and glycogen and protein synthesis. Insulin is not required for glucose entry during exercise.
- In fat cells insulin promotes glucose entry, activity of LPL, glycolysis (to produce glycerol-3-phosphate) and TG synthesis. It inhibits TG breakdown and FFA release by Hormone Sensitive Lipase (HSL). The dependence on insulin-mediated glucose entry for glycerol generation ensures that TG synthesis and storage occurs only when blood glucose is sufficiently high (fed state, when extra glucose is present). Thus, storage of dietary fatty acids (taken up from chylomicrons by LPL) occurs only when blood glucose and insulin are sufficiently high.

Phase II: Early fasting state [few hours (4–10 hours) after meal] (Fig. 12.4)

- Hepatic glycogenolysis maintains blood glucose levels.
- Lactate, alanine and pyruvate are diverted from oxidation and fatty acid synthesis to gluconeogenesis, Cori's cycle and alanine cycle becomes active (Fig. 12.5).

Phase III: Fasting state (10–12 hours of fasting to 2–3 days) (Fig. 12.7)

- No dietery fuel, and little glycogen left after 10–12 hours of fasting.
- Hepatic gluconeogenesis supplies glucose to brain.
- Cori and alanine cycles play important role but cannot provide carbon for net synthesis of glucose. This is because the glucose formed from them in liver merely replaces the glucose used to produce them in muscles and other peripheral tissues (Fig. 12.5).

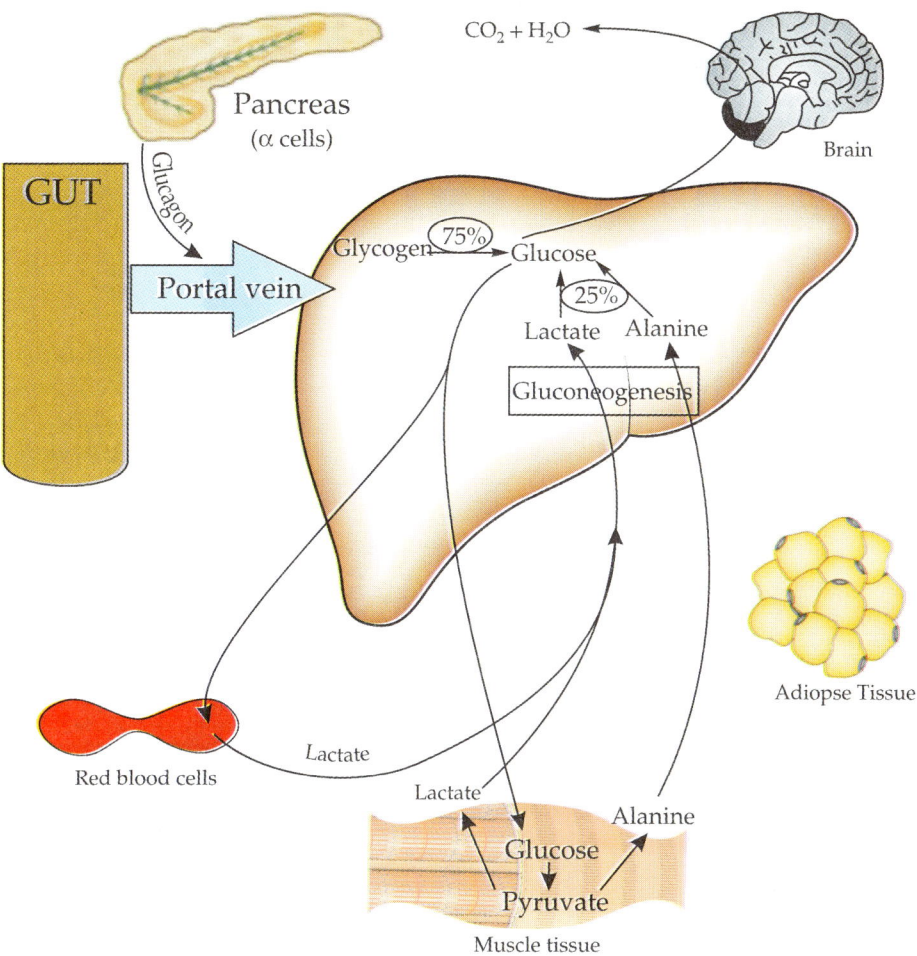

Fig. 12.4. The early fasting state. 75% of glucose output from liver is derived from glycogen and 25% from gluconeogenesis from alanine and lactate.

- As brain oxidises glucose to CO_2 and H_2O, net glucose synthesis from other carbon source is required. Amino acids from skeletal muscle proteins are the most important source followed by glycerol and odd chain fatty acids from adipose tissue.
- Proteins are broken in muscles and most amino acids are partially metabolized. Alanine and glutamine are released in largest amounts. Other amino acids are metabolized to α-ketoglutarate and pyruvate from which glutamine and alanine are made for export. Branched chain amino acids are a major source of ammonia for production of alanine and glutamine from pyruvate and α-ketoglutarate. Their α-keto acids are also released in blood and taken up by liver to produce glucose from α-keto acid of valine and leucine and ketone bodies from α-keto acid of isoleucine and leucine.
- Part of glutamine released by muscles is used by intestinal epithelium, lymphocytes and macrophages, as shown in Fig. 12.6, to produce energy and for pyrimidine and purine synthesis. Partial oxidation of Gln to Ala or Asp is used to generate ATP from TCA.

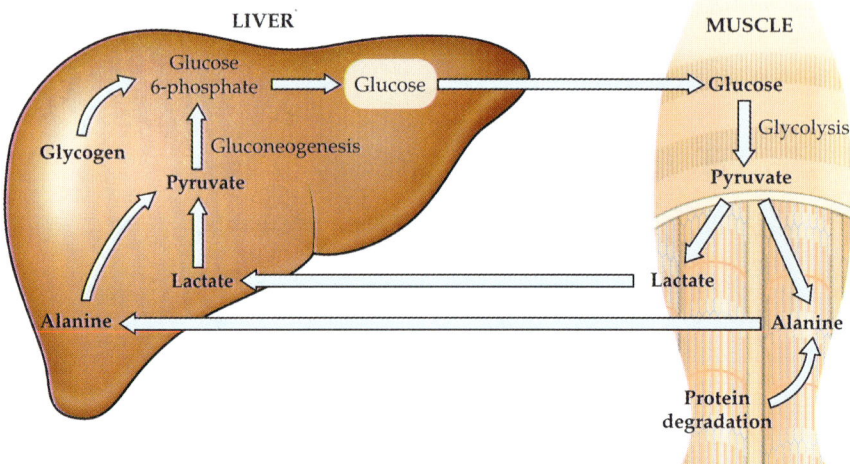

Fig. 12.5. The Cori's and alanine cycles.

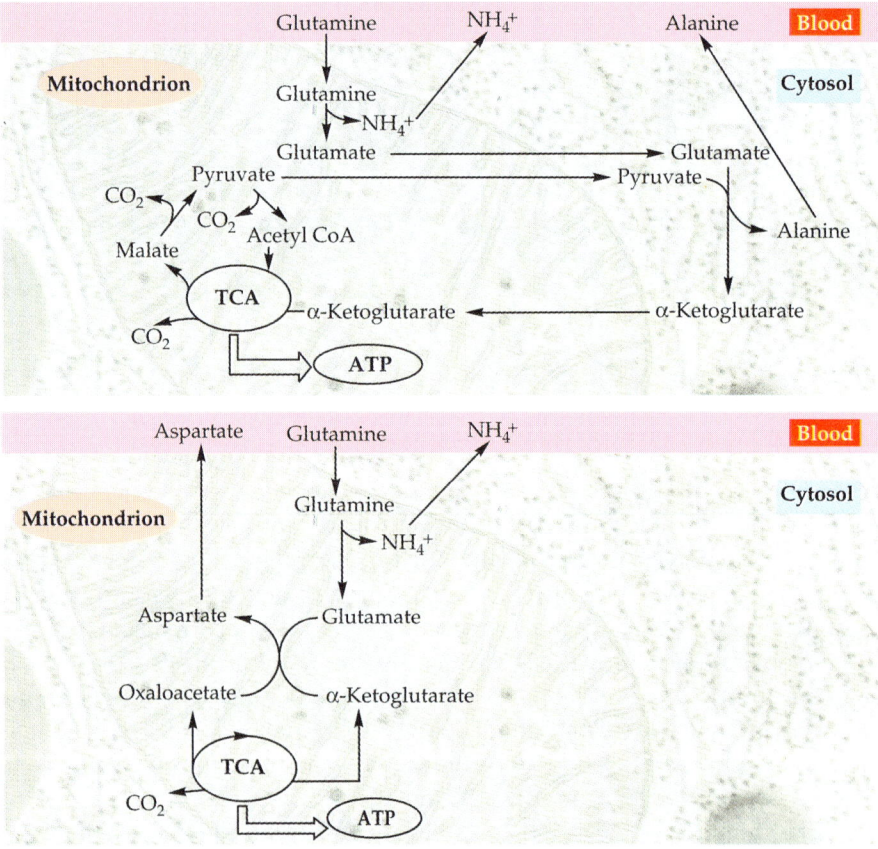

Fig. 12.6. Glutaminolysis in intestinal epithelium, lymphocytes and macrophages. Partial oxidation of Gln to Ala or Asp is used to generate ATP from TCA.

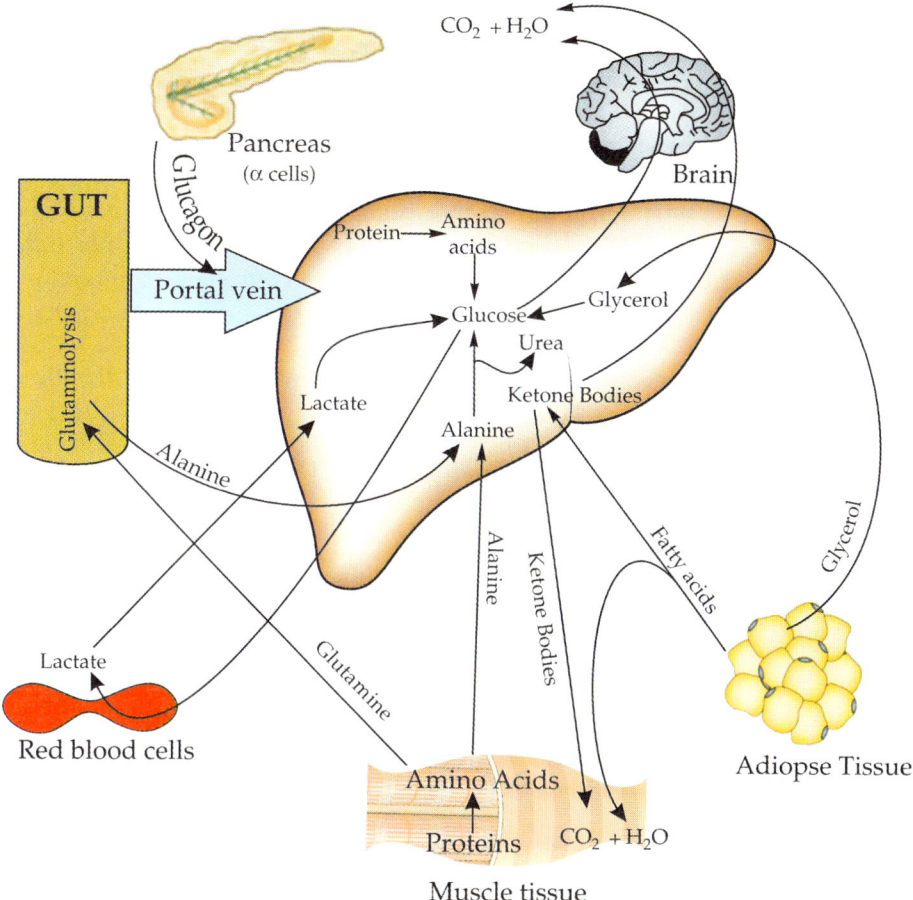

Fig. 12.7. The prolonged fasting state.

- Urea synthesis occurs simultaneously when hepatic gluconeogenesis occurs (urea bicycle) to excrete the ammonia group while carbon skeleton is used for gluconeogenesis and ketone production (free fatty acids).

- Hormone-sensitive lipase (HSL) releases FFA and glycerol from adipose tissues in large amounts. FFA are used preferentially over glucose as fuel in most tissues like heart and muscles (β-oxidation inhibits glycolysis and pyruvate dehydrogenase, acetyl CoA and NADH from β-oxidation activate PDH kinase allosterically to phosphorylate and inactivate PDH, this is called the glucose–fatty acid cycle). In liver FFA oxidation provides most ATP and energy needed for various processes including gluconeogenesis. The supply of FFA to liver is far greater than that required for energy by liver. The remaining FFA after β-oxidation converts to ketone bodies rather than going into TCA. Ketone bodies are exported as alternate fuel and used by β-oxidation in other tissues, again being preferred over glucose oxidation. Even brain can get upto 70% of energy from them in very prolonged starvation, while FFA cannot enter brain. Use of ketone bodies and FFA by most tissues spares precious glucose for brain.

- Ketone bodies and FFA by supplying energy, suppress proteolysis and branched chain amino acid oxidation in muscles, and decrease alanine release for alanine cycle. This prevents muscle wasting and loss of precious muscle protein as well as decreases burden on hepatic gluconeogenesis for a long time.
- Ketone bodies are water soluble and easily transported in blood. During prolonged starvation their oxidation contributes to 90% of the total body oxygen consumption.
- Thus, the energy stored in fat reserve is channeled all over the body while sparing and maintaining glucose levels for brain. As long as glucose levels are maintained some insulin is released and it also works to keep proteolysis in muscles at minimum.
- Thus, liver makes glucose to maintain levels using substrate from muscles and energy from fats.
- Fasting also reduces T_4 to T_3 conversion lowering the basal metabolic rate and energy requirement by upto 25%.

Early refed state
- Availability of dietary fuel after fasting.
- TG is metabolised as in fed state.
- Liver continues to use glucose (now from diet) poorly, remaining in gluconeogenic mode for a few hours. This allows the glucose to restore glycogen stores in muscles which are much greater than liver stores.
- The hepatic gluconeogenesis provides glucose-6-phosphate for replenishing liver glycogen.
- Lactate from peripheral tissues and amino acids from GIT also are used to produce glucose-6-phosphate and glycogen.
- After the rate of gluconeogenesis declines dietary glucose is used to make glycogen in liver.

5 phases of glucose homeostasis

Glucose homeostasis is tightly controlled in all phases of fed state as well as prolonged starvation, as glucose levels lower than 30 mg/dL lead to coma and death as glucose is essential for brain. Acute hyperglycemia must be avoided to prevent loss of glucose in urine (above 180 mg/dL, renal threshold) which will lead to dehydration. Very high levels of glucose can cause hyperosmolarity causing brain cells to shrink leading to coma and death (hyperosmolar coma). Chronic hyperglycemia can also lead to various complications of diabetes mellitus. The levels of FFA and ketones fluctuate over 10 to 100 times in starvation states as compared to the narrower fluctuations in glucose levels. The levels of various metabolites and hormones in different phases of starve–feed cycle are shown in Table 12.1.

The 5 phases of glucose homeostasis were determined from obese patients undergoing long-term starvation for weight loss (Fig. 12.8 and Table 12.2).

- **Phase I** – Well-fed state.
- **Phase II** – Hepatic glycogen breakdown maintains blood glucose, gluconeogenesis starts as glycogen dwindles.
- **Phase III** – Hepatic gluconeogenesis from amino acids and glycerol maintains blood glucose. Ketogenesis occurs. This phase is fully active by around 20 hrs after beginning of last meal, depending on previous hepatic glycogen content.

Table 12.1. Substrate and hormone levels in different phases of starve–feed cycle

Hormone or substrate (units)	Very well fed	Post-absorptive 12 h	Fasted 3 days	Starved 5 weeks
Insulin ($\mu U\ mL^{-1}$)	40	15	8	6
Glucagon ($pg\ mL^{-1}$)	80	100	150	120
Insulin/glucagon ratio ($\mu U\ pg^{-1}$)	0.50	0.15	0.05	0.05
Glucose (mM)	6.1	4.8	3.8	3.6
Fatty acids (mM)	0.14	0.6	1.2	1.4
Acetoacetate (mM)	0.04	0.05	0.4	1.3
β-Hydroxybutyrate (mM)	0.03	0.10	1.4	6.0
Lactate (mM)	2.5	0.7	0.7	0.6
Pyruvate (mM)	0.25	0.06	0.04	0.03
Alanine (mM)	0.8	0.3	0.3	0.1
ATP equivalents (mM)	313	290	380	537

Table 12.2. 5 phases of glucose homeostasis

Phase	Origin of blood glucose	Tissues using glucose	Major fuel of brain
I	Exogenous	All	Glucose
II	Glycogen Hepatic gluconeogenesis	All except liver Muscle and adipose tissue at diminished rates	Glucose
III	Hepatic gluconeogenesis Glycogen	All except liver Muscle and adipose tissue at rates intermediate between II and IV	Glucose
IV	Gluconeogenesis, hepatic and renal	Brain, RBCs, renal medulla. Small amount by muscle	Glucose, ketone bodies
V	Gluconeogenesis, hepatic and renal	Brain at a diminished rate, RBCs, renal medulla	Ketone bodies, glucose

- **Phase IV** – Starts with several days of fasting, dependence on gluconeogenesis decreases, ketone bodies are main fuel. By now ketone body levels have risen sufficiently to enter brain and contribute to its energy demand. Renal gluconeogenesis also becomes significant.
- **Phase V** – Occurs only after prolonged starvation in extremely obese individuals and is characterized by even less dependence on gluconeogenesis, energy need of almost every tissue is met largely by FFA or ketone bodies. As long as ketone body concentrations are high and glucose levels are maintained, proteolysis stays within limits and muscle proteins and enzymes are conserved. This continues till all fat is used up. Then there is no alternative but to use muscle protein for gluconeogenesis. The person does not survive long enough for all protein to be catabolized. Table 12.3 shows the fuel metabolism at 40th day of starvation as compared to the 3rd day of starvation.

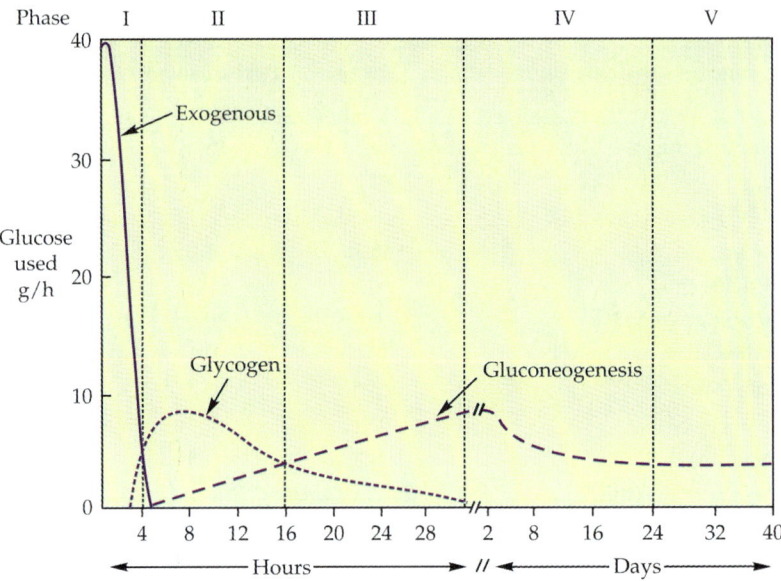

Fig. 12.8. The 5 phases of glucose homeostasis.

Table 12.3. Fuel metabolism in starvation

Fuel exchanges and consumption	Amount formed or consumed in 24 hours (grams)	
	3rd day	40th day
Fuel use by the brain		
Glucose	100 →	40
Ketone bodies	50 →	100
All other use of glucose	50	40
Fuel mobilization		
Adipose tissue lipolysis	180	180
Muscle protein degradation	75 →	20
Fuel output of the liver		
Glucose	150 →	80
Ketone bodies	150	150

Females are more resistant to adverse effects of starvation. They have a lower BMR and therefore need less food per day than males. Evolutionary pressure has been greater on females of most species in time of food deprivation and famines. In most species many females can mate with one male and males are not needed during pregnancy and lactation, further they compete for food with offspring. Thus, survival of males is less important during long periods of food shortage. Thus, evolution has naturally selected genes which confer greater resistance to starvation in females. Mitochondria from females are more highly differentiated and have more enzymes for oxidative phosphorylation.

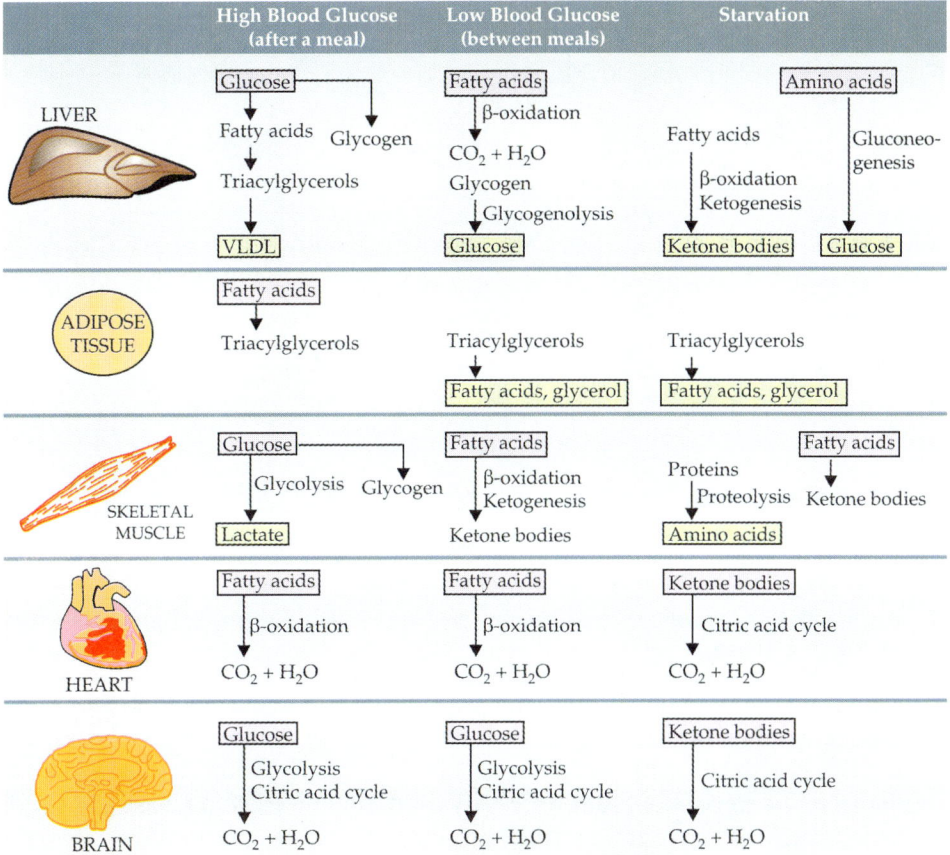

Fig. 12.9. Summary of the metabolism in various organs in different phases of feed–starve cycle.

Q. 3. What is the significance of AMP-activated protein kinase?

Ans. AMP-activated protein kinase (AMPK) is the cellular energy sensor. Due to the nature of the adenylate kinase equilibrium, AMP levels increase exponentially as ATP levels decrease (Fig. 12.10).

AMP is an allosteric activator of AMPK, whereas ATP at high levels acts as an allosteric inhibitor by displacing AMP from the allosteric site. Thus, competition between AMP and ATP for binding to the AMPK allosteric sites determines the activity of AMPK. So:
- When cellular energy levels are high, as signalled by high ATP concentrations, AMPK is inactive.
- When cellular energy levels are depleted, as signalled by high [AMP], AMPK is allosterically activated and phosphorylates many targets.

AMPK is an $\alpha\beta\gamma$-heterotrimer. The γ-subunit is the regulatory subunit which has AMP/ATP binding sites. These sites are located toward the C-terminus in the form of four CBS domains. The CBS domains act in pairs to form structures known as Bateman modules. The Bateman modules provide the binding sites for the allosteric ligands, AMP and ATP. AMP binding to Bateman modules is highly cooperative. Binding of AMP to one module markedly enhances AMP-binding at the other. This co-operativity makes AMPK very sensitive to changes in AMP concentration. When AMP binds to the Bateman modules, conformational

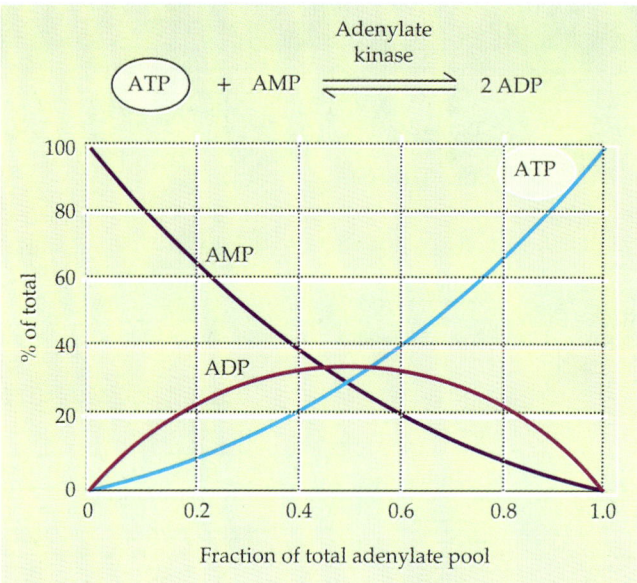

Fig. 12.10. The adenylate kinase reaction and the relative changes in concentration of ATP, ADP and AMP with ATP use.

changes in the γ-subunit displace the pseudosubstrate sequence from the catalytic site on α-subunit, freeing it to act. AMP activates AMPK in two ways: first, it is an allosteric activator; second, AMP binding favours phosphorylation of Thr172 within the α-subunit kinase domain. Phosphorylation of Thr172 is necessary for α-subunit protein kinase activity. Both of these actions by AMP are reversed if ATP displaces AMP from the allosteric site. AMP binding to AMPK increases its protein kinase activity by more than 1000-fold.

Activated AMPK targets key enzymes in energy production and consumption (Figs. 12.11 and 12.12)

1. Stimulates catabolic pathways leading to ATP synthesis. Enzymes involved in energy production that are activated upon phosphorylation by AMPK include:
   – Phosphofructokinase-2 (PFK-2) – stimulates glycolysis
   – Glycogen phosphorylase – activates glycogen breakdown
   – Malonyl CoA decarboxylase – increases β-oxidation and inhibits fatty acid synthesis.
2. Inhibits anabolic pathways which consume ATP. Enzymes involved in energy consumption that are down-regulated upon phosphorylation by AMPK include:
   – Glycogen synthase – glycogen synthesis
   – Fructose 1,6-bisphosphatase – gluconeogenesis
   – Acetyl-CoA carboxylase – committed and regulated step in fatty acid biosynthesis
   – 3-Hydroxy-3-methylglutaryl-CoA reductase – regulatory reaction in cholesterol biosynthesis.

Inhibition of acetyl CoA carboxylase and activation of malonyl CoA decarboxylase decreases malonyl CoA and thus inhibits fatty acid synthesis as well as relieves inhibition of CPT-1 to allow β-oxidation to increase (Fig. 12.12).

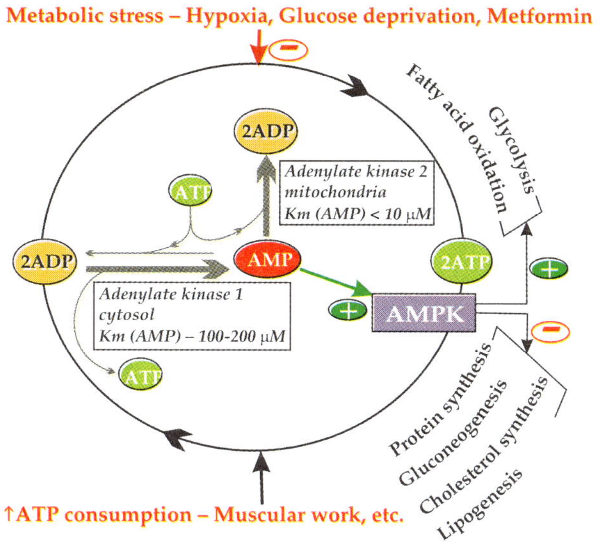

Integration of Metabolism and Endocrinology

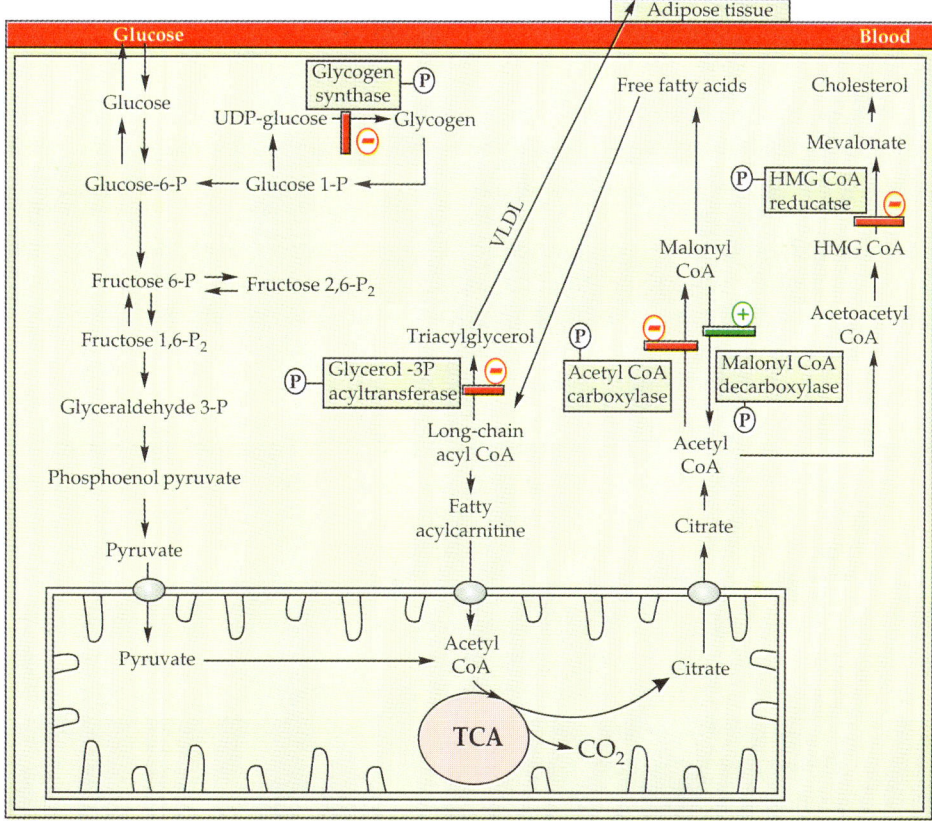

Fig. 12.11. AMPK inhibits ATP-requiring processes and activates ATP-producing processes.

Fig. 12.12. Enzymes regulated by AMPK in liver. 1. Glycogen synthase; 2. Glycerol-3-phosphate acyltransferase; 3. Acetyl CoA carboxylase; 4. Malonyl CoA decarboxylase; 5. HMG CoA reductase.

AMPK controls whole body energy homeostasis

AMPK also plays a central role in energy balance in multicellular organisms:

1. AMPK in skeletal muscle is activated by hormones such as adiponectin and leptin, and by physical activity (exercise). Skeletal muscle AMPK activates glucose uptake (stimulates transport of vesicles with GLUT 4 to plasma membrane to increase glucose entry), fatty acid oxidation, and mitochondrial biogenesis through phosphorylation of metabolic enzymes and transcription factors that control expression of genes involved in energy production and consumption.
2. AMPK's actions in the liver lead to lowered ATP (energy) consumption through down-regulation of fatty acid synthesis, cholesterol synthesis, and gluconeogenesis.
3. AMPK blocks insulin secretion by pancreatic β-cells.
4. AMPK is also a master regulator of eating behaviour through its activity in the hypothalamus.
5. Leptin and adiponectin improve insulin sensitivity by directly enhancing the activity of the AMP-activated protein kinase (AMPK) in liver and skeletal muscles.
6. Metformin, a widely used drug for the treatment of type 2 diabetes, activates AMPK and thus lowers blood glucose levels through inhibition of liver gluconeogenesis.

Q. 4. What is the biochemical basis of harmful effects of obesity?

Ans. Obesity has many significant adverse effects on health. Obesity is associated with a 50–100% increased risk of death from all causes compared to normal-weight individuals, mostly due to cardiovascular causes. Mortality rates rise as obesity increases, particularly when obesity is associated with increased intra-abdominal fat. Life expectancy of a moderately obese individual could be shortened by 2–5 years, and a 20- to 30-year-old male with a BMI > 45 may lose 13 years of life. The degree to which obesity affects particular organ systems is influenced by susceptibility genes that vary in the population.

Intra-abdominal fat or central obesity is more harmful. Visceral fat is composed of several adipose depots including mesenteric, epididymal white adipose tissue (EWAT) and perirenal fat. An excess of visceral fat is known as central obesity, the "pot belly" or "beer belly" effect, in which the abdomen protrudes excessively. This body type is also known as "apple shaped," as opposed to "pear-shaped," in which fat is deposited on the hips and buttocks. Central obesity (abdominal fat) is more likely to be linked with insulin resistance than are peripheral (gluteal/subcutaneous) fat depots as:

- Central adipose tissue is more "lipolytic" than peripheral sites
- Visceral fat cells will release their metabolic by-products in the portal circulation, where the blood goes straight to the liver. Thus, the excess of fatty acids secreted by the visceral fat cells will go into the liver and accumulate there. This is known as lipotoxicity.
- Abdominal fat is especially active hormonally, secreting more adipokines that create insulin resistance.

Besides being a storage depot for fat, adipose cell is also an endocrine cell that releases numerous molecules in a regulated fashion (Fig. 12.13). These are responsible for the harmful consequences of obesity.

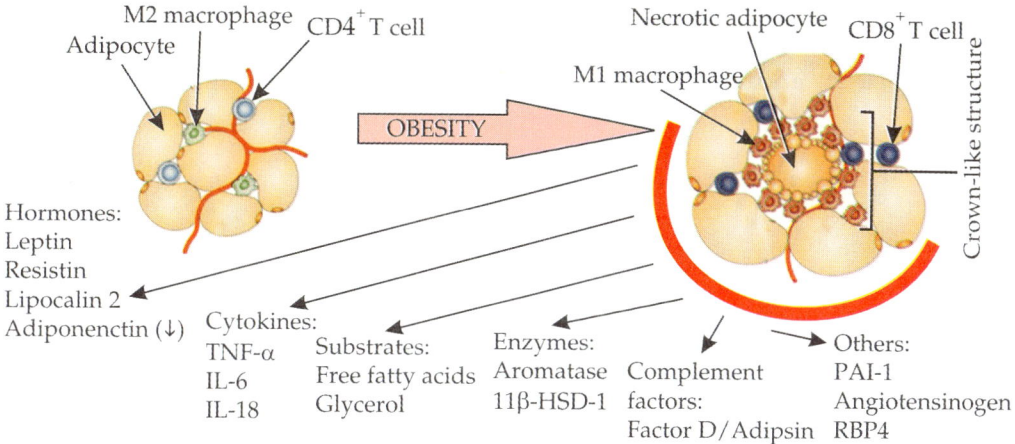

Fig. 12.13. Factors released by adipose tissues responsible for consequences of obesity.

Consequences of obesity and their biochemical basis

1. Insulin resistance and hyperinsulinemia (Fig. 12.14)

It is defined as the failure of target tissues (muscle, liver and fat) to respond normally to insulin. It leads to:
- decreased uptake of glucose in muscle;
- inability to suppress hepatic gluconeogenesis;
- increased release of free fatty acids from adipose tissue (lack of inhibition of hormone-sensitive lipase); and
- reduced glycolysis and hence fatty acid oxidation in the liver.

Functional defects in the insulin signalling pathway in states of insulin resistance include reduced tyrosine phosphorylation and increased serine phosphorylation of the insulin receptor and IRS (insulin receptor substrate) proteins, which attenuate signal transduction. Post-receptor defects in insulin-regulated phosphorylation/dephosphorylation play predominant role in insulin resistance. Insulin resistance is present even in simple obesity unaccompanied by hyperglycemia, indicating a fundamental abnormality of insulin signalling in states of fatty excess. Molecular mechanisms of obesity and insulin resistance in fat, muscle, and liver include:

- **Free fatty acids or non-esterified fatty acids (NEFAs):** Excess intracellular NEFAs overwhelm the fatty acid oxidation pathways, leading to accumulation of cytoplasmic intermediates like diacylglycerol (DAG) and ceramide. These "toxic" intermediates can activate serine/threonine kinases, which cause aberrant serine phosphorylation of the insulin receptor and IRS proteins. Phosphorylation at serine instead of tyrosine residues attenuates insulin signalling. Excess NEFAs also compete with glucose for oxidation, leading to feedback inhibition of glycolytic enzymes, decreasing glucose utilization.

- **Intracellular lipid accumulation:** Level of intracellular triglycerides is markedly increased in muscle and liver tissues of obese individuals because excess circulating NEFAs are deposited in these organs. The accumulation of lipid within skeletal myocytes impairs mitochondrial oxidative phosphorylation and reduces insulin-stimulated mitochondrial ATP production. Impaired fatty acid oxidation and lipid accumulation within skeletal myocytes also generate reactive oxygen species such as lipid peroxides.

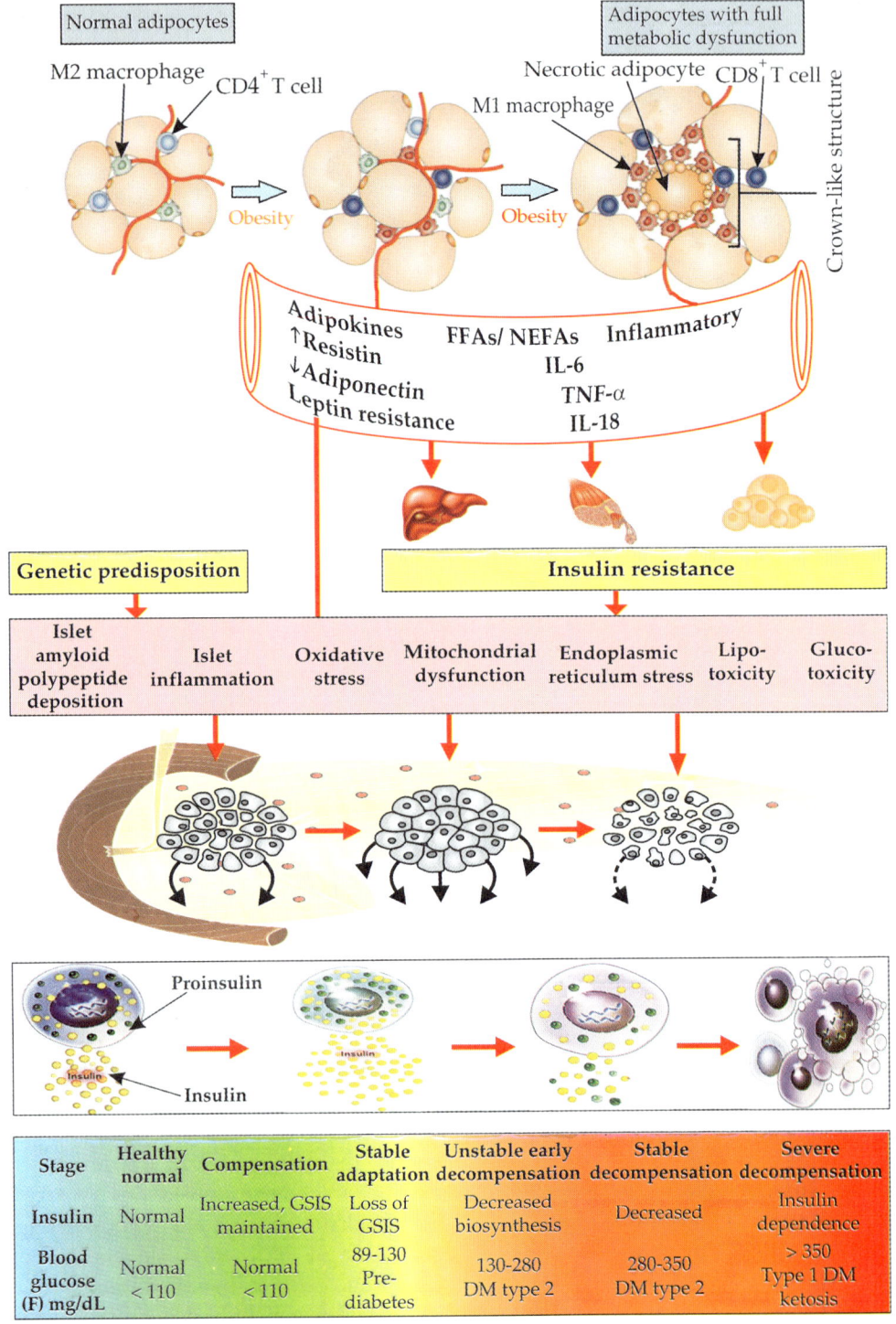

Fig. 12.14. Obesity, insulin resistance and diabetes.

- **Circulating peptides produced by adipocytes:** Resistin and retinol-binding protein 4 [RBP4] are pro-hyperglycemic adipokines and leptin and adiponectin are anti-hyperglycemic adipokines.

    Leptin and adiponectin improve insulin sensitivity by directly enhancing the activity of the AMP-activated protein kinase (AMPK) in liver and skeletal muscle. Adiponectin decreases gluconeogenesis, increases glucose uptake, increases β-oxidation and triglyceride clearance, protects from endothelial dysfunction, increases insulin sensitivity, and up-regulates uncoupling proteins. Adiponectin levels are reduced in obesity, contributing to insulin resistance.

    Although, leptin reduces appetite as a circulating signal, obese individuals generally exhibit an unusually high circulating concentration of leptin. These people are resistant to the effects of leptin. The sustained high concentrations of leptin from the enlarged adipose stores may cause leptin desensitization.

    Resistin and RBP4 promote insulin resistance. Resistin also increases inflammation, increases LDL production and decreases LDL clearance by decreasing LDL receptor in liver.

- **Obesity-linked inflammation:** Infiltration of macrophages into tissues including fat, and induction of the endoplasmic reticulum stress response, leads to insulin resistance. Adipose tissue also secretes a variety of pro-inflammatory cytokines like tumor necrosis factor, interleukin-6, and macrophage chemoattractant protein-1, attracting macrophages to fat deposits. These cytokines induce insulin resistance by increasing cellular "stress", which, in turn, activates multiple signalling cascades that antagonize insulin action on peripheral tissues.

- **Insulin itself:** In obesity, glucose tolerance remains near-normal, despite insulin resistance, because the pancreatic beta cells compensate by increasing insulin output. However, hyperinsulinemia can induce receptor downregulation. Insulin receptor levels and tyrosine kinase activity in skeletal muscle are reduced due to hyperinsulinemia.

2. Type 2 diabetes

As insulin resistance and compensatory hyperinsulinemia progress, the pancreatic islets in some individuals are unable to sustain the hyperinsulinemic state. Impaired glucose tolerance (elevated postprandial glucose) then develops. A further decline in insulin secretion and an increase in hepatic glucose production lead to diabetes with fasting hyperglycemia. Beta cell mass is decreased by approximately 50% in individuals with long-standing type 2 diabetes. Despite the prevalence of insulin resistance, most obese individuals do not develop diabetes, suggesting that diabetes requires an interaction between obesity-induced insulin resistance and other genetic and environmental factors which impair insulin secretion and damage β cells (Fig. 12.14). Obesity, however, is the major risk factor for diabetes, and as many as 80% of patients with type 2 diabetes mellitus are obese. Weight loss and exercise, even of modest degree, increase insulin sensitivity and often improve glucose control in diabetes. Obesity also leads to β cell dysfunction. Chronic hyperglycemia paradoxically impairs islet function ("glucose toxicity") and leads to a worsening of hyperglycemia. Improvement in glycemic control is often associated with improved islet function. In addition, elevation of free fatty acid levels ("lipotoxicity") and dietary fat may also worsen islet function.

3. Male hypogonadism

In men whose weight is > 160% ideal body weight, plasma testosterone and sex hormone-binding globulin (SHBG) are reduced, and estrogen levels are increased. Estrogen is derived from conversion of adrenal androgens in adipose tissue which produce aromatase and 11β-hydroxysteroid dehydrogenase. Gynecomastia can occur. However, masculinization, libido, potency, and spermatogenesis are preserved in most of these individuals. Free testosterone may be decreased in morbidly obese men whose weight is > 200% ideal body weight.

4. Menstrual abnormalities in women and PCOS

Particularly in women with upper body obesity. Common findings are increased androgen production, decreased SHBG, and increased peripheral conversion of androgen to estrogen (by aromatase produced by adipocytes). Most obese women with oligomenorrhea have the polycystic ovarian syndrome (PCOS), with its associated anovulation and ovarian hyperandrogenism; while 40% of women with PCOS are obese. Most non-obese women with PCOS are also insulin-resistant, suggesting that insulin resistance, hyperinsulinemia, or the combination of the two are causative or contribute to the ovarian pathophysiology in PCOS in both obese and lean individuals. In obese women with PCOS, weight loss or treatment with insulin-sensitizing drugs often restores normal menses. The increased conversion of androstenedione to estrogen, which occurs to a greater degree in women with obesity, contributes to the increased incidence of uterine cancer in postmenopausal women with obesity.

5. Hypertension

Measurement of blood pressure in the obese requires use of a larger cuff size to avoid artifactual increases. Adipocytes produce angiotensinogen and obesity-induced hypertension is associated with increased peripheral resistance and cardiac output, increased sympathetic nervous system tone, increased salt sensitivity, and insulin-mediated salt retention. It is often responsive to modest weight loss.

6. Obesity

Obesity tilts the balance in favour of thrombosis in hemostatic pathway. Adipocytes produce plasminogen activator inhibitor 1, which inhibits activation of plasminogen and thus clot lysis. This increases risk of arterial blockade in atherosclerosis.

7. Cardiovascular disease

Obesity is an independent risk factor for cardiovascular disease in men and women (including coronary disease, stroke, and congestive heart failure). Obesity, especially abdominal obesity, is associated with dyslipidemia and an atherogenic lipid profile, with increased low-density lipoprotein cholesterol, very low density lipoprotein, and triglyceride, and with decreased high density lipoprotein cholesterol and decreased levels of the vascular protective adipokine adiponectin. Not all insulin signal transduction pathways are resistant to the effects of insulin (e.g., those controlling cell growth and differentiation using the mitogenic-activated protein kinase pathway). Consequently, hyperinsulinemia increases the insulin action through these pathways, accelerating atherosclerosis. Obesity is associated with persistent mild chronic inflammation (increased cytokine and CRP production by adipocytes) which contributes to atherosclerosis.

8. Hepatobiliary disease

Obesity is frequently associated with the common disorder – nonalcoholic fatty liver disease (NAFLD). This hepatic fatty infiltration of NAFLD can progress to inflammatory non-alcoholic steatohepatitis (NASH) and more rarely to cirrhosis and hepatocellular carcinoma. This occurs due to the excessive supply of FFA from fat cells to liver due to insulin resistance as well as increased levels of inflammatory cytokines. Obesity is associated with enhanced biliary secretion of cholesterol, supersaturation of bile, and a higher incidence of gallstones, particularly cholesterol gallstones. A person 50% above ideal body weight has about a six-fold increased incidence of symptomatic gallstones. Steatosis has been noted to improve following weight loss, diet control or bariatric surgery.

9. Cancer

Obesity in males is associated with higher mortality from cancer, including cancer of the esophagus, colon, rectum, pancreas, liver, and prostate; obesity in females is associated with higher mortality from cancer of the gallbladder, bile ducts, breasts, endometrium, cervix, and ovaries. These may be due to increased rates of conversion of androstenedione to estrone in adipose tissue of obese individuals. Possible links between obesity and cancer are hormones like insulin, leptin, adiponectin, and IGF-1 and the state of chronic low grade inflammation occurring in obesity. Insulin, leptin and IGF-1 have mitogenic activity, i.e. they promote cell proliferation.

10. Bone, joint, and cutaneous disease

Increased risk of osteoarthritis, due to the trauma of added weight bearing and activation of inflammatory pathways by cytokines secreted by fat cells. Among the skin problems associated with obesity is acanthosis nigricans, manifested by darkening and thickening of the skinfolds on the neck, elbows, and dorsal interphalangeal spaces. Acanthosis reflects the severity of underlying insulin resistance and diminishes with weight loss. Friability of skin may be increased, especially in skinfolds, enhancing the risk of fungal and yeast infections. Venous stasis is also increased in the obesity.

11. Pulmonary disease

Reduced chest wall compliance, increased work of breathing, increased minute ventilation due to increased metabolic rate, and decreased functional residual capacity and expiratory reserve volume. Severe obesity may be associated with obstructive sleep apnea and the "obesity hypoventilation syndrome" also called the 'Pickwickian syndrome' with attenuated hypoxic and hypercapnic ventilatory responses. Sleep apnea can be obstructive (most common), central, or mixed and is associated with hypertension. Sleep apnea is a component of metabolic syndrome and is itself also known to promote insulin resistance. Weight loss (10–20 kg) can bring substantial improvement.

Q. 5. Why there is hyperlipoproteinemia in DM when there is lack of insulin (or insulin resistance) as insulin increases lipid synthesis? What are the differences in metabolic abnormalities in type 1 DM and type 2 DM?

Ans. **Metabolic abnormalities in type 2 DM** (Fig. 12.15)
- Type 2 DM patients are mostly obese and obesity is responsible for the insulin resistance. Patients in initial years have compensatory hyperinsulinemia and over many years insulin

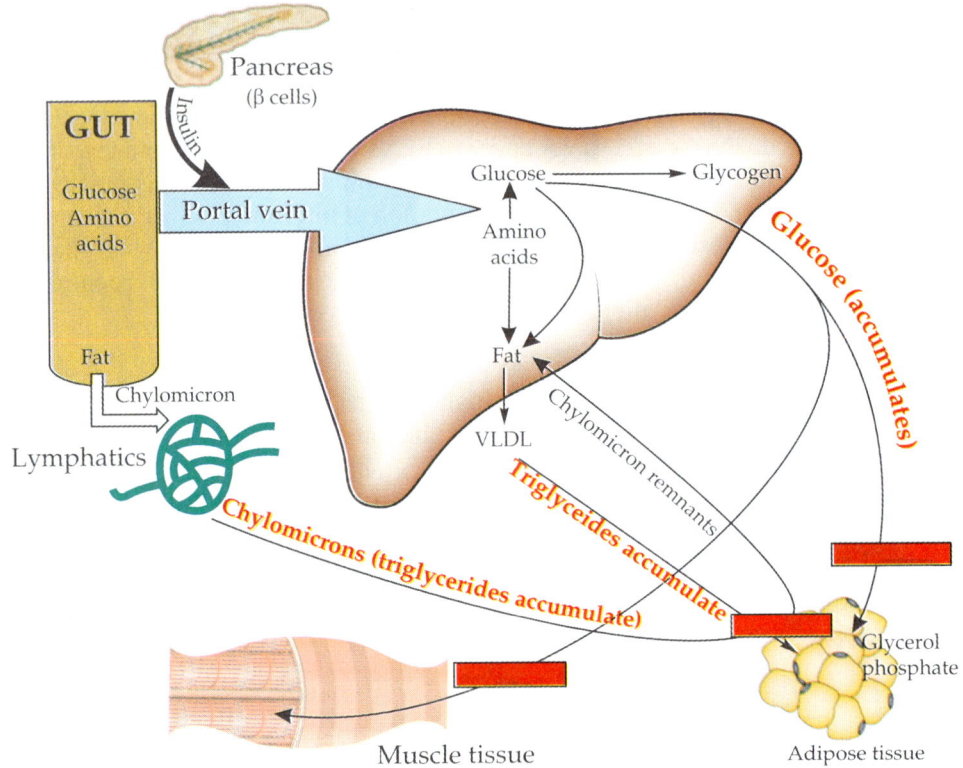

Fig. 12.15. Metabolic abnormalities in type 2 DM.

levels decrease due to decrease in β-cell mass when finally patients may convert to type 1 DM requiring exogenous insulin. Most patients are > 40 years of age though DM type 2 is now very common in young obese too.

- Thus, type 2 DM has insulin resistance with hyperinsulinemia.
- The dyslipidemia seen in type 2 DM characterized by insulin resistance is mainly due to increase in VLDL production in liver while chylomicrons remain normal. Due to increased VLDL, IDL and LDL are also increased as they are derived from VLDL.
- Type 2 DM is characterized by decreased inhibition of hormone sensitive lipase in adipose cells due to insulin resistance. This increases lipolysis and FFA flux to liver which can use it for ATP production to a limited extent. Rest of incoming FFA in liver must undergo re-esterification, VLDL synthesis and export or ketone body synthesis depending on relative insulin and glucagon concentrations. Increased TG and VLDL synthesis occur in liver in type 2 DM along with the increased lipolysis in adipose tissue.
- This anomaly results from a state of mixed insulin resistance in insulin signalling pathways. Not all actions of insulin have same defect. A defect in the pathway (PI_3 kinase pathway) inhibiting gluconeogenesis results in excessive hepatic glucose production. While the pathway controlling fatty acid and TG synthesis is more responsive leading liver to overproduce VLDL from the incoming flux of FFA. Thus, more fatty acids and TG are synthesized de novo from glucose too in liver.
- Extra TG in liver also leads to lipid storage or steatosis in the liver and may lead to non-alcoholic fatty liver disease.

- Although body produces more insulin it is not sufficient to promote glucose uptake in skeletal muscles. Transport of GLUT 4 to membrane from vesicles is decreased in both skeletal muscles and fat cells.
- Increased hepatic glucose output (from gluconeogenesis) predominantly accounts for increased fasting plasma glucose (FPG) levels, whereas decreased peripheral glucose usage results in postprandial hyperglycemia. In skeletal muscle, there is a greater impairment in nonoxidative glucose usage (glycogen formation) than in oxidative glucose metabolism through glycolysis.
- Glucose metabolism in insulin-independent tissues is not altered in type 2 DM.
- Ketoacidosis rarely develops as sufficient insulin is available to suppress excessive uncontrolled release of FFA from adipose tissue and FFA in liver are directed to TG synthesis, rather than ketone synthesis by the available insulin.
- Hyperinsulinemia plays role in complications like atherosclerosis and increased risk of cancer due to its mitogenic (cell proliferating and growth promoting) effect.
- Diet, exercise and weight control can reverse most changes unless there is significant β-cell loss in pancreas.

Type 1 DM (Fig. 12.16)

- It is an autoimmune disease with gradual destruction of β-cells leading to complete insulin deficiency. Most patients are young lean and thin individuals though the autoimmune disease can occur at any age.
- As insulin always remains absent and insulin/glucagon ratio cannot increase, liver always remains in gluconeogenic and ketogenic mode.
- Liver contributes to hyperglycemia in both fed and fasted states.

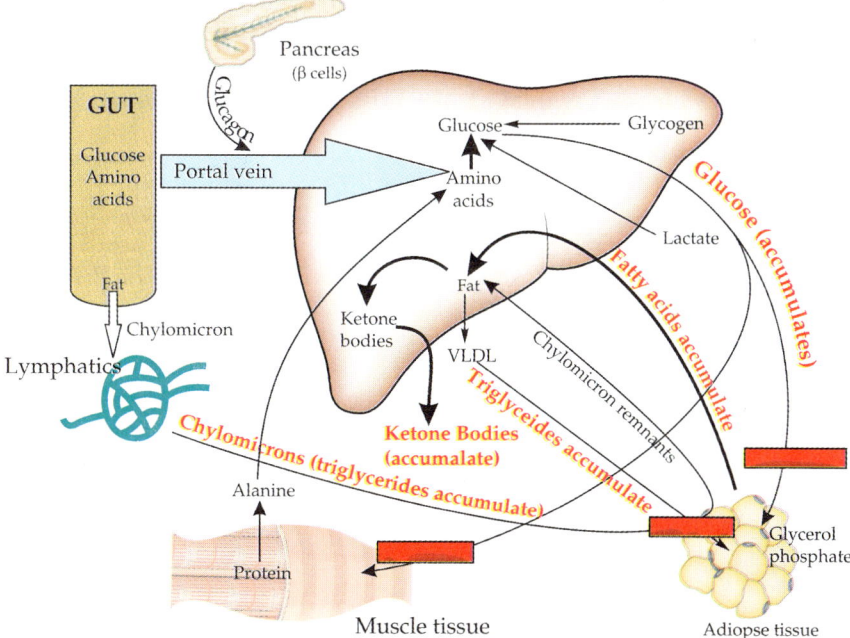

Fig. 12.16. Metabolic abnormalities in type 1 DM.

- Uncontrolled gluconeogenesis occurs from muscle protein amino acids, and there is lack of insulin to inhibit proteolysis. There is muscle wasting.
- Uncontrolled and continuous lipolysis in adipose tissue increases plasma FFA and ketone body, production in liver. There is not sufficient insulin to inhibit hepatic ketogenesis. Thus diabetic ketoacidosis occurs frequently unlike in type 2 DM.
- Even with fatty acid oxidation and ketone body production the excessive supply of FFA from fat cells cannot be disposed of by liver and the remaining FFA flood the pathway for TG and VLDL synthesis. This is an example of substrate level regulation by substrate concentrations overriding the hormonal controls. Further, due to complete absence of insulin to activate LPL the TG in extra VLDL and chylomicrons from diet are not cleared from blood. LPL expression depends on insulin. Thus, there is hypertriglyceridemia, increased VLDL and LDL though due to different mechanism from type 2 DM.
- In type 1 DM every tissue is in catabolic state like in starvation in spite of adequate fuel availability from diet. Thus, there is severe wasting and ultimately death if exogenous insulin is not given as therapy.

Q. 6. What are calcimimetics? What is their mechanism of action and use?

Ans. In parathyroid cells, extracellular ionized calcium activates the CaSR (Calcium sensing receptor) and decreases the release of PTH that is stored within secretory granules (Fig. 12.17). Thus, high ionized calcium levels inhibit PTH release and low ionized calcium levels increase PTH releases. The primary action of PTH is to maintain ionized calcium levels in a narrow range in plasma and plasma-ionized calcium is the major regulator of PTH secretion. An inverse sigmoidal curve describes the relationship between ionized calcium and PTH concentrations (Fig. 12.17). CaSR is a G protein-coupled seven transmembrane domain or serpentine receptor. Its activation activates phospholipase C producing IP3 and DAG which mediate PTH release (Fig. 12.18).

Changes in PTH release that are mediated through the CaSR occur within seconds or minutes, whereas other regulators of PTH secretion lower plasma PTH levels over many

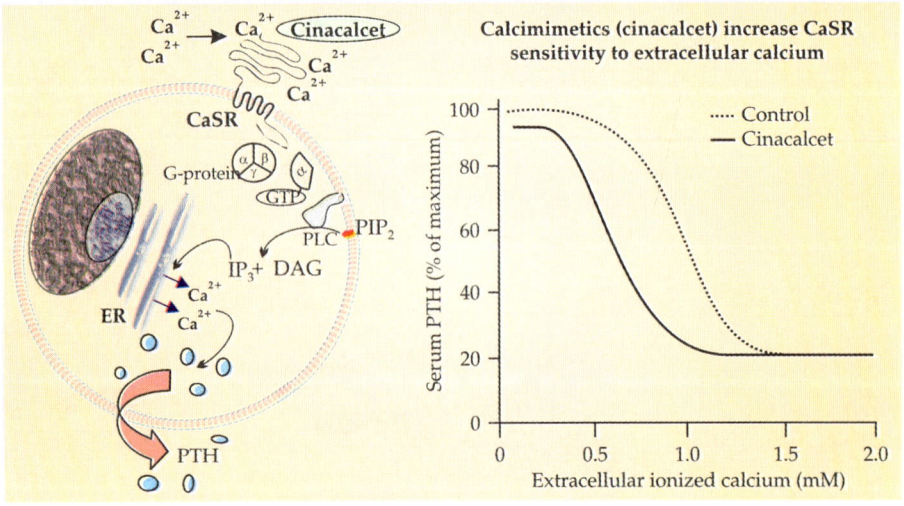

Fig. 12.17. Relation between calcium and PTH release.

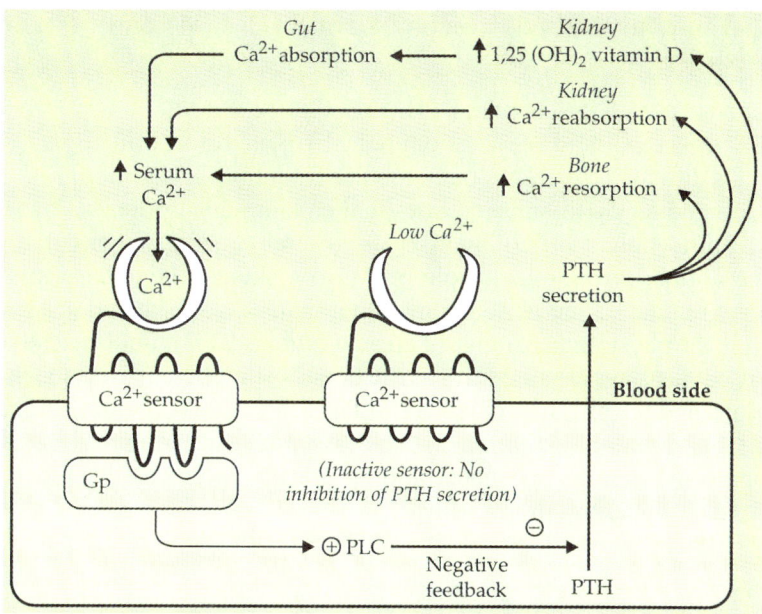

Fig. 12.18. Calcium inhibits PTH release via CaSR.

hours or several days. Both vitamin D and calcium inhibit pre-pro-PTH gene transcription directly by interacting with distinct upstream negative regulatory elements within DNA. The exogenous administration of vitamin D or calcium can also diminish PTH secretion indirectly by raising serum calcium concentrations, but the effects of these interventions on serum calcium and plasma PTH levels typically occur over several days.

Calcimimetic drugs are small organic molecules that act as allosteric activators of the CaSR in the parathyroid glands and other tissues. They lower the threshold for CaSR activation by extracellular calcium ions and diminish PTH release from parathyroid cells. Calcimimetic compounds lower the set point for calcium-regulated PTH release rendering parathyroid cells more sensitive to the inhibitory action of calcium. The calcium PTH curve shifts to left and downwards. Calcimimetic agents alter signal transduction by inducing conformational changes in the CaSR. They neither compete with calcium for binding to the extracellular domain of the CaSR nor do they activate the receptor in the absence of extracellular calcium ions. They abruptly lower plasma PTH levels without any preceding rise in serum calcium concentration. Cinacalcet (brand name Sensipar) is the only drug of this class.

Calcimimetics can effectively reduce PTH secretion in all forms of hyperparathyroidism and are especially used for treating secondary hyperparathyroidism due to renal failure. When given repeatedly and/or in sufficiently large doses to humans, calcimimetic compounds not only lower plasma PTH levels but also reduce blood calcium concentrations. Decreases in serum calcium occurs due to the decline in plasma PTH levels. In patients with secondary hyperparathyroidism, blood calcium concentrations reach lowest levels by 4–8 h after individual doses. Apart from their effect to diminish PTH secretion, calcimimetic compounds also influence the process of parathyroid gland hyperplasia. Calcium, acting through the CaSR, is a more important determinant of parathyroid gland hyperplasia than vitamin D. Calcimimetic agents by inhibiting signalling through the CaSR can provide a means for controlling parathyroid hyperplasia, particularly during the course of progressive renal disease.

Q. 7. Explain how teriparatide (recombinant PTH 1-34) can be used for treatment of osteoporosis.

Ans. In response to hypocalcaemia, PTH (Fig. 12.19):
- increases calcium release from bone by bone resorption;
- acts directly to increase renal tubular calcium reabsorption;
- acts indirectly to enhance intestinal calcium absorption via its stimulatory action on renal 1-cholecalciferol hydroxylase (thereby increasing circulating calcitriol).

The normal physiological role of PTH on skeletal homeostasis is more complex, and serves to regulate bone remodelling rather than overall skeletal mass (Fig. 12.19).
- Within the physiological range of concentrations, PTH stimulates the bone-forming activity of osteoblasts at the same level as the bone-losing activity of osteoclasts. Normal concentrations and the pulsatile character of PTH secretion support the bone-formation process.
- Osteoclastic bone resorption and free osseous calcium ion release into the extracellular fluid occur when PTH concentration is constantly elevated, as seen in both primary and secondary hyperparathyroidism.

PTH can act through 2 receptors: PTH receptor type 1 and type 2 receptor for PTH.

PTH receptor type 1

The primary biological activity of endogenous PTH (1–84) depends on the N-terminal fragment sequence, which is why the shortened, N-terminal, 34-amino acid hPTH analogue (1–34) (teriparatide) has the main activities of the entire molecule. The majority of PTH actions, as well as of the actions of its evolutional analogue, a parathormone-related peptide (PTHrP), are mediated by PTH receptor type 1 (PTH-receptor-PTHrP, a G protein coupled receptor, increases cAMP) which is activated by the above-mentioned N-terminal sequence of amino acids. The PTH receptor is present on the osteoblast surface only. Thus, the primary physiological activity of PTH, i.e. maintaining normal calcium levels by enhancing

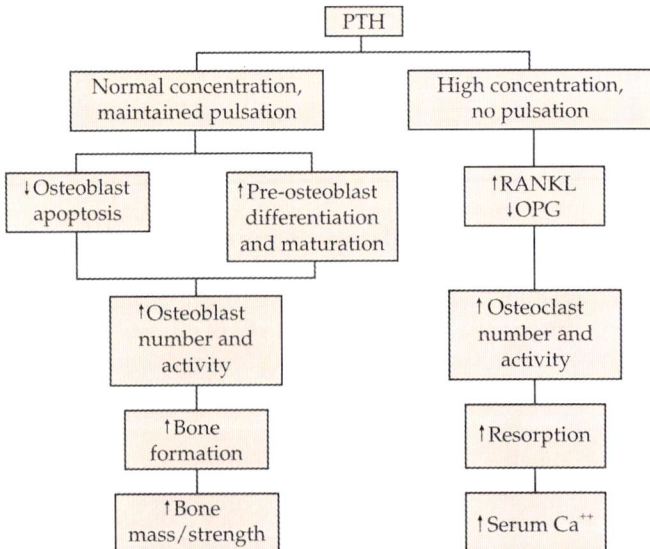

Fig. 12.19. PTH activity, anabolic or catabolic, depending on secretion rate and character.

osteoclastic bone resorption and releasing the free calcium ion into the extracellular space, is an indirect effect.

Effect on osteoclasts is indirect

- In pre-osteoblasts, PTH amplifies the production of RANKL (Receptor Activator of NFkappaB Ligand) cytokine, belonging to the superfamily of tumour necrosis factors (TNF), while simultaneously decreasing the release of osteoprotegerin (OPG), a soluble, decoy receptor for RANKL which inhibits RANKL action.
- It increases the accessibility of RANKL for the functional RANK receptor on the surface of the monocyte/macrophage-osteoblast development line cells. In this way, RANKL enhances the proliferation/differentiation/fusion/maturation and metabolic activity of osteoclasts, so leading to intensification of osteolysis.

Effects on osteoblasts

- PTH simultaneously activates cAMP-dependent protein kinase and calcium-dependent C protein kinase, as well as MAP kinase and phospholipase A & D, all important for osteoblast activity.
- The PTH-receptor complex also undergoes internalisation into osteoblasts and thus has significant gene transcription controlling activity.
- PTH demonstrates mitogenic activity towards osteoblasts, inhibiting their apoptosis, thus increasing number of osteoblasts.
- PTH induces the synthesis of the insulin-like growth factor 1 (IGF-1), a strong bone anabolic factor, in bone tissue.
- PTH suppresses the expression of sclerostin. Sclerostin, an osteocyte-derived protein, blocks the activity of the Wnt-β-catenin pathway responsible for promotion of transcription of many genes. Sclerostin has catabolic effect on bone metabolism. Wnt-β-catenin pathway decreases bone formation.
- PTH helps in bone surface preparation, by increasing bone matrix metaloproteinase synthesis.
- PTH modulates secretion of locally secreted paracrine factors (TGF-β, transforming growth factor beta), enzymes and other substances (including prostaglandins), participating in cell replication processes and osteogenesis stimulation.

Type 2 receptor for PTH

- Activated by the C-terminal section of PTH (1–84), as well as by C-terminal fragments of PTH, either directly released from the parathyroid glands or produced as a result of peripheral degradation.
- The C-terminal fragments of PTH enhance the apoptosis of osteocytes.
- So, it is possible that the therapeutic activity of the whole PTH molecule (1–84) may slightly differ from teriparatide activity, which may lack the inhibitory activity on osteocytes mediated by C-terminal fraction of full PTH.

Teriparatide

Teriparatide, the N-terminal 1–34 fragment of the human parathormone (rhPTH (1–34), teriparatide), obtained via recombinant DNA technology is administered intermittently and promotes new bone formation and bone weight increase much more effectively than antiresorptive agents.

Q. 8. How hormones effect gene expression? What are HREs? What are nuclear receptors and nuclear receptors with special ligands? Describe their characteristic structural features.

Ans. The expression of eukaryotic protein-coding genes (also called class II or structural genes) can be regulated at several steps, including transcription initiation and elongation, and mRNA processing, transport, translation, and stability. Most of the regulation, however, occurs at the level of transcription initiation. In eukaryotes, transcription of protein-coding genes is performed by RNA polymerase II. Genes transcribed by RNA polymerase II typically contain two types of transcriptional regulatory DNA elements:

(a) Promoter – responsible for basal level of expression and includes the core promoter and the upstream element (Fig. 12.20).
- The core "promoter", often composed of the TATA box and/or Inr and/or DPE elements, directs RNA polymerase II to the correct site (fidelity). In certain genes that lack TATA, the so-called TATA-less promoters, an initiator (Inr) and/or DPE elements may direct the polymerase to this site.
- The upstream elements specify the basal frequency of initiation; such elements can either be proximal (50–200 bp) or distal (1000–10^5 bp) to the promoter. Among the best studied of the proximal elements is the CAAT box, but several other elements (bound by the transactivator proteins Sp1, NF1, AP1, etc.) may be used. Thus, various genes have a core promoter and nearby (proximal) regulatory elements – responsible for the basal level of transcription.

(b) Distal regulatory elements – enhance or repress expression above or below the basal level (Fig. 12.20):
- Include enhancers, silencers, insulators, or locus control regions (LCR).
- Mediate the response to various signals, including hormones, heat shock proteins, heavy metals, and chemicals.
- Responsible for tissue-specific expression of genes.
- These transcriptional regulatory elements contain recognition sites for DNA-binding transcription factors, which function either to enhance or repress transcription over the basal level produced by the action of promoter.

Thus, action of RNA polymerase for transcription can be regulated by:
- Altering the specificity and hence binding of RNA polymerase for a particular gene promoter or set of gene promoters.
- Repressor proteins bind to the non-coding sequences on the DNA strand (known as operators/promoter-dependent silencers) that are close to or overlap the promoter region, impeding RNA polymerase's progress along the strand.
- General transcription factors: These help position RNA polymerase at the correct position on DNA, i.e. at the start of a protein-coding sequence, i.e. help in recognition of start sites. They help in formation of the pre-initiation and the transcription complex (Fig. 12.21).
- Activators/inducers – bind to regions on DNA known as enhancer sites and enhance the interaction between RNA polymerase and a particular promoter, increasing the expression of the gene over basal level achieved by the polymerase and general transcription factors. They increase the rate of formation of the initiation complex or assembly of general transcription factors (Fig. 12.21).

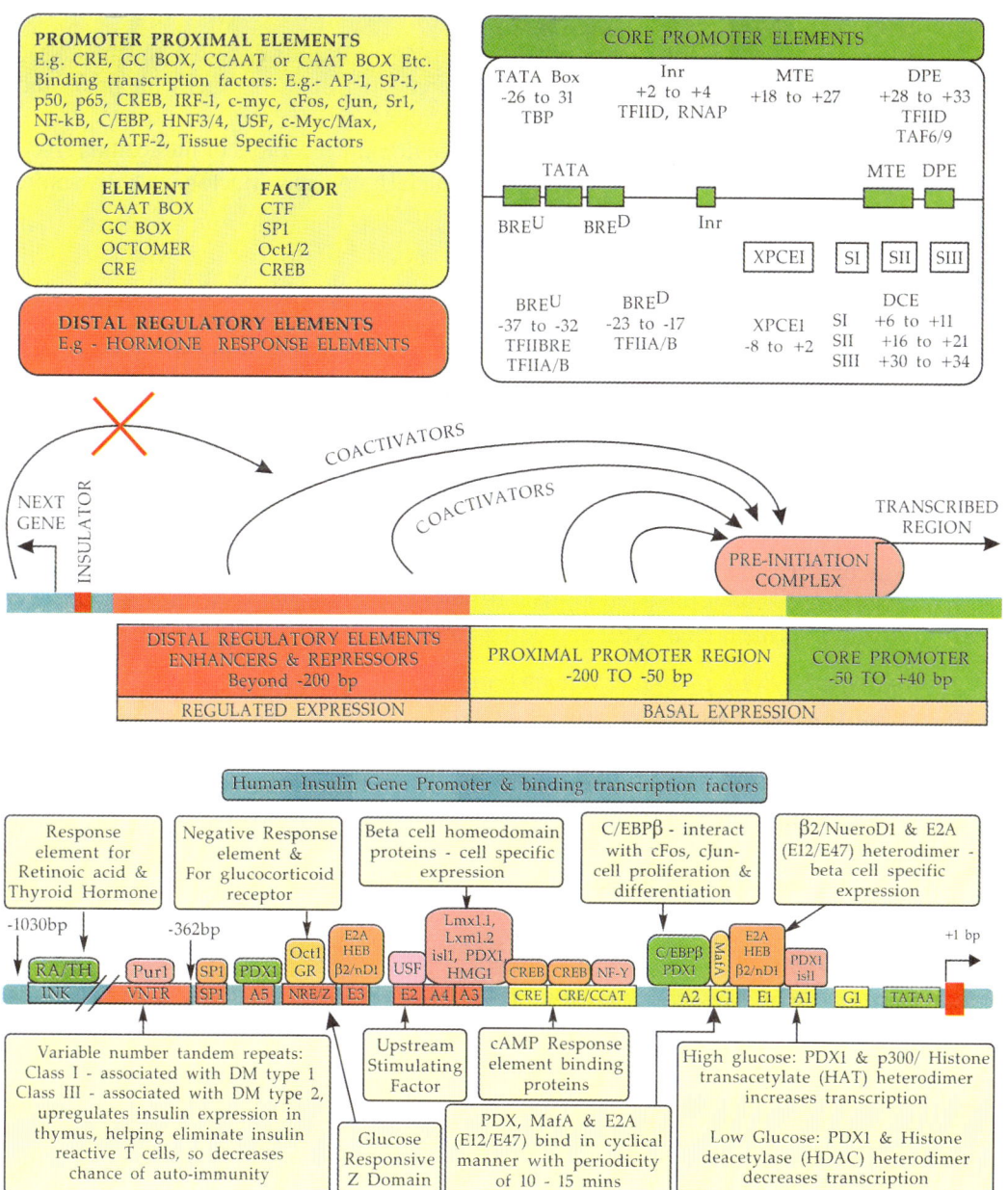

Fig. 12.20. Regulation and control of transcription, e.g., regulation of insulin transcription.

- Similarly, repressors may bind silencers to decrease rate of formation of the transcription complex.
- Chromatin remodelling through specific use of miRNA: Euchromatin, typically associated with transcriptional activity, is converted to hetereochromatin, reducing transcription.
- Histone modification like acetylation, etc.

Hormones can effect transcription by:
- The hormone–receptor (intracellular receptors) complex can go to the nucleus, acting as a activator or repressor by binding to enhancers or silencers. Such enhancers and silencers on DNA are called Hormone response elements (HRE) (Fig. 12.22).
- Hormone-generated signals (from either membrane receptors or intracellular receptors) can modify the location, amount, or activity of general transcription factors or activators or repressors.

The intracellular receptors for steroid hormones and thyroid hormones (which easily cross cell membrane) are a part of a large superfamily of nuclear receptors (which act by binding to regulatory element on DNA) because of the extensive similarities in their DNA-binding domains (DBDs). These nuclear receptors need to interact with another large group of co-regulatory molecules to bring about the changes in the transcription of specific genes. Further, there are AFE or Accessory factor-binding elements on DNA which bind accessory transcription factors and interact with the HRE-Rec-Hormone complex and co-regulators to integrate the whole process. They may have DNA modifying activity allowing DNA to bend and loop (Fig. 12.22).

HRE

Glucocorticoids, progestins, mineralocorticoids, and androgens have vastly different physiologic actions but have similar HRE as shown in Table 12.4. Still they can have specific effects with the help of AFE and coregulators.

Family of nuclear receptor proteins (Fig. 12.23)

There is a large family of nuclear receptor proteins. The nuclear receptor superfamily consists of a diverse set of transcription factors that were discovered because of a sequence similarity in their DBDs. This family, now with > 50 members, includes the nuclear hormone receptors and a number of other receptors whose ligands were discovered after the receptors were

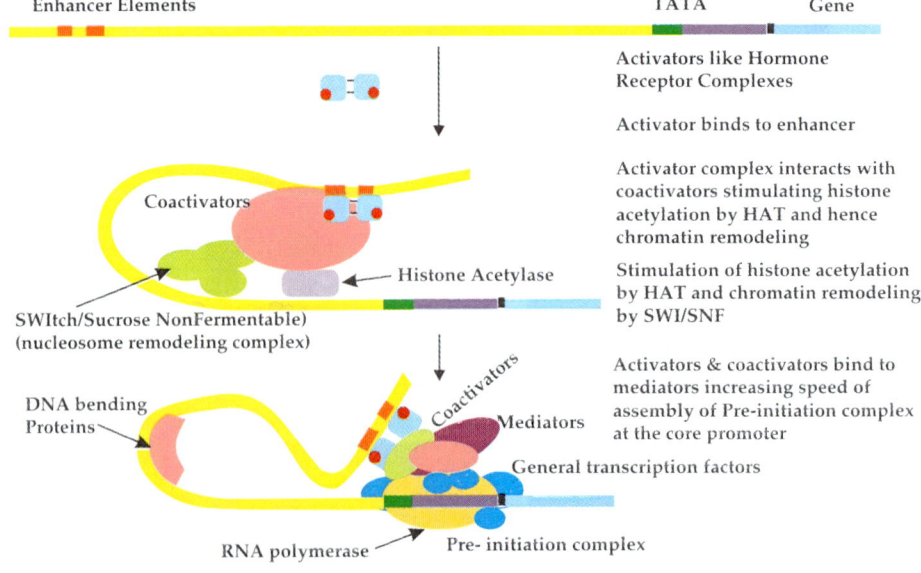

Fig. 12.21. How enhancers work.

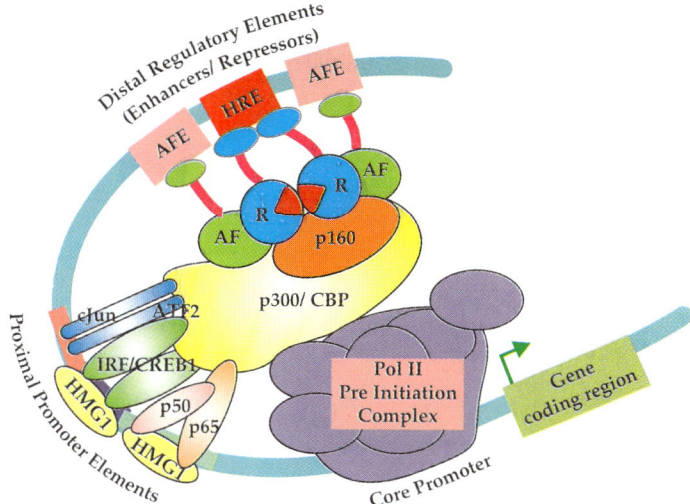

Fig. 12.22. HRE, AFE, the hormone receptor complex, and the coregulators (p160 and p300) which interact with the basal transcription machinery. R = Hormone receptor, AF = Accessory factor.

identified (then called orphan receptors) and many putative or orphan receptors for which a ligand has yet to be discovered.

Common structural features of nuclear receptors (Fig. 12.23)

These nuclear receptors have several common structural features:
- All have a centrally located DBD that allows the receptor to bind with high affinity to a response element. The DBD contains two zinc finger-binding motifs that direct binding either as homodimers, or as heterodimers (usually with a retinoid X receptor [RXR] partner), or as monomers.
- The target HRE consists of one or two DNA half-site consensus sequences arranged as an inverted or direct repeat. The spacing between them helps determine binding specificity.
- A multifunctional ligand-binding domain (LBD) is located in the carboxyl terminal half of the receptor. The LBD binds to the specific hormones or metabolites.
- Hinge region: Highly variable, separates the DBD from the LBD, provides flexibility to the receptor; so, it can assume different DNA-binding conformations and interact with hormone and DNA simultaneously.
- AF2 domain: Interacts with coactivators, thus a transactivator domain.
- AF-1 region: Transactivation domain, provides for distinct physiologic functions through the binding of different coregulator proteins. A hormone can have many isoforms of its receptor with different AF-1 domains generated by the use of different promoters, alternative splice sites, or multiple translation initiation sites. These subtypes can mediate different effects of a hormone in different tissues, e.g. estrogen receptor α and β.

Classification of nuclear receptors (Fig. 12.23)

- Classic hormone receptors for glucocorticoids (GR), mineralocorticoids (MR), estrogens (ER), androgens (AR), and progestins (PR) bind as homodimers to inverted repeat sequences on DNA (HRE).
- Other hormone receptors such as thyroid (TR), retinoic acid (RAR), and vitamin D (VDR) and nuclear receptors with special ligands bind as heterodimers, with retinoid X receptor (RXR) as a partner (Table 12.5).

Table 12.4. The DNA sequences of several Hormone Response Elements (HREs) and hormones acting through HRE

Hormone or Effector	HRE	DNA Sequence of HRE
Glucocorticoids	GRE	GGTACA NNN TGTTCT
Progestins	PRE	
Mineralocorticoids	MRE	
Androgens	ARE	
Estrogens	ERE	AGGTCA—TGACCT
Thyroid hormone	TRE	AGGTCA N1-5 AGGTCA
Retinoic acid	RARE	
Vitamin D	VDRE	
cAMP	CRE	TGACGTCA

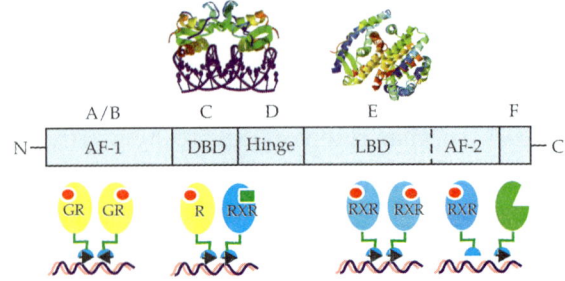

Receptors	Steroid class	RXR partnered	Orphans
Binding	Homodimers	Heterodimers	Homodimers/Monomer
Ligand	Steroids	9-Cis RA + (X)	?
DNA	Inverted repeat	Direct repeats	Direct repeats
Examples	GR, MR, PR AR, ER	TR, RAR, VDR, PPARα, β, γ	COUP-TF, Tr2, GEN8 HNF-4, TLX, GCNF, SF-1,ERR, ROR, NGFI-B

Fig. 12.23. The nuclear receptor superfamily. See also Table 12.5.

Table 12.5. Nuclear receptors with special ligands

Receptor	Partner		Ligand	Process affected
Peroxisome proliferator-activated receptor	PPARα	RXR (DR1)	Fatty acids	Peroxisome proliferation
	PPARβ		Fatty acids	
	PPARγ		Fatty acids, eicosanoids, thiazolidinediones	Lipid and carbohydrate metabolism
Farnesoid X	FXR	RXR (DR4)	Farnesol, bile acids	Bile acid metabolism
Liver X	LXR	RXR (DR4)	Oxysterols	Cholesterol metabolism
Xenobiotic X	CAR	RXR (DR5)	Androstanes, pheno-barbital, xenobiotics	Protection against certain drugs, toxic metabolites, and xenobiotics
	PXR	RXR (DR3)	Pregnanes, xenobiotics	

- Another group of orphan receptors that as yet have no known ligand bind as homodimers or monomers to direct repeat sequences on DNA (Fig. 12.23).

Nuclear receptors with special ligands are receptors that bind various metabolite ligands as shown in Table 12.5.

Hormones with cell surface receptors can also regulate transcription

Hormones having cell membrane receptors can also regulate gene transcription by modifying the location, amount, or activity of general transcription factors or activators or repressors (Fig. 12.24). For example:
- JAK/STAT pathway used by many hormones (growth hormone, prolactin, etc.) and cytokines.
- Regulation of NFκB pathway by TNF, steroids, etc.
- cAMP regulates activity of CREB (cAMP response element binding protein) which is a transcription factor.
- Insulin and EGF, etc. regulate activity of AP-1 transcription factor by MAP kinase pathway.

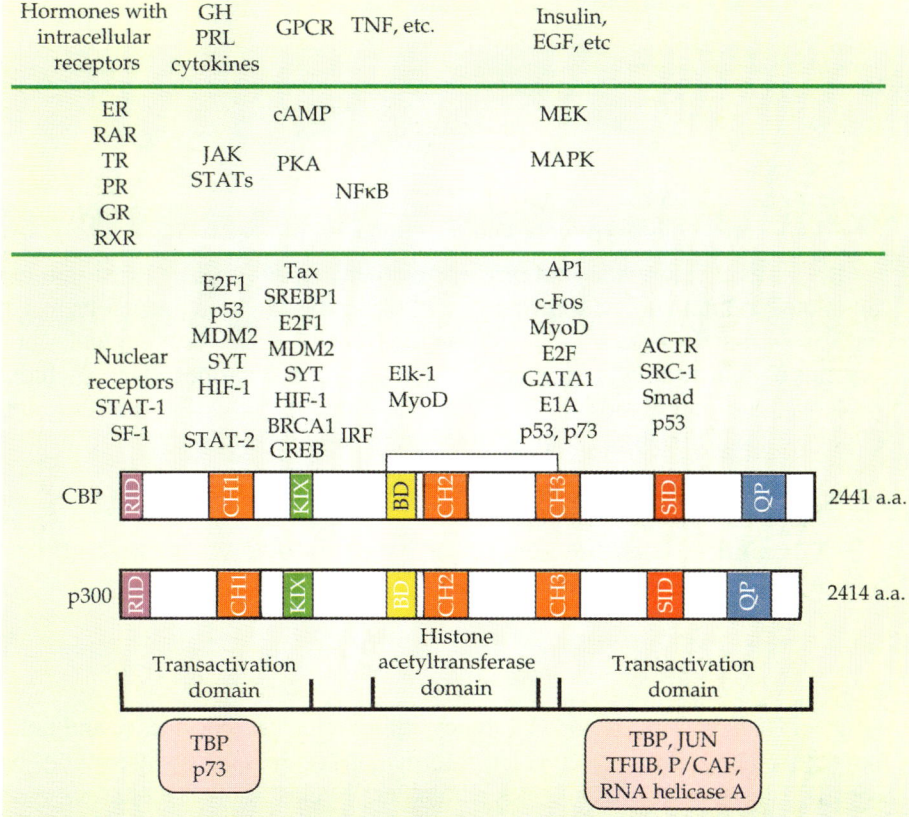

Fig. 12.24. Hormones with cell surface receptors also regulate transcription. Many types of signals modulate transcription by using different transcription factors but common coregulators CBP and p300. Group I hormones have intracellular nuclear receptors. GPCR = G protein coupled receptor, EGF = Epidermal growth factor, GH = Growth hormone, Prl = Prolactin.

Glycoproteins, ECM and Protein Trafficking

Chapter 13

Q. 1. What is sugar code of life or how carbohydrates can carry biological information?

Ans. Besides being the important fuel (glucose and glycogen), carbohydrates serve important role as:
- Structural components
- Information-containing molecules
- In 3-dimensional structure and function of proteins.

Because carbohydrates and proteins by themselves serve in a vast number of biological functions, it should not be surprising that linking the two together results in a macromolecule with an extremely large number of functions (Fig. 13.1). Glycoconjugates are conjugates of proteins or lipids with oligosaccharide chains or polysaccharides. These include glycoproteins, proteoglycans and glycolipids (glycosphingolipids). 50% of all proteins are glycosylated. Glycosylation is the most abundant post-translational modification (Fig. 13.1).

- **Glycome:** It is the entire collection of sugars or carbohydrates, free or part of complex molecules present in an organism.
- **Glycomics:** It is the comprehensive study of glycomes including their genetic, physiologic, pathologic and other aspects.

Information coding in sugars

Sugar code of life

Oligosaccharide chains encode biological information as the sequence and linkage of the eight possible sugars in glycoproteins. The information is expressed via interactions binding between specific sugars, in glycoconjugates with other proteins or other molecules. As shown in Figs. 13.2–13.5, the actual size and proportions of glycans in a glycoprotein make them prominent contributors to protein function. Functional proteomics can only be described with glycomics.

Glycoproteins, ECM and Protein Trafficking

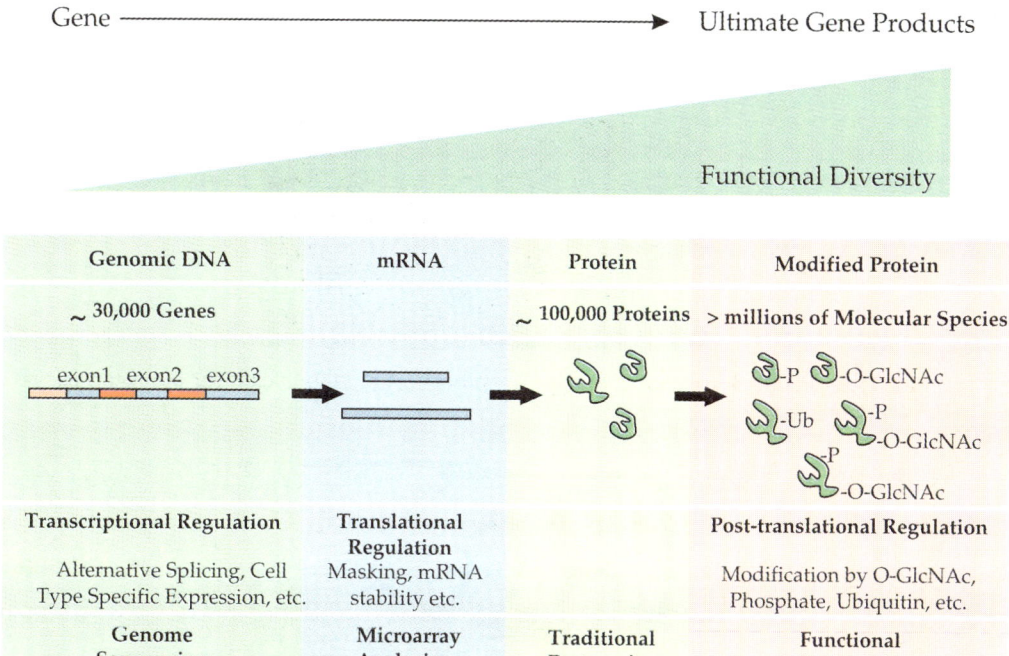

Fig. 13.1. Glycosylation is the most abundant post-translational modification and greatly increases the functional diversity of proteins.

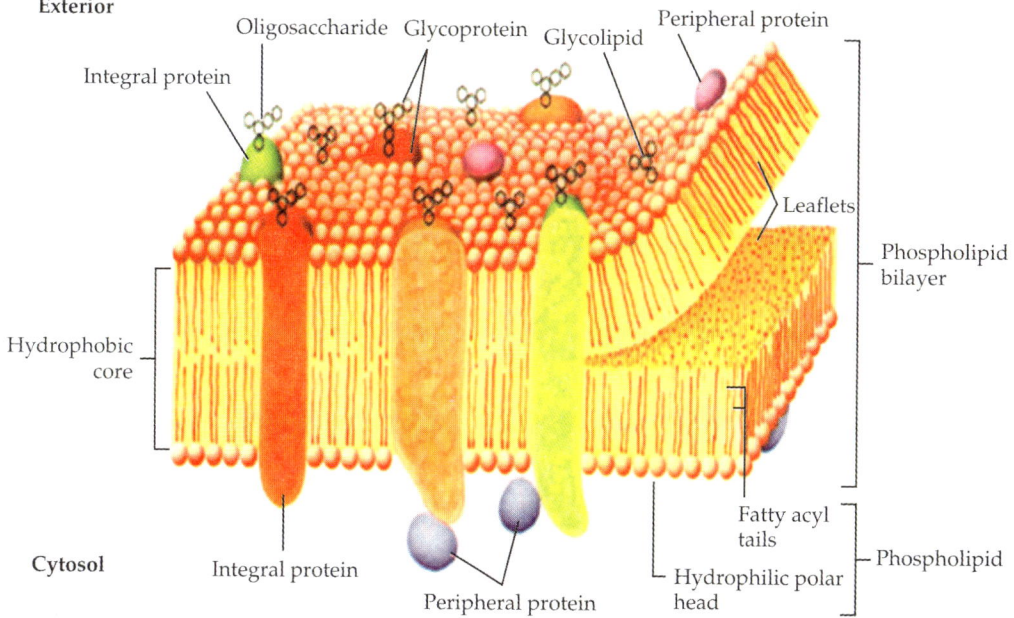

Fig. 13.2. Artist's misconception of the cell surface.

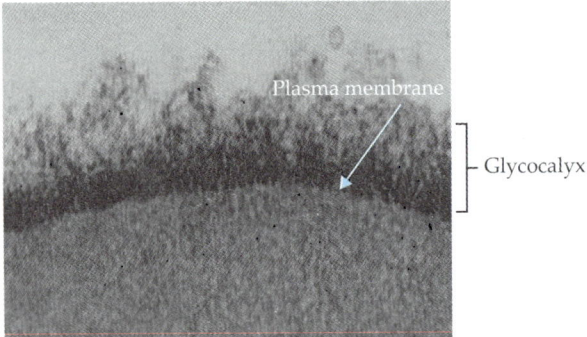

Fig. 13.3. Actual glycocalyx of human erythrocyte. Note the thick layer of glycan chains above the plasma membrane.

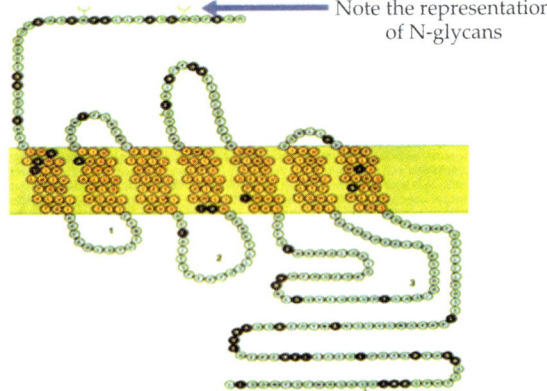

Fig. 13.4. Misleading depiction of β-adrenergic receptor. Note the representation of N-glycans.

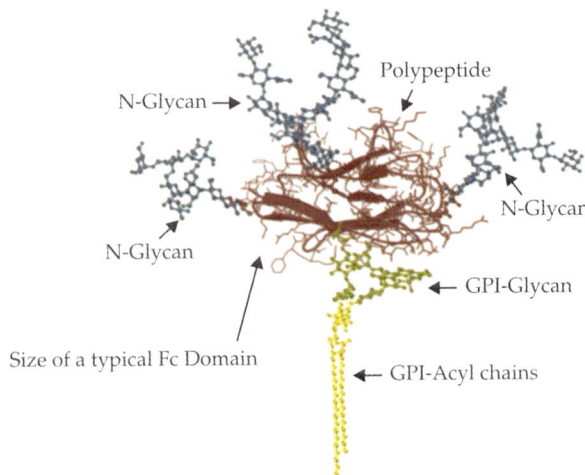

Fig. 13.5. Actual proportion of complex glycans in a glycoprotein – Rivalling the size of the polypeptides to which they are attached.

Glycoproteins, ECM and Protein Trafficking

There are a total of 13 monosaccharides and 8 amino acids producing at least 41 types of glycosidic linkages between them. This variety allows the glycans to code specific information and participate in signalling pathways.

Carbohydrates as part of proteins
- Modulate physicochemical properties, for example, solubility, viscosity, charge, conformation, denaturation, and binding sites for various molecules, bacteria, viruses, and some parasites.
- Protect against proteolysis. Removal of sialic acid residue from many plasma proteins makes them good ligand for liver asialoglycoprotein receptor which binds and endocytose them leading to degradation in lysosomes. Thus, sialic acid regulates half-life and metabolism of these proteins.
- Affect proteolytic processing of precursor proteins to smaller products.
- Involved in biologic activity, for example, of human chorionic gonadotropin (hCG).
- Affect insertion into membranes, intracellular migration, protein sorting, trafficking and secretion.
- Affect cell adhesion and cell–cell interaction.
- Proteins and cells can be 'tagged' or labelled by the projecting oligosaccharide and sugars. Interaction of these with lectins (carbohydrate-binding proteins) help recognize these 'tags' for different purposes.
- Affect embryonic development and differentiation.
- May affect sites of metastases selected by cancer cells.

All these features are highlighted by the different functions served by glycoproteins and proteoglycans.

Q. 2. Describe the general structure and classification of proteoglycans and their functions.

Ans. **Proteoglycans** (also known as mucopolysaccharides or mucoproteins)
- Proteoglycans are a type of glycoconjugates (conjugate of carbohydrate and proteins) composed of proteins and glycosaminoglycan (heteropolysaccharide) chains.
- The carbohydrate content in proteoglycans is much greater than in glycoproteins and may comprise upto 90–95% of weight of total macromolecule. They vary by tissue distribution, nature of protein, attached glycosaminoglycans and functions.
- They are also known as mucopolysaccharides or mucoproteins because they were first found in mucous secretion. These terms are now considered obsolete because it implies that they are confined to mucous secretion; whereas they are found almost everywhere.
- Components:
  - Proteins: Core and link proteins
  - Glycosaminoglycans (GAG): Linear heteropolysaccharides.
- The glycosaminoglycan chains are much larger than the oligosaccharide chains of glycoproteins. Therefore, the properties of the glycosaminoglycans tend to dominate the chemical properties of proteoglycan molecules.

Glycosaminoglycans are linear heteropolysaccharides. They are polymers of disaccharide building blocks made up of:

Hexosamine (amino sugar, *N*-acetylglucosamine, or *N*-acetylgalactosamine)

and

Hexuronic acid (glucuronic acid or iduronic acid) or hexose – galactose

There are 7 types of GAG and they are listed in Table 13.1.

Table 13.1. Types of GAG

Name	Hexuronic acid/Hexose	Hexosamine	Linkage of GAG–protein	Unique features and distribution
1. Chondroitin sulphate (CS)	GlcUA or GlcUA(2S)	GalNAc or GalNAc(4S/6S/4,6S)	Xyl-Ser	Most prevalent GAG. Cartilage, bone, cornea
2. Dermatan sulphate (DS)	GlcUA or IdoUA or IdoUA(2S)	GalNAc or GalNAc(4S/6S/4,6S)	Xyl-Ser	Wide distribution
3. Keratan sulphate I (KS-I)	Gal or Gal(6S)	GlcNAc or GlcNAc(6S)	GlcNAc-Asn	Cornea
4. Keratan sulphate II (KS-II)	Gal or Gal(6S)	GlcNAc or GlcNAc(6S)	GalNAc-Thr	May be fucosylated. Loose connective tissue
5. Heparin	GlcUA or IdoUA(2S)	GlcNAc or GlcNS or GlcNAc(6S) or GlcNS(6S)	Xyl-Ser	Highest negative charge density of any known biological molecule. Mast cells
6. Heparan sulphate (HS)	GlcUA or IdoUA or IdoUA(2S)	GlcNAc or GlcNS or GlcNAc(6S) or GlcNS(6S)	Xyl-Ser	Highly similar to heparin, but heparan sulfate's disaccharide units are organised into distinct sulfated and non-sulfated domains. Skin fibroblasts, aortic wall
7. Hyaluronan/ Hyaluronic acid (HA)	GlcUA	GlcNAc	None (non-covalent interaction with link proteins)	The only GAG that is exclusively non-sulfated. Synovial fluid, vitreous humour, loose connective tissue.

(S) = sulphate

General structure of simple proteoglycans

Consists of glycosaminoglycan chains linked covalently with a core protein with the help of a link trisaccharide as shown in Fig. 13.6. While the diagram represents a general structure of proteoglycans, a large variation occurs due to:
- Large number of core proteins.
- Each can be attached with one or two types of GAG chains.

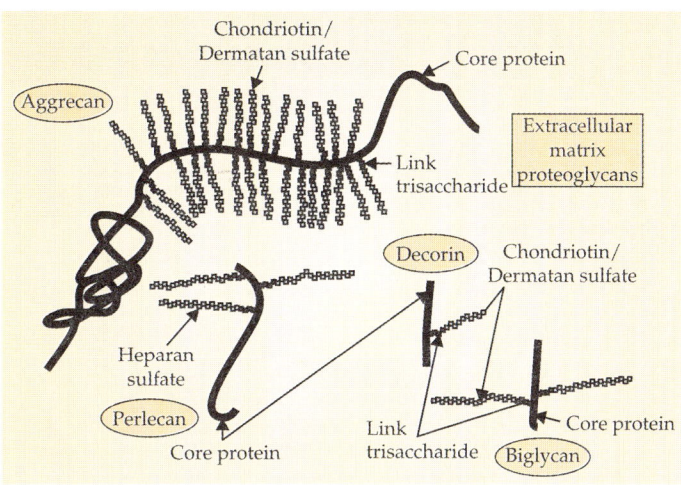

Fig. 13.6. General structure of simple proteoglycans: GAG linked covalently to core protein. Brown- core protein, yellow- CS/DS, blue- HS, green- link trisaccharide.

- Variation in number of GAG chains from few (decorin) to hundreds (aggrecan).
- Not all attachment sites for GAGs may be used.
- Proteoglycans can be "part time", that is, they may exist with or without a glycosaminoglycan chain or with only a truncated oligosaccharide. A given proteoglycan present in different cell types often exhibits differences in the number of glycosaminoglycan chains, their lengths, and the arrangement of sulfated residues along the chains.

Linkage between GAG and core protein

These are of 3 types:

1. An *O*-glycosidic bond between xylose (Xyl) and Ser – found only in proteoglycans. A link trisaccharide of Gal-Gal-Xyl is there, with Xyl forming the *O*-glycosidic bond with Serine and GAG chain grows on the Gal (Fig. 13.7).
2. An *O*-glycosidic bond forms between GalNAc (*N*-acetylgalactosamine) and Ser (Thr) – present only in keratan sulfate II (Fig. 13.7).
3. An *N*-glycosylamine bond between GlcNAc (*N*-acetylglucosamine) and the amide nitrogen of Asparagine (Asn) – similar to that in *N*-linked glycoproteins (Fig. 13.7).

Classification of proteoglycans

It is based on structural components, location and function. The major classes of proteoglycans based on location and functions are:

   1. **ECM/Interstitial proteoglycans and the aggrecan family:** These include SLRPs and aggrecan family (aggrecan, versican, brevican, and neurocan).

- Found in ECM, act as ground substance or cementing substance. They are associated with each other and also with the other major structural components of the matrix-collagen and elastin, fibronectin and laminin. Proteoglycans containing CS and DS chains have large capacity to bind water and form hydrated matrices. Thus, these molecules fill the space between cells. In cartilage, the aggregates of proteoglycans and hyaluronan provide a

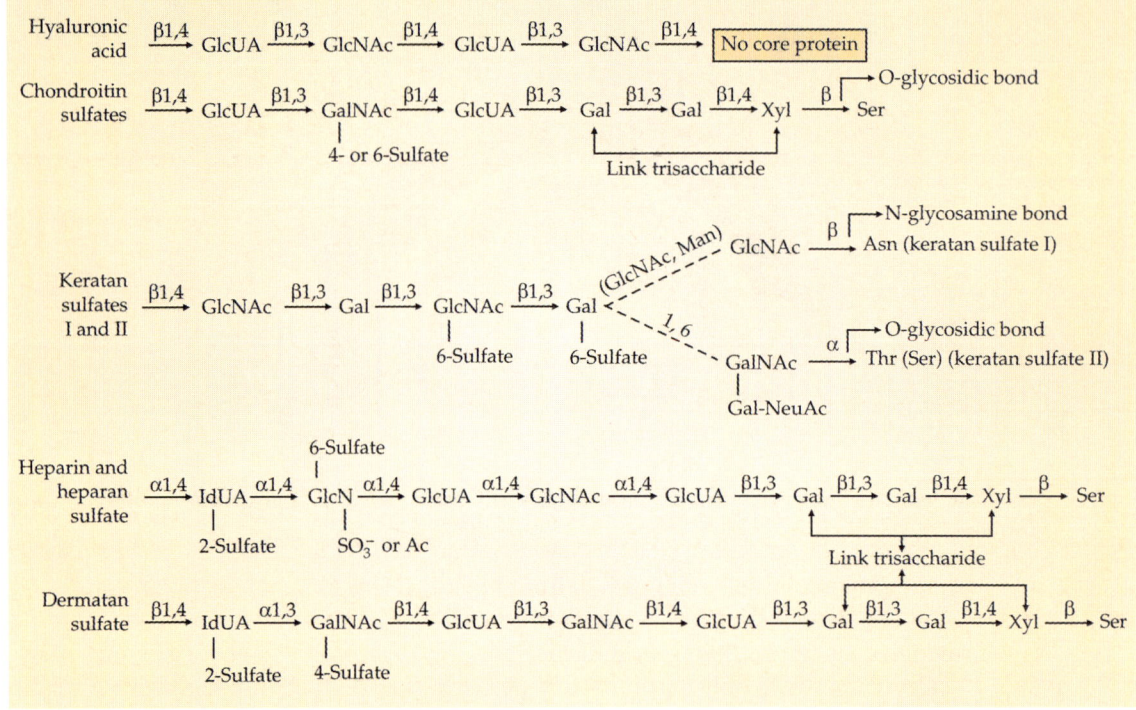

Fig. 13.7. The structure of 7 types of GAGs listed in Table 13.1 and their covalent linkages with amino acid of proteins.

stable matrix capable of absorbing high compressive loads by water desorption and resorption. The GAGs present in the proteoglycans are polyanions and hence bind polycations and cations such as Na^+ and K^+. This latter ability attracts water by osmotic pressure into the extracellular matrix and contributes to its turgor.

- Small leucine-rich proteoglycans (SLRPs) – help to stabilize and organize collagen fibres, for example, in tendons.
  - In the cornea, KS proteoglycans maintain the arrangement of collagen fibres and the space between them required for transparency. Defects in sulfation (macular corneal dystrophy) or chain formation (keratoconus) cause distortions in fibril organization and corneal opacity. The presence of dermatan sulfate in the sclera may also play a role in maintaining the overall shape of the eye.
  - Proteoglycans like decorin in the ECM can bind cytokines, chemokines, growth factors, and morphogens, protecting them against proteolysis. Decorin can bind transforming growth factor β (TGF-β), serving as a sink to keep the growth factor sequestered in the matrix surrounding most cells. These interactions provide a depot/reserve of regulatory factors that can be liberated by selective degradation of the matrix (Figs. 13.8 and 13.9). The released growth factors help in tissue repair after inflammation and damage and stimulate new bone formation after resorption of bone by osteoclasts for remodelling. They are also involved in pathology of aortic aneurysms due to GLUT 10 mutations (Figs. 13.8 and 13.9).

Glycoproteins, ECM and Protein Trafficking

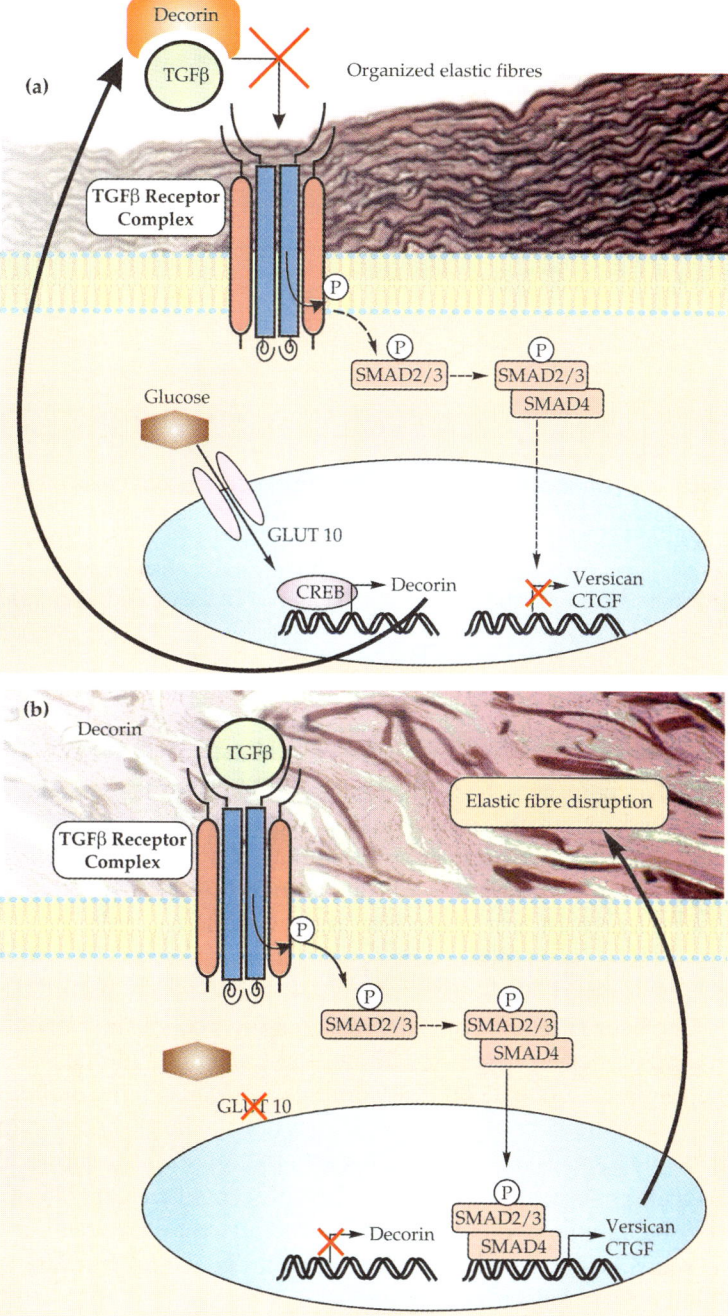

Fig. 13.8. Decorin and TGFβ action: (a) Glucose transported into smooth muscle cell nucleus by GLUT10 activates decorin transcription via cAMP response element binding protein (CREB). Decorin binds to TGFβ and blocks its binding to its receptor. (b) Loss of GLUT10 decreases decorin production. The now-free-to-act TGFβ activates its receptor leading to production of connective tissue growth (CTGF) factor and versican, both of which disrupt the elastic fibre network in vessels causing aortic weakness (aortic aneurysm).

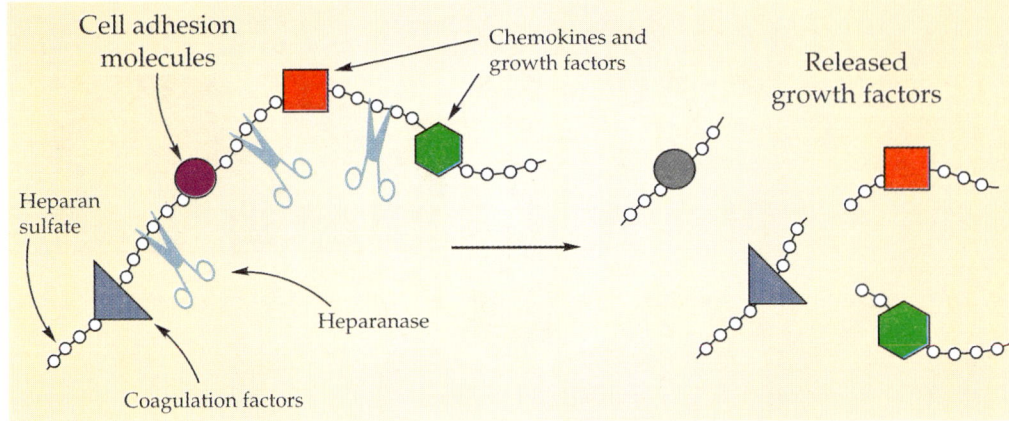

Fig. 13.9. Coagulation factors, chemokines, growth factors, etc. are bound to heparan sulftae of proteoglycans and thus stay inactive. Destruction of ECM or heparanse enzyme cleaves HS, releasing the growth factors which become free to act on cell surface receptors. Invading microbes and WBC secrete heparanse which cleaves the proteoglycan helping cells move in ECM. The released chemokines and growth factors attract WBC and macrophages to fight microbes and stimulate growth factors to stimulate ECM production helping in repair of tissue after damage.

- The aggrecan family of proteoglycans consists of aggrecan, versican, brevican, and neurocan. In all four members, the core protein moiety contains an amino-terminal domain capable of binding hyaluronan non-covalently through a link protein, a central region that contain covalently bound CS chains, and a carboxy-terminal domain containing a C-type lectin domain
    - Aggrecan represents the major proteoglycan in cartilage. It contains as many as 100 CS chains and, in humans, it contains KS chains as well. It is very large (about 2×10^3 kDa with its overall structure resembling that of a bottle brush (Fig. 13.10). It contains a long strand of hyaluronic acid (one type of GAG) to which link proteins are attached noncovalently. In turn, these later interact noncovalently with core protein molecule from which chains of other GAGs (keratan sulfate and chondroitin sulfate) project.

    Aggrecan provides intervertebral disc and cartilage with the ability to resist compressive loads (Fig. 13.11). The localized high concentrations of aggrecan provide the osmotic properties necessary for normal tissue function with the GAGs producing the swelling pressure that counters compressive loads on the tissue. The retention of water due to large number of negative charges and the bottle brush shape shown in Fig. 13.1 allows it to act as very good shock absorber or suspension.
    - Versican undergoes alternative splicing events that generate a family of proteins of differing complexity that may have a role in neural crest cell and axonal migration.
    - Neurocan is expressed in the late embryonic central nervous system (CNS) and can inhibit neurite outgrowth.
    - Brevican is expressed in the terminally differentiated CNS, particularly in perineuronal nets
- GAGs also gel at relatively low concentrations. Because of the long extended nature of the polysaccharide chains of GAGs and their ability to gel, the proteoglycans can act a sieves, restricting the passage of large macromolecules into the ECM but allowing relatively free diffusion of small molecules.

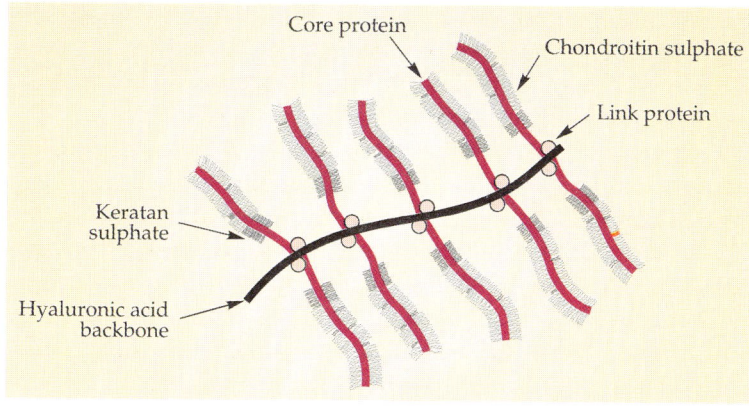

Fig. 13.10. The structure of aggrecan.

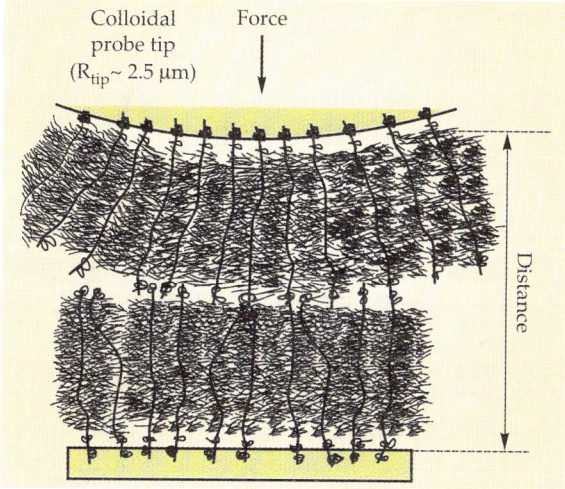

Fig. 13.11. Aggrecan molecules help cartilage to act as a shock absorber. The turgor due to the osmotically-held water, repulsion between the negative charges on GAG and the bottle brush structure, all help in the shock absorbing and lubricating function of cartilage.

- Hyaluronic acid is especially high in concentration in embryonic tissues and is thought to play an important role in permitting cell migration during morphogenesis and wound repair. Its ability to attract water into the extracellular matrix and thereby "loosen it up" is important in this regard.
- Chondroitin sulfates are located at sites of calcification in endochondral bone and are also found in cartilage. They are also located inside certain neurons and may provide an endoskeletal structure, helping to maintain their shape.

2. **Secretory granule proteoglycan:** Secreted along with other secretory products in secretory vesicles. Secretory granule proteoglycans are thought to help sequester and regulate the availability of positively charged components, such as proteases and bioactive amines, through interaction with the negatively charged glycosaminoglycan chains. For example:

- Serglycin is the major proteoglycan present in cytoplasmic secretory granules in endothelial, endocrine, and hematopoietic cells.
- Heparin is a highly sulfated form of heparan sulphate and is made exclusively on serglycin present in connective tissue-type mast cells.
- Chromogranin A, part-time proteoglycan, is secreted in vesicles from neuroendocrine cells and chromaffin cells of adrenal medulla, intestines and pancreatic β cells.

Proteoglycans in secretory vesicles have a role in packaging granular contents, maintaining proteases in an active state, and regulating various biological activities after secretion, such as coagulation, host defence, and wound repair.

3. **Basement membrane proteoglycan:** The basement membrane is an organized layer of the ECM that lies very closely against epithelial cells and consists largely of laminin, nidogen, collagens, and proteoglycans.

Basement membranes contain at least four types of proteoglycans depending on type of tissue: perlecan, agrin, and collagen type XVIII (which carries HS chains) and leprecan (which carries CS chains).

- Perlecan has a role in embryogenesis and tissue morphogenesis and a particularly important role in cartilage development.
- Agrin acts in neuromuscular junctions (where it aggregates acetylcholine receptors) and in renal tubules (where it has an important role in determining the filtration properties of the glomerulus).

Proteoglycans help to organize basement membranes, thus providing a scaffold for epithelial cell migration, proliferation, and differentiation. They can regulate the permeability properties of specialized basement membranes like glomerular basement membrane.

The attachment of cells to their substratum in culture is mediated at least in part by the heparan sulfate. It is also found in the basement membrane of the kidney along with type IV collagen and laminin, where it plays a major role in determining the charge selectiveness of glomerular filtration.

4. **Membrane-bound proteoglycan:** Transmembrane or peripheral proteins attached by GPI anchors. Have a single membrane-spanning domain or a glycosylphosphatidylinositol (GPI) anchor (Fig. 13.12).

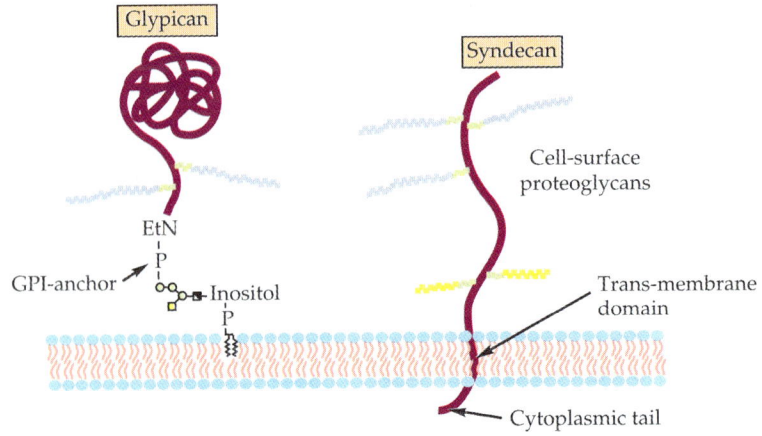

Fig. 13.12. Membrane-bound proteoglycans.

- Syndecan family consists of four members, each with a short hydrophobic domain that spans the membrane.
  - Syndecan 1–4 are expressed in a tissue-specific manner and facilitate cellular interactions with a wide range of extracellular ligands, such as growth factors and matrix molecules.
  - Because of their membrane-spanning properties, the syndecans can transmit signals from the extracellular environment to the intracellular cytoskeleton via their cytoplasmic tails.
  - For example, binding of a ligand to the HS (heparan sulphate) chain can induce oligomerization of syndecans at the cell surface, which leads to recruitment of factors at their cytoplasmic tails, such as kinases (e.g., c-Src), PDZ-domain proteins, or cytoskeletal proteins. The recruitment of cytoplasmic proteins in turn triggers a signal that affects actin assembly. Syndecan binding ligands include fibroblast growth factor (FGF), vascular endothelial growth factor (VEGF), fibronectin, and antithrombin-1. These ligands can also be released from ECM proteoglycans and hence activated by heparanse enzyme (Fig. 13.9).
  - Proteolytic cleavage of the syndecans occurs by matrix metalloproteases, resulting in shedding of the extracellular part bearing the glycosaminoglycan chains. These ectodomains can have potent biological activity as well by binding the same ligands.
- Glypican family has a GPI anchor attached at the carboxyl terminus which embeds these proteoglycans in the outer leaflet of the plasma membrane. Thus, the glypicans do not have a cytoplasmic tail like the syndecans.
  - Six glypican family members exist in mammals. Humans lacking functional GPC3 exhibit Simpson–Golabi–Behmel syndrome, characterized as an overgrowth disorder. The overgrowth phenotype suggests that GPC3 normally functions to inhibit cell proliferation by binding to IGF-II.
- The CS proteoglycan NG2 is a surface marker expressed on stem cell populations, cartilage chondroblasts, myoblasts, endothelial cells of the brain, and glial progenitors.
- CD44, a transmembrane cell-surface receptor present on leukocytes and other cells, has a role in processes as diverse as immune cell trafficking and function, axon guidance, and organ development. Only certain splice forms of CD44 carry a glycosaminoglycan chain, and, like the aggrecan family, it can bind hyaluronan.
- Phosphacan is expressed as three different splice variants in the CNS, and, depending on the isoform, it can carry KS or CS chains. One splice variant is present in the ECM, whereas two other forms represent short- and full-length versions of a protein-tyrosine-phosphatase type of transmembrane receptor.
- Membrane proteoglycans can act as coreceptors for various growth factor receptors, lowering the threshold or changing the duration of signalling reactions (e.g. Fig. 13.13).
- Membrane proteoglycans cooperate with integrins and other cell adhesion receptors to facilitate cell attachment, cell–cell interactions, and cell motility. Proteoglycans in the ECM can regulate cell migration as well.
- Certain proteoglycans (e.g., heparan sulfate) are associated with the plasma membrane of cells, with their core proteins spanning that membrane. Thus, they may act as receptors and may also participate in the mediation of the cell growth and cell–cell communication.

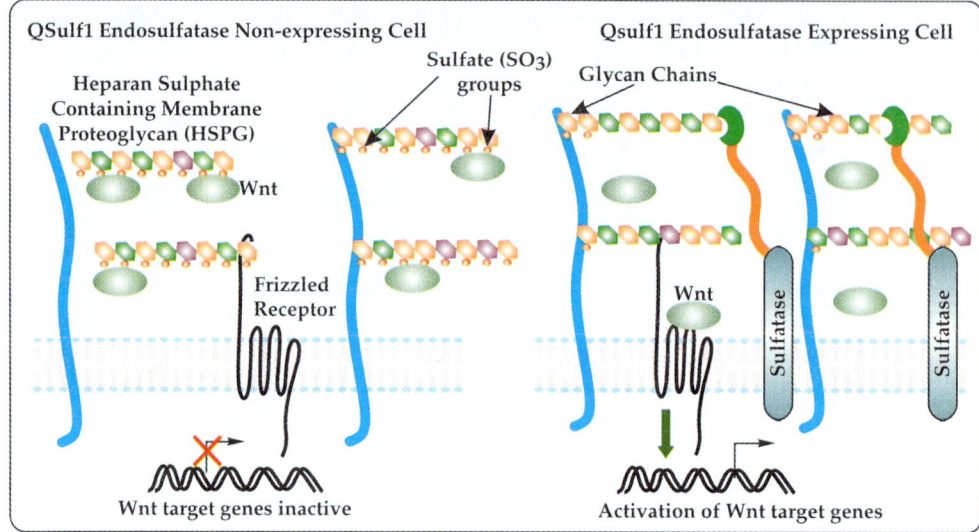

Fig. 13.13. Modulation of growth factor signalling by heparan sulphate containing membrane proteoglycan (HSPG). (A) In endosulfatase (QSulf1) nonexpressing embryonic cells, HS chains on cell surface HSPGs are in a 6-O-sulfated state, which binds with high affinities to catch Wnt ligands, preventing functional interactions of these bound Wnts with their Frizzled receptors (G protein coupled receptor). (B) In QSulf1-expressing cells, selective 6-O desulfation activity of QSulf1 removes 6-O sulfates from HS chains on cell surface HSPGs to convert HS to a low affinity binding state for Wnts. 6-O-desulfated HS then can present Wnt ligands to Frizzled receptor and can form functionally active Wnt-HS-Frizzled receptor complexes for initiation of Wnt signal transduction.

Classification based on composition of GAG

1. Chondroitin sulfate proteoglycans

Proteoglycan	Tissue distribution
Aggrecan family	
Aggrecan	Secreted; cartilage
Versican/PG-M	Secreted; connective tissue cells, aorta, brain
Neurocan	Secreted; brain
Brevican	Secreted; brain
SLRPs (Small leucine rich proteins)	
Decorin	Secreted; connective tissue cells
Biglycan	Secreted; connective tissue cells
Other examples	
Leprecan	Secreted; basement membranes
Type IX collagen, α_2 chain	Secreted; cartilage, vitreous humor
Phosphacan	Membrane bound; brain
Thrombomodulin	Membrane bound; endothelial cells
CD44	Membrane bound; lymphocytes
NG2	Membrane bound; neural cells
Invariant chain	Membrane bound; antigen-processing cells
Serglycin	Intracellular granules; myeloid cells

2. Keratan sulfate proteoglycans

Proteoglycan	Type	Tissue distribution
SLRPs		
Lumican	KS I	Secreted; broad
Keratocan	KS I	Secreted; broad, but sulfated only in cornea
Fibromodulin	KS I	Secreted; broad
Mimecan	KS I	Secreted; broad, but sulfated only in cornea
Other examples		
SV2	KS I	Membrane bound; synaptic vesicles
Claustrin	KS II	Membrane bound; CNS
Aggrecan (human)	KS II	Secreted; cartilage

3. Heparan sulfate proteoglycans

Proteoglycan	Tissue distribution
Perlecan	Secreted; basement membranes, cartilage
Agrin	Secreted; neuromuscular junctions
Collagen type XVIII	Secreted; basement membranes
Syndecans 1–4	Membrane bound; epithelial cells and fibroblasts
Betaglycan	Membrane bound; fibroblasts
Glypicans 1–6	Membrane bound; epithelial cells and fibroblasts
Serglycin	Intracellular granules; mast cells

To a large extent, the biological functions of proteoglycans depend on the interaction of the glycosaminoglycan chains with different protein ligands. Examples of proteins that bind to sulfated glycosaminoglycans are given in Table 13.2 and also classified according to the function.

Table 13.2. Proteins binding to sulfated glycosaminoglycans

Cell/matrix interactions	Coagulation/ fibrinolysis	Lipolysis	Inflammation	Growth factors and morphogens
Laminin	Antithrombin	Lipoprotein lipase	Cytokines (IL-2, IL-7, IL-8)	FGFs and FGF receptors
Fibronectin	Heparin cofactor II	Hepatic lipase		HGF, scatter factor
Vitronectin	Tissue factor pathway inhibitor	apoE	Chemokines (e.g., MIP-1β, SDF-1, etc.)	VEGF
Thrombospondin		apoB		TGF-β
Tenascin	Thrombin	apoA-V		BMPs
Various collagens	Protein C inhibitor		TNF-α	Hedgehogs
Amyloid proteins	tPA and PAI-1		L and P selectins, superoxide dismutase, microbial adhesins	Wnts

Proteoglycans and diseases

- **Tumor cell migration:** Hyaluronic acid may be important in permitting tumor cells to migrate through the ECM. Tumor cells can induce fibroblasts to synthesize greatly increased amounts of this GAG, thereby facilitating their own spread. Some tumor cells have less heparan sulfate at their surfaces, and this may play a role in the lack of adhesiveness to neighbouring cells that these cells display.
- **Atherosclerosis:** The intima of the arterial wall contains hyaluronic acid and chondroitin sulfate, dermatan sulfate, and heparan sulfate proteoglycans. Dermatan sulfate binds plasma low-density lipoproteins.
- **Arthritis:** In various types of arthritis, proteoglycans may act as autoantigens, thus contributing to the pathologic features of these conditions. The amount of chondroitin sulfate in cartilage diminishes with age, whereas the amounts of keratan sulfate and hyaluronic acid increase. These changes may contribute to the development of osteoarthritis. Increased activity of the enzyme aggrecanase, which acts to degrade aggrecan, also contributes.
- **Skin ageing:** Changes in the amounts of certain GAGs in the skin are observed with aging and account for the characteristic changes noted in the elderly.

Q. 3. Differentiate between heparin and heparan sulphate.

Ans. Heparin is made solely as a serglycin proteoglycan by connective tissue-type mast cells, whereas heparan sulphate is made by virtually all cells. The repeating disaccharide of heparin contains glucosamine (GlcN) and either of IdUA or GlcUA. Most of the amino groups of the GlcN residues are N-sulfated, but a few are acetylated. The GlcN also carries a sulfate attached to carbon 6. Approximately 90% of the uronic acid residues are IdUA. Initially, all of the uronic acids are GlcUA, but a 5′-epimerase converts approximately 90% of the GlcUA residues to IdUA after the polysaccharide chain is formed. The protein molecule of the heparin proteoglycan is unique, consisting exclusively of serine and glycine residues (hence called serglycin). Approximately two-thirds of the serine residues contain GAG chains, usually of 5–15 kDa but occasionally much larger.

Heparin is an anticoagulant. Injection of heparin into the bloodstream results in rapid anticoagulation (because of binding and activation of antithrombin), release of lipoprotein lipase, transient blockade of P and L selectins, displacement of growth factors and chemokines etc. Heparin is used as an anticoagulant therapeutically. It binds with factors IX and XI, but its most important interaction is with plasma antithrombin. Antithrombin-heparin interaction depends on a specific pentasaccharide sequence. Heparin can also bind specifically to lipoprotein lipase present in capillary walls, causing a release of this enzyme into the circulation. Heparan sulfate can also contain anticoagulant activity, but typical preparations are much less active than heparin.

Heparan sulphate is present on many cell surfaces as a proteoglycan and is extracellular. It contains GlcN with fewer N-sulfates than heparin, and, unlike heparin, its predominant uronic acid is GlcUA. Differences between heparin and heparan sulfate are given in Table 13.3.

Heparin derived from porcine and bovine entrails is prepared commercially by selective precipitation and is sold by pharmaceutical companies as an anticoagulant due to its capacity to bind to antithrombin.

Glycoproteins, ECM and Protein Trafficking

Table 13.3. Differences between heparin and heparan sulfate

Characteristics	Heparan sulphate	Heparin
Soluble in 2 M potassium acetate (pH 5.7, 4°C)	Yes	No
Size	10–70 kD	7–20 kD
Sulfate/hexosamine ratio	0.8–1.8	1.8–2.6
$GlcNSO_3$	40–60%	≥ 80%
Iduronic acid	30–50% (GLcUA)	≥ 70% (IdUA)
Binding to antithrombin	0–0.3%	~ 30%
Site of synthesis	Virtually all cells, skin fibroblasts, aortic wall	Connective tissue-type mast cells
Core protein	Many	Serglycin
	Highly similar to heparin, but heparan sulfate's disaccharide units are organised into distinct sulfated and non-sulfated domains.	Highest negative charge density of any known biological molecule.

Low molecular weight heparins (LMWH) are derived from commercial unfractionated heparin (UFH) by chemical and enzymatic cleavage, depending on the brand. The active sequence is a pentasaccharide, which is now sold as a purely synthetic anticoagulant. Selectively desulfated forms of heparin are also commercially available, some of which lack anticoagulant activity, but still retain other potentially useful properties (e.g., inhibition of inflammation and cell proliferation, and antimetastatic activity).

Q. 4. Describe role of oligosaccharides in protein folding.

Ans. 50% of all proteins are glycoproteins. Proteins synthesized on ER-bound ribosomes are soluble (secreted) or membrane proteins and most of these are glycoproteins. During their synthesis (translation) they are simultaneously inserted into the lumen of ER where they undergo co-translational and post-translational modifications and also achieve their active natural conformation. Modifications include:

- Signal peptide cleavage
- GPI anchor addition
- Disulphide bond formation
- N-linked glycosylation

Even though environment in ER is strictly controlled to help achieve proper folding, misfolding occurs frequently. Hence the need of a process that allows misfolded proteins to refold correctly (to save precious proteins) and also to degrade permanently misfolded proteins (prevent their accumulation). This is known as folding assistance and quality controls of proteins. This is achieved with the help of two glycoproteins and the process critically depends on the N-linked oligosaccharide chains of the newly formed glycoproteins. The process is known as Calnexin/Calreticulin cycle (Fig. 13.14).

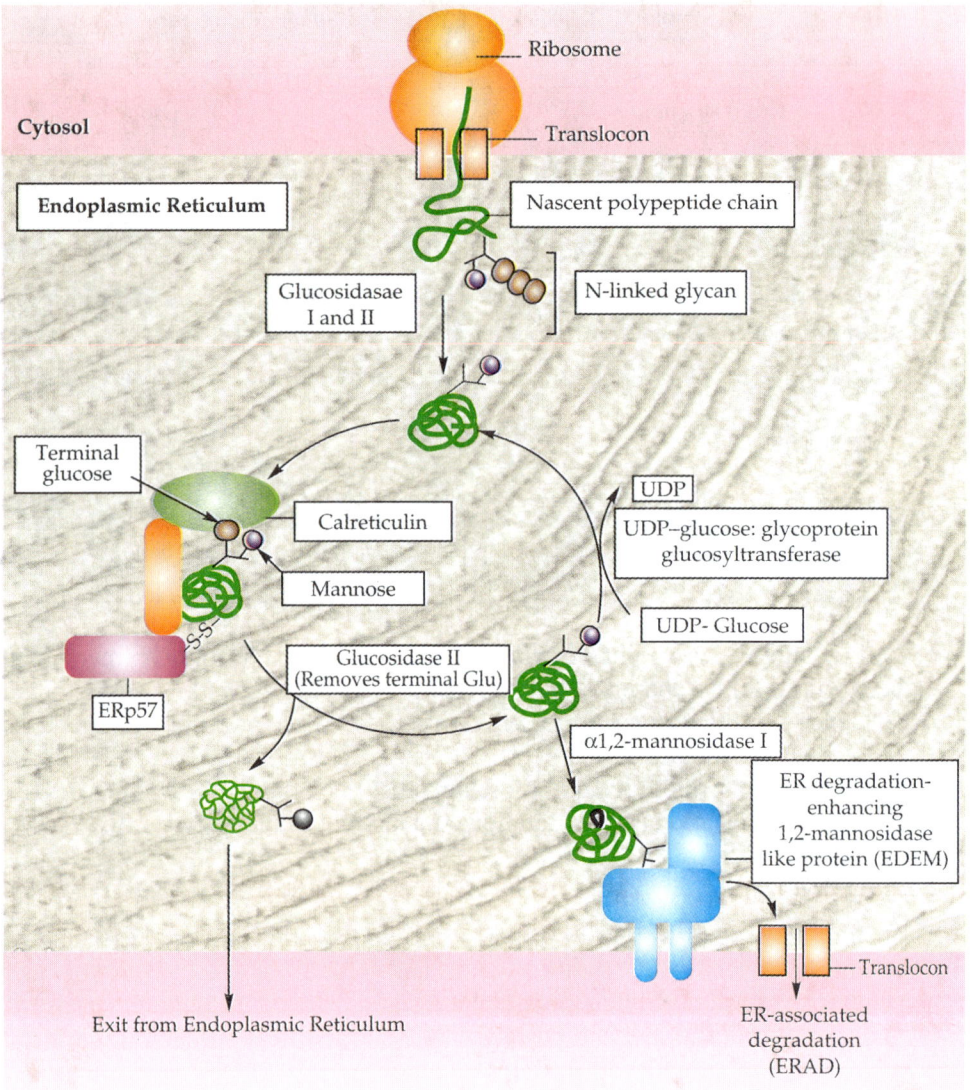

Fig. 13.14. The calnexin/calreticulin cycle.

Calnexin (a transmembrane protein in ER) and calreticulin (soluble protein in ER lumen) are themselves glycoproteins that can also bind to carbohydrates (oligosaccharide or glycan chain) on glycoproteins, hence acting as lectins. By binding to the glycan chains of newly formed glycoproteins they help in their correct folding thus acting as chaperones.

- As a new growing polypeptide chain enters the ER, certain Asn residues (contained in the consensus sequence Asn-any-Ser/Thr of newly synthesized polypeptides) are glycosylated by addition of $Glc_3Man_9GlcNAc_2$.
- The outermost two molecules of glucose are removed via the actions of glucosidases I and II.

- This exposes the innermost molecule of glucose (monoglycosylated structure), which is recognized by the lectin sites of calnexin and calreticulin. In their ATP-bound state, calnexin and calreticulin bind to the monoglucosylated oligosaccharide (via their lectin sites) as well as to hydrophobic segments of the unfolded glycoprotein (via their polypeptide binding or chaperone sites).
- Binding to calnexin prevents a glycoprotein from aggregating. Binding with the glycan part rather than peptide chain allows the peptide to change conformations easily during folding and refolding.
- Calnexin and the bound glycoprotein form a complex with ERp57, which catalyzes disulfide bond interchange (protein disulfide isomerase), facilitating proper folding.
- Only if the glycoprotein is completely folded in the ER, the terminal glucose is removed by glucosidase-II (thus also senses the proper folding) and the glycoprotein is released from the CNX/CRT chaperone cycle.
- However, if the glycoprotein is not properly folded, the terminal glucose is once again attached by the action of UDP-glucose: glycoprotein glucosyltransferase (UGGT), which discriminates between folded and unfolded substrates. It acts only on misfolded proteins. This causes rebinding to the calnexin-ERp57 complex. The reglucosylated glycoprotein can then rebind to the ATP form of calnexin/calreticulin. Thus, both the glucosyltransferase and calnexin/calreticulin act as folding sensors. If now properly folded, the glycoprotein is again deglucosylated by glucosidase II and leaves the ER.
- If the protein is permanently misfolded or cannot be refolded correctly by this process the mannose residue in the middle branch of the oligosaccharide is removed by ER α-1,2-mannosidase I. This leads to recognition by the ER degradation-enhancing 1,2-mannosidase-like protein (EDEM), which targets glycoproteins for ER-associated degradation (ERAD). It is translocated out of the ER into the cytoplasm for proteosomal degradation.
- This is so-called calnexin cycle. In this way, calnexin retains certain partly folded (or misfolded) glycoproteins and releases them when further folding has occurred. The glucosyltransferase, by sensing the folding of the glycoprotein and only reglucosylating misfolded proteins, is a key component of the cycle.
- This cycle of binding and release has three functions: It prevents glycoprotein aggregation; it retains non-native conformers in the ER until a native structure is acquired (quality control); and binding to calnexin/calreticulin brings ERp57 into proximity with the non-native glycoprotein. ERp57 catalyzes disulfide bond formation and isomerization within the glycoprotein substrate, assisting it to assume its native conformation. As a final defence mechanism, unfolded or aberrantly-folded proteins are degraded by the cytoplasmic proteasome complex.
- In spite of similar sugar-binding specificity, CNX and CRT bind to a variety of distinct target proteins. Gene knockout studies demonstrated that CRT-knockout mice were lethal, and CNX-knockout mice showed early death with severe neural abnormalities, indicating that CNX and CRT could not compensate each other's function in development. These suggest that CNX and CRT play distinct biological roles in the cell.
- Stress (such as through heat shock) stimulates ER chaperone activity. Non-native forms of some proteins that "escape" this surveillance system can accumulate and result in diseases like Alzheimer's and Parkinson's disease.

Q. 5. What are lectins, their significance and applications?

Ans. Lectins (themselves glycoproteins) are carbohydrate-binding proteins. The term "lectin" is a general term that encompasses several families of proteins of non-immune origin that bind to glycoconjugates. Also known as agglutinins since original discoveries used agglutination of red blood cells (recognition of surface sugars) as a criteria.

- They may bind to a soluble carbohydrate or to a carbohydrate moiety that is a part of a glycoprotein or glycolipid.
- A lectin molecule contains at least two sugar-binding sites; sugar-binding proteins with a single site will not agglutinate or precipitate structures that contain sugar residues, so are not classified as lectins.
- The specificity of a lectin for binding carbohydrate is usually defined by the monosaccharides or oligosaccharides that are best at inhibiting the agglutination or precipitation caused by the lectin.
- Lectins occur in many types of organisms; they may be soluble or membrane-bound.
- Sugar-specific enzymes, transport proteins and toxins may qualify as lectins if they have multiple-sugar binding sites.

Lectins perform recognition on the cellular and molecular levels and play numerous roles in biological recognition phenomena involving cells, carbohydrates, and proteins.

Classification of lectins

- **C-type lectins:** Characterized by a Ca^{2+}-dependent carbohydrate recognition domain (CRD); includes the mammalian asialoglycoprotein receptor, the selectins, and the mannose-binding protein.
- **S-type lectins:** β-Galactoside-binding animal lectins with roles in cell–cell and cell–matrix interactions.
- **P-type lectins:** Mannose-6-P receptor, role in protein trafficking to lysosomes.
- **L-type lectins:** Members of the immunoglobulin superfamily, for example, sialoadhesin-mediating adhesion of macrophages to various cells.

Biological functions of lectins

- Lectins present on microbes mediate their attachment and binding of bacteria and viruses to human host cells.
  – HIV can bind to both Langerhans and dendritic cells in the epithelium. HIV binds to dendritic cells via a lectin called DC-SIGN (CD209 or C-type lectin receptor).

Examples of glycan receptors for viruses

Virus	Lectin	Glycan receptor specificity	Site of infection
Myxoviruses			
Influenza A and B (human)	Hemagglutinin	Neu5Acα2-6Gal	Upper respiratory tract mucosa
Influenza A and B (avian and porcine)	Hemagglutinin	Neu5Acα2-3Gal	Intestinal mucosa
Influenza C	Hemagglutinin esterase	9-O-acetyl-Neu5Acα-	

(Contd.)

Virus	Lectin	Glycan receptor specificity	Site of infection
Newcastle disease	Hemagglutinin neuraminidase	Neu5Acα2-3Gal-	
Sendai	Hemagglutinin neuraminidase	Neu5Acα2-8Neu5Ac-	
Papoviruses			
Polyoma		Neu5Acα2-3Gal-, Neu5Acα2-3Galβ1-3 (Neu5Acα2-6)GalNAc- (e.g., gangliosides GD1α, GT1aα, GQ1bα)	
Herpesviruses			
Herpes simplex	Glycoproteins gB, gC, gD	3-O-sulfated heparan sulfate	Mucosal surfaces of mouth, eyes, genital and respiratory tracts
Picornaviruses			
Foot-and-mouth disease	Caspid proteins	Heparan sulfate	
Retroviruses			
HIV	gp120 V3 loop	Heparan sulfate	CD4 lymphocytes
Flaviviruses			
Dengue	Envelope protein	Heparan sulfate	Macrophages

Examples of glycan receptors for parasites

Microorganism	Adhesin/Lectin	Glycan receptor sequence	Target tissue
Entamoeba histolytica	260-kD receptor	Terminal Gal/GalNAc residues	Small intestinal mucosa
Plasmodium falciparum	EBA175; circumsporozoite (CS) protein	Sialic acid-containing glycans (Neu5Acα2-3Galβ-); heparan sulfate	Erythrocytes (infected cells bind to placental vasculature); hepatocytes
Trypanosoma cruzi		Sialic acid-containing glycans; heparan sulfate	Blood
Leishmania amazonensi		Heparan sulfate	Macrophages, fibroblasts, epithelium
Cryptosporidium parvum		Terminal Gal-GalNAc	Intestinal epithelium
Giardia lamblia		Mannose-terminated oligosaccharides	

Examples of receptors for bacterial toxins

Microorganism	Toxin/Lectin	Glycan receptor sequence	Target tissue
Bacillus thuringiensis	Crystal toxins	Galβ1–3/6Galβ/β1-3(±Glcβ1-6) GalNAcβGlcNAcβ1-3Manβ1-4GlcβCer	Intestinal epithelia of insects
Clostridium botulinum	Botulinum toxins (A–E)	Gangliosides GT1b, GQ1b	Nerve membrane
Clostridium difficile	Toxin A	GalNAcβ1–3Galβ1-4GlcNAcβ1-3Galβ1-4GlcβCer	Large intestine
Clostridium tetani	Tetanus toxin	Ganglioside GT1b	Nerve membrane
Escherichia coli	Heat-labile toxin	GM1	Intestine
Shigella dysenteriae	Shiga toxin	Galα1-4GalβCer Galα1-4Galβ1-4GlcβCer	Large intestine
Vibrio cholera	Cholera toxin	GM1	Small intestine

- Lectins in immunity:
  - The innate immune system protein, mannose-binding lectin (MBL), recognizes a broad range of molecular patterns on a broad range of infectious agents and is able to distinguish them from self. MBL is a liver-derived serum protein and is secreted into the serum, where it can activate an immune response before the induction of antigen-specific immunity.
  - Mannose-binding lectin (MBL) and ficolin are lectins composed of a lectin domain attached to collagenous region. However, they use a different lectin domain: a carbohydrate recognition domain (CRD) is responsible for MBL and a fibrinogen-like domain for ficolin. These two collagenous lectins are pattern recognition receptors, and upon recognition of the infectious agent, they trigger the activation of the lectin-complement pathway through attached serine proteases, MBL-associated serine proteases (MASPs).
  - C type lectins (including the mannose receptor, CLEC5A, CLEC9A, and DC-SIGN), contribute to immunity against fungi, bacteria, viruses, and parasites.
- Regulation of cell adhesion:
  - Sialoadhesin-mediating adhesion of macrophages to various cells.
  - Selectins are lectins specific for leukocyte-endothelium interactions
    - Participate in leukocyte rolling and adhesion
    - Each type of selectin binds to specific oligosaccharide sequence
    - P-selectin on endothelial cells binds to sialyl-Lewis^X antigen – sequence present on leukocytes.

Molecule	Cell	Ligands (glycoproteins)
Selectins		
L-selectin	PMN, lymphs	CD34, Gly-CAM-1, sialyl-Lewis^X, and others (present on endothelial cells)
P-selectin	EC, platelets	P-selectin glycoprotein ligand-1 (PSGL-1), sialyl-Lewis^X, and others (present on endothelial cells)
E-selectin	EC	Sialyl-Lewis^X and others (on leucocytes)

EC = endothelial cells

- Control of protein levels in the blood: The mammalian asialoglycoprotein receptor is involved in clearance of certain glycoproteins from plasma by hepatocytes. Proteins losing the terminal NeuAc residue have exposed subterminal Gal residues that is recognised by the receptor leading to endocytosis and degradation in liver. Thus, glycosylation regulates half life of proteins in blood. Liver cells contain a mammalian asialoglycoprotein receptor that recognizes the Gal moiety of many desialylated plasma proteins and leads to their endocytosis.
- A lectin receptor (mannose-6-P receptor) recognizes hydrolytic enzymes containing mannose-6-phosphate, and targets these proteins for delivery into lysosomes. I-cell disease is one type of defect in this particular system. There is defect in the GlcNAc phosphotranferase which phosphorylates mannose to mannose-6-PO_4 on N-linked glycoproteins in Golgi apparatus. Due to lack of M-6-PO_4 the hydrolytic enzymes for breakdown of oligosaccharides, lipids and GAG cannot be targeted to reach lysosomes. Thus, these substances cannot be digested in lysosomes leading to inclusion cell or I-cell disease.

Uses of lectins in medicine and medical research

- Purified lectins are important in a clinical setting because they are used for blood typing. Some of the glycolipids and glycoproteins on an individual's red blood cells can be identified by lectins.
    - A lectin from Dolichos biflorus is used to identify cells that belong to the A1 blood group.
    - A lectin from Ulex europaeus is used to identify the H blood group antigen.
    - A lectin from Vicia graminea is used to identify the N blood group antigen.
    - A lectin from Iberis amara is used to identify the M blood group antigen.
    - A lectin from coconut milk is used to identify Theros antigen.
    - A lectin from Dorex is used to identify R antigen.
- In neuroscience, the anterograde labelling method is used to trace the path of efferent axons with PHA-L, a lectin from the kidney bean.
- A lectin (BanLec) from bananas inhibits HIV-1 *in vitro*.
- Use in studying carbohydrate recognition by proteins: Lectins from legume plants, such as PHA or concanavalin A, have been widely used as model systems to understand the molecular basis of how proteins recognize carbohydrates, because they are relatively easy to obtain and have a wide variety of sugar specificities. The crystal structures of legume lectins have led to a detailed insight of the atomic interactions between carbohydrates and proteins.
- Concanavalin A and other commercially available lectins have been widely used in affinity chromatography for purifying glycoproteins.
- Biochemical warfare agent ricin: The protein ricin is isolated from seeds of the castor oil plant and comprises two protein domains. Abrin from the jequirity pea is similar. It also has two domains. One domain is a lectin that binds cell surface galactosyl residues and enables the protein to enter cells. The second domain is an *N*-glycosidase that cleaves nucleobases from ribosomal RNA, resulting in inhibition of protein synthesis and cell death.
- Lectins have been incorporated into genetically engineered crops to transfer traits such as resistance to pests and resistance to herbicides.

Nutrition and lectins

Foods with high concentrations of lectins, such as beans, cereal grains, seeds, nuts, and potatoes, may be harmful if consumed in excess in uncooked or improperly cooked form. Adverse effects may include nutritional deficiencies, and immune (allergic) reactions. Possibly, most effects of lectins are due to gastrointestinal distress through interaction of the lectins with the gut epithelial cells. Lectin damage may occur by interfering with the repair of already-damaged epithelial cells. Lectins are considered a major family of protein anti-nutrients (ANCs). The toxicity of lectins has been identified by consumption of food with high lectin content, which can lead to diarrhoea, nausea, bloating, vomiting, even death (as from ricin). Many legume seeds have been proven to contain high lectin activity, termed hemagglutinating activity. Soybean is the most important grain legume crop, the seeds of which contain high activity of soybean lectins (soybean agglutinin or SBA). SBA is able to disrupt small intestinal metabolism and damage small intestinal villi via the ability of lectins to bind with brush border surfaces (via *N*-acetylgalactosamine, GalNAc) in the distal part of small intestine and promotes inflammation. Heat processing can reduce the toxicity of lectins, but low temperature or insufficient cooking may not completely eliminate their toxicity, as some plant lectins are resistant to heat. It is believed that undercooking red kidney beans (*rajma*) increases toxicity. In addition, lectins can result in irritation and over-secretion of mucus in the intestines, causing impaired absorptive capacity of the intestinal wall.

Chapter 14

Organ Function Tests

Q. 1. What is serum–ascites albumin gradient?

Ans. Serum and ascitic fluid albumin levels are measured simultaneously to permit calculation of the serum-ascites albumin gradient (SAAG). It is calculated by subtracting the ascitic albumin from the serum albumin and does not change with diuresis.

According to Starling's law:
- The force which will promote flow of fluid from serum to peritoneal space will be
 (Hydrostatic pressure in capillaries – Hydrostatic pressure in peritoneum)
- The force which favours flow of fluid from peritoneum to serum will be the osmotic gradient in favour of serum, reflected by
 (Serum albumin – Peritoneal fluid albumin)

Thus, fluid will accumulate in peritoneal cavity causing ascites if:
- Pressure in capillaries is raised due to high venous pressure in the portal circulation.
- Osmotic gradient favouring fluid movement from peritoneal space to serum (which normally has much higher albumin) is reduced – either due to decreased serum albumin protein or due to increased albumin in peritoneal fluid (exudative inflammation).

A high SAAG implies that if despite high osmotic gradient favouring fluid movement from peritoneum to serum ascites has developed, the pressure in portal circulation is high. Portal hypertension is defined as the elevation of the hepatic venous pressure gradient (HVPG) to > 5 mmHg. Thus, according to Starling's law, a high SAAG reflects the oncotic pressure that counterbalances the portal pressure. The SAAG is useful for distinguishing ascites caused by portal hypertension from non-portal hypertensive ascites. It reflects the pressure within the hepatic sinusoids and correlates with the hepatic venous pressure gradient.

- A SAAG ≥ 1.1 g/dL reflects the presence of portal hypertension and indicates that the ascites is from an increased pressure in the hepatic sinusoids. Possible causes include cirrhosis, cardiac ascites, sinusoidal obstruction syndrome (venoocclusive disease), massive liver metastasis, or hepatic vein thrombosis (Budd-Chiari syndrome) (Fig. 14.1).
- A SAAG < 1.1 g/dL indicates that the ascites is not related to portal hypertension as in tuberculous peritonitis, peritoneal carcinomatosis, or pancreatic ascites (Fig. 14.1).

- For high-SAAG (≥ 1.1) ascites, the ascitic protein level can provide further clues to the etiology (Fig. 14.1).
  - An ascitic protein level of 2.5 g/dL indicates that the hepatic sinusoids are normal and allows passage of protein into the ascites, as occurs in cardiac ascites, sinusoidal obstruction syndrome, or early Budd-Chiari syndrome.
  - An ascitic protein level < 2.5 g/dL indicates that the hepatic sinusoids have been damaged and scarred and no longer allow passage of protein, as occurs with cirrhosis, late Budd-Chiari syndrome, or massive liver metastases.

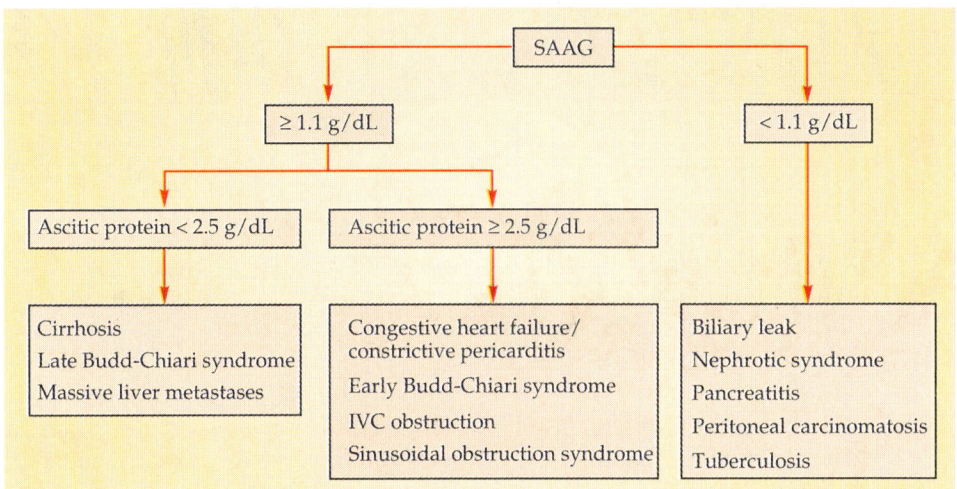

Fig. 14.1. SAAG and ascetic fluid protein levels can help in differential diagnosis of ascites.

Q. 2. What is the biochemical basis of development of ascites in cirrhosis?

Ans. Cirrhosis leads to ascites due to following reasons (Fig. 14.2):
- The presence of portal hypertension: There is an increase in intrahepatic resistance, causing increased portal pressure, but there is also vasodilation of the splanchnic arterial system (vasodilating factors such as nitric oxide are responsible for the vasodilatory effect), which, in turn, results in an increase in portal venous inflow. Both of these abnormalities result in increased production of splanchnic lymph and increased hydrostatic pressure gradient from capillaries to peritoneum.
- Hypoalbuminemia and reduced plasma oncotic pressure also contribute to the loss of fluid from the vascular compartment into the peritoneal cavity. Hypoalbuminemia is due to decreased synthetic function in a cirrhotic liver.
- All these hemodynamic changes result in fluid accumulation into the peritoneal fluid. As intravascular fluid and pressure fall activation of the renin-angiotensin-aldosterone system (RAS) occurs with the development of hyperaldosteronism. Underfilling of the arterial circulation secondary to arterial vasodilation in the splanchnic vascular bed also activates the RAS system. The renal effects of increased aldosterone lead to sodium retention and also contribute to the development of ascites. Sodium retention causes fluid accumulation and expansion of the extracellular fluid volume, which results in the formation of peripheral

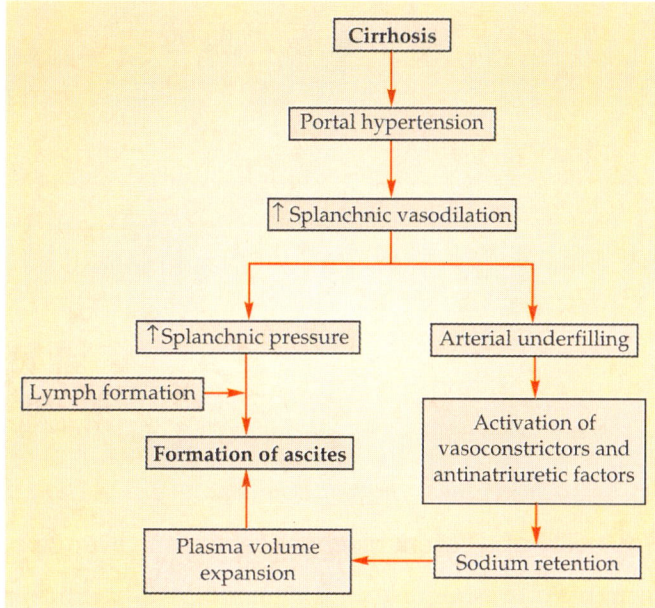

Fig. 14.2. Pathogenesis of ascites due to cirrhosis.

edema and ascites. Because the retained fluid is constantly leaking out of the intravascular compartment into the peritoneal cavity, the sensation of vascular filling is not achieved, and the process continues with increasing ascites and peripheral edema.

Q. 3. How to distinguish pleural or other fluids as transudate or exudate by biochemical tests?

Ans. In cases of pleural effusion or accumulation of fluid in other such dead spaces in body the first step is to determine whether the effusion is a transudate or an exudate.
- A transudative pleural effusion occurs when systemic factors that influence the formation and absorption of pleural fluid are altered or it is due to alterations in the Starling forces governing movement of fluid between pleural space and capillaries. The leading causes of transudative pleural effusions are left ventricular failure and cirrhosis.
- An exudative pleural effusion occurs when local factors that influence the formation and absorption of pleural fluid are altered or there is inflammation with increased extravasation of fluid, plasma proteins and cells (leukocytes and RBCs) from capillaries (blood) into the pleural space. The leading causes of exudative pleural effusions are bacterial pneumonia, malignancy, viral infection, and pulmonary embolism.

Additional diagnostic procedures are required with exudative effusions to define the cause of the local inflammation and pathology.

The distinction between exudate and transudate can be made by measuring pleural fluid and serum protein and LDH levels as shown in Fig. 14.3. Higher ratios suggest exudate in which plasma proteins leak into the pleural fluid due to inflammation. Similar formulae can be used for other fluids also.

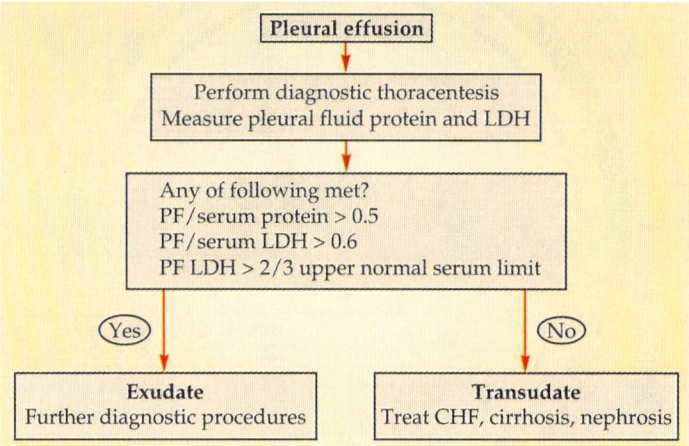

Fig. 14.3. Differentiation between transudate and exudate by biochemical tests.

Q. 4. Describe the utility of different biochemical tests in liver diseases.

Ans. Several biochemical tests are useful in the evaluation and management of patients with hepatic dysfunction. These tests are useful to:
- detect the presence of liver disease;
- distinguish among different types of liver disorders;
- study the extent of liver damage; and
- follow the response to treatment.

Tests based on detoxification and excretory functions

1. Serum bilirubin

- Bilirubin is a product of RBC turnover (heme breakdown), extracted from blood and biotransformed in liver to bilirubin diglucoronide.
- Excreted in bile as glucoronides (90% as diglucoronide and 10% as monoglucoronide). These are hydrolysed by β-glucoronidase from liver, intestinal epithelium and gut bacteria.
- The unconjugated bilirubin so produced is reduced by anaerobic bacteria in intestines to three compounds – collectively called urobilinogens (includes stercobilinogen, mesobilinogen and urobilinogen). 20% are reabsorbed and undergo enterohepatic recirculation. 2–5% of the reabsorbed urobilinogen appears in urine.
- In lower intestines the three urobilinogens are spontaneously oxidized to form stercobilin, mesobilin and urobilin, responsible for the orange-brown colour of stool.
- About 50% of conjugated bilirubin excreted in bile is metabolized to various products and excreted.
- The unconjugated fraction is insoluble in water and is bound to albumin in the blood. The conjugated bilirubin fraction is water-soluble and can therefore be excreted by the kidney. Normally conjugated bilirubin is at very low levels in blood and absent from urine when measured by routine methods.
- Measured by the Van den Bergh (diazo) reaction (used routinely in clinical labs) in which direct bilirubin is an approximate measure of conjugated bilirubin and indirect of unconjugated bilirubin.

- As the Van den Bergh method overestimates conjugated bilirubin as direct bilirubin (as some unconjugated bilirubin can react even in absence of methanol), if the direct-acting fraction is less than 15% of the total, the bilirubin can be considered to be all unconjugated (indirect).
- The 4 fractions – α-bilirubin (unconjugated), β-bilirubin (monoconjugated), γ-bilirubin (diconjugated) and δ-bilirubin (monoconjugated bilirubin bound covalently to lysine of albumin) can be accurately measured by HPLC.
- Elevation of the unconjugated fraction of bilirubin is rarely due to liver disease. An isolated elevation of unconjugated bilirubin is seen primarily in hemolytic disorders and in genetic conditions such as Crigler-Najjar and Gilbert's syndromes (Fig. 14.4).
- Conjugated hyperbilirubinemia almost always implies liver or biliary tract disease. The rate-limiting step in bilirubin metabolism is not conjugation of bilirubin, but rather the transport of conjugated bilirubin into the bile canaliculi. Thus, elevation of the conjugated fraction may be seen in any type of liver disease.
- In most liver diseases, both conjugated and unconjugated fractions of the bilirubin tend to be elevated. Thus, except in the presence of a purely unconjugated hyperbilirubinemia, fractionation of the bilirubin is rarely helpful in determining the cause of jaundice.
- In viral hepatitis, the higher the serum bilirubin, the greater the hepatocellular damage.
- Higher levels of total serum bilirubin correlates with poor outcomes in alcoholic hepatitis.
- It is also a critical component of the Model for Endstage Liver Disease (MELD) score, a tool used to estimate survival of patients with end-stage liver disease. An elevated total serum bilirubin in patients with drug-induced liver disease indicates more severe injury.

2. Urine bilirubin

- Unconjugated bilirubin always binds to albumin in the serum and is not filtered by the kidney. Therefore, any bilirubin found in the urine is conjugated bilirubin; the presence of bilirubinuria implies the presence of liver disease. Urine bilirubin reflects the increased plasma concentration of conjugated bilirubin.
- A urine dipstick test (Icto test) can theoretically give the same information as measuring direct and indirect serum bilirubin. This test is almost 100% accurate. Phenothiazines may give a false-positive reading with the Ictotest tablet.
- In patients recovering from jaundice, the urine bilirubin clears prior to the serum bilirubin. This is because of formation of δ-bilirubin (monoconjugated bilirubin bound covalently to lysine of albumin) in blood which has a half-life of 17–19 days and thus clears slowly. It reacts as conjugated bilirubin in Van den Bergh test.

3. Blood ammonia

Ammonia is produced in the body during normal protein metabolism and by intestinal bacteria, primarily those in the colon. The liver converts ammonia to urea, which is excreted by the kidneys.

Ammonia levels can be raised in the following situations:
- **Genetic defects:** Urea cycle defects, inborn errors in metabolism of dibasic amino acids lysine and ornithine, inborn errors in metabolism of organic acids like propionic acid, methylmalonic acid, isovaleric acid, etc.
- **Acquired diseases:** Advanced liver diseases – severe or chronic liver failure, cirrhosis and fulminant hepatitis, renal failure, Reye's syndrome.

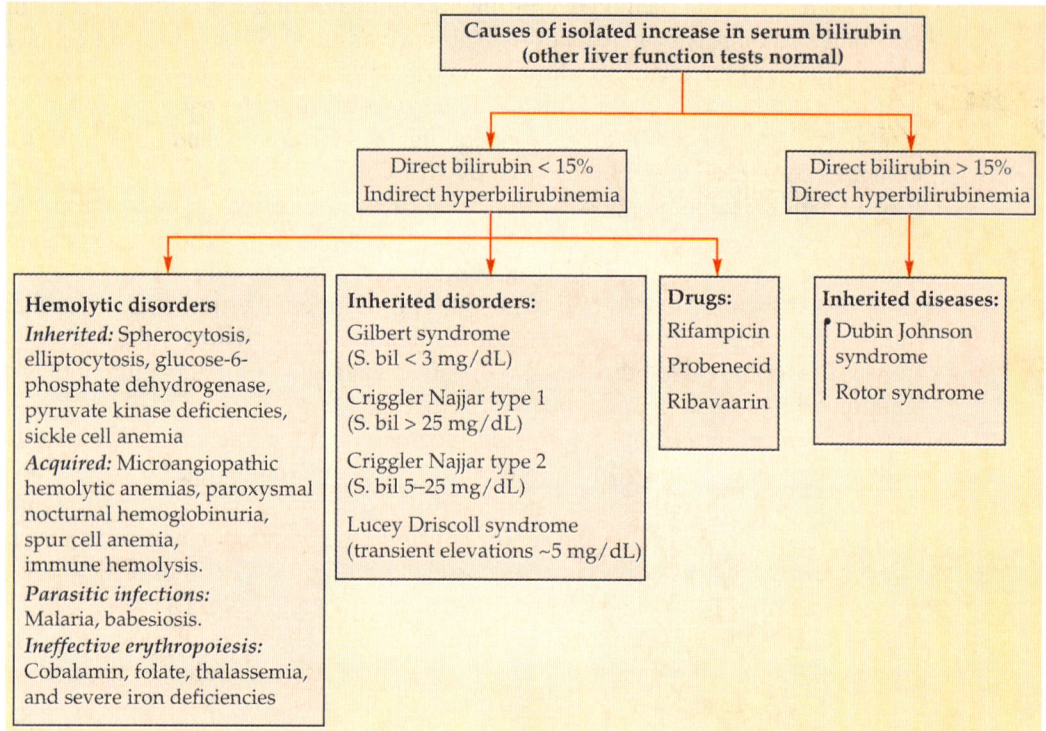

Fig. 14.4. Causes of isolated increase in serum bilirubin with other liver function tests normal.

Significance of blood ammonia levels

- Elevated ammonia levels are toxic to brain and lead to encephalopathy. Ammonia entry into CNS is dependent on blood pH as ammonia crosses blood-brain barrier more readily than ammonium ion. About 3% of total ammonia exists as NH_3 at normal pH of 7.4. This increases by 67% to 5% of total ammonia at pH 7.6 (alkalosis).
- Fasting venous plasma concentration of ammonia is useful in distinguishing cause of encephalopathy as due to liver disease. It can be occasionally useful for identifying occult liver disease in patients with mental status changes.
- It is very useful in diagnosis of Reye's syndrome, inborn errors of metabolism, and increased ammonia levels due to drug toxicity of salicylates and valproate, etc.
- In acute liver injury, ammonia concentrations > 200 μmol/L are associated with cerebral edema and poor prognosis.
- It is not useful in patients with known chronic liver failure.
- There is very poor correlation between either the presence or the severity of encephalopathy and elevation of blood ammonia.
- There is also a poor correlation of the blood serum ammonia and hepatic function.
- Ammonia concentration actually better reflects the presence of shunting of blood around the portal veins than degree of liver dysfunction. Thus, ammonia can be elevated in patients with severe portal hypertension and portal blood shunting around the liver even in the presence of normal or near-normal hepatic function.

4. Bile acids

- Are produced from cholesterol and secreted actively in bile to help in digestion and absorption of fat and fat-soluble vitamins.
- Help maintain cholesterol homeostasis (cholesterol excretion).
- Undergo enterohepatic recirculation.
- Four major bile acids are known. Cholic and chenodeoxycholic acid are primary bile acids made in liver from cholesterol. Primary bile acids are metabolized in intestines to secondary bile acids – deoxycholic acid and lithocholic acid. Bile acids are conjugated with glycine and taurine in liver.
- In cholestatic or obstructive jaundice there is decreased delivery of primary bile acids to intestine and increased regurgitation into blood. Thus, there is increased concentration, increased ratio of primary to secondary bile acid in blood and appearance of bile acids in urine.
- In intestinal bypass surgeries, increased fecal loss of bile acids leads to decreased blood bile acids (both primary and secondary), and decreased cholesterol levels (more is converted to bile acids).
- Although, abnormal in many clinical conditions, they add little to standard tests of liver function and are rarely used in clinical medicine.

5. Xenobiotic metabolism and excretion

- Rates of metabolism of xenobiotics are used as quantitative liver function tests as they gradually worsen as liver disease progresses.
- Their measurement adds only slightly to the information given by the routine liver function tests like bilirubin, albumin and prothrombin time.
- Are not very sensitive and specific for different stages of liver disease.
- Include dye excretion tests (bromosulphthalein and indocyanin green clearance tests), and drug clearance test (aminopyrine, caffeine, lidocaine), e.g., a single dose of caffeine 3.5 mg/kg (max. 200 mg) is given dissolved in water, juice or milk orally. Blood or salivary samples are taken before administration and at timed intervals after dosage and caffeine is estimated by immunoassay or HPLC. Caffeine is rapidly absorbed by GIT and undergoes N-demethylation by hepatic mixed function oxidase system. Clearance is normally 2 mL/min/kg in adults and 10 mL/min/kg in children and is prolonged in chronic hepatitis and cirrhosis.

Tests that measure biosynthetic function of the liver

1. Plasma proteins

- All plasma proteins except γ-globulins are synthesized in liver. Factors which effect plasma protein levels include:
  - Decreased availability of amino acids: malnutrition (PEM), maldigestion, malabsorption
  - Catabolic states: hyperthyroidism, Cushing's syndrome, burns, post-surgery recovery
  - Protein losing states: nephrotic syndrome and protein losing enteropathy
  - Actions of cytokines like IL-6: decrease in transport proteins such as albumin, transferrin and lipoproteins but increase in inflammatory response modifiers like ceruloplasmin, $\alpha 1$-antitrypsin, $\alpha 2$-macroglobulin.

- Actions of hormones like estrogen, cortisol, androgens, and thyroid hormones to increase or decrease specific proteins.
- Congenital deficiency states – Wilson's disease and α1-antitrypsin deficiency, etc.
• Liver has an extensive reserve capacity, preventing protein concentration from falling unless liver damage is extensive. The pattern of protein alterations seen in liver disease depends on type, severity and duration of liver damage.
• In acute hepatic dysfunction, little change is seen in plasma protein profile or total protein levels.
• In fulminant hepatic failure or acute severe liver injury concentrations of short half-life proteins (transthyretin and prothrombin) fall quickly, while proteins with longer half-life (albumin) are normal or minimally changed.
• In cirrhosis, concentration of all liver synthesized proteins decreases and that of γ-globulins increases leading to reversal of A : G ratio (albumin to globulin ratio). In cirrhosis, the increased serum gamma globulin concentration is due to the increased synthesis of antibodies, some of which are directed against intestinal bacteria. This occurs because the cirrhotic liver fails to clear bacterial antigens that normally reach the liver through the hepatic circulation.
• Globulins: Diffuse polyclonal increases in IgG levels are common in autoimmune hepatitis; increases > 100% should alert the clinician to this possibility. Increases in the IgM levels are common in primary biliary cirrhosis, while increases in the IgA levels occur in alcoholic liver disease.
• Serial determination of plasma proteins provides prognostic information, e.g. worsening of prothrombin time during acute hepatitis suggests a poor prognosis.
• Albumin:
  - Exclusively made by liver.
  - Rate of synthesis depends on age, nutritional status and hormonal environment.
  - Hypoalbuminemia is not specific for liver disease and may occur in protein malnutrition of any cause, as well as protein-losing enteropathies, nephrotic syndrome, and chronic infections that are associated with prolonged increases in levels of serum interleukin 1 (IL-1) and/or tumor necrosis factor, cytokines that inhibit albumin synthesis.
  - Decreased in cirrhosis, autoimmune hepatitis, alcoholic hepatitis.
  - Serum albumin has a long half-life, 18–20 days, with 4% degraded per day.
  - Because of this slow turnover, the serum albumin is not a good indicator of acute or mild hepatic dysfunction.
  - Only minimal changes in the serum albumin are seen in acute liver conditions such as viral hepatitis, drug-related hepatoxicity, and obstructive jaundice.
  - In hepatitis, albumin levels < 3 g/dL suggest chronic liver disease.
  - Hypoalbuminemia is more common in chronic liver disorders such as cirrhosis and usually reflects severe liver damage and decreased albumin synthesis.
  - Exceptions are the patients with ascites in whom synthesis may be normal or even increased, but levels are low because of the increased loss into ascitic fluid.
• Coagulation factors and prothrombin time:
  - With the exception of factor VIII, which is produced by vascular endothelial cells, all the blood clotting factors are made exclusively in hepatocytes.

- Their serum half-lives are much shorter than albumin, ranging from 6 h for factor VII to 5 days for fibrinogen.
- Because of their rapid turnover, measurement of the clotting factors is the single best accurate measure of hepatic synthetic function and helpful in both the diagnosis and assessing the prognosis of acute liver disease.
- Useful for this purpose is the serum prothrombin time, which collectively measures factors II, V, VII, and X.
- Biosynthesis of factors II, VII, IX, and X depends on vitamin K. Thus, prothrombin time may be elevated in hepatitis and cirrhosis as well as in disorders that lead to vitamin K deficiency such as obstructive jaundice or fat malabsorption of any kind.
- PT not corrected in a few days by parenteral injection of 10 mg vitamin K (water-soluble menadione), or absence of rise of PIVKA (proteins induced by vitamin K antagonists – non-carboxylated clotting factors) indicates hepatic cause rather than vitamin K deficiency.
- Marked prolongation of the prothrombin time, > 5 s above control, and non-correction by intravenous vitamin K administration is a poor prognostic sign in acute viral hepatitis and other acute and chronic liver diseases.
- The INR-PT, along with the total serum bilirubin and creatinine, are components of the MELD score which is used to allocate organs for liver transplantation.

2. Urea

Patients with end-stage liver disease have low urea levels; plasma ammonia is elevated. Low levels also occur in urea cycle defects along with hyperammonemia.

3. Glucose

Liver produces glucose by gluconeogenesis. Hypoglycaemia is a common complication in certain liver diseases like Reye's syndrome, fulminant hepatic failure, advanced cirrhosis, and hepatocellular carcinoma. However, routine measurements of carbohydrates do not have any role in diagnosis of liver diseases.

Serum Enzymes

These are actually mistakenly called 'liver function test' as they do not tell about any function of liver, though their evaluation is very important in diagnosis and prognosis of liver diseases. The liver contains thousands of enzymes, some of which are also present in the serum in very low concentrations. These enzymes have no known function in the serum. The level of a given enzyme activity in the serum depends on entry into blood from cell turnover and damage and its clearance by macrophages and the reticuloendothelial system and kidney. Elevation in levels is thought to primarily reflect its increased rate of entry into serum from damaged liver cells.

Serum enzyme tests can be grouped into three categories:

1. Hepatocellular damage: Enzymes whose elevation in serum reflects damage to hepatocytes.
2. Cholestasis: Enzymes whose elevation in serum reflects obstruction to flow of bile.
3. Mixed pattern: Enzyme tests that do not fit precisely into either pattern.

1. Enzymes that reflect damage to hepatocytes

Aminotransferases or transaminases – alanine transaminase (ALT) and aspartate transaminase (AST)

- AST is found in the liver, cardiac muscle, skeletal muscle, kidneys, brain, pancreas, lungs, leukocytes, and erythrocytes in decreasing order of concentration. It has both cytosolic and mitochondrial isoenzymes which are genetically different enzymes. Mitochondrial enzyme accounts for 5–10% of serum activity.
- ALT is found primarily in the liver and kidney and is therefore a more specific indicator of liver injury. Also ALT elevations persist longer than that of AST. ALT is exclusively cytosolic.
- These are sensitive indicators of liver cell injury and are most helpful in recognizing acute hepatocellular diseases such as hepatitis.
- Normally, present in the serum in low concentrations. These enzymes are released into the blood in greater amounts when there is damage to the liver cell membrane resulting in increased permeability. Liver cell necrosis is not essential for the release of the aminotransferases, and there is a poor correlation between the degree of liver cell damage and the level of the aminotransferases.
- Thus, the absolute elevation of the aminotransferases is of no prognostic significance in acute hepatocellular disorders.
- The normal range is 10–40 U/L.
- Any type of liver cell injury can cause modest elevations in the serum aminotransferases. Levels of up to 300 U/L are nonspecific and may be found in any type of liver disorder.
- Minimal ALT elevations in asymptomatic blood donors rarely indicate severe liver disease; fatty liver disease is the most likely explanation.
- Striking elevations, i.e., aminotransferases > 1000 U/L, occur almost exclusively in disorders associated with extensive hepatocellular injury such as viral hepatitis, ischemic liver injury (prolonged hypotension or acute heart failure), or toxin- or drug-induced liver injury.
- In viral hepatitis, levels are raised even before clinical jaundice appears. 10–40 times elevations are commonly seen, levels may go up to 100 times the normal range. The sensitivity and specificity for diagnosing acute liver injury is > 95% if levels are more than 7 times the normal. Peak activity occurs by 7th to 12th days and has no relation with prognosis. Levels reach normal by 3rd to 5th week in case of uneventful recovery.
- Persistence of elevated ALT beyond 6 months after episode of acute hepatitis is diagnostic of chronic hepatitis.
- In toxic hepatitis like acetaminophen-induced liver damage peak is more than 85 times the normal range in 90% of cases. Levels peak early and fall rapidly.
- Other main cause of elevation is non-alcoholic fatty liver disease and metabolic syndrome.
- In most liver diseases ALT activity > AST, except in alcoholic hepatitis, cirrhosis and liver cancer.
- Though AST : ALT ratio is < 1 in chronic hepatitis, as cirrhosis develops this ratio rises to greater than 1. This occurs due to decreased ALT production in a damaged liver, and reduced clearance of AST in advancing liver fibrosis. AST : ALT ratio > 1 has > 90% positive predictive value for diagnosing advanced fibrosis in patients with chronic hepatitis

- An AST : ALT ratio > 2 : 1 is suggestive, while a ratio > 3 : 1 is highly suggestive of alcoholic liver disease. The AST in alcoholic liver disease is rarely > 300 U/L, and the ALT is often normal. This is due to associated deficiency of PLP (B6) required for enzyme activity, decreased ALT production in liver cytoplasm and increase in mitochondrial fraction of AST. Mitochondrial AST is increased in patients with extensive liver cell degeneration and necrosis (cell death).
- Ratio between m-AST and total AST can be used for diagnosing alcoholic hepatitis. It seems to identify the liver cell 'necrotic type' condition characterized by moderate increase in total enzyme levels but relatively high activity of mitochondrial enzymes. It is typical of alcoholic hepatitis.
- The aminotransferases are usually not greatly elevated in obstructive jaundice. One notable exception occurs during the acute phase of biliary obstruction caused by the passage of a gallstone into the common bile duct. In this setting, the aminotransferases can briefly be in the 1000–2000 U/L range. However, aminotransferase levels decrease quickly, and the pattern of liver function tests rapidly evolve into one typical of cholestasis.

Glutamate dehydrogenase

- Mitochondrial enzyme in liver, heart muscle and kidneys and small amounts in other tissues like brain, etc.
- As an exclusive mitochondrial enzyme it is released form necrotic cells, thus levels are higher in disorders with extensive necrosis. Release is much less than ALT in diffuse inflammatory conditions.
- Like m-AST, it is of value in estimating severity of liver cell damage.

2. Enzymes that reflect cholestasis

The activities of three enzymes – alkaline phosphatase, 5′-nucleotidase, and glutamyl transpeptidase (GGT) – are usually elevated in cholestasis.

- Alkaline phosphatase and 5′-nucleotidase are found in or near the bile canalicular membrane of hepatocytes, while GGT is located in the endoplasmic reticulum and in bile duct epithelial cells. With obstruction to bile flow, the surfactants (bile acids) in the accumulated bile dissolves or removes these enzymes from bile canalicular membrane into interstitial space and blood.
- Reflecting its more diffuse localization in the liver, GGT elevation in serum is less specific for cholestasis than are elevations of alkaline phosphatase or 5′-nucleotidase.
- ALP is present in many organs and cells and has many isoenzymes and isoforms.
- The normal serum alkaline phosphatase consists of many distinct isoenzymes found in the liver, bone, placenta, and, less commonly, small intestine. In healthy adults ALP present in serum is mostly of hepatic origin, rest is from bones.
- As intestinal ALP may be released after meals (especially fatty meals); levels should be measured in fasting samples only.
- ALP is non-pathologically elevated in children and adolescents undergoing rapid bone growth, because of bone alkaline phosphatase, and late in normal pregnancies due to the placental alkaline phosphatase.
- Elevation of liver-derived alkaline phosphatase is not totally specific for cholestasis, and a less than three-fold elevation can be seen in almost any type of liver disease.

- Alkaline phosphatase elevations greater than four times normal occur primarily in patients with cholestatic liver disorders, infiltrative liver diseases such as cancer and amyloidosis, and bone conditions characterized by rapid bone turnover (e.g., Paget's disease).
- In bone diseases, the elevation is due to increased amounts of the bone isoenzymes. In liver diseases, the elevation is due to increased amounts of the liver isoenzyme.
- Isoenzyme measurement by immunoassay or electrophoresis can help. If an elevated serum alkaline phosphatase is the only abnormal finding in an apparently healthy person, or if the degree of elevation is higher than expected in the clinical setting, identification of the source of elevated isoenzymes is helpful. A good alternative is to measure serum 5'-nucleotidase or GGT. These enzymes are rarely elevated in conditions other than liver disease.
- In biliary obstruction, liver responds by synthesizing more ALP; some of the newly synthesized ALP enters the serum, increasing the levels.
- Elevations are higher in extrahepatic than intrahepatic cholestasis and in complete obstruction than partial obstruction.
- Serum levels may reach 10–12 times upper normal limit and return to normal after surgical removal of obstruction.
- In the absence of jaundice or elevated aminotransferases, an elevated alkaline phosphatase of liver origin often suggests early cholestasis and, less often, hepatic infiltration by tumor or granulomata. Other conditions that cause isolated elevations of the alkaline phosphatase include Hodgkin's disease, diabetes, hyperthyroidism, congestive heart failure, amyloidosis, and inflammatory bowel disease.
- The level of serum alkaline phosphatase elevation is not helpful in distinguishing between intra-hepatic and extrahepatic cholestasis. There is no difference among the values found in obstructive jaundice due to cancer, common duct stone, sclerosing cholangitis, or bile duct stricture.
- Values are similarly increased in patients with intrahepatic cholestasis due to drug-induced hepatitis, primary biliary cirrhosis, rejection of transplanted livers, and, rarely, alcohol-induced steatohepatitis.
- Values are also greatly elevated in hepatobiliary disorders seen in patients with AIDS (e.g., AIDS, cholangiopathy due to cytomegalovirus or cryptosporidial infection and tuberculosis with hepatic involvement).
- γ-GGT or γ-glutamyltransferase: Though found in many tissues, serum levels come mainly from liver. It is present in cytoplasm (microsomes/ER) and mainly in cell membrane. It is a sensitive indicator of hepatobiliary disease. It is increased in most patients regardless of the cause. Highest increase is in intra- or post-hepatic obstruction, primary or metastatic liver neoplasia. High levels in hepatitis C patients predict poor response to interferon treatment. Levels are increased by alcohol, anticonvulsant drugs like phenytoin and phenobarbital due to new enzyme production in endoplasmic reticulum.

Enzyme with mixed pattern

Glutathione S transferase

An emerging marker of liver disease, found predominantly in periportal hepatocytes, is evenly distributed across the liver acinus and thus released in all types of liver injury. May be more helpful than AST in detecting early rejection episodes in liver transplant patients.

Other diagnostic tests

Percutaneous liver biopsy

Percutaneous biopsy of the liver is a safe procedure that can be easily performed at the bedside with local anesthesia and ultrasound guidance. Liver biopsy is of proven value in the following situations:

1. Hepatocellular disease of uncertain cause
2. Prolonged hepatitis with the possibility of chronic active hepatitis
3. Unexplained hepatomegaly
4. Unexplained splenomegaly
5. Hepatic filling defects by radiologic imaging
6. Fever of unknown origin
7. Staging of malignant lymphoma.

Ultrasonography

Ultrasonography is the first diagnostic test to use in patients whose liver tests suggest cholestasis, to look for the presence of a dilated intrahepatic or extrahepatic biliary tree or to identify gallstones. In addition, it shows space-occupying lesions within the liver, enables the clinician to distinguish between cystic and solid masses, and helps perform direct percutaneous biopsies. Ultrasound with Doppler imaging can detect the patency of the portal vein, hepatic artery, and hepatic veins and determine the direction and pressure of blood flow.

Uses of liver function tests

- The severity of liver cell damage is assessed by serial measurement of serum total bilirubin, albumin, transaminase and prothrombin time after vitamin K administration (intravenous).
- The diagnosis of minimal hepatocellular damage may be suspected by noting minimally elevated serum transaminase values and sometimes serum bilirubin. Causes will include alcoholic liver damage [where serum γ-glutamyl transpeptidase (γ-GT) is of particular value], and well compensated cirrhosis, although similar changes may be seen in heart failure and fever.
- Quantitative methods of assessment of liver function using substrates for a specific hepatic pathway (like galactose, caffeine and lignocaine) give a better measure of hepatic function rather than damage.
- Fibrosis may be assessed by serum markers, including procollagen type III peptide.
- Quantification of the asialoglycoprotein receptor provides a measure of the 'functional mass' of the liver.
- The pattern of conventional tests (bilirubin, enzymes) indicate which more specialist tests are likely to be valuable (Fig. 14.5).

Grading and staging of liver disease

- Grading refers to an assessment of the severity or activity of liver disease (of inflammation) – active or inactive; and mild, moderate, or severe.
- Though liver biopsy is the most accurate means of assessing severity, particularly in chronic liver disease, serum aminotransferase levels are used as convenient and noninvasive means to follow disease activity.

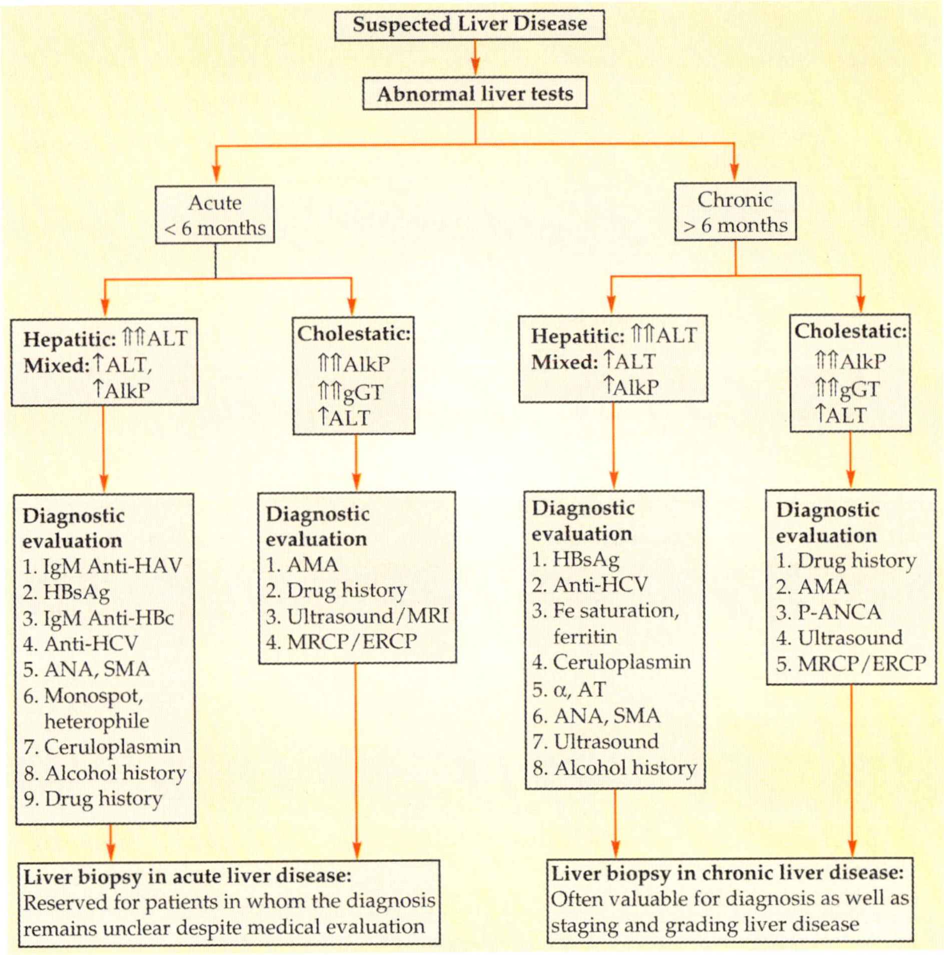

Fig. 14.5. Evaluation of abnormal liver function tests.

- Liver biopsy is also the most accurate means of assessing stage of disease as early or advanced; precirrhotic, and cirrhotic. Noninvasive tests that suggest advanced fibrosis include mild elevations of bilirubin, prolongation of prothrombin time, slight decreases in serum albumin, and mild thrombocytopenia (which is often the first indication of worsening fibrosis).
- Cirrhosis can also be staged clinically. A reliable staging system is the modified Child-Pugh classification with a scoring system of 5–15: scores of 5 and 6 being Child-Pugh class A (consistent with "compensated cirrhosis"), scores of 7–9 indicating class B, and 10–15 indicating class C (Table 14.1).
  - Helpful to stratify patients into risk groups prior to undergoing portal decompressive surgery.
  - Reliable predictor of survival in many liver diseases and predicts the likelihood of major complications of cirrhosis such as bleeding from varices and spontaneous bacterial peritonitis.
  - Assess prognosis in cirrhosis and to provide the standard criteria for assessing suitability for liver transplantation (Child-Pugh class B).

Organ Function Tests

Table 14.1. Child-Pugh classification of cirrhosis

Factor	Units	1	2	3
Serum bilirubin	mol/L	< 34	34–51	> 51
	mg/dL	< 2.0	2.0–3.0	> 3.0
Serum albumin	g/L	> 35	30–35	< 30
	g/dL	> 3.5	3.0–3.5	< 3.0
Prothrombin time	seconds	0–4	4–6	> 6
	prolonged INR	< 1.7	1.7–2.3	> 2.3
Ascites		None	Easily controlled	Poorly controlled
Hepatic encephalopathy		None	Minimal	Advanced

Recently, the Child-Pugh system has been replaced by the model for end-stage liver disease (MELD) score for assessing the need for liver transplantation. The MELD score is a scoring system designed to predict prognosis of patients with liver disease and portal hypertension. It is calculated using three noninvasive variables – the prothrombin time expressed as international normalized ratio (INR), serum bilirubin, and serum creatinine. A similar system using bilirubin, prothrombin time, serum albumin, age, and nutritional status is used for children below the age of 12 years [pediatric end-stage liver disease (PELD)].

Q. 5. Describe the cell-based model of coagulation. How is it different and better than the 'Waterfall' or Cascade model? Why haemophiliacs suffer bleeding even though he extrinsic pathway of coagulation is intact? What is the role of high dose FVIIa therapy to control bleeding?

Ans. Hemostasis is a protective mechanism responsible for preventing blood loss by sealing the sites of injury in the vascular system. It must also be regulated so that blood does not clot within the vasculature and obstruct normal blood flow.

The Cascade/Waterfall Model (Fig 14.6)

- Consists of a sequence of steps where enzymes cleave zymogen substrates (also known as proenzymes) to generate the next enzyme in the cascade.
- The majority of the steps in the cascade occur on phospholipid membrane surfaces and require calcium. Exception: Cleavage of fibrinogen by thrombin.
- Coagulation factors were named after their discoverer, or after the first patient described with a deficiency of that factor, and numbered in order of their discovery.
- Divided into the familiar extrinsic and intrinsic pathway
- The extrinsic system is localized outside (or extrinsic from) the blood, and consists of Tissue Factor (TF) and FVIIa.
- The intrinsic system is localized within the blood (or intrinsic to) and is initiated by the contact activation of FXII on negatively charged surfaces.
- Either pathway can activate FX to FXa, which then (with its cofactor FVa) activates prothrombin to thrombin. Thrombin cleaves fibrinogen to form fibrin (common pathway).
- Cross-interactions between different components (factor VIIa can activate factor IX).

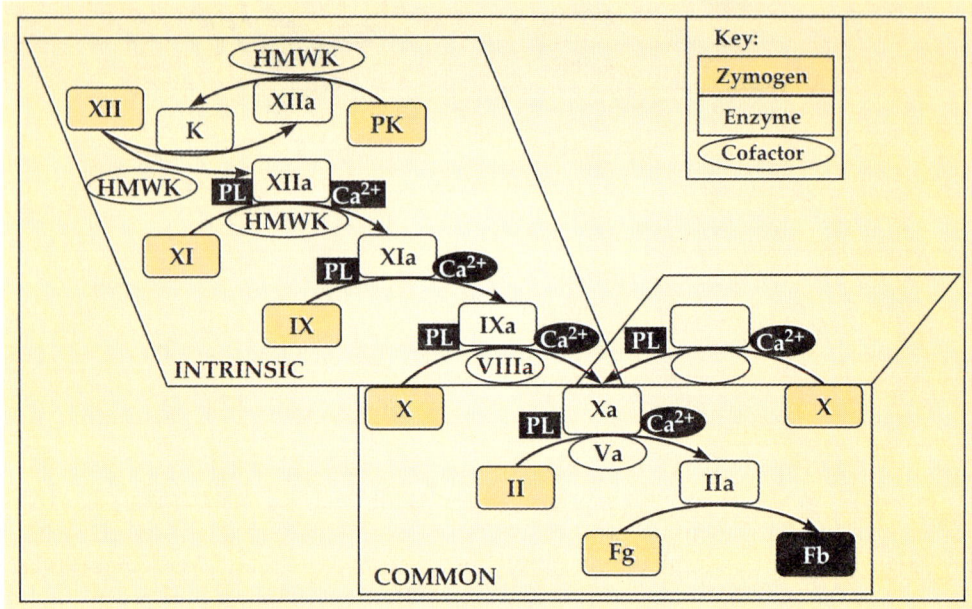

Fig. 14.6. The cascade or waterfall model of coagulation.

Utility of cascade model
- Prevention of coagulation in blood collection using calcium chelators.
- Deficiencies in the extrinsic or common pathways are identified using the prothrombin time
- Deficiencies in the intrinsic or common pathways are reflected with prolongation of the activated partial thromboplastin time (aPTT).
- Tests such as the Russell's viper venom time, the thrombin time, and assays for function of specific factors allowed for further isolation of the exact site of coagulation defects.

Deficiencies in the cascade model
- Does not fully explain the hemostatic process as it occurs *in vivo*.
- Suggests that the extrinsic and intrinsic pathways operate as independent and redundant pathways, while clinical manifestations of individual factor deficiencies clearly contradict this concept:
  - Deficiencies in the initial components of the intrinsic pathway (FXII, HMWK, or PK) cause marked prolongation of the aPTT, but they are not associated with a tendency for bleeding.
  - FXII is clearly not required for normal hemostasis because some mammalian species (such as whales and dolphins) do not have this protein.
  - Deficiency of the next downstream enzyme of intrinsic pathway FXI (hemophilia C) is associated with variable hemostatic deficits in humans, with some individuals experiencing bleeding.
  - Deficiency in either of the next downstream components of the intrinsic pathway (FVIII and FIX) results in the serious bleeding tendencies seen with hemophilia A and B,

despite the fact that these patients have an intact extrinsic pathway. The extrinsic pathway is not able to compensate for lack of FVIII or FIX in haemophiliacs.
– Similarly, deficiency of the primary enzyme of the extrinsic pathway (FVII) is associated with bleeding manifestation, despite the presence of an intact intrinsic pathway.

The Cell-based Model of Coagulation

Salient features

- Coagulation is regulated by the properties of cell surfaces.
- Specific cellular receptors (on platelets, etc.) act as binding sites for coagulation proteins.
- Different cells with different array of receptors can play different role in regulating hemostasis.
- The ability of cells to control the nature of their membrane surface constitutes a powerful method of regulating coagulation reactions.
- Role of microparticles.
- Some coagulation factors (like thrombin) also have roles besides hemostasis, such as in regulating inflammation, vessel wall function, and cell proliferation.
- Coagulation occurs not as a 'cascade', but in three overlapping phases or stages:
  1. *Initiation*
  2. *Amplification*
  3. *Propagation*

Role of cell surfaces

- In the inactive resting membrane state, neutral phospholipids (primarily phosphatidylcholine, sphingomyelin, and sugar-linked sphingolipids) are located on the external leaflet of the membrane, and phosphatyldserine (PS) and phosphatidylethanolamine (PE) are localized to the inner surface of the membrane. This membrane asymmetry is essential and tightly controlled by ATP dependent enzymes under normal conditions.
- When a cell is activated or injured (such as occurs when platelets are exposed to platelet activators, or when other cell types are stimulated to undergo apoptosis) the enzyme scramblase actively shuffles the phospholipids between the two surfaces in response to increased concentrations of calcium in the cytosol. This results in the appearance of PS and PE on the external membrane surface (they increase from almost none to 12% of membrane lipids).
- The expression of PS with PE on the external leaflet turns the cell membrane into a procoagulant surface. Presence of PS on the membrane markedly increases the speed of coagulation reactions (four thousand times). Less PS is required for maximum speed when PE is present.
- The speed of many enzymatic reactions of coagulation is significantly affected by the presence of an appropriate membrane surface. Localization to a membrane surface helps properly align the participating proteins speeding up the proteolysis reactions.
- TF is the only coagulation protein that is permanently attached to the membrane surface.
- Other coagulation proteins (e.g., FVII, FIX, FX, prothrombin, protein C, protein S, protein Z) contain carboxylated glutamic acid (Gla) residues that allow for binding of the protein to a membrane surface via interaction between calcium and negatively charged phospholipids (phosphatyldserine and phosphatidylethanolamine).

- Gla proteins preferentially bind to PS clusters on the membrane surface, and that PE aids in grouping PS into these clusters.
- Some cofactors (FV and FVIII) also have other regions that interact with phospholipids of membranes, allowing for formation of the fully functional enzymatic complex on the membrane surface.
- Because coagulation reactions occur very slowly on membranes that do not contain PS, resting cells are essentially incapable of supporting the coagulation cascade.

Role of microparticles

- Microparticles (MPs) are intact vesicles derived from cells. They vary in size from 2% to 20% of the size of a RBC and arise when activated or apopototic cells shed bits of membrane.
- Cytokines (such as tumor necrosis factor and interleukin-6), thrombin, shear stress, and hypoxia can stimulate MP formation.
- MPs contain cell surface proteins similar to those found on their parent cell (e.g., ultra large vWF monomers on endothelial cell-derived MPs, P-selectin on platelet-derived MPs, TF on monocyte-derived MPs) that can participate in coagulation reactions, especially when the MP expresses a procoagulant membrane.
- Normally MPs are primarily derived from endothelial cells, platelets, and monocytes, but in certain disease states, MPs may arise from granulocytes and erythrocytes.
- The quantity of circulating MPs is increased in certain illnesses such as diabetes mellitus, sepsis, and cardiovascular disease and contribute to pathologic coagulation in a variety of disorders.

Cell surface receptors decide the role of particular cells and help in localization of coagulation

- Specialized cellular features are critical to localizing, and controlling, the coagulation process. These include surface expression of protein receptors, lipid composition of the outer leaflet of the plasma membrane, cell surface expression of glycosaminoglycans and synthesis or storage of coagulation proteins.
- The activated factors that are surface bound are relatively protected from plasma protease inhibitors, while proteases in the solution phase are more rapidly inactivated. Thus, under usual conditions, activated factors tend to express their activity on or very near the surface on which they are activated.
- The plasma proteins are available to any cell that comes into contact with blood. The cells can "choose" which of the proteins they will utilize by binding them to selective sites on their surfaces.
- Both unactivated and activated platelets have several receptors or binding sites for thrombin: Glycoprotein (GP) Ib/IX, protease activated receptors (PAR) and others. PARs transduces a signal for activation to the platelet.
- GPIb/IX is the receptor for vWF. It also binds thrombin and plays a role in platelet activation by thrombin. GPIb/IX seems primarily to localize thrombin to the surface of the platelet, where it can activate other procoagulant factors and cofactors.
- GPIb/IX promotes adhesion of unactivated platelets at sites of vascular injury through vWF. Adhesion of platelets through GPIb/IX and vWF promotes at least partial platelet activation.

- vWF is the also the carrier protein for plasma factor VIII. Binding of vWF to GPIb/IX localizes FVIII to the platelet surface, where it is most efficiently activated by thrombin. By this mechanism the relatively unstable activated form of FVIII is produced directly on the surface where its activity is needed to support the coagulation reactions.
- Binding site exists for factor IX/IXa on platelets.
- Effector protease receptor-1 (EPR-1) may be the protein receptor on platelets for factor Xa and serves to coordinate assembly of the prothrombinase (FXa/Va) complex.
- Receptors for other coagulation factors are yet to be identified.
- Endothelial cells express a number of the same receptors as platelets in a regulated fashion, including GPIb, vWF, FV, thrombin receptor (PAR), and P-selectin (discussed below).
- As TF is the primary initiator of coagulation, the amount of TF exposure decides whether clotting occurs or not. TF expression is necessary for initiation of coagulation or thrombosis, but it is not sufficient. Additional factors determine whether an effective procoagulant signal is produced or not, e.g. many different types of cancer cells express TF, but their tendency to cause thrombosis does not necessarily correlate with TF activity.

Resting/normal endothelial cells regulate and prevent inappropriate coagulation by expression of many anticoagulant proteins and receptors on membrane surface

- Heparan sulfated proteoglycans (HSPGs): Produced by endothelial cells, these are expressed on luminal side in contact with flowing blood. Binds to antithrombin which on binding to HSPG becomes activated and inhibits any active thrombin near it. Soluble non-membrane bound heparin used as a drug acts similarly.
- Thrombomodulin (TM): Thrombin, once bound to TM, converts from a procoagulant to an anticoagulant protein because the thrombin-TM complex rapidly activates protein C (aPC). Protein C is localized to endothelial surfaces by an endothelial protein C receptor (EPCR-1), that facilitates its activation by thrombin/TM. aPC (with its cofactor protein S [ProS]) then irreversibly cleaves FVa and FVIIIa, preventing their further participation in generation of additional new thrombin molecules. aPC-ProS also inactivates an important inhibitor of fibrinolysis (plasminogen activator inhibitor 1, PAI-1) which ultimately increases lysis of any fibrin that is formed. Expression of TM is 100-fold higher in capillary endothelium as compared with endothelium in the major vessels. Thus, any thrombin circulating in large vessels will be quickly extracted when the blood passes through a capillary.
- Tissue factor pathway inhibitor (TFPI): It prevents additional thrombin generation by acting as an upstream inhibitor of FXa and FVIIa. It irreversibly binds to FXa, then forms a quaternary complex between TFPI, FXa, FVIIa, and TF, preventing further participation of these protein molecules in the generation of additional thrombin.
- Endothelial cells also express cell-surface ADPase activity (CD39): This enzyme metabolizes ADP released from activated platelets, resulting in blockade of the aggregation response when the platelets are in close proximity to healthy endothelium.
- Injury or inflammatory cytokines can induce endothelial cells to decrease expression of TM, and increase expression of TF and surface adhesion molecules. This is probably an adaptive defense mechanism that facilitates hemostasis at sites of injury. However, these mechanisms can contribute to thrombosis in a number of disease states, such as atherosclerosis, thrombophlebitis and vasculitis.

Phases/Stages of Coagulation in the Cell-based Model (Fig. 14.7)

Initiation

It takes place on TF-bearing cells, like fibroblast. If the procoagulant stimulus is sufficiently strong, enough factors Xa, IXa and thrombin are formed to successfully initiate the coagulation process.

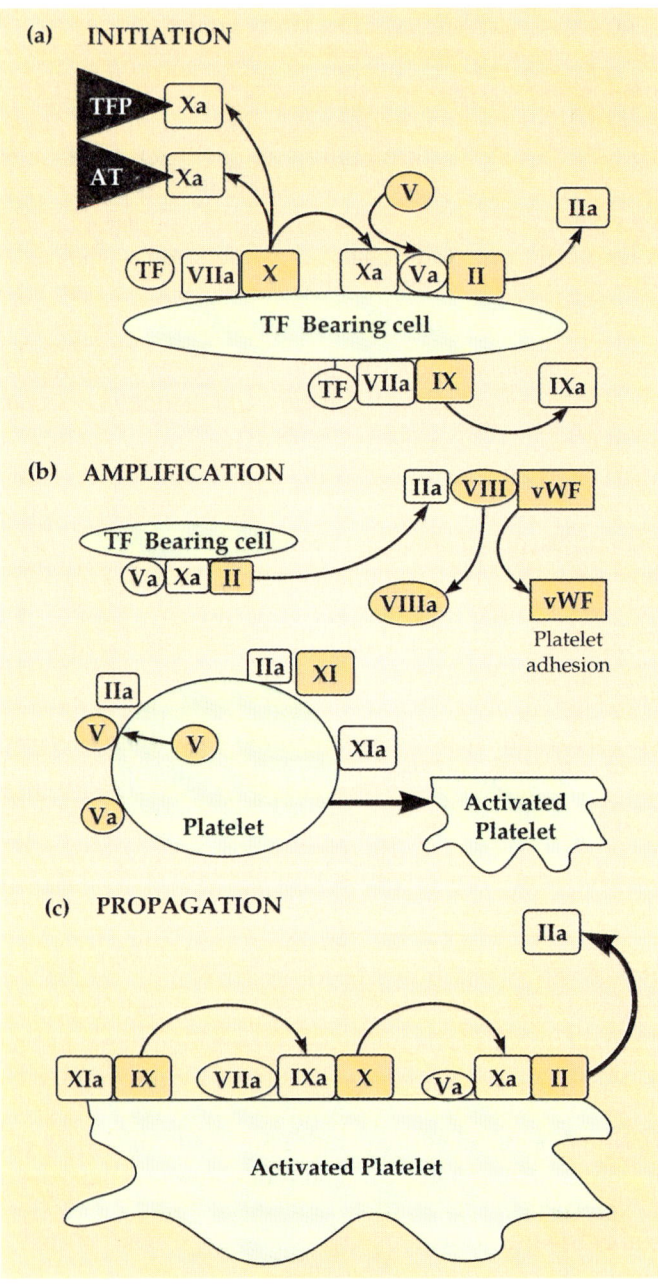

Fig. 14.7. Phases of coagulation – the cell-based model of coagulation.

- TF is the sole relevant initiator of coagulation *in vivo*.
- Cells expressing TF are localized outside the vasculature, which prevents initiation of coagulation under normal flow circumstances with an intact endothelium.
- Some circulating cells (e.g., monocytes or tumor cells) and MPs express TF on their membrane surface, but this TF under normal conditions is inactive due to additional bonds or because the membrane surface on which it resides is not a PS-containing procoagulant membrane.
- Once an injury occurs and the flowing blood is exposed to a TF-bearing cell, FVIIa rapidly binds to the exposed TF.
- FVIIa is the only coagulation protein that routinely circulates in the blood in its active enzyme form, with approximately 1% of total FVII circulating as FVIIa. All other coagulation proteins circulate solely as zymogens.
- The TF-FVIIa complex then activates additional FVII to FVIIa, allowing for even more TF-FVIIa complex activity, which then activates small amounts of FIX and FX.
- FV can be activated directly by FXa although very slowly.
- The FXa generated by TF-FVIIa binds to the few generated molecules of its cofactor FVa to form the prothrombinase complex, which subsequently cleaves prothrombin (FII) and generates a small amount of thrombin (FIIa).
- Any FXa that dissociates from the membrane surface of the TF-bearing cell is rapidly inactivated by either TFPI or AT.
- The FXa generated is effectively restricted to the surface of the TF-bearing cell on which it was generated.
- However, the FIXa generated can dissociate and move to the surface of nearby platelets or other cells. FIXa is not inhibited by TFPI, and much more slowly inhibited by AT than is FXa.
- TF is always expressed in the perivascular space. Any FVIIa that leaves the vasculature through minor breaks in the endothelial barrier will bind to TF and potentially initiate coagulation. The gaps in the endothelial barrier under normal conditions are very small. Most of the upstream coagulation proteins are relatively small (e.g., FVII: 50,000 Da) whereas some of the downstream proteins are much larger (e.g., FV: 330,000 Da; fibrinogen: 340,000 Da). This means that platelets and large proteins are sequestered from the extravascular space. Thus, progresses of coagulation beyond the generation of the small amount of thrombin occurring with the initiation phase can occur only when the injury allows platelets and larger proteins to leave the vascular space and adhere to the TF-bearing cells in the extravascular area.
- Bringing FVIIa/TF activity into close proximity to activated platelet surfaces is a key step in effective initiation of hemostatic coagulation (or thrombosis).

Amplification

It occurs as the "action" moves from the TF-bearing cell to the platelet surface. The procoagulant stimulus is amplified as platelets adhere, are activated and accumulate activated cofactors on their surfaces.
- The small amount of thrombin generated on the surface of a TF-bearing cell (the initiation phase) diffuses away from the TF-bearing cell and is available for activation of platelets that have leaked from the vasculature at the site of injury.

- Binding of thrombin to platelet surface receptors (PAR, protease-activated receptor) causes extreme changes in the surface of the platelet, resulting in shape change, shuffling of membrane phospholipids to create a procoagulant membrane surface, and release of granule contents that provide additional fuel for the fire.
- Platelet granules contain a large number of proteins and other substances that include raw materials for clotting reactions and agonists to induce further platelet activation. Calcium may induce clustering of PS (increasing the procoagulant nature of the membrane), and promotes binding of coagulation proteins to the activated membrane surface.
- During activation, platelets release FV from alpha granules onto their surfaces in a partially activated form. Factor Va is then fully activated by thrombin or FXa
- In addition to activating platelets, the thrombin generated in the initiation phase cleaves FXI to FXIa and activates FV to FVa on the platelet surface. Thrombin also cleaves von Willebrand factor off FVIII (they circulate bound together), releasing it to mediate platelet adhesion and aggregation. The released FVIII is subsequently activated by thrombin to FVIIIa3.
- Some of the thrombin bound to non-PAR receptors, such as GPIb/IX, remains active and can activate other coagulation factors on the platelet surface. von Willebrand factor (vWF)/ FVIII binds to platelets and is efficiently cleaved by thrombin to activate FVIII and release it from vWF. The FVIIIa remains bound to the platelet surface. Now that the platelets have been activated and have activated cofactors V and VIII bound to their surfaces, assembly of the procoagulant complexes and large-scale thrombin generation begins.

Thus, thrombin acts on the platelet surface to "set the stage" for procoagulant complex assembly.

Propagation

- Once a few platelets are activated in the amplification phase, the release of the granule contents results in recruitment of additional platelets to the site of injury. The propagation phase occurs on the surface of these platelets.
- Expression of ligands on their surface results in cell–cell interactions that lead to aggregation of platelets. FIXa that was generated by TF-FVIIa in the initiation phase can bind to FVIIIa (generated in the amplification phase) on the platelet surface. Additional FIXa is generated due to cleavage of FIX by FXIa that was generated during amplification on the platelet surface.
- Once the intrinsic tenase complex forms (FIXa– FVIIIa) on the activated platelet surface, it rapidly begins to generate FXa on the platelet.
- FXa was also generated during the initiation phase on the TF-bearing cell surface. As this FXa is rapidly inhibited if it moves away from the TF-bearing cell surface, it cannot easily reach the platelet surface. The majority of FXa must therefore be generated directly on the platelet surface through cleavage by the intrinsic tenase complex.
- The FXa generated on platelets then rapidly binds to FVa (generated by thrombin in the amplification phase) and cleaves prothrombin to thrombin.
- This prothrombinase activity results in a burst of thrombin generation leading to cleavage of fibrinopeptide A from fibrinogen.
- When enough thrombin is generated with enough speed to result in a critical mass of fibrin, these soluble fibrin molecules will spontaneously polymerize into fibrin strands, resulting in an insoluble fibrin matrix.

Additional steps
- Generation of enough thrombin to result in a clot is not, however, the end of coagulation.
- Approximately 95% of the thrombin generation occurs after the time of fibrin gel formation.
- Routine plasma-based clotting assays such as the prothrombin time and aPTT detect fibrin gel formation. As 95% of thrombin is generated after the time of fibrin gel formation, these assays are unable to detect abnormalities associated with hemostasis that are due to deficiencies in hemostatic function that occur following initial fibrin polymerization.
- Thrombin generation subsequent to fibrin polymerization plays many important roles in the structure of the clot that is formed.
- In addition to the cleavage site for fibrinopeptide A, fibrinogen contains a site where thrombin cleaves off fibrinopepetide B. While removal of fibrinopeptide B is not strictly required for fibrin polymerization, its removal results in changes in the structure of the fibrin that is formed.
- Thrombin additionally activates FXIII to FXIIIa. This enzyme modifies the polymerized fibrin to form cross-links between fibrin strands. Cross-link formation drastically impacts the strength and elasticity of the fibrin clot that is formed. The importance of crosslinking in clot structure is demonstrated by the bleeding phenotype observed in with FXIII deficiency. FXIII deficiency is associated with persistent bleeding from the umbilical stump a few days after it falls off (seen in about 80% of cases of factor XIII deficiency) and bleeding in soft tissues which takes the form of bruises (accumulation of blood under the skin).
- Some of the thrombin generated will bind to TM on the endothelial cell surface. TM bound thrombin can activate thrombin activatable fibrinolysis inhibitor. This acts to modify the fibrin molecules by removing their terminal lysine residues. As lysine residues are the necessary binding site for several fibrinolytic proteins, fibrin that has been acted on by activated thrombin activatable fibrinolysis inhibitor becomes markedly more resistant to fibrinolysis.
- TM bound thrombin has additional role in termination of coagulation due to its activation of protein C. aPC forms a complex with its cofactor ProS, which cleaves FVa and FVIIIa, preventing further cofactor activity of either of these proteins. Activity of aPC-ProS consequently shuts down generation of new thrombin molecules.

The limitation of spread of coagulation beyond site of injury
- Inevitably, some proteases diffuse away from the vicinity of the activated platelets and are carried downstream. The lack of a procoagulant membrane on resting endothelial cells that are located away from the site of injury prevents efficient generation of thrombin by any FXa that diffuses away from the cell surface and is carried through the vasculature.
- FXa and thrombin are also effectively inhibited by the endothelial cell surface associated anticoagulant systems including AT and TFPI.
- Thrombin generation is limited because aPC/ProS is a much better inactivator of FVa on the endothelial cell surface than on the platelet surface. This means that aPC/ProS is efficient at limiting thrombin generation on healthy resting endothelial cells, but not efficient at inhibiting generation of thrombin on activated platelets.

Thrombin plays a central role in all the phases of coagulation (Fig 14.8).

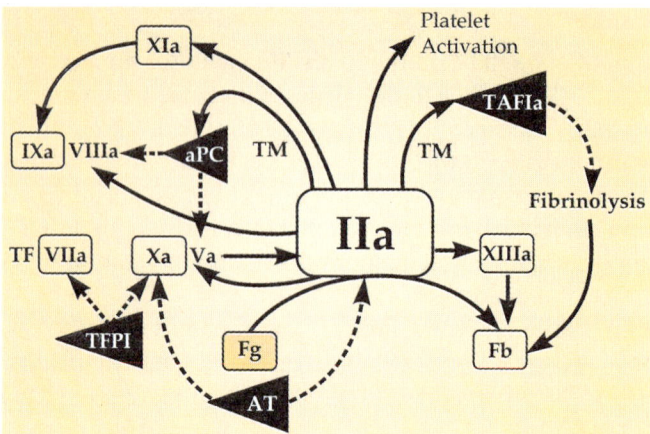

Fig. 14.8. The central role of thrombin. Thrombin is generated in small quantities during the initiation phase which occurs on the TF-bearing cell, then in larger quantities on the platelet surface in the propagation phase. Thrombin becomes anticoagulant via thrombomodulin-mediated activation of the protein C system. Thrombin also impacts clot structure through activation of cross-linker FXIII, and fibrinolysis inhibitor thrombin activatable fibrinolysis inhibitor.

Advantages of the cell-based model
- This model adequately explains the bleeding defects observed with FXI, FIX, and FVIII deficiencies, because these proteins are required for generation of FXa (and subsequently thrombin) on platelet membranes.
- For coagulation to occur effectively, thrombin must be generated directly on the activated platelet surface, not just on the surface of the TF-bearing cell.
- This model suggests that the extrinsic and intrinsic systems are in fact parallel generators of FXa that occur on different cell surfaces, rather than redundant pathways.

Haemophilia
- The cascade model of coagulation does not explain why the "extrinsic" pathway cannot produce enough FXa to (at least partially) compensate for a lack of factor VIII or IX in haemophiliacs.
- The problem in hemophilia is not that enough FXa isn't made, but that it is made on the wrong cell surface.
- Factor Xa made on a TF-bearing cell cannot reach the platelet surface without being inhibited by either ATIII or TFPI. These two inhibitors, at their normal plasma levels, inhibit FXa so efficiently that it has a half life of a minute or less in the solution phase.
- By contrast, factor IXa is inhibited much less rapidly by ATIII and not at all by TFPI. Therefore, FIXa can move from the TF-bearing cell to the activated platelet surface to form the platelet tenase complex.
- In order for FXa to be incorporated efficiently into prothrombinase complexes, it must be formed on the platelet surface (i.e. by FIXa/VIIIa) in close proximity to FVa.
- In hemophilia there is a failure specifically of platelet-surface FX activation leading to a failure of platelet-surface thrombin generation.

FVIIA provides hemostasis in hemophilia

- Hemophilia has a failure of platelet surface FXa generation on platelet surface.
- High-dose FVIIa is very efficient in promoting hemostasis in hemophiliacs. The doses of FVIIa, used clinically, produce plasma levels that are several thousand times greater than the K_d for binding of FVIIa to TF. Thus it is unlikely that FVIIa works via TF. Also FVIIa has very little proteolytic activity in the absence of its cofactor.
- FVIIa can bind to activated platelets (but not unactivated platelets). Then FVIIa can activate FX. The amount of FXa generated by this mechanism is sufficient to support near normal levels of thrombin generation. Platelet surface thrombin generation fails in hemophilia, high levels of FVIIa restores the platelet surface thrombin generation.
- This also explains why high dose FVIIa is effective in establishing hemostasis in patients with thrombocytopenia and platelet function defects.

Immunology

Chapter 15

Q. 1. Describe the antiviral defence of innate immune system.

Ans. Antiviral defence is a part of the innate immune system and consists of a cytokine-mediated reaction in which cells acquire resistance to viral infection and killing of virus-infected cells by NK cells. The major way by which the innate immune system deals with viral infections is to induce the expression of type I interferons, whose most important action is to inhibit viral replication.

Viruses contain single- and double-stranded DNA unique to them. These are their pathogen-associated molecular patterns recognised by the Cell-Associated Pattern Recognition Receptors present in cells of the innate immune system. As these are also essential to viral action, they cannot evade the innate immune response by altering them (Fig. 15.1).

The Toll-like receptors (TLRs), NOD-like receptors (NLRs) and Rig-like receptors (RLRs) present on cell membrane and in cytoplasm of dendritic cells, phagocytes, B cells, endothelial cells, epithelial cells and many other cells recognise the unique viral nucleic acids (Fig. 15.1). On binding to them they generate signals that stimulate IFN-α and IFN-β (type 1 interferons) gene expression in many different cell types (Fig. 15.2). The type I interferons are secreted from these cells and act on other cells to prevent spread of viral infection. In adaptive immunity, antigen-activated T cells stimulate mononuclear phagocytes to synthesize type I interferons.

Type I interferons are a large family of structurally related cytokines that mediate the early innate immune response to viral infections. The term interferon derives from the ability of these cytokines to interfere with viral infection. There are many type I interferons, all of which have considerable structural homology and are encoded by genes in a single cluster on chromosome 9. The most important type I interferons in viral defence are IFN-α (which actually includes 13 different closely related proteins) and IFN-β, which is a single protein.

Plasmacytoid dendritic cells are the major sources of IFN-α but it may also be produced by mononuclear phagocytes. IFN-β is produced by many cells. The most potent stimuli for type I interferon synthesis are viral nucleic acids which are recognized by toll-like receptors

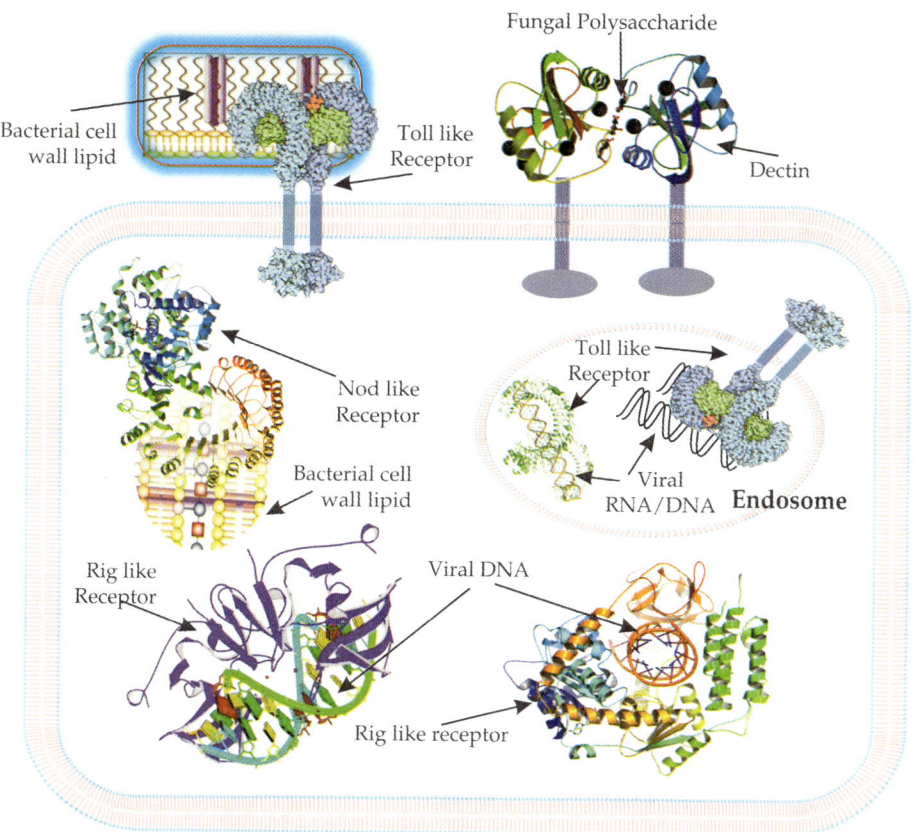

Fig. 15.1. The toll-like receptors: Cell surface TLRs recognize pathogen-associated molecular patterns like fungal polysaccharides, bacterial cell wall lipids while cytosolic and endosomal TLRs recognize and bind to viral RNA and DNA.

The antiviral action of type I interferon is primarily a paracrine action in that a virally infected cell secretes interferon to act on and protect neighbouring cells that are not yet infected. Interferon secreted by an infected cell may also act in an autocrine fashion to inhibit viral replication in that cell.

Actions of type I interferons

- The receptor for type I interferons, which binds both IFN-α and IFN-β, is a heterodimer of two structurally related polypeptides, IFNAR1 and IFNAR2, expressed on all nucleated cells. This receptor signals to activate STAT1, STAT2, and IRF9 transcription factors, which induce expression of several different genes that have many antiviral effects.
- The type I interferon-induced genes include (Fig. 15.3):
  - double-stranded RNA-activated serine/threonine protein kinase (PKR), which blocks viral transcriptional and translational events;
  - 2′,5′-oligoadenylate synthetase and RNase L18, 19, which promote viral RNA degradation.
  - Large dynamin like GTPases (Mx GTPases) which block assembly of virus particles.

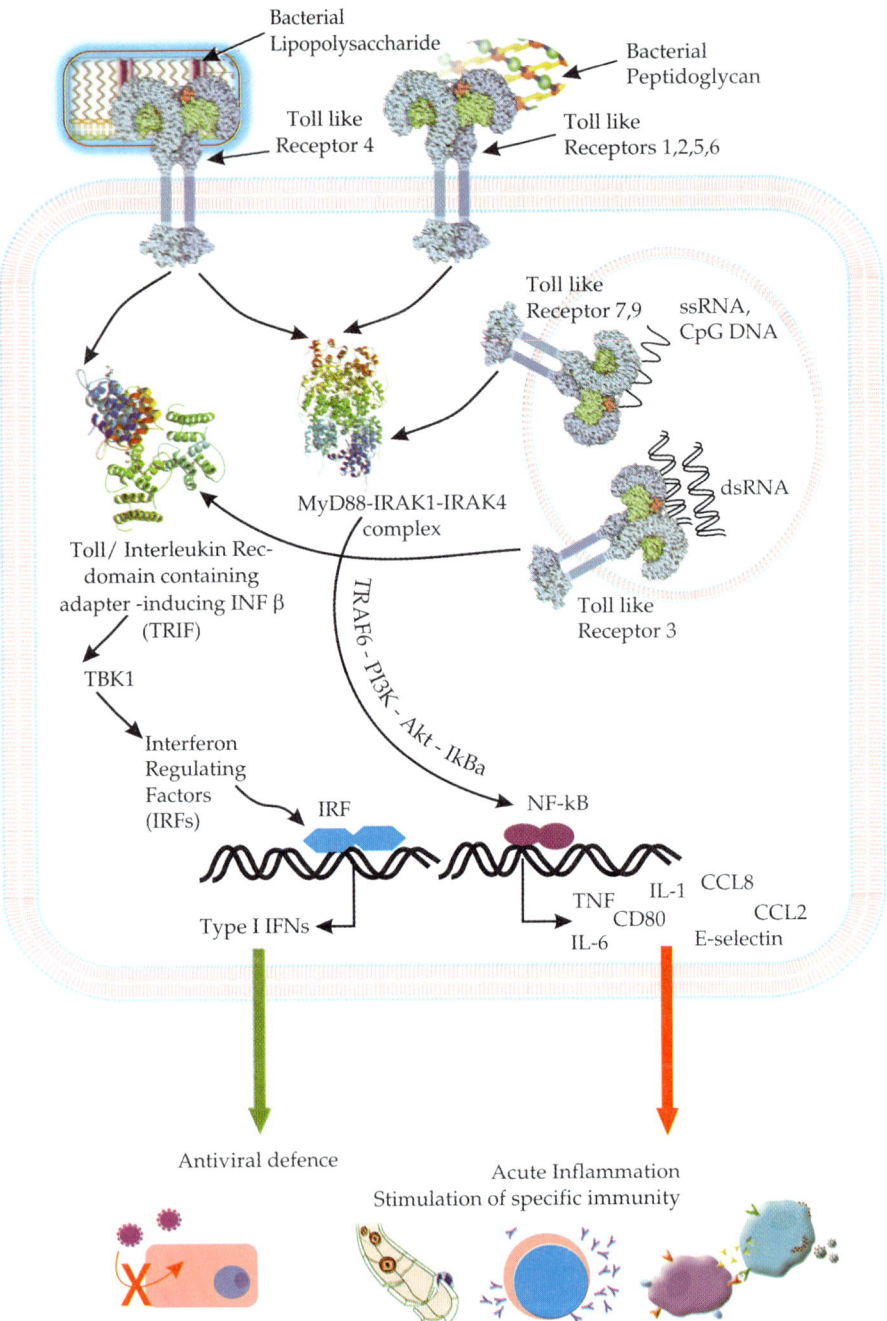

Fig. 15.2. The structure and function of toll-like receptors (TLR) in innate and adaptive immunity. C binding to various PAMP i.e. pathogen-associated molecular patterns they activate expression o type I interferons (antiviral defence) and NF-κB activity which causes synthesis of cytokine chemokines, cell adhesion molecules, co-stimulatory molecules to promote acute inflammation ar stimulate adaptive immunity.

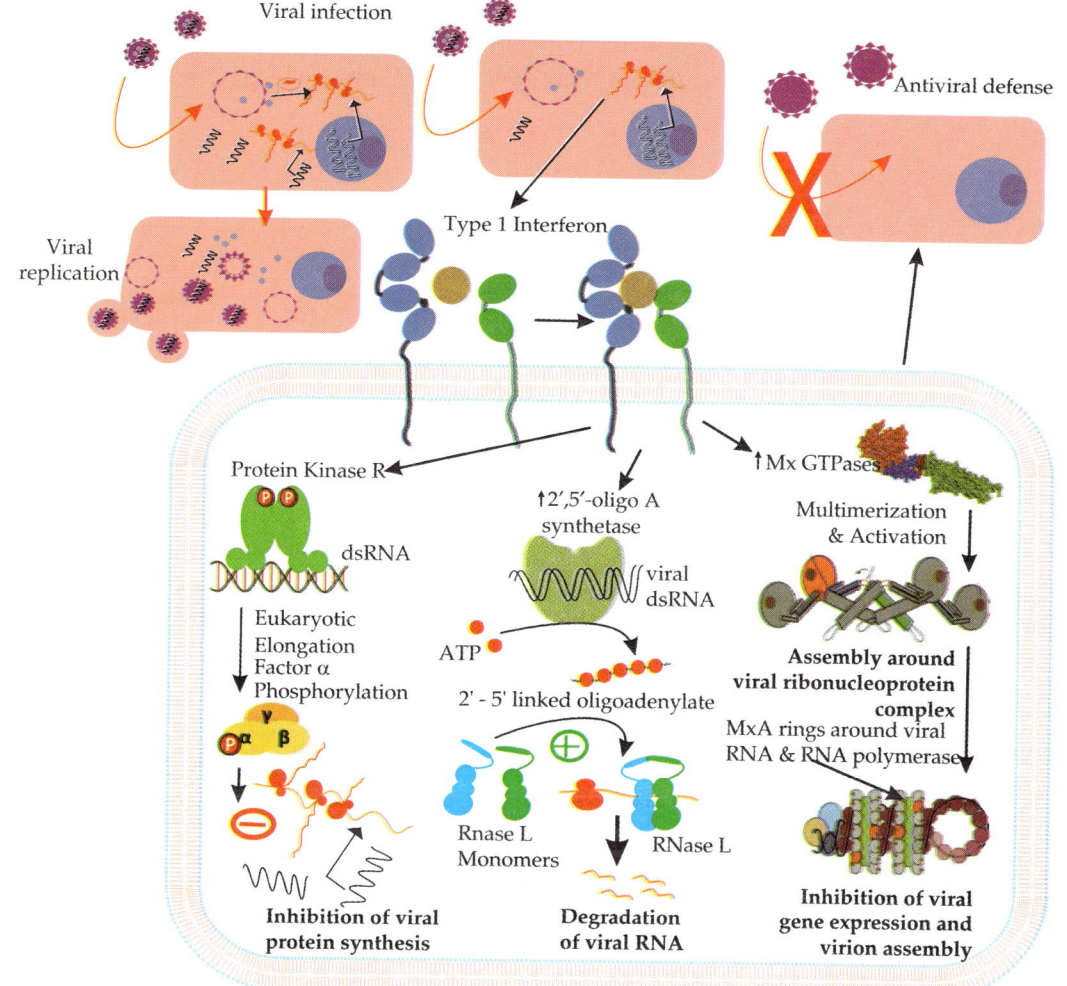

Fig. 15.3. Actions of type 1 interferons.

- Type I interferons cause sequestration of lymphocytes in lymph nodes, thus maximizing the opportunity for encounter with microbial antigens. The mechanism for this effect of type I interferons is the induction of a molecule on the lymphocytes, called CD69, that forms a complex with and reduces surface expression of the sphingosine-1-phosphate (S1P) receptor S1PR1. Binding of sphingosine-1-PO_4 to S1PR1 stimulates movement of lymphocytes out of lymph nodes.

- Type I interferons increase the cytotoxicity of NK cells and CD8+ CTLs and promote the differentiation of naive T cells to the T_H1 subset of helper T cells. These effects of type I interferons enhance both innate and adaptive immunity against intracellular infections, including viruses and some bacteria.

- Type I interferons upregulate expression of class I MHC molecules and thereby increase the probability that virally infected cells will be recognized and killed by CD8+ CTLs of adaptive immune system. Virus-specific CD8+ CTLs recognize peptides derived from viral proteins bound to class I MHC molecules on the surface of infected cells. The end result is the killing of cells that support viral replication, which is needed to eradicate viral infections.

Other antiviral defences in innate immunity

- Protection against viruses is also due to the activation of intrinsic apoptotic death pathways in infected cells and enhanced sensitivity to extrinsic inducers of apoptosis leading to apoptosis of virally infected cells.
- Virally infected cells can sense abnormal DNA replication and abnormal glycoprotein synthesis, leading to initiation of p53-dependent or endoplasmic reticulum-dependent apoptotic pathways, respectively. Virally infected cells are sensitized to TNF-induced apoptosis. Abundant TNF is made by plasmacytoid dendritic cells and macrophages in response to viral infections, in addition to type I interferons.
- NK cell activity: Virally infected cells of body are stressed and have decreased MHC expression (MHC I inhibits NK cell activity) and increased expression of activating ligands for NK cells. When NK cells are activated, exocytosis releases granule proteins adjacent to the target cells. One NK cell granule protein, called perforin, facilitates the entry of other granule proteins, called granzymes, into the cytoplasm of target cells. The granzyme are enzymes that initiate the sequence of apoptosis. This action removes the reservoirs of viral infection.

Knockout mice lacking the receptor for type I interferons are susceptible to viral infections. IFN-α is in clinical use as an antiviral agent in certain forms of viral hepatitis. IFN-α is also used for the treatment of some tumors, perhaps because it boosts CTL activity or interfere with cell growth. IFN-β is used as a therapy for multiple sclerosis.

Q. 2. Explain the biochemical basis of tolerance. Give some therapeutic applications of the phenomena of tolerance.

Ans. Immunologic tolerance is defined as unresponsiveness to an antigen that is induced by previous exposure to that antigen. When specific lymphocytes encounter antigens, the lymphocytes may be activated, leading to immune responses, or the cells may be inactivate or eliminated, leading to tolerance. Tolerance to self-antigens, also called self-tolerance, is fundamental property of the normal immune system, and failure of self-tolerance results in immune reactions against self (autologous) antigens.

Whether lymphocytes that recognize antigens become activated or tolerant is determine by the properties of the antigens, the state of maturation of the antigen-specific lymphocytes and the types of co-stimuli received when these lymphocytes encounter the antigens (Table 15.1).

All individuals inherit the same antigen receptor gene segments for T and B cell receptor Recombination and hypermutation of these segments during maturation of B and T cell from stem cells produce the large diversity or the capability to recognise 10^7 distinct antigen. The specificities of the receptors encoded by the recombined genes are random, and are not affected by what is foreign or self. Thus, during this process of generating a large and diverse antigen-binding capacity, some developing T and B cells in every individual may express

Table 15.1. Factors that determine the immunogenicity and tolerogenicity of protein antigens

Factor	Features that favour stimulation of immune responses	Features that favour tolerance
Persistence	Short-lived (eliminated by immune response)	Prolonged
Portal of entry; location	Subcutaneous, intradermal; absence from generative organs	Intravenous, mucosal; presence in generative organs
Presence of adjuvants	Antigens with adjuvants: stimulate helper T cells	Antigens without adjuvants: non-immunogenic or tolerogenic
Properties of antigen-presenting cells	High levels of costimulators	Low levels of costimulators and cytokines

receptors capable of recognizing normal molecules in that individual (i.e., self-antigens). Therefore, there is a risk for lymphocytes to react against that individual's cells and tissues, causing disease. Normal individuals are tolerant of their own (self) antigens because these lymphocytes that recognize self-antigens are killed or inactivated or the specificity of these lymphocytes is changed. This is achieved by two mechanisms:
- Central tolerance
- Peripheral tolerance

Central tolerance (Fig. 15.4)

- Central tolerance develops during the maturation of lymphocytes in the central lymphoid organs – thymus and bone marrow, where all developing lymphocytes (immature lymphocytes) pass through a stage at which strong binding with any antigen may lead to cell death or replacement of the reactive antigen receptor with a new one. At this stage they are exposed to most possible self-antigens and thus lymphocytes capable of reacting with self-antigens are deleted or modified.
- T cell tolerance:
  – In T lymphocytes, central tolerance (negative selection) occurs when immature T-cells with high-affinity receptors for self-antigens recognize self antigens in the thymus. Some of them die and others develop into FoxP3+ regulatory T lymphocytes, which function to control responses to self- antigens in peripheral tissues.
  – Self-proteins are processed and presented in association with MHC molecules on thymic antigen-presenting cells (dendritic cells). The antigens that are present in the thymus include many circulating and cell-associated proteins that are widely distributed in tissues. The thymus also has an unusual mechanism for expressing protein antigens that are present only in certain peripheral tissues.
  – Some of the peripheral tissue antigens are expressed in thymic medullary epithelial cells under the control of the auto-immune regulator (AIRE) protein. Mutations in the AIRE gene are the cause of a multiorgan autoimmune disease called the autoimmune polyendocrine syndrome (APS).
- B cell tolerance:
  – In B lymphocytes, central tolerance is induced when immature B cells recognize multivalent self-antigens in the bone marrow.

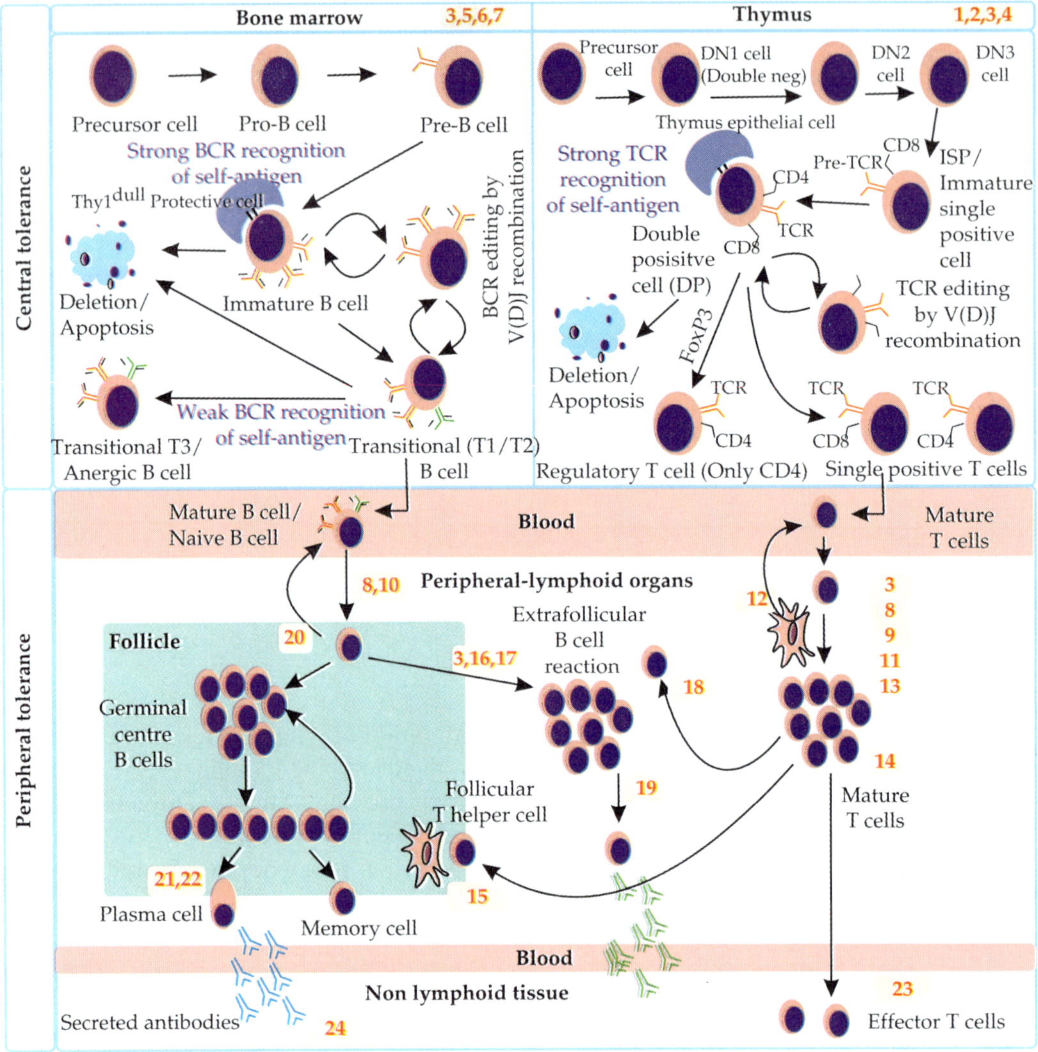

Tolerance mechanisms in central lymphoid organs:
(1) TCR editing by V(D)J recombination
(2) Thymic negative selection
(3) B and T cell anergy and inhibitory signaling
(4) FoxP3+ T regulatory cell differentiation
(5) Immature B cell maturation arrest
(6) BCR editing by V(D)J recombination
(7) Immature B cell deletion

Tolerance mechanisms in target tissues:
(23) Control of effector T cell functions in tissues (inhibition by PD-1 ligands, dependence on MHC upregulation by interferons, and inhibition by Treg cells and TGF-β)
(24) Control of antibody extravasation and inflammation in tissues

Tolerance mechanisms in peripheral lymphoid organs:
(3) B and T cell anergy and inhibitory signaling
(8) TCR or BCR induction of BIM

(9) T cell competition for IL-2, IL-7, IL-15, and peptide/MHC
(10) B cell competition for the survival cytokine BAFF
(11) T cell growth dependence on CD28 ligands and other costimulatory molecules
(12) Elimination of antigen-bearing dendritic cells by activated T cells producing perforin or FasL
(13) Suppression of T and B cells by Treg cells and TGF-β
(14) T cell death by FasL
(15) Regulation of T follicular helper cell differentiation and function
(16) B cell growth dependence on extrafollicular T cell help (CD40L, IL-2, IL-4, etc.)
(17) B cell growth dependence on TLR ligands
(18) B cell death by FasL from T cells
(19) BCR inhibition of plasma cell differentiation
(20) B cell follicular exclusion
(21) BCR-induced death of germinal centre B cells
(22) Germinal centre B cell growth/survival dependence on follicular helper T cells (CD40L, IL-21).

Fig. 15.4. Central and peripheral tolerance.

- *Receptor editing:* Encounter with self-antigens leads to reactivation of RAG1 and RAG2 genes and initiation of new round of VJ recombination in immunoglobulin genes. The result is the acquisition of a new specificity, called receptor editing.
- *Deletion:* If editing fails, the immature B cells may be deleted (apoptosis).
- *Anergy:* If developing B cells recognize self-antigens weakly (e.g., if the antigen is soluble and does not cross-link many antigen receptors or if the B cell receptors recognize the antigen with low affinity), the cells become functionally unresponsive (anergic) and exit the bone marrow in this unresponsive state. Anergy is due to downregulation of antigen receptor expression as well as a block in antigen receptor signalling.

Peripheral tolerance (Fig. 15.4)

- Peripheral tolerance occurs when, as a consequence of recognizing self-antigens, mature lymphocytes become incapable of responding to that antigen, or are induced to die by apoptosis, or mature T cells are actively suppressed by regulatory T cells.
- Peripheral tolerance is most important for maintaining unresponsiveness to self-antigens that are expressed in peripheral tissues and not in the generative lymphoid organs and for tolerance to self-antigens that are expressed only in adult life, after mature lymphocytes have been generated.
- Peripheral mechanisms may also serve as a back-up for the central mechanisms, which may not eliminate all self-reactive lymphocytes.
- Peripheral T cell tolerance (Fig. 15.5):
  - *Anergy/Functional unresponsiveness:* Exposure of mature CD4+ T cells to an antigen in the absence of costimulation (interaction of B7 on antigen presenting cell or APC with CD28 on T cell) or innate immunity may make the cells incapable of responding to that antigen. Anergic cells show a block in TCR-induced signal transduction. Self-antigen recognition may activate cellular ubiquitin ligases, which ubiquitinate TCR-associated proteins and target them for proteolytic degradation in proteasomes or lysosomes. When T cells recognize self-antigens, they may engage inhibitory co-receptors of the CD28 family (CTLA-4 and PD-1) with B7 on APC, whose function is to terminate T cell responses.
  - *Suppression of self-reactive lymphocytes by regulatory T cells:* A transcription factor called FoxP3 is critical for the development and function of the majority of regulatory T cells. A rare autoimmune disease in humans called IPEX (immune dysregulation, polyendocrinopathy, enteropathy, X-linked syndrome) is also associated with deficiency of regulatory T cells (caused by mutations in the FoxP3 gene).

    Regulatory T cells produce IL-10 and TGF-β both of which inhibit immune responses. Regulatory T cells inhibit the ability of APCs to stimulate T cells. CTLA-4 on regulatory cells binds to B7 molecules on APCs like dendritic cells and blocks them from interacting with T cells.
  - *Clonal deletion:* T cells that recognise self-antigens may receive signals that promote their death by apoptosis.
  - *Activation-induced cell death:* T lymphocytes that recognize self-antigens without inflammation or that are repeatedly stimulated by antigens die by apoptosis. T cells that recognize self-antigens in the absence of costimulation may activate Bim, resulting in

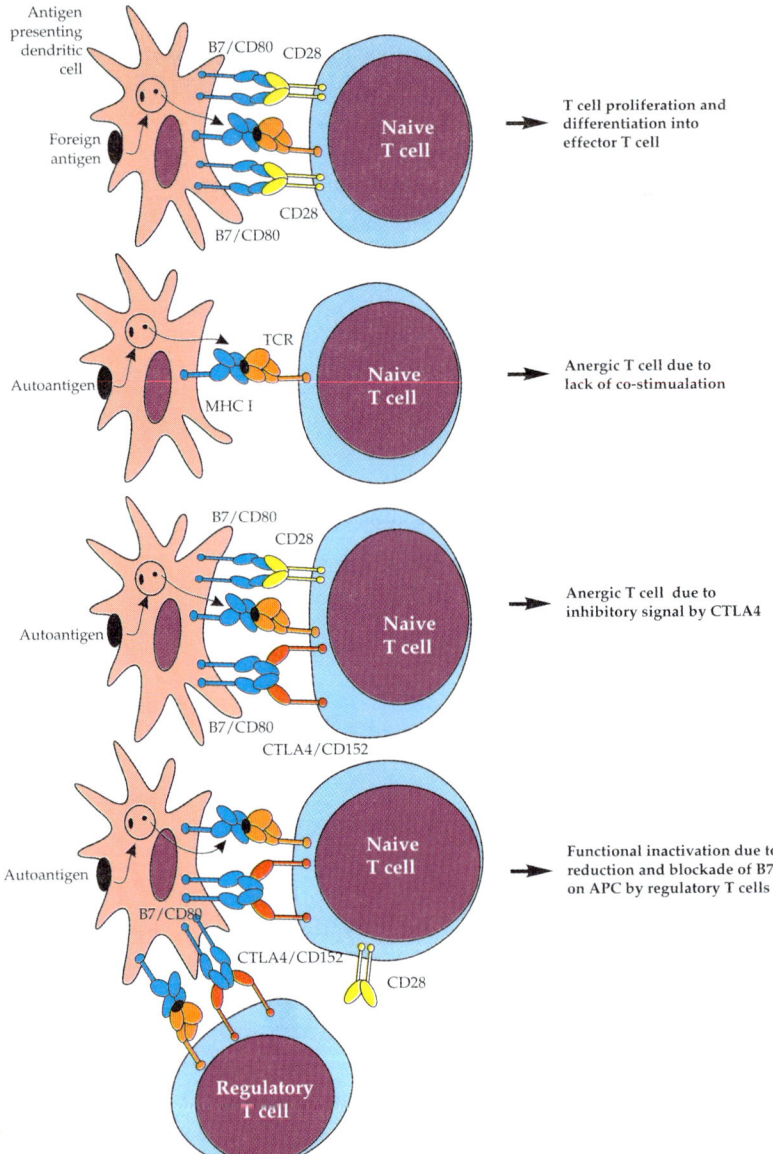

Fig. 15.5. T cell anergy due to lack of co-stimulatory signal or interaction of B7 with CTLA-4 instead of CD28.

apoptosis by the mitochondrial pathway. Repeated stimulation of T cells results in the coexpression of death receptors and their ligands, and engagement of the death receptors triggers apoptotic death.
- Peripheral B cell tolerance: Mature B cells that recognize self-antigens in the periphery in the absence of T cell help may be rendered anergic and ultimately die by apoptosis or become functionally unresponsive.
  - *Anergy and deletion:* Some self-reactive B cells that are repeatedly stimulated by self-antigens become unresponsive to further activation. These cells require high levels of

the growth factor BAFF/BLys for survival and cannot compete efficiently with less BAFF-dependent normal naive B cells for survival in lymphoid follicles. As a result, these B cells that have encountered self-antigens have a shortened life span and are eliminated more rapidly than cells that have not recognized self-antigens. B cells that bind with high avidity to self-antigens in the periphery may also undergo apoptotic death by the mitochondrial pathway.
- *Signalling by inhibitory receptors:* B cells that recognize self-antigens with low affinity may be prevented from responding by the engagement of various inhibitory receptors.
- **Ignorance:** Some self-antigens may be ignored by the immune system. Some antigens may be anatomically sequestered from the immune system and thus cannot engage antigen receptors.

Tolerance induced by foreign protein antigens and its clinical applications

Foreign antigens may be administered in ways that preferentially induce tolerance rather than immune responses.

- **Oral tolerance:** The oral administration of a protein antigen often leads to suppression of systemic humoral and cell-mediated immune responses to immunization with the same antigen.
- **Clonal exhaustion:** Some systemic infections (e.g., with viruses) may initiate an immune response, but the response is impaired before the virus is cleared, resulting in a state of persistent infection. In this situation, virus-specific T cell clones are present but do not respond normally and are unable to eradicate the infection. The antigen-specific lymphocyte clones make an initial response but then become anergic, or "exhausted". Clonal exhaustion is due to upregulation of inhibitory receptors such as PD-1 on virus-specific CD8+ T cells seen in patients infected with the human immunodeficiency virus (HIV).

Applications

- **Effective immunization:** Foreign antigens in the absence of costimulatory signals may inhibit immune responses by inducing tolerance in specific lymphocytes. Effective immunization methods are designed to enhance the immunogenicity of antigens by administering them in ways that promote lymphocyte activation and prevent tolerance induction.
- **Evasion of immune system by microbes and tumors:** Some microbes and tumors may also evade immune attack by inducing unresponsiveness in specific lymphocytes.
- **Treating autoimmune diseases and preventing graft rejection:** The induction of immunologic tolerance can be exploited as a therapeutic approach for preventing harmful immune responses to treat autoimmune and allergic diseases and to prevent the rejection of organ transplants.
- **Prevention of immune reactions to the products of newly expressed genes:** Tolerance induction may also be useful for preventing immune reactions to the products of newly expressed genes in gene therapy protocols, for preventing reactions to injected proteins in patients with deficiencies of these proteins (e.g., haemophiliacs treated with factor VIII), and for promoting acceptance of stem cell transplants.

Q. 3. Explain biochemical basis of autoimmunity, give examples of some autoimmune diseases.

Ans. Autoimmunity is inappropriate immune response to self-antigens. A disease is called auto-immune disease when:
- there is presence of autoimmune reaction;
- autoimmune reaction is not secondary to tissue damage; and
- there is absence of another cause of the disease.

Autoimmunity results from a failure of the mechanisms of self-tolerance in T or B cells. Some of the general mechanisms that are associated with autoimmune reactions are the following:

- Failure of self-tolerance:
  - Defects in deletion (negative selection) of T or B cells or receptor editing in B cells during the maturation of these cells in the generative lymphoid organs.
  - Defective numbers and functions of regulatory T lymphocytes.
  - Defective apoptosis of mature self-reactive lymphocytes.
  - Inadequate function of inhibitory receptors.
- Activation of antigen presenting cells, which overcomes regulatory mechanisms and results in excessive T cell activation.
- Molecular mimicry.
- Release of sequestered antigens.

The major factors that contribute to the development of autoimmunity are (Fig. 15.6):

- Genetic susceptibility
- Environmental triggers – infections and local tissue injury.

Genetic basis of autoimmunity

- Most autoimmune diseases are complex polygenic traits, in which affected individuals inherit multiple genetic polymorphisms that contribute to disease susceptibility and these genes act with environmental factors to cause the diseases.
- The strongest associations are with MHC genes. Particular variants of MHC may be leading to failure of self-tolerance as all antigens are presented to T and B cells on MHC complex by APCs (Table 15.2).
- Polymorphism in non-MHC gene mutations can also increase risk of autoimmune diseases. These are mainly involved in costimulation, cytokine regulation, tolerance mechanisms, etc. (Table 15.3).
- Some single gene mutations lead to autoimmune diseases (Table 15.4).

Environmental triggers

- Role of infections in autoimmunity
  - Polyclonal activation of B cells: Generalized activation of B cells due to certain infections leads to production of antibodies against self-antigens causing hemolytic anemia, etc. For example:
    - Polyclonal activators like Epstein Barr virus (EBV), cytomegalovirus (CMV), and Gram –ve bacteria stimulate B cells reactive to self-antigen.

Table 15.2. Association of autoimmune diseases with MHC/HLA alleles

Disease	HLA allele	Relative risk
Rheumatoid arthritis (anti-CCP Ab positive)	DRB1, 1 SE allele DRB1, 2 SE alleles	4 12
Type 1 diabetes	DRB*0301-DQA1*0501-DQB1*0201 haplotype DRB1*0401-DQA1*0301-DQB1*0302 haplotype DRB1*0301/0401 heterozygotes	4 8 35
Multiple sclerosis	DRB1*1501	3
Systemic lupus erythematosus	DRB1*0301 DRB1*1501	2 1.3
Ankylosing spondylitis	B*27 (mainly B*2705 and *2702)	100–200
Celiac disease	DQA1*0501-DB1*0201 haplotype	7

Table 15.3. Polymorphisms in non-MHC genes associated with autoimmune diseases

Gene	Function	Diseases
Genes involved in immune regulation		
PTPN22	Protein tyrosine phosphatase; role in T and B cell receptors signalling	Rheumatoid arthritis, type 1 diabetes mellitus, inflammatory bowel disease
CD2/CD58	Costimulation of T cells	Rheumatoid arthritis, multiple sclerosis
IL23R	Component of IL-23 receptor; role in generation and maintenance of T_H17 cells	Inflammatory bowel disease, psoriasis, multiple sclerosis
IL10	Downregulates expression of co-stimulators, MHC molecules, IL-12 in dendritic cells; inhibits T_H1 responses	Inflammatory bowel disease, systemic lupus erythamatosus, type 1 diabetes mellitus
CTLA4	Inhibitory receptor of T cells, effector molecule of regulatory T cells	Type 1 diabetes mellitus, rheumatoid arthritis
IL2/IL21	Growth and differentiation factors for T cells; IL-2 is involved in maintenance of functional Tregs	Inflammatory bowel disease, celiac disease, rheumatoid arthritis, type 1 diabetes mellitus, multiple sclerosis
IL12B	p40 subunit of IL-12 (T_H1-inducing cytokine) and IL-23 (T_H17-inducing cytokine)	Inflammatory bowel disease, psoriasis
BLK	B lymphocyte tyrosine kinase, involved in B cell activation	Systemic lupus erythamatosus, rheumatoid arthritis
IL2RA	IL-2 receptor a chain (CD25); role in T cell activation and maintenance of regulatory T cells	Multiple sclerosis, type 1 diabetes mellitus
Genes involved in responses to microbes		
NOD2	Cytoplasmic sensor of bacteria (TLR)	Inflammatory bowel disease
ATG16	Autophagy (destruction of microbes, maintenance of epithelial cell integrity)	Inflammatory bowel disease
IRF5, IFIH1	Type 1 interferon responses to viruses	Systemic lupus erythamatosus

Table 15.4. Single gene mutations leading to autoimmune diseases

Gene	Mechanism of failure of tolerance	Human disease
AIRE	Failure of central tolerance	Autoimmune polyendocrine syndrome (APS)
C4	Defective clearance of immune complexes; failure of B cell tolerance	SLE (systemic lupus erythematosus)
CTLA-4	Failure of anergy in CD4+ T cells; defective function of regulatory T cells	CTLA-4 polymorphisms associated with several autoimmune diseases
Fas/FasL	Defective deletion of anergic self-reactive B cells; reduced deletion of mature CD4+ T cells	Autoimmune lymphoproliferative syndrome (ALPS)
FoxP3	Deficiency of regulatory T cells	IPEX (immune dysregulation, poly-endocrinopathy, enteropathy)

AIRE = Autoimmune regulatory gene.

- Infectious mononucleosis: Production of autoantibodies against T cells, B cells and nuclear components occurs.
- AIDS-autoantibodies to RBCs and platelets are produced.
– Microbes may activate the APCs to express costimulators, and when these APCs present self-antigens, the self-reactive T cells are activated rather than rendered tolerant (Fig. 15.7).
– Molecular mimicry: Some microbial antigens may cross-react with self-antigens (molecular mimicry) (Figs. 15.7 and 15.8). Therefore, immune responses initiated by the microbes may activate T cells specific for self-antigens, e.g. post-rabies vaccination encephalitis. Vaccine is made by growing rabies virus in rabbit brain cultures. Rabbit brain Ag induces antibody in vaccinated person which cross-reacts with human brain antigens leading to encephalitis. Some other examples of molecular mimicry are Polio virus – Acetylcholine receptor, Rabies virus protein – Insulin receptor, HIV-p24 antigen – immunoglobulin IgG, and Measles virus p3 protein – corticotropin.
- Release of sequestered antigen: Certain antigens are usually anatomically hidden and self-tolerance to them does not develop. On exposure, due to tissue damage, they lead to immune response (Fig. 15.9). For example:
  – Sperms after vasectomy
  – Lens proteins after eye damage
  – Myelin basic protein (MBP) – causes multiple sclerosis.
- Tissue injury/trauma/excessive inflammation or viral infections: Leads to inappropriate MHC expression. Expression of MHC on non-APCs leads to sensitization of T_H cells to host proteins causing autoimmune reaction. Trauma or viral infection causing excessive inflammation produces increased amounts of IFN-γ which induces high MHC-II expression on non-APC causing inappropriate T_H cell activation.

Various effector mechanisms are responsible for tissue injury in different autoimmune diseases. These are:
- Immune complexes: Type III hypersensitivity reactions
- Circulating autoantibodies: Type II hypersensitivity
- Auto-reactive T lymphocytes.

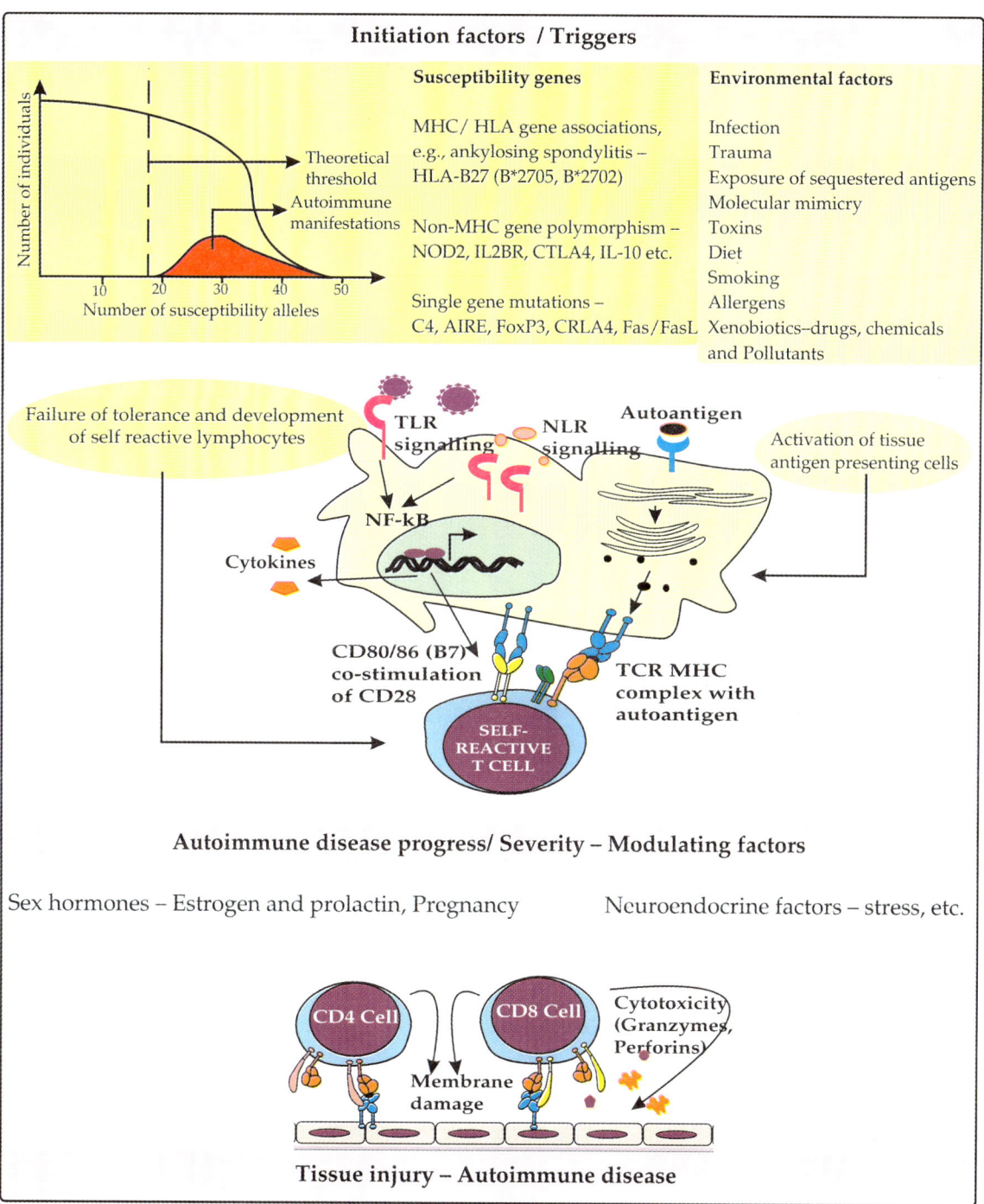

Fig. 15.6. Development of autoimmunity.

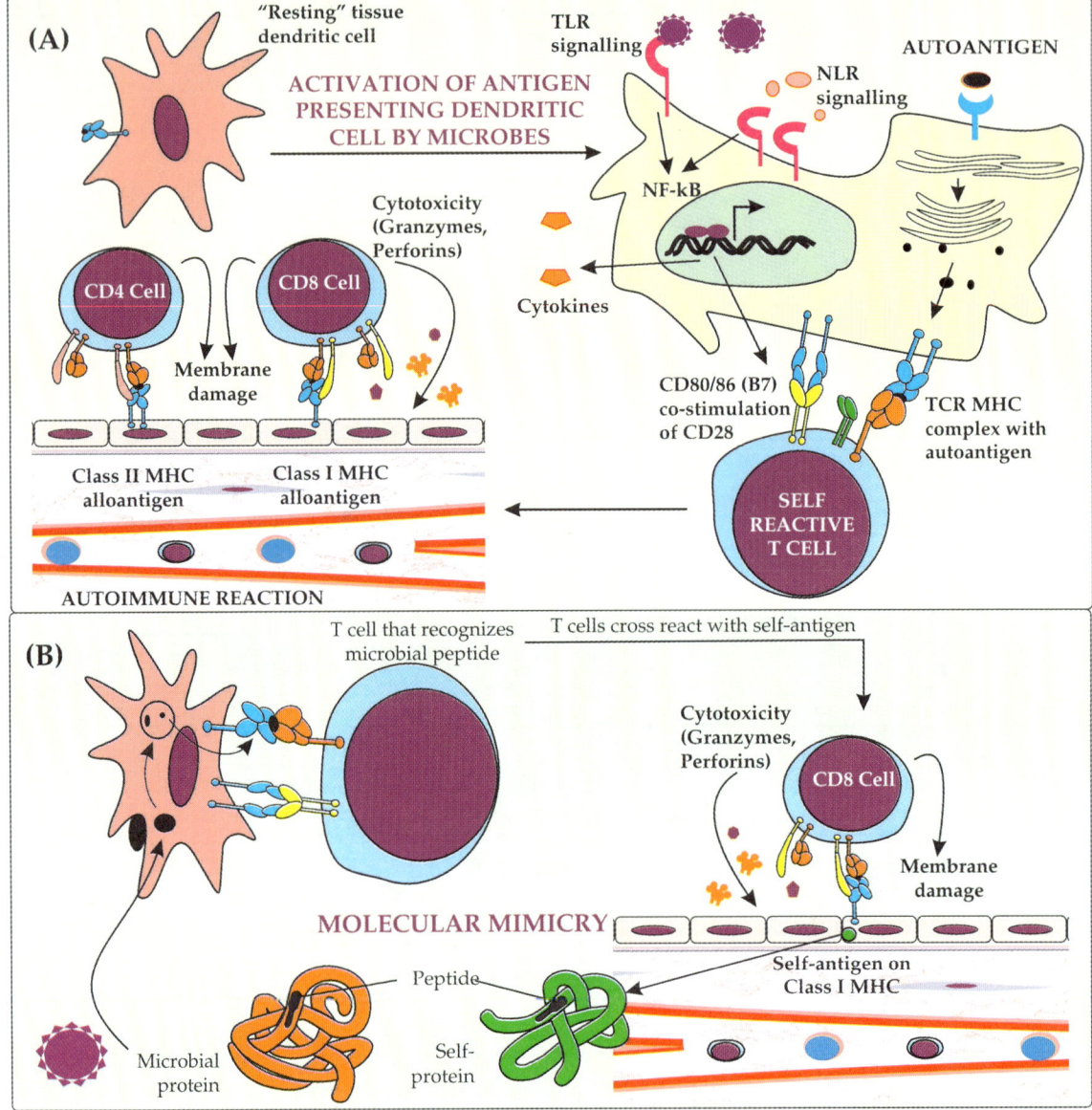

Fig. 15.7. (a) Microbial infections can activate dendritic cells (DC) presenting self-antigens to express co-stimulatory signals. (b) Molecular mimicry.

Autoimmune diseases tend to be chronic, progressive, and self-perpetuating because:
- Tissue damage due to immune system further exposes some sequestered and intracellular antigens usually not exposed to immune system leading to production of secondary autoantibodies to the damaged tissues.
- Excessive inflammation, T and B cell activation.
- As failure of self-tolerance is the basic mechanism, it can go on producing immune response to multiple self-antigens.

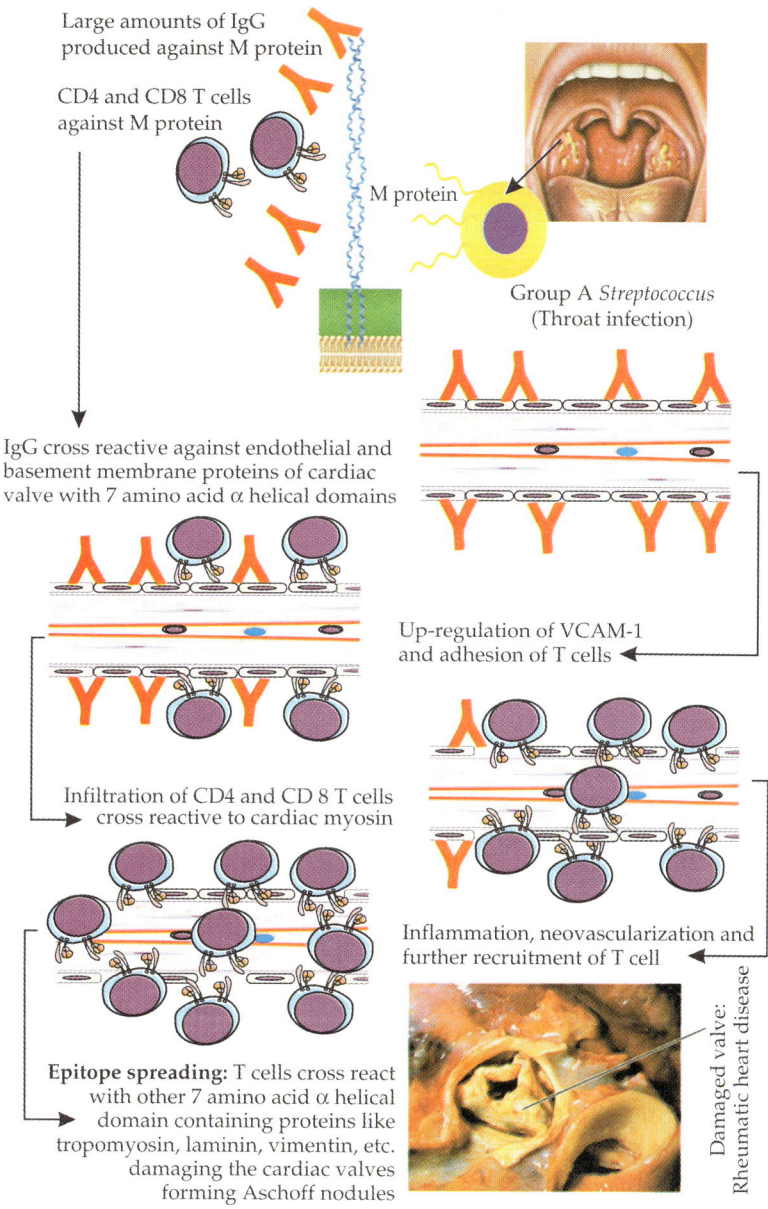

Fig. 15.8. Rheumatic heart disease due to molecular mimicry.

Autoimmune diseases can be organ-specific or multiorgan/systemic (Tables 15.5 and 15.6).

Systemic autoimmune disease:
- Tissue damage widespread.
- Against widely present antigens like RBCs, platelets, DNA, myelin, connective tissue.
- Defect of immune regulation.
- More common in females.

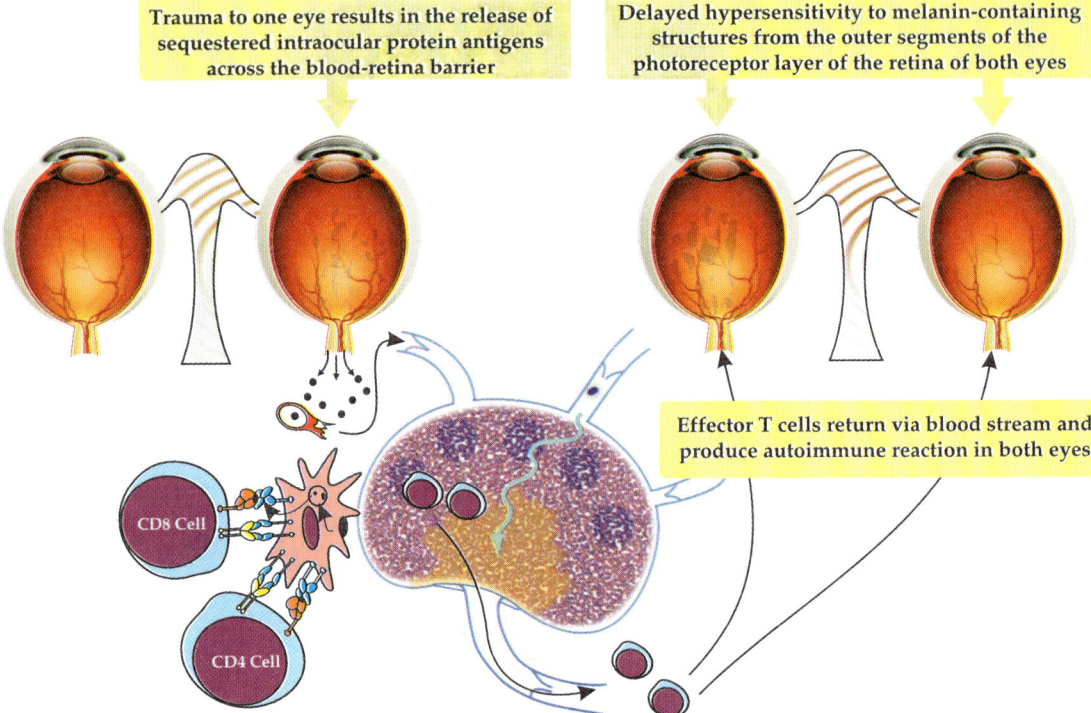

Fig. 15.9. Sympathetic ophthalmia.

Females are more susceptible to autoimmune diseases because of hormonal influence:
- Estrogen: Acts as an immunostimulatory hormone.
- Prolactin: Profound influence on immune responses. In mice, removal of the anterior pituitary results in a severe immunosuppression which can be entirely reversed by treatment with exogenous prolactin. Prolactin receptors are present on peripheral T and B cells in humans. Prolactin may tend to turn cells towards T_H1-dominated immune responses.

Q. 4. How are transplant grafts rejected? Explain the immune mechanisms and describe the methods used to prevent graft rejection.

Ans. Types of transplanted tissues include:
- Autograft – Within same individual
- Isograft – Monozygotic donor/syngenic animal
- Allograft – Genetically different member of the same species
- Xenograft – Different species.

Graft rejection occurs when the host immune system finds the antigens on the graft as foreign or non-self and mounts a specific immune response against them. Most grafts are allografts and the antigens on them recognised as non-self or foreign by the host are called alloantigens. All individuals of the same species have similar genetic material and proteins

Table 15.5. Organ-specific autoimmune diseases

Disease	Self-antigen	Immune response
Addison's disease	Adrenal cells	Auto-antibodies
Autoimmune hemolytic anaemia	RBC membrane proteins	Auto-antibodies
Goodpasture's syndrome	Renal and lung basement membranes	Auto-antibodies
Graves' disease	Thyroid-stimulating hormone receptor	Auto-antibody (stimulating)
Hashimoto's thyroiditis	Thyroid proteins and cells	T_{DTH} cells, auto-antibodies
Idiopathic thrombocytopenia purpura	Platelet membrane proteins	Auto-antibodies
Insulin-dependent diabetes mellitus	Pancreatic beta cells	T_{DTH} cells, auto-antibodies
Myasthenia gravis	Acetylcholine receptors	Auto-antibody (blocking)
Myocardial infarction	Heart	Auto-antibodies
Pernicious anaemia	Gastric parietal cells, intrinsic factor	Auto-antibody
Poststreptococcal glomerulonephritis	Kidney	Antigen-antibody complexes
Spontaneous infertility	Sperm	Auto-antibodies

Table 15.6. Systemic autoimmune diseases

Disease	Organ affected	Immune response
Ankylosing spondylitis	Vertebrae	Immune complexes
Multiple sclerosis	Brain or white matter	T_H1 cells and T_C cells, auto-antibodies
Rheumatoid arthritis	Connective tissue, IgG	Auto-antibodies, immune complexes
Scleroderma	Nuclei, heart, lungs, gastrointestinal tract, kidney	Auto-antibodies
Sjogren's syndrome	Salivary gland, liver, kidney, thyroid	Auto-antibodies
Systemic lupus erythematosus (SLE)	DNA, nuclear protein, RBC and platelet membranes	Auto-antibodies, immune complexes

with same primary and 3D structure. Immune response can occur only against proteins which are different between two individuals or in other words are polymorphic (different alleles). As humans have two sets of chromosomes these polymorphic proteins can have maximum of two types in an individual (heterozygous).

Most important allogenic antigens are the polymorphic MHC or the HLA proteins and are responsible for almost all strong rejection reactions. Others include major and minor blood group antigens like ABO, Rh, MN, etc. and are more important for blood transfusion.

The normal function of MHC molecules is to present peptides derived from protein antigens in a form that can be recognized by T cells. The B and T cells of an individual are self MHC-restricted i.e. they recognise antigens presented on own MHC molecules only.

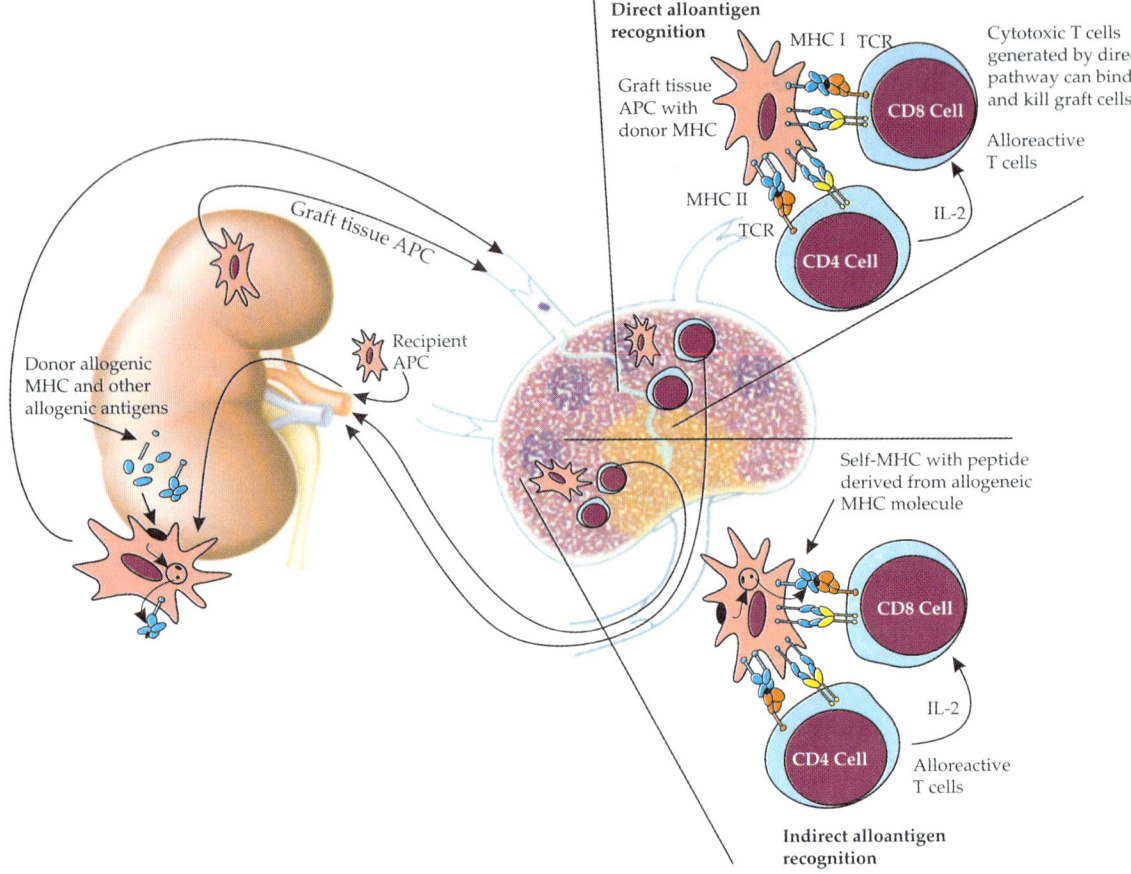

Fig. 15.10. Direct and indirect alloantigen presentation.

Allogeneic MHC molecules of a graft may be presented for recognition by the T cells of the recipient in two fundamentally different ways, called direct and indirect (Fig. 15.10).

1. Direct

An intact MHC molecule is displayed on the donor antigen-presenting cells (APCs) in the graft and is recognized by recipient T cells without a need for host APCs. This may seem puzzling that T cells that are normally selected during their maturation to be self MHC-restricted are capable of recognizing foreign (allogeneic or xenogeneic) MHC molecules. However, the frequency of T cells in a normal individual that can recognize a single allogeneic MHC molecule is as high as 1% to 2% of all T cells, which is 100 to 1000 times greater than the frequency of T cells specific for any microbial peptide displayed by self MHC molecules. This is because:

- The structure of all T cell receptors (TCRs) is inherently designed to recognize MHC molecules, even before selection in the thymus. During T cell development in the thymus, positive selection results in survival of T cells with weak self MHC reactivity, and among these T cells, there may be many with strong reactivity to allogeneic MHC molecules.

Negative selection in the thymus eliminates T cells with high affinity for self MHC, but it does not necessarily eliminate T cells that bind strongly to allogeneic MHC molecules, simply because these molecules are not present in the thymus. The result is that the mature T cells have an intrinsic weak affinity for self MHC molecules and includes many T cells that bind allogeneic MHC molecules with high affinity.
- The structure of an allogeneic MHC molecule is similar enough to self MHC that many self MHC-restricted T cells recognize the foreign MHC molecule.
- Since one MHC can present many processed peptides from many antigens, a single MHC can be recognized by large number of T-cells.
- Even though body's T cells do not recognize self-antigens presented with self-MHC (due to negative selection) these same antigens (same as self-peptides) in the graft tissue when present on foreign MHC (i.e. on graft APC) can be recognized by the recipient's T cells. In other words, T cells may respond to non-polymorphic human proteins when present on foreign MHC.

Direct allorecognition can generate both CD4+ and CD8+ T cells that recognize graft antigens and contribute to rejection.

2. Indirect presentation of alloantigens

Donor (allogeneic) MHC molecules are captured and processed by recipient APCs that enter graft tissue, and peptides derived from the allogeneic MHC molecules are presented in association with self MHC molecules. Peptides from the allogeneic MHC molecules are displayed by host APCs on self MHC I or II and are recognized by T cells like conventional foreign protein antigens. Because allogeneic MHC molecules have amino acid sequences different from those of the host, they can generate foreign peptides associated with self MHC molecules on the surface of host APCs. MHC molecules are the most polymorphic proteins in the genome; therefore, each allogeneic MHC molecule may give rise to multiple foreign peptides, each recognized by different T cells. This pathway can generate both activated CD4 and CD8 cells. Polymorphic alloantigens other than MHC are also presented by this pathway.

Activation of alloreactive lymphocytes and graft rejection

- The T cell response to an organ graft is initiated in the lymph nodes that drain the graft.
- Donor APCs migrate to regional lymph nodes and present, on their surface, unprocessed allogeneic MHC molecules to the recipient's T cells (the direct pathway of allorecognition).
- Host dendritic cells from the recipient migrate into the graft, pick up graft alloantigens, and transport these back to the draining lymph nodes, where they are displayed (the indirect pathway).
- Naive lymphocytes that normally move through the lymph node encounter these allo-antigens and are induced to proliferate and differentiate into effector cells. This process is called sensitization to alloantigens.
- Effector T cells migrate back into the graft and mediate rejection.
- As many as 1% to 2% of an individual's T cells are capable of recognizing and responding to a single foreign MHC molecule, and this high frequency of T cells reactive with allogeneic MHC molecules is the reason that allografts elicit strong immune responses. The usual frequency of T cells reactive with any foreign (e.g., microbial) antigen is only 1 in 10^5 or 10^6.

- Many of the T cells that respond to an allogeneic MHC molecule, even on first exposure, are memory T cells. These memory cells were generated during previous exposure to other foreign (e.g., microbial) antigens and cross-react with allogeneic MHC molecules. Memory cells are more resistant to immunosuppression than naive lymphocytes, and the presence of large numbers of memory cells leads to poor outcomes of transplantation.
- Alloreactive CD4+ and CD8+ T cells that are activated by graft alloantigens cause rejection by many mechanisms (Fig. 15.11). The CD4+ helper T cells differentiate into cytokine-producing effector cells that damage grafts by cytokine-mediated inflammation, similar to a delayed-type hypersensitivity (DTH) reaction. Alloreactive CD8+ T cells differentiate into cytotoxic T lymphocytes (CTLs), which kill nucleated cells in the graft that express the allogeneic class I MHC molecules. CTLs also secrete inflammatory cytokines, which can contribute to graft damage (Fig. 15.11).

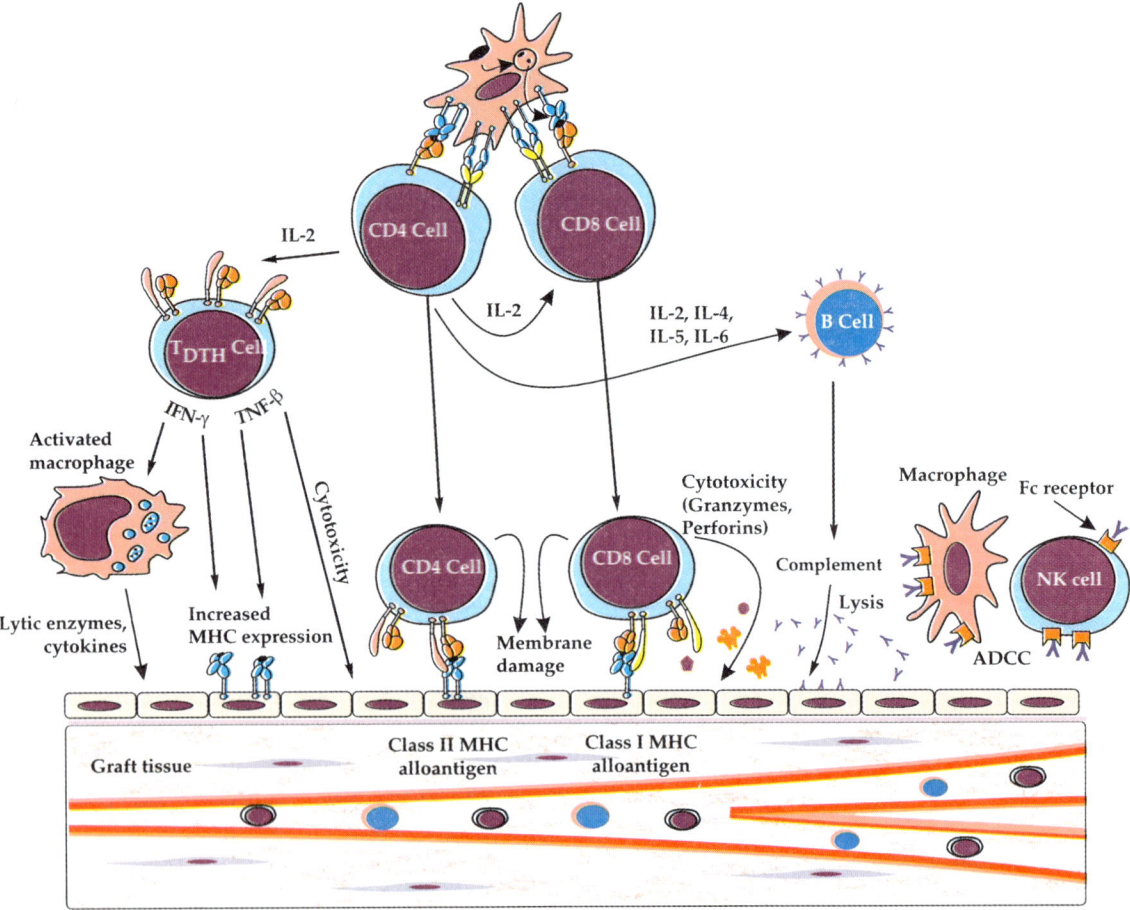

Fig. 15.11. Effector mechanisms of graft damage. Only CD8+ T cells and NK cells can kill directly. Other cells cause cytokine-mediated damage. Antibodies kill by ADCC (antibody-dependent cell cytotoxicity) and by complement-mediated lysis.

- Only CTLs that are generated by direct allogeneic MHC recognition can recognize, bind and directly kill graft cells, whereas CTLs or helper T cells generated by either direct or indirect alloantigen recognition can cause cytokine-mediated damage to grafts only (Fig. 15.11). CD8+ CTLs that are generated by the indirect pathway are self MHC restricted, and so they cannot bind and kill the foreign graft cells which do not express 'self' MHC alleles of the recipient.
- CD8+ CTLs induced by direct recognition of alloantigens are most important for acute cellular rejection of allografts, in which killing of graft cells is a prominent component, whereas CD4+ effector T cells stimulated by the indirect pathway play a greater role in chronic rejection (Fig. 15.11).
- Most high-affinity alloantibodies are produced by helper T cell-dependent activation of alloreactive B cells. The antigens most frequently recognized by alloantibodies in graft rejection are donor HLA molecules, including both class I and class II MHC proteins. Naive B lymphocytes recognize foreign MHC molecules, internalize and process these proteins, and present peptides derived from them to helper T cells that were previously activated by the same peptides presented by dendritic cells. Activation of alloreactive B cells is an example of indirect presentation of alloantigens. Anti-HLA antibodies contribute significantly to allograft rejection.

Patterns/types of rejections (Fig. 15.12)

1. Hyperacute rejection
2. Acute rejection
3. Chronic rejection

1. Hyperacute rejection

Mediated by preexisting antibodies in the host circulation that bind to donor endothelial cell antigens. Pre-existing antibodies may be there because of previous sensitization to foreign MHC due to:

- Repeated blood transfusion
- Repeated pregnancies
- Previous transplant

The pre-existing antibodies bind to the MHC antigens on the endothelial cells of graft vessels causing activation of complement and then clotting and thrombosis. Occlusion of the graft vasculature begins within minutes to hours after host blood vessels are anastomosed to graft vessels and leads to ischaemic cell death of the graft. It can occur due to IgM antibodies directed to ABO blood group antigens or now more commonly due to IgG antibodies to alloantigens like MHC.

2. Acute rejection

Acute rejection is a process of injury to the graft parenchyma and blood vessels mediated by alloreactive T cells and antibodies. Occurs over few weeks. The delayed time of onset of acute rejection is because alloreactive effector T cells and antibodies take time to be generated from naive or resting memory T cells in response to the graft. In current clinical practice, episodes of acute rejection may occur at much later times, even years after transplantation, if immunosuppression is reduced for any reason.

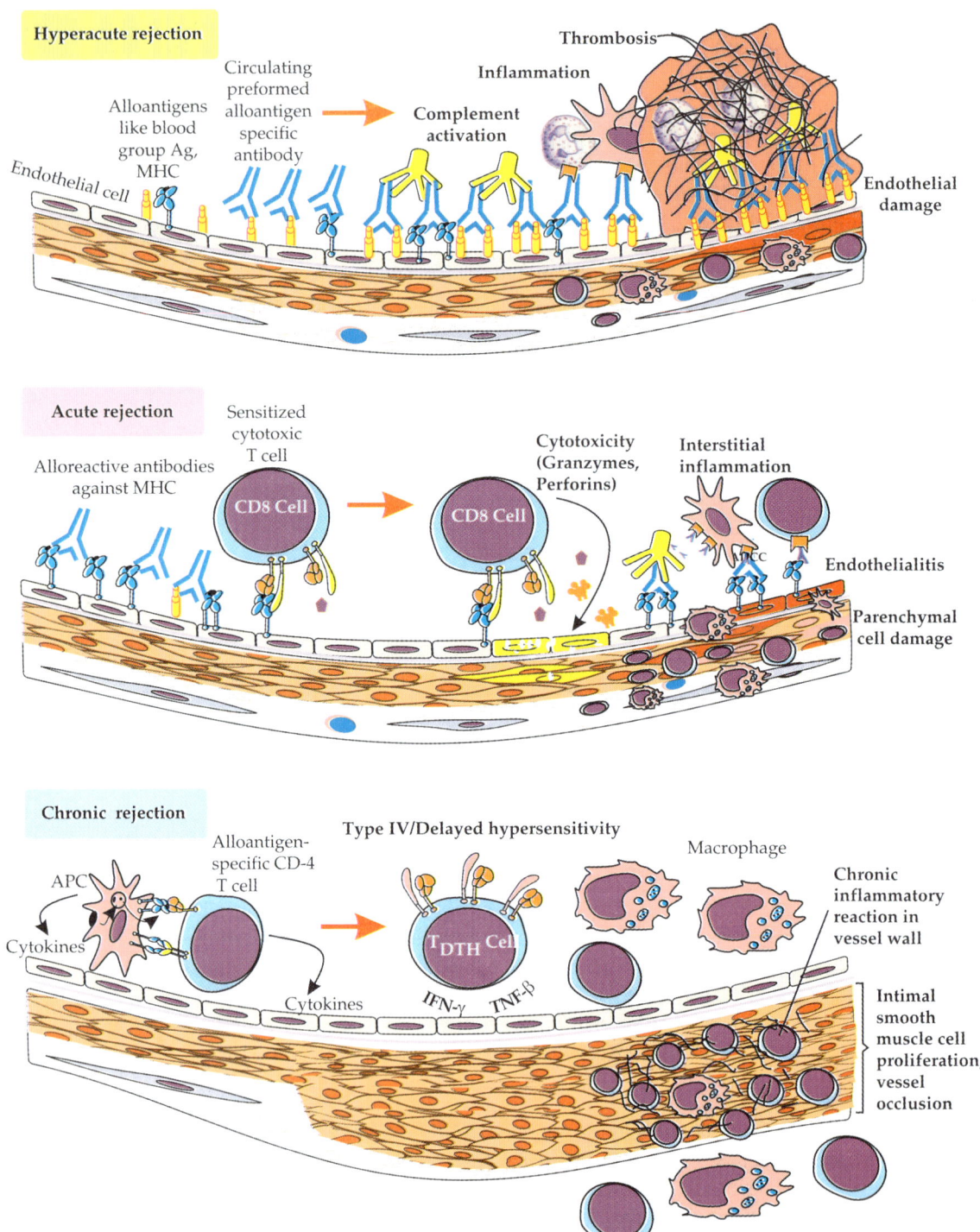

Fig. 15.12. Patterns of graft rejection.

- Acute cellular rejection: The principal mechanism of acute cellular rejection is CTL-mediated killing of cells of the graft.
- Acute antibody-mediated rejection: Alloantibodies cause acute rejection by binding to alloantigens, mainly HLA molecules, on vascular endothelial cells, causing endothelial injury and intravascular thrombosis that results in graft destruction.

Usually both mechanisms co-exist.

3. Chronic rejection

As therapy for acute rejection has improved, it has become the major cause of the failure of vascularized organ allografts.

It is characterized by arterial occlusion as a result of the proliferation of intimal smooth muscle cells, and the grafts eventually dies because of the ischemic damage. Occurs over months to years.

Graft vasculopathy is frequently seen in failed cardiac and renal allografts and can develop in any vascularized organ transplant within 6 months to a year after transplantation. The pathogenesis of the lesions involves a combination of immunologic and nonimmunologic processes. The mechanisms are:

- Activation of alloreactive T cells and secretion of cytokines that stimulate proliferation of vascular endothelial and smooth muscle cells.
- Repair with fibrosis after repeated bouts of acute antibody T-cell-mediated damage.
- Consequences of perioperative ischemia, toxic effects of immunosuppressive drugs, and even chronic viral infections.

As the arterial lesions of graft arteriosclerosis progress, blood flow to the graft parenchyma is compromised, and the parenchyma is slowly replaced by nonfunctioning fibrous tissue. This process leads to congestive heart failure or arrhythmias in cardiac transplant patients or loss of function in glomeruli and ischemic renal failure in renal transplant patients.

Prevention of graft rejection

- Reducing graft immunogenicity: HLA typing and cross-matching.
- Immunosuppression: Immunosuppressive drugs that inhibit or kill T lymphocytes are the principal agents used to treat or prevent graft rejection.
- Induction of tolerance (experimental approach under research).

Reducing graft immunogenicity: HLA typing and cross-matching

In human transplantation, the major strategy is to minimize alloantigenic differences between the donor and recipient. Several clinical laboratory tests are routinely performed to reduce the risk for immunologic rejection of allografts. These include:

- ABO blood typing: Avoids hyperacute rejection.
- HLA typing: Determination of HLA alleles expressed on donor and recipient cells, called tissue typing. Donors with same HLA alleles as recipient are chosen.
- Detection of preformed antibodies in the recipient that recognize HLA and other antigens representative of the donor population. In the panel reactive antibody test, patients waiting for organ transplants are screened for the presence of preformed antibodies that react with allogeneic HLA molecules prevalent in the population.

- Cross-matching: Detection of preformed antibodies in the recipient that bind to antigens of an identified donor's leukocytes. In a potential donor the cross-matching test will determine whether the patient has antibodies that react specifically with that donor's cells. The test is performed by mixing the recipient's serum with the donor's blood lymphocytes. Complement-mediated cytotoxicity tests or flow cytometric assays can then be used to determine if antibodies in the recipient serum have bound to the donor cells.
- Mixed lymphocyte reaction: The response of alloreactive T cells to foreign MHC molecules can be analyzed in an *in vitro* reaction called the mixed lymphocyte reaction (MLR) (Fig. 15.13). The MLR is used as a predictive test of T cell-mediated graft rejection. The MLR is induced by culturing mononuclear leukocytes (which include T cells, B cells, natural

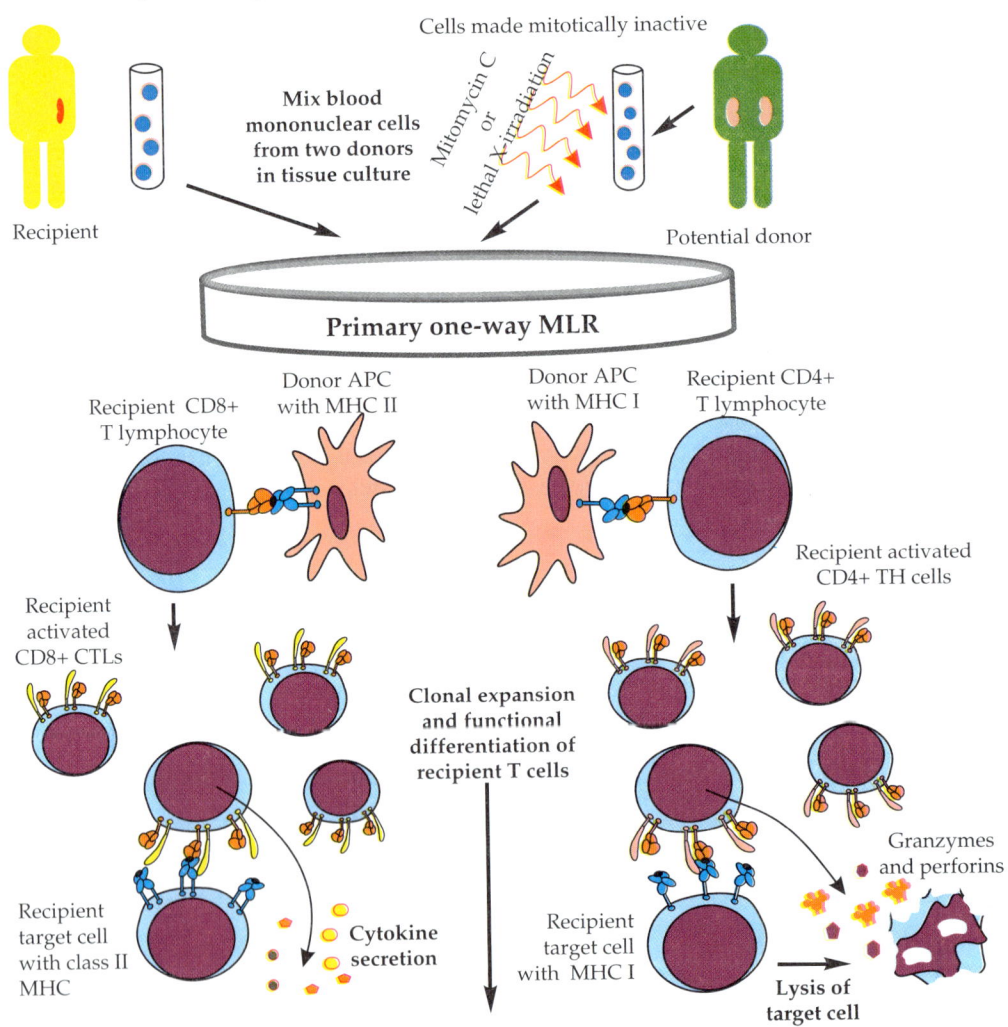

Fig. 15.13. One-way MLR.

killer [NK] cells, mononuclear phagocytes, and dendritic cells) from one individual with mononuclear leukocytes derived from another individual. If the two individuals have differences in the alleles of the MHC genes, a large proportion of the mononuclear cells will proliferate during a period of 4 to 7 days. This proliferative response is called the allogeneic MLR. If cells from two MHC-disparate individuals are mixed, each can react against the other and both will proliferate, thus resulting in a two-way MLR. In one-way MLR, the mononuclear cells from potential donors are made mitotically inactive so that after mixing only mononuclear cells from recipient can react against alloantigens on donor cells (Fig. 15.13).

Methods to induce donor-specific tolerance under research

Allograft rejection may be prevented by making the host tolerant to the alloantigens of the graft by various approaches:

- Costimulatory blockade: Inhibits immune responses to the allograft but do not induce long-lived tolerance, and patients have to be maintained on the therapy.
- Hematopoietic chimerism: Transfusion of donor blood cells into recipient inhibits rejection. The transfused donor hematopoietic stem cells survive for extended periods in the recipient, and the recipient becomes a chimera (mixed population of lymphocytes). Hematopoietic chimerism with long-term allograft tolerance has also been achieved in a small number of renal allograft patients by doing a bone marrow cell transplant from the donor at the same time as the organ allograft.
- Transfer or induction of regulatory T cells: Generation of donor-specific regulatory T cells in culture and to transfer these into graft recipients. It has been tried with some success in hematopoietic stem cell transplantation to decrease graft vs host disease.

Immunosuppression

Generalized immunosuppressant therapy

- Mitotic inhibitors like azathioprine, methotrexate: All rapidly-dividing cells including T and B cells and epithelial cells, bone marrow cells are affected due to block in synthesis of nucleotides.
- Corticosteroids: Cause lympholysis, decrease T cell activation by inhibiting NF-kb, reduce phagocytic activity of macrophages.

Specific immunosuppression (Fig. 15.14)

- Inhibitors of T cell signalling pathways:
  - Cyclosporine: The calcineurin inhibitors cyclosporine and FK506 (tacrolimus) inhibit transcription of certain genes in T cells, including those encoding for cytokines such as IL-2.
  - Calcineurin is required to activate the transcription factor NFAT (nuclear factor of activated T cells); cyclosporine inhibits NFAT activation and the transcription of IL-2 and other cytokine genes.
  - The immunosuppressive drug rapamycin (sirolimus) inhibits growth factor-mediated T cell proliferation.

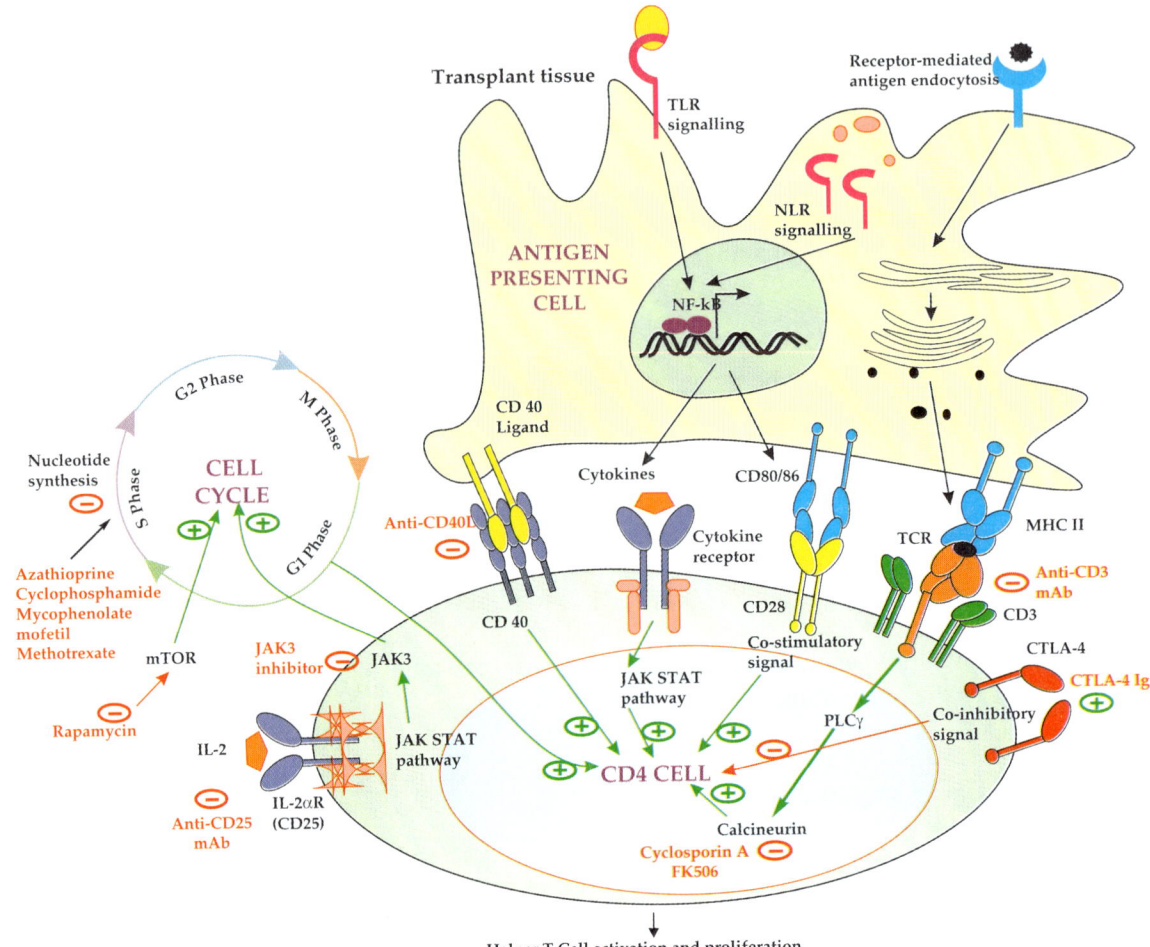

Fig. 15.14. Drugs used to prevent graft rejection and their mechanisms of action.

- Antimetabolites:
  - Metabolic toxins that kill proliferating T cells are used in combination with other drugs to treat graft rejection.
  - The most widely used drug in this class is mycophenolate mofetil (MMF).
  - MMF is metabolized to mycophenolic acid, which blocks a lymphocyte-specific isoform of inosine monophosphate dehydrogenase, an enzyme required for *de novo* synthesis of guanine nucleotides.
  - Because MMF selectively inhibits the lymphocyte-specific isoform of this enzyme; it has relatively few toxic effects on other cells.
- Function-blocking or depleting antilymphocyte antibodies:
  - Antibodies that react with T cell surface structures and deplete or inhibit T cells are used to treat acute rejection episodes.
  - One widely used antibody is a mouse monoclonal antibody called OKT3 that is specific for human CD3 (part of T cell receptor complex).

- Monoclonal antibodies specific for CD25, the α subunit of the IL-2 receptor.
- Costimulatory blockade:
  - Drugs that block T cell costimulatory pathways reduce acute allograft rejection.
  - A soluble high-affinity form of CTLA-4 fused to an IgG Fc domain binds to B7 molecules on APCs and prevents them from interacting with T cell CD28.
- Drugs targeting alloantibodies and alloreactive B cells:
  - Intravenous immune globulin (IVIG) therapy, for acute antibody-mediated rejection. Pooled IgG from normal donors is injected intravenously into a patient. Mechanism of action involves binding of the injected IgG to the patient's Fc receptors on various cell types, thereby reducing alloantibody production and blocking effector functions of the patient's own antibodies. IVIG also enhances degradation of the patient's antibodies by competitively inhibiting their binding to the neonatal Fc receptor.
  - A monoclonal antibody specific for the B cell surface protein CD20 very effectively depletes mature B cells from the circulation and secondary lymphoid organs.
- Inhibitors of leukocyte migration:
  - Fingolimod (FTY720), works by binding to and blocking sphingosine-1-phosphate (S1P) receptors on lymphocytes.
  - Anti-integrin antibodies have proved to be effective treatments for some autoimmune diseases because they block leukocyte recruitment from the circulation into inflamed tissues.
- TLI – Total lymphoid irradiation: Used in bone marrow transplantation. Recipient's lymphoid tissues are irradiated before grafting. Transplanted lymphoid cells proliferate and renew the circulating lymphocytes.

Q. 5. What are superantigens?

Ans. When the immune system encounters a conventional T-dependent antigen, only a small fraction of the T cell population is able to recognize the antigen and become activated. However, some antigens can polyclonally activate a large fraction of the T cells, setting off massive immune response. These antigens are called superantigens. Superantigens stimulate up to 10% of T cells to respond whereas an antigen would normally stimulate only 0.001–0.01% of T cells to respond. Superantigens (SAgs) are the most powerful T cell mitogens ever discovered. Concentrations of less than 0.1 pg/ml of a bacterial superantigen are sufficient to stimulate the T lymphocytes in an uncontrolled manner resulting in fever, shock and death. SAgs bind as intact molecules to the class II major histocompatibility complex (MHC) outside the peptide-binding groove and then bind the T cell receptor (TcR) via the variable region of the TcR β-chain (TCR Vβ, Figs. 15.15). Superantigens are presented to T cells by binding to nonpolymorphic regions of class II MHC molecules on APCs, and they interact with conserved regions of TCR Vβ domains. The β chain V domain contains a fourth hypervariable region – CDR4 (besides the antigen-binding hypervariable regions CDR 1–3) that does not appear to participate in antigen recognition but is the binding site for superantigens.

Each SAg can bind a particular TCR Vβ type and as there are only 57 types of Vβ domains, each SAg can activate a substantial number of T cells. This can be as high as 20% of all T cells compared with only 1 in 10^5–10^6 naive T cells that are responsive to a

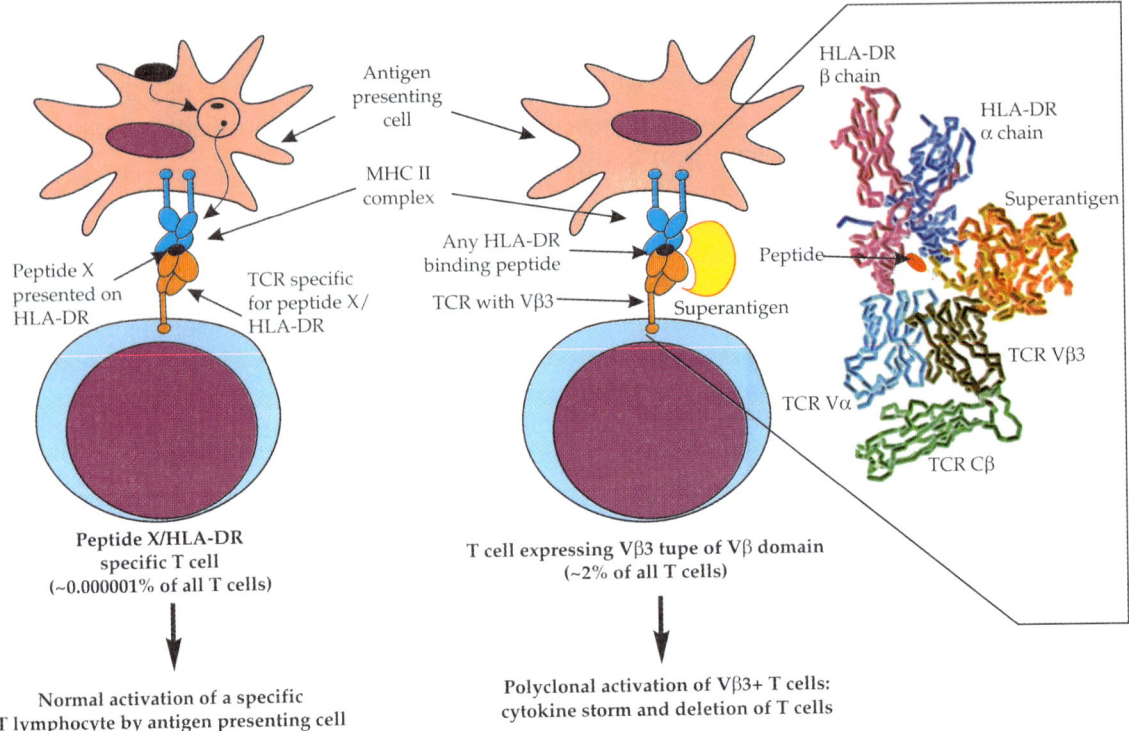

Fig. 15.15. Mechanism of T cell activation by 'normal' antigens and superantigens.

conventional peptide antigen which binds to a particular TCR through CDR1,2,3 (peptide-binding cleft) on the variavle domains of α and β chains. This results in massive systemic release of pro-inflammatory cytokines, such as tumour necrosis factor-alpha (TNF-α), interleukin-1beta (IL-1β) and IL-2, which can lead to fever and shock.

Examples of superantigens include:
- Staphylococcal enterotoxins
- Staphylococcal toxic shock toxin (TSST-1)
- Streptococcal pyrogenic exotoxins (exotoxin A and exotoxin B)
- Mouse mammary tumour virus (retrovirus), which causes breast cancer in mice.

Superantigens are considered virulence factors; the stimulated T cells respond by secreting cytokines that suppress specific immune responses. Superantigen also induces apoptosis in the superantigen-binding CD4 T cells, so T cells that can respond to the pathogen are deleted. Certain bacterial toxins stimulate all the T cells in an individual that express a particular type of Vβ T cell receptor (TCR) gene. Such toxins are called superantigens because they resemble antigens in that they bind to TCRs and to class II MHC molecules (although not to the peptide-binding clefts) but activate many more T cells than do conventional peptide antigens. Their importance lies in their ability to activate many T cells, with the subsequent production of large amounts of cytokines that can also cause a systemic inflammatory syndrome.

Superantigens in human disease

Food poisoning

The staphylococcal superantigens SEA-SEE and SEG-SEI are potent gastrointestinal toxins responsible for staphylococcal food poisoning. Quantities of less than 1 µg of toxin are sufficient to trigger vomiting in humans.

Toxic shock syndrome (TSS)

Toxic shock syndrome (TSS) is an inflammatory response syndrome produced by Toxic shock syndrome toxin-1 producing strains of *S. aureus*, characterized by fever, rash, nausea, vomiting, diarrhoea, hypotension and multiorgan involvement. TSS has been typically associated with tampon use in healthy menstruating women. The disease is now known to also occur in men, neonates, and nonmenstruating women in conditions including post-operative wound infection or post-influenza staphylococcal infection. In contrast to other staphylococcal SAgs, TSST has the ability to cross the mucosa.

Streptococcal toxic shock syndrome (STSS)

STSS, caused by *S. pyogenes*, is the most severe form of invasive streptococcal disease, with mortality rates of up to 50%. The clinical symptoms are very similar to those in TSS, but STSS is often associated with bacteraemia, myositis or necrotizing fasciitis. Streptococcal SAgs have been implicated in STSS.

Acute rheumatic fever (ARF)

ARF, a post-infection sequelae, is the leading cause of preventable paediatric heart disease. It usually occurs in school-age children and young adults after pharyngeal infection with *S. pyogenes*. ARF is a cross-reactive immune response to the host's cardiac tissue and it has been proposed that the reactive T cells might be driven by SAgs.

Kawasaki disease (KD)

KD is an acute multi-system vasculitis of unknown aetiology that affects mainly young children and is now recognized as the leading cause of acquired heart disease in children in the developed world. KD is associated with marked activation of T cells and monocytes and there is a remarkable similarity among KD, TSS, STSS and scarlet fever in the clinical symptoms. Intravenous immunoglobulin therapy is highly effective when given early, suggesting that the causative agent is a toxin. Selective expansion of T cells bearing the Vβ2-1 TcR occurs, which points towards a SAg involvement in the disease. A potential association between KD and the *Y. pseudotuberculosis* mitogenic factor (YPM) a superantigen has also been described.

Q. 6. What are isotypes, allotypes and idiotypes?

Ans. **Isotypes**

Immunoglobulin isotype refers to the genetic variations or differences in the constant regions of the heavy and light chains. Isotypes are antigenic determinants formed by the unique sequences located in constant regions of heavy and light chains of Ig molecule (Fig. 15.16). Antibody isotypes are the same as antibody classes. There are 5 major isotypes: IgM, IgD, IgG, IgE, and IgA. The difference between these isotypes lies in the heavy chain (Mu, Delta,

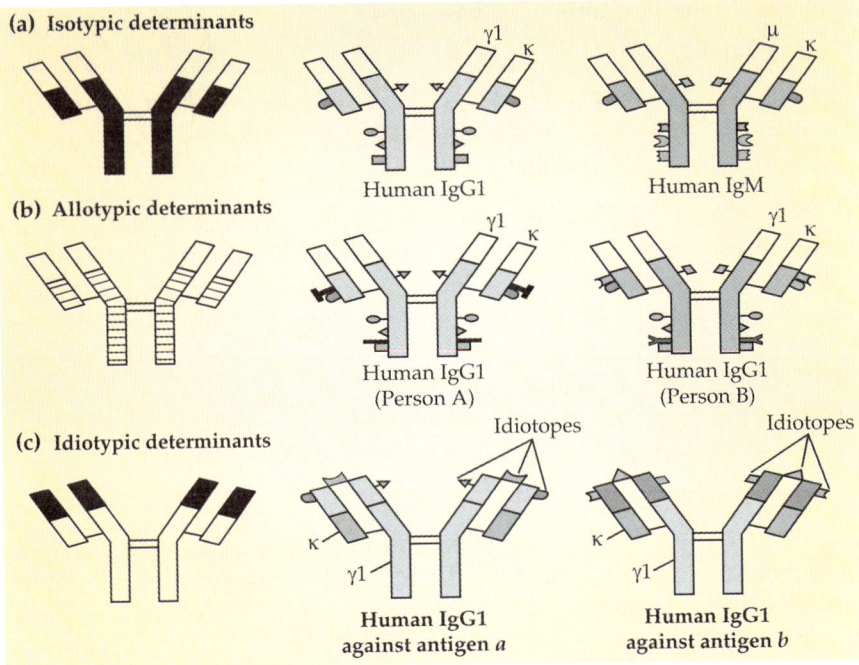

Fig. 15.16. Isotype, allotype and idiotype determinants of an antibody. Location on antibody structure and examples.

Gamma, Epsilon, or Alpha). Either kappa or lambda light chains can occur with any of these isotypes. All isotypes can be readily found in normal sera of any individual. Each isotype is encoded by a separate constant region gene. In humans, the most plentiful isotype is IgG; the least plentiful one is IgE. IgG1 and IgG2 subclasses of IgG are also isotypes. Similarly IgGκ and IgGλ are also isotypes. Immunoglobulin class switching can be used to change the class of the heavy chain, but not of the light chain.

Allotypes

Allotypes represent the genetically determined differences in antibodies between different people. While two different people both have IgG, their IgGs are very slightly different, by a 1-4 amino acids in the constant region of the heavy or light chains. An immunoglobulin allotype is the allele of the antibody chains found in the individual. Thus, the antigenic determinants present in constant regions of heavy and light chains and encoded by polymorphic alleles are called allotypes (Figs. 15.17 and 15.18). The word allotype comes from two Greek roots, *allo* meaning 'other or differing from the norm' and *typos* meaning 'mark'. Thus allotype refers to the idea that each immunoglobin has unique sequences particular to the individual's genome in its constant region. The most important types are Gm (heavy chain) and km (light chain).

Allotypes are known for all four subclasses of IgG and subclass IgA2. No allotypes exist for other classes and subclasses. They are named in a characteristic manner, e.g.

G1m(2) – 2nd allotype of the IgG1 subclass
A2m(1) – 1st allotype of IgA2 subclass

There are in all 25 Gm markers belonging to different subclasses. IgA2 has only two allotypes – A2(m)1 and A2m(2). The κ light chain has three allotypes: km(1), km(2) and km(3). Antibodies to allotypes can arise due to pregnancy and blood transfusion. Allotypes can be used as genetic markers for resolving paternity disputes.

Idiotypes

Idiotypic determinants are present in the hypervariable regions of the V_H and V_L domains of antibodies (Figs. 15.17 and 15.18). Thus all anitbodies having a common epitope-binding region or paratope will belong to one idiotype. Due to large diversity of paratopes in any individual lot of idotypes are present and body does not produce antibodies against the different variable regions of antibodies due to their small individual concentration and number. However, when injected into another person of the same species antibodies may be produced against them. Thus, even if an antibody of the same isotype and allotype but different idiotype is injected into another person antibodies are produced against it as it has a unique and different hypervariable region or the paratope.

An idiotype is a shared characteristic between a group of immunoglobulin or T cell receptor (TCR) molecules based upon the antigen-binding specificity and therefore structure of their variable region. The word idiotype comes from two Greek roots, *idio* meaning 'private, distinctive, peculiar' and *typos* meaning 'mark'. Thus, idiotype describes the distinctive sequence and region (variable region) that makes any immunoglobulin/TCR unique from others of the same type. The variable region of antigen receptors of T cells (TCRs) and B cells (immunoglobulins) contain complementarity determining regions (CDRs) with unique amino acid sequences. They define the surface and properties of the variable region, determining the antigen specificity and therefore the idiotope of the molecule. Antibody idiotype diversity is produced by:

- Gene rearrangement
- Junctional diversity
- P-nucleotides (palindromic nucleotides at sites of single-strand breaks)
- N-nucleotides
- Somatic hypermutations.

The term idiotype is sometimes used to describe the collection of multiple idiotopes, and therefore overall antigen binding capacity, possessed by an antibody. Idiotypes are antibodies that recognize different specific epitopes.

Q. 7. What are cryoglobulins and cold agglutinins?

Ans. Cryoglobulins

Cryoglobulins are either immunoglobulins or a mixture of immunoglobulins and complement components which can precipitate at temperature less than the body temperature (37°C) or on refrigeration of serum and plasma. Cryoglobulins form complexes and precipitate out of serum at low temperatures and redissolve upon warming. The temperature at which cryoglobulins precipitate varies with the total protein concentration. Higher concentrations of protein in a sample increases the temperature at which the cryoglobulins precipitate. Due to some unique sequence of amino acids present in them they can polymerize at low temperatures. They can precipitate alone as homogeneous complexes or at even lower temperatures can form heterogeneous complexes with fironectin and fibrin. The precipitation phenomenon at low temperatures is a result of the physicochemical properties of the cryoglobulin molecule itself unrelated to the specific antibody-antigen binding.

Excess of cryoglobulins cause cryoglobulinemia. Cryoglobulinemia without an associated disease has been known as essential, or idiopathic, cryoglobulinemia. Cryoglobulinemia associated with a particular disease (lymphoproliferative disorder, autoimmune disease, infectious disease) is known as secondary cryoglobulinemia.

- The precipitation of their immune complexes causes systemic inflammation most commonly affecting kidney and skin (glomerulonephritis, chronic vasculitis).
- Complement activation: Complement fragments (C3a, C5a) that act as chemotactic mediators of inflammation can be generated.
- Intravascular cryoglobulin deposits can cause plugging and thrombosis of small arteries and capillaries in the extremities (gangrene) and glomeruli (acute renal failure).
- Circulating large molecular-weight cryoprotein complexes, even when unprecipitated *in vivo*, can lead to clinical hyperviscosity syndrome.
- Clinical manifestations vary according to type and range but the classical triad (Meltzer's triad) is purpura, weakness and arthralgia.

Cryoglobulins and their associated disorders are classified into three types based on their composition of cryoglobulins (Table 15.7).

- Specific clinical manifestations associated with type I cryoglobulinemia are related to hyperviscosity and thrombosis, due to high concentrations of immunoglobulins and limited interference with complement function. These manifestations include acrocyanosis, retinal hemorrhage, severe Raynaud's disease with digital ulceration, livedo reticularis, purpura, and arterial thrombosis.
- Specific clinical manifestations associated with types II and III cryoglobulinemia include joint involvement (usually arthralgias in the proximal interphalangeal [PIP] joints, metacarpophalangeal [MCP] joints, knees, and ankles), fatigue, myalgias, renal immune-complex disease, cutaneous vasculitis, and peripheral neuropathy.

Cold aglutinins

Autoimmune haemolytic anaemia (AIHA) is an acquired hemolytic anemia in which destruction of red blood cells (RBCs) is mediated by autoantibodies directed against antigens on the patient's RBCs. Two types of autoantibodies are produced in AIHA:

- IgG antibodies that generally react with protein antigens on the RBC surface at body temperature. Thus, they are called "warm agglutinins" even though IgG can rarely directly agglutinate the RBCs. Rarely, IgM antibodies can be the cause and readily agglutinate red cells.
- IgM antibodies that generally react with polysaccharide antigens on the RBC surface only at temperatures below that of the core temperature of the body. They are called "cold agglutinins". Rarely, IgG antibodies can cause such reaction either alone or with IgM antibodies.

Table 15.7

Type	Composition	Description	Disorders
Type I	Isolated monoclonal immunoglobulins	These are composed of a single monoclonal immunoglobulin paraprotein IgM or IgG (usually IgM). Sometimes, these are represented by light chains only and can be excreted in the urine; or, they may accumulate in blood in the event of renal failure. Concentration is usually high (> 5 mg/mL).	• Waldenstrom's macroglobulinemia – hyperviscosity of the blood, cold urticaria, Raynaud's phenomenon, purpura, and cutaneous vasculitis with or without ulcerative retinal hemorrhage. • Paroxysmal cold hemoglobinuria – Type I cryoglobulin gets attached to complement at low temperatures and lyses red blood cells when temperature rises to 37°C. The antibody specificity is directed against the red blood cell antigen P3. • Idiopathic non-malignant monoclonal cryoglobulinemia – genetic disease with high rate of synthesis of cryoglobulins in nonmalignant B cells.
Type II	Immune complexes formed by monoclonal IgM and polyclonal IgG	Consist of monoclonal IgM or IgA and a polyclonal IgG. The monoclonal component, IgM or IgA, has a rheumatoid factor activity. The IgM can recognize intact IgG; either the Fab region or Fc region of IgG fragments. This is why most type II cryoglobulins are IgM–IgG complexes. Concentrations are usually > 1 mg/ml.	• Essential Mixed Cryolobulinemia or (EMC). It is characterized by purpura, weakness, arrhythmia, hepatosplenomegaly and glomerulonephritis. Treatment for EMC includes plasma exchange, steroids, and use of cytotoxic drugs.
Type III	Immune complexes formed by polyclonal IgM (mixed cryoglobulins that lack a monoclonal component)	Consists of two or more immunoglobulins of different classes (polyclonal IgM and IgG molecules). Their concentration is usually < 1 mg/ml. Have very similar function to the type II cryoglobulins.	• Type III cryoglobulin disorders: – Very rare and get resolved when the precipitate dissolves.

Cold agglutinin disease

This is a rare blood disorder, a type of Autoimmune Hemolytic Anemia. All individuals have circulating antibodies directed against red blood cells, but their concentrations are often too low to trigger disease (titres under 64 at 4°C). In individuals with cold agglutinin disease, these antibodies are in much higher concentrations (titres over 1000 at 4°C). At peripheral body temperatures of 28–31°C (encountered during winter months) and occasionally at body temperatures of 37°C, antibodies (generally IgM) bind to the polysaccharide region of glycoproteins on the surface of red blood cells (typically the I antigen, i antigen, and Pr antigens). Binding of antibodies to red blood cells activates the classical pathway of the complement system. If the complement response is sufficient, red blood cells are damaged by the membrane attack complex. In the formation of the membrane attack complex, several complement proteins are inserted into the red blood cell membrane, forming pores that lead to membrane instability and intravascular hemolysis (destruction of the red blood cells within the blood vessels). If the complement response is insufficient to form membrane attack complexes, then extravascular lysis will be favoured over intravascular red blood cell lysis. Instead of the membrane attack complex, complement proteins (particularly C3b and C4b) are deposited on red blood cells. This opsonization enhances the clearance of red blood cell by phagocytes in the liver, spleen, and lungs, a process termed extravascular hemolysis. When the rate of destruction exceeds the ability of the bone marrow to produce an adequate number of oxygen-carrying red cells, then anaemia occurs. Many people with CAD also can be affected by two conditions called Raynaud's phenomenon and acrocyanosis.

The temperature, at which the agglutination (clumping) takes place, varies from patient to patient. The thermal amplitude, defined as the highest temperature at which the antibody will react with the antigen, appears to be more important than the titre with respect to the pathogenicity.

There are two forms of cold agglutinin disease:

- Primary form is by definition idiopathic, a disease for which no cause is known. 50% of CAD patients are said to have primary CAD. It is now believed that 10% of those with primary CAD are idiopathic (no known cause) and 90% are considered to have a low grade lymphoproliferative bone marrow disorder.
- Secondary cold agglutinin disease is a result of an underlying condition. In adults, this is typically due to a lymphoproliferative disease such as lymphoma and chronic lymphoid leukemia, or infection. In children, cold agglutinin disease is often secondary to an infection, such as mycoplasma pneumonia, mononucleosis, and HIV, etc.

Both Primary and Secondary Cold Agglutinin Diseases are acquired conditions, not inherited. One can have both warm and cold agglutinins at the same time. Warm antibody disease is easier to treat. Occasionally, IgM macroglobulin acts as both cryoglobulin and cold agglutinin. Not all cryoglobulins are cold agglutinins because they do not share some of the antibody characteristics of cold agglutinins.

Xenobiotic Metabolism, Antioxidants and Biochemistry of Ageing

Chapter 16

Q. 1. What are xenobiotics? How are they metabolized and what is the importance of their biotransformation?

Ans. Xenobiotics (Gk *xenos* "stranger") are chemical substances that are foreign to the biological system. Xenobiotics are chemicals not naturally belonging to or originating from a particular organism or an ecosystem. They include:

- Food components (methyl glyoxal, coffee, etc.)
- Food additives and contaminants (preservatives, aflatoxin B1, etc.)
- Drugs
- Cosmetics
- Environmental pollutants
- Cigarette smoke (benzopyrene, NNK – nocotine-derived nitrosamine ketone)
- Chemicals of abuse (ethanol, tobacco, etc.)
- Agrochemicals (fertilizers, insecticides, herbicide, etc.)
- Industrial chemicals (solvents, dyes, monomers, polymers, vinyl chloride, etc.)

Xenobiotic metabolism describes the total fate of a xenobiotic which includes absorption, distribution, biotransformation and excretion (Figs. 16.1 and 16.2). More than 200,000 manufactured environmental chemicals exist.

Depending on the chemical nature xenobiotics may be hydrophilic or lipophilic. Hydrophilic (polar) compounds are water soluble, difficult to transport through membranes and rapidly eliminated with the urine. Lipophilic (nonpolar, hydrophobic) compounds are poorly soluble in water, need a blood transporter (albumin), freely diffuse through membranes, can be stored in membranes and are only slowly eliminated from the body.

Absorption

They may be absorbed through GIT (mostly), skin or lungs. Those entering through GIT first pass through the liver by portal circulation (first pass metabolism, Fig. 16.1).

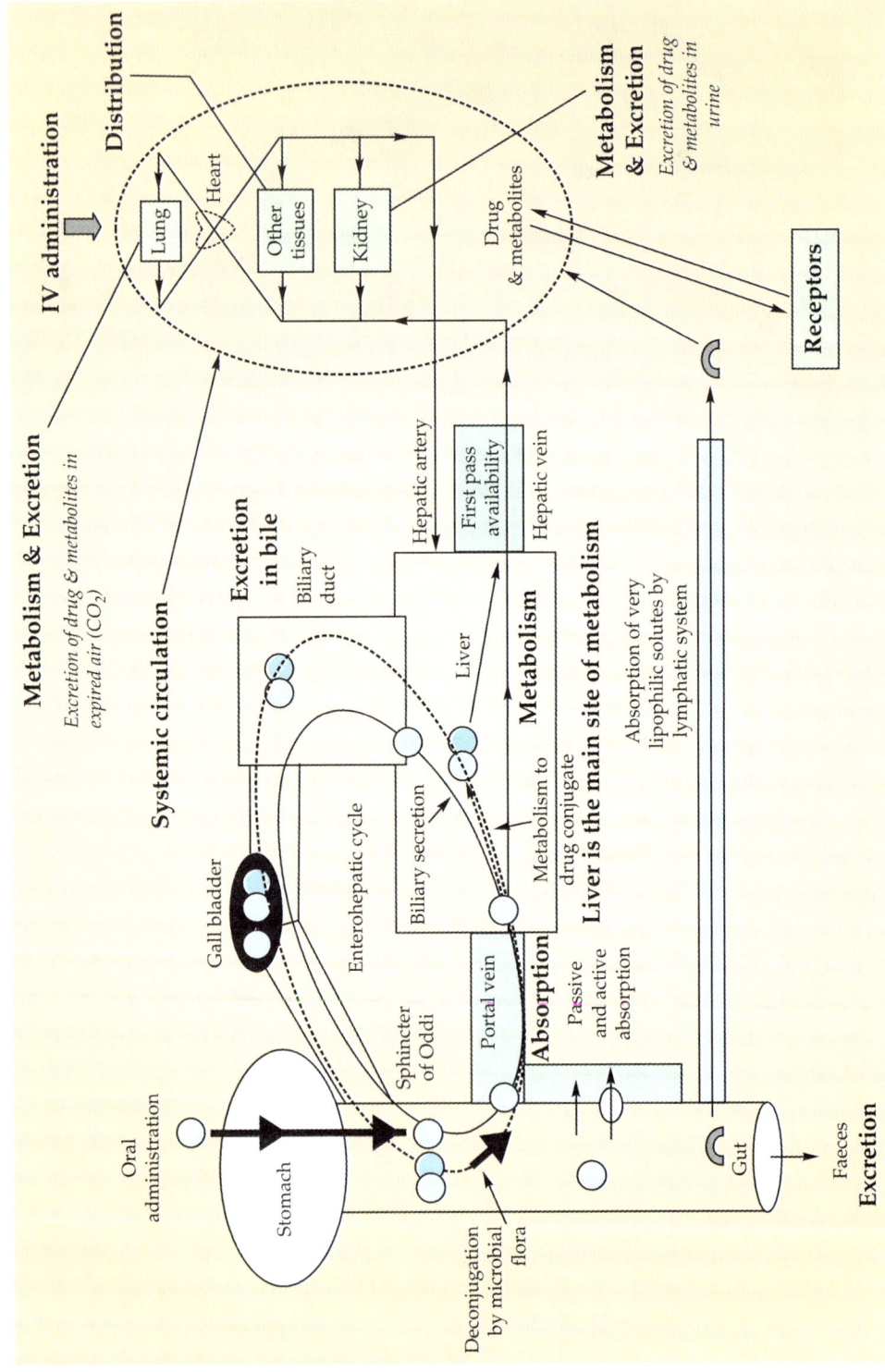

Fig. 16.1. Xenobiotic metabolism – entry, distribution, first pass metabolism, circulation, metabolism and excretion.

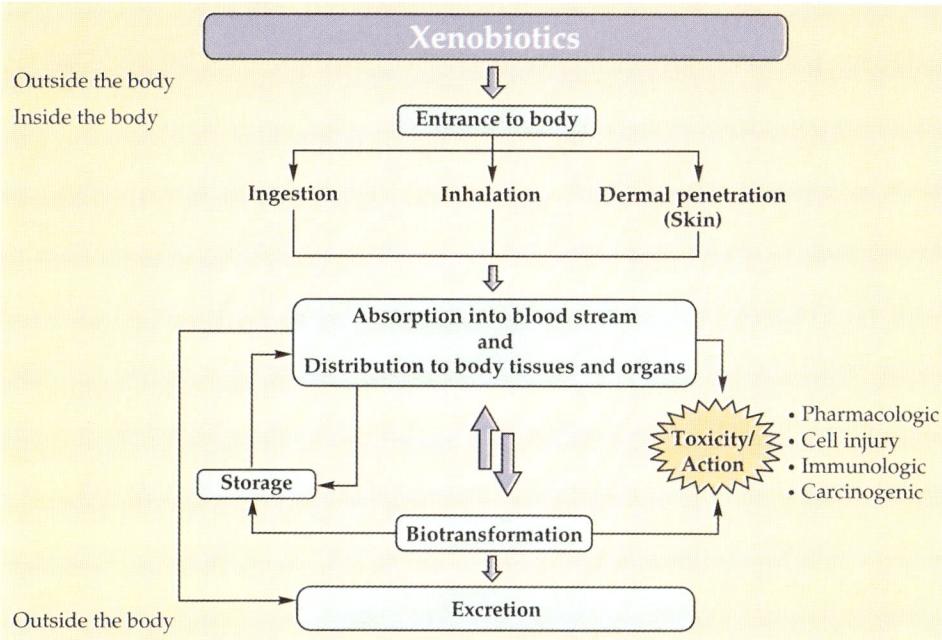

Fig. 16.2. Overview of metabolism of xenobiotics.

Distribution

After the compound is absorbed into the bloodstream, it rapidly circulates through the body. Most compounds don't spread out evenly through the body. Some drugs are distributed widely in all extracellular compartments while others concentrate in specific tissues such as liver and kidneys. Some bind tightly to blood protein and leave the bloodstream very slowly while others leave bloodstream quickly into other tissues and intracellular fluid. Thus, xenobiotics may distribute to only blood, or both blood and extracellular fluid, or to total body water (ECF + ICF), or be concentrated in particular tissues. The protein binding is reversible and depends on ionic and hydrophobic interactions. Competition of compounds for binding to blood proteins can lead to drug interactions. Only free fraction of the xenobiotic is biologically active and the binding to proteins tends to decrease elimination of the xenobiotic from the body.

Biotransformation

It is the process by which a drug is chemically altered by the body. The liver is the principal, but not the only, site of drug metabolism.

Excretion

It refers to the processes by which the body eliminates a drug. The kidneys are the major organs of excretion. They are particularly effective in eliminating water-soluble drugs and their metabolites. The kidneys filter drugs from the bloodstream and excrete them into the urine. The liver excretes some drugs through bile. These drugs enter the GI tract and end up in the faeces if they are not reabsorbed into the bloodstream or decomposed. Small amounts of drugs are also excreted in saliva, sweat, breast milk, and even in exhaled air.

Importance of biotransformation

1. **Inactivation or activation:** The products of biotransformation or metabolism are called metabolites. Metabolites may be inactive or they may have similar, lower or higher therapeutic activity or toxicity than the original drug.
2. **Increased solubility to help in excretion:** Biotransformation helps to make lipophilic compounds more soluble to aid excretion. During the process of biotransformation, the molecular structure of a drug is changed from one that is absorbed (lipophilic, or capable of crossing the lipid core of membranes) to one that can be readily eliminated from the body (incapable of crossing the lipid core of membranes, or hydrophilic). If lipophilic drugs are not metabolized, they will remain in the body for longer than intended, and their cumulative biological effects will eventually cause harm. Thus, the formation of water-soluble metabolites not only enhances drug elimination but also converts them to compounds that are generally pharmacologically inactive and relatively nontoxic.

Knowledge of the metabolism of xenobiotics is basic to a rational understanding of pharmacology and therapeutics, pharmacy, toxicology, management of cancer, and drug addiction. All these areas involve administration of, or exposure to, xenobiotics.

Q. 2. What can be the harmful effects of xenobiotics?

Ans. Xenobiotics and drugs or their active metabolites can have multiple effects like:

1. Enzyme or receptor activation or inhibition to produce therapeutic or toxic effects or drug interactions.
2. Covalent binding to macromolecules like proteins, RNA and DNA. Binding to proteins can lead to cell injury and immune response. While binding to DNA can lead to DNA damage and mutation which can cause cell injury, apoptosis or cancer (genotoxicity).

    If the macromolecule to which the reactive xenobiotic binds is essential for short-term cell survival, for example, a protein or enzyme involved in some critical cellular function such as oxidative phosphorylation or regulation of the permeability of the plasma membrane, then severe effects on cellular function could become evident quite rapidly.

    The reactive species of a xenobiotic may bind to a protein, altering its antigenicity. The xenobiotic is then said to act as a hapten, that is, a small molecule that by itself does not stimulate antibody synthesis but will combine with antibody once formed. The resulting antibodies can then damage the cell (Fig. 16.3).
3. Increased generation of oxidants – reactive oxygen or nitrogen species and lipid peroxidation

Q. 3. How are xenobiotics metabolized?

Ans. Metabolism of xenobiotics occurs mainly in liver and involves at least 30 different types of enzymes. Other sites include the gut, lungs, skin and kidneys. Many endogenous lipophilic compounds also use these enzymes for metabolism.

Biotransformation involves two phases of reactions (Fig. 16.4).

Phase I Reactions

Convert parent compound into a more polar (=hydrophilic) metabolite by adding or unmasking functional groups (–OH, –SH, –NH$_2$, –COOH, etc.). Main function of phase I

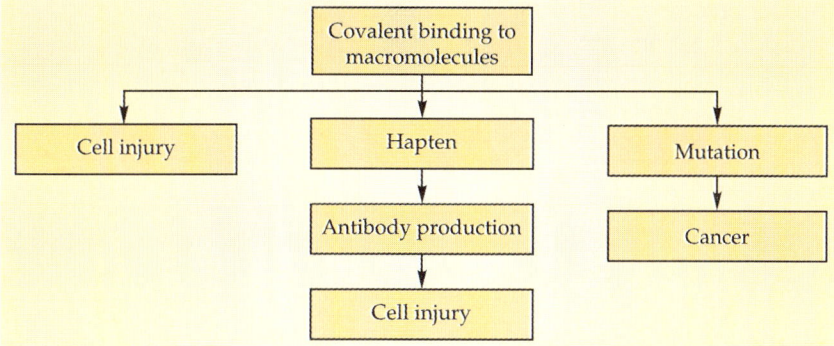

Fig. 16.3. Consequences of covalent binding of xenobiotics to cellular macromolecules.

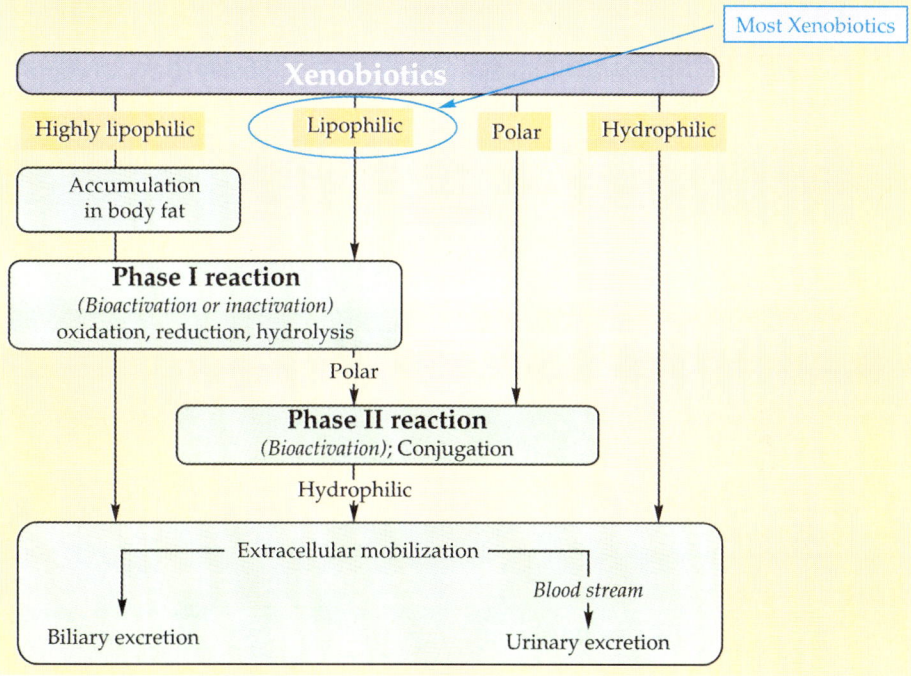

Fig. 16.4. Metabolism and excretion of xenobiotics.

reactions is to prepare chemicals for phase II metabolism (true detoxification step) and subsequent excretion. The reactions include:

- Oxidation (most xenobiotics and most common)
- Reduction (azo/nitro compunds, reduce aldehydes and ketones to hydroxyl compounds)
- Hydrolytic cleavage (esters and amides)
- Alkylation (methylation)
- Dealkylation
- Ring cyclization
- N-carboxylation

- Dimerization
- Isomerization
- Transamidation
- Decarboxylation

Oxidation

Oxidation is the most common and an important route of metabolism of most xenobiotics. There are two types of oxidation reactions:
- Oxygen is incorporated into the drug molecule (hydroxylation)
- Oxidation causes the loss of a part of the drug molecule (oxidative deamination, dealkylation, dehydrogenation).

Main enzymes involved in oxidation are: Mixed function oxidases or Cytochrome P450s (P450s), Aldehyde oxidase (AO), Xanthine oxidase (XO), Monoamine oxidases (MAOs) and Flavin-containing monooxygenases (FMOs).

Mixed function oxidases or monooxygenases are the most common and important enzymes for oxidation and can incorporate one oxygen atom in the parent compound. These are found in the smooth endoplasmic reticulum or microsomes of liver cells. The system is composed of two enzymes – Flavoprotein containing NADPH-cytochrome P450 reductase and cytochrome P450. The reaction uses 1 molecule of O_2; one atom is reduced to water, the other is incorporated into substrate to form –OH group (hydroxylation) (Fig. 16.5), e.g.
- Aromatic hydroxylation: lignocaine, analine, chlorobenzene (Fig. 16.6)
- Aliphatic hydroxylation: pentobarbitone (Fig. 16.7)

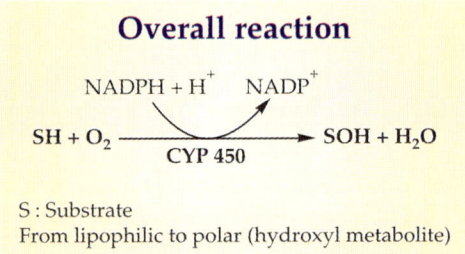

Fig. 16.5. Overall reaction of CYP450.

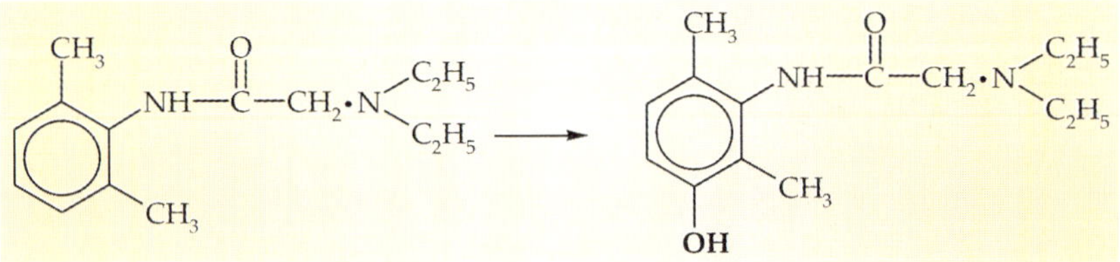

Fig. 16.6. 3-hydroxylation of lignocaine by CYP450.

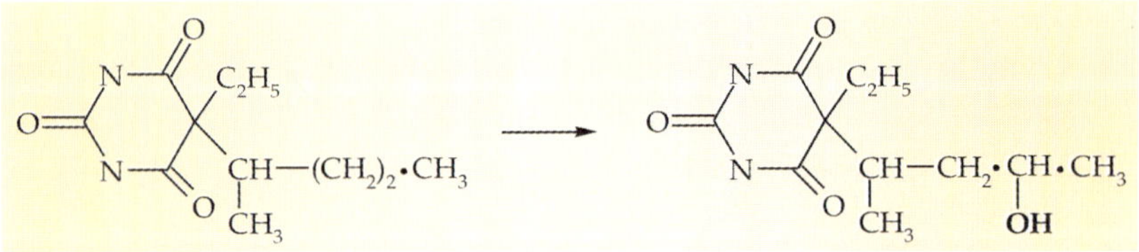

Fig. 16.7. Side chain hydroxylation of pentobarbitone.

- Epoxidation: benzopyrene (Fig. 16.8)
- N-demethylation of diazepam with production of HCHO (formaldehyde)
- Demethylation of codeine with production of HCHO (formaldehyde)
- S-demethylation of S-methylthiopurine with production of HCHO (formaldehyde)
- N-oxidation of 3-methylpyridine
- N-hydroxylation of 2-acetylaminofluorene (Fig. 16.9).

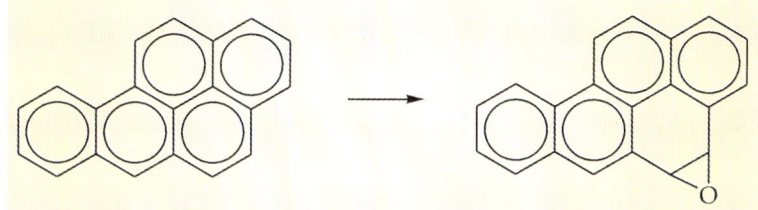

Fig. 16.8. Formation of benzo[a]pyrene-4,5-epoxide.

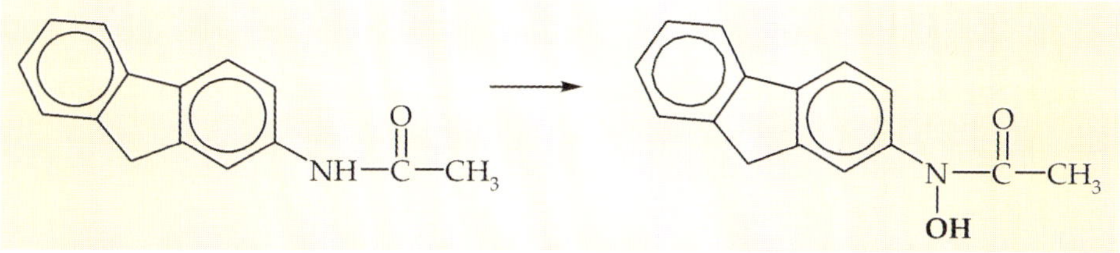

Fig. 16.9. N-hydroxylation of 2-acetylaminofluorene, a carcinogenic compound.

Oxidation reactions not catalyzed by Cytochrome P450 include:

- Flavin-containing monoxygenase system: Present mainly in liver but some is expressed in gut and lung, located in smooth endoplasmic reticulum, oxidizes compounds containing sulfur and nitrogen and uses NADH and NADPH as cofactors, e.g. cimetidine reduction.
- Alcohol dehydrogenase (cytosol).
- Aldehyde oxidation (cytosol).
- Xanthine oxidase.
- Amine oxidases.
- Monoamine oxidase (nerve terminals, mitochondria): Found in neurons, GIT, platelets and liver and primarily involved in oxidation of catecholamines.

Examples of other phase 1 reactions

- Azo and nitro reduction of prontosil and chloramphenicol
- Reduction of quinones
- Reductive cleavage of zonisamide and ziprasidone
- Hydrolysis, e.g. procaine and procainamide.

Phase II Reactions

Involve conjugation with endogenous substrate to further increase aqueous solubility. They include:

- Glucuronidation by UDP-glucuronosyltransferase (on –OH, –COOH, –NH$_2$, –SH groups)
- Sulfation by sulfotransferase (on –NH$_2$, –SO$_2$NH$_2$, –OH groups)
- Acetylation by acetyltransferase (on –NH$_2$, –SO$_2$NH$_2$, –OH groups)
- Amino acid conjugation (on –COOH groups)
- Glutathione conjugation by glutathione-S-transferase (to epoxides or organic halides)
- Fatty acid conjugation (on –OH groups)
- Condensation reactions
- Methylation (CH$_3$ donor – SAM)

Glucuronidation (Fig. 16.10)

Conjugation to α-d-glucuronic acid requires enzyme UDP-glucuronosyltransferase (UGT) and UDP-glucuronic acid. Quantitatively, glucuronidation is the most important and most frequent phase II pathway for drugs and endogenous compounds. Products are excreted in the bile. Enterohepatic recycling may occur due to gut glucuronidases (Fig. 16.10). Substrates include bilirubin, simple phenols, carboxylic acid, primary amines and opioids. There are 16 isoforms of UGT in humans classified under UGT1 and UGT2 groups. Examples: N-glucoronidation of sulfanilamde and cyproheptidine, O-glucoronidation of morphine, chloramphenicol, salicylic acid and ibuprofen, S-glucoronidation of methimazole, C-glucoronidation of phenylbutazone.

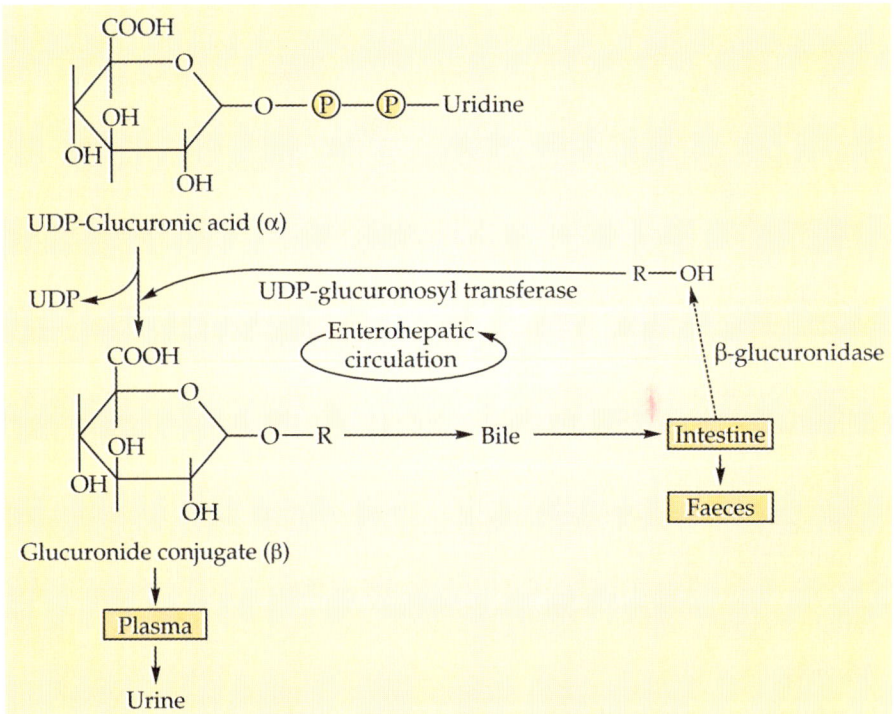

Fig. 16.10. Glucoronidation of a xenobiotic R and enterohepatic circulation.

Sulfation (Fig. 16.11)

Major pathway for phenols but also occurs for alcohols, amines and thiols. PAPS (3'-phosphoadenosine-5'-phosphosulfate) acts as the donor of sulphate groups. Sulfotransferases (=SULTs) catalyze transfer of sulfate to substrates. Phenol, alcohol and arylamine sulfotransferases are fairly non-specific while steroid sulfotransferases are very specific. Sulfation and glucuronidation are competing pathways. Sulfation predominates at low substrate concentrations while glucuronidation predominates at higher concentrations of xenobiotics. There is relatively less PAPS (75 nM) in cell cytosol compared to UDP-glucuronic acid (350 nM).

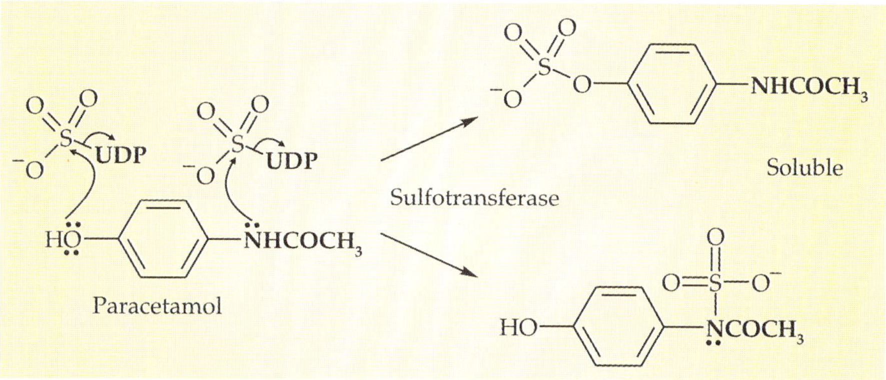

Fig. 16.11. Sulfation of paracetamol.

Acetylation

- Common reaction for aromatic amines and sulfonamides
- Requires co-factor acetyl-CoA
- Responsible enzyme is N-acetyltransferase (NAT)
- Takes place mainly in the liver
- Important in sulfonamide metabolism because acetyl-sulfonamides are less soluble than the parent compound and may cause renal toxicity due to precipitation in the kidney.

Genetic polymorphisms in N-acetylation enzymes have been identified in humans and other species. The human population is segregated into slow acetylators and fast acetylators based on the rates of acetylation of the drug isoniazid. The slow acetylator phenotype is the result of polymorphisms in the NAT2 gene. Slow acetylators are predisposed to toxicity of drugs that are inactivated by acetylation such as isoniazid and dapsone. This enzyme also acetylates aromatic amine dyes such as benzidine dyes, 4-aminobiphenyl, and o-toluidine to which workers are exposed in industries. Workers in the acrylamine dye industry who are slow acetylators have been shown to have an increased risk of bladder cancer. The low activity of NAT2 in the liver of slow acetylators may make the aromatic amines more available for hydroxylation. The resulting hydroxylamines then accumulate in the bladder acting as carcinogens.

Methylation

Catalysed by methyltransferases and SAM acts as the methyl donor. Methylation reactions are mainly involved with endogenous compounds such as melatonin, histamine, serotonin, dopamine, etc.), and with some xenobiotics like thiouracil, nicotine, 6-mercaptopurine and dopamine, etc. Acetylation and methylation do not improve solubility of xenobiotics but rather they reduce their pharmacological activity.

Glutathione conjugation (Fig. 16.12)

The tripeptide glutathione (GSH) is found in virtually all mammalian tissues and it contains a potent nucleophilic thiol group. The enzymes catalyzing GSH conjugation reactions are called glutathione S-transferases and are present in high amounts in liver cytosol and in lower amounts in other tissues. A variety of glutathione S-transferases are present in human tissue. Glutathione function as a scavenger of harmful electrophilic compounds ingested or

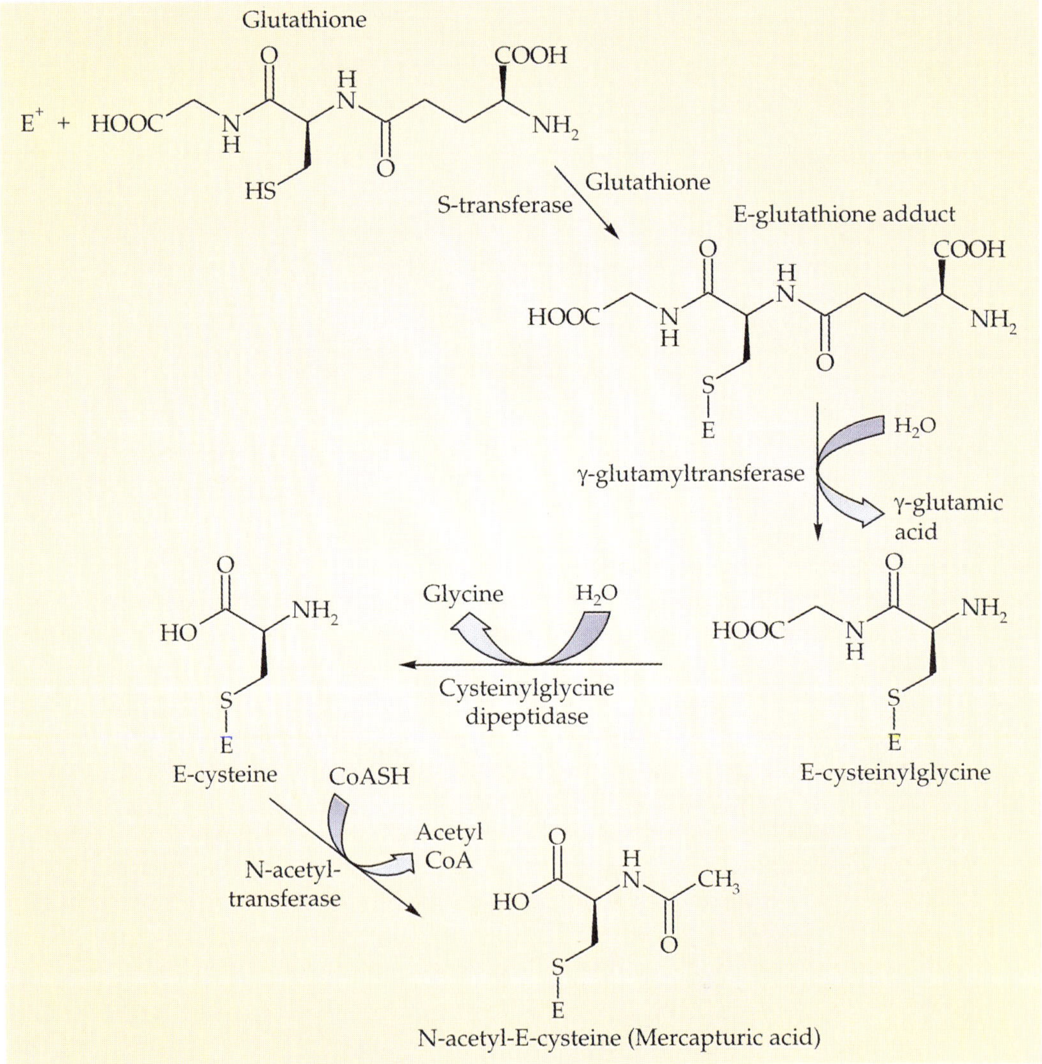

Fig. 16.12. Conjugation of an electrophile (E) glutathione and subsequent conversion to E-mercapturic acid conjugate.

produced by metabolism. Xenobiotics that are conjugated with glutathione are either highly electrophilic as such or are first metabolized to an electrophilic product prior to conjugation. Drug toxicity can result from the reaction of cellular nucleophiles with electrophilic metabolites if glutathione does not first intercept these reactive compounds. If the potentially toxic xenobiotics were not conjugated to GSH, they would be free to combine covalently with DNA, RNA, or cell protein and could thus lead to serious cell damage. GSH is therefore an important defence mechanism against toxic compounds, such as some drugs and carcinogens. If the levels of GSH in a tissue such as liver are lowered then that tissue can be shown to be more susceptible to injury by various chemicals that would normally be conjugated to GSH.

GSH conjugates are rarely excreted in urine due to their high molecular weight, they are excreted in the bile. Glutathione conjugates are subjected to further metabolism before excretion. The glutamyl and glycinyl groups belonging to glutathione are removed by specific enzymes, and an acetyl group (donated by acetyl-CoA) is added to the amino group of the remaining cysteinyl moiety. The resulting compound is a mercapturic acid, a conjugate of L-acetylcysteine, which is then excreted in the urine. This is also sometimes referred to as a phase III reaction (Fig. 16.12).

Glutathione has other important functions in human cells apart from its role in xenobiotic metabolism.

- It participates in the decomposition of potentially toxic hydrogen peroxide in the reaction catalyzed by glutathione peroxidase.
- It is an important intracellular reductant and antioxidant, helping to maintain essential SH groups of enzymes in their reduced state.
- A metabolic cycle involving GSH as a carrier is involved in the transport of certain amino acids across membranes in the kidney and GIT (Miester cycle).

Fatty acid conjugation

Stearic and palmitic acids are conjugated to drug by esterification reaction which occurs in liver endoplasmic reticulum, e.g. cannabinols are metabolized in this fashion.

Conjugation with amino acids

Carboxylic acids, particularly aromatic acids and arylacetic acids, are conjugated with polar endogenous amino acids. The quantity of amino acid conjugation is minute because of the limited availability of amino acids in the body and competition with glucuronidation for carboxylic acid substrates. Amino acids conjugation of carboxylic acids leads to amide bond formation. Glycine conjugates are the most common amino acid conjugates in animals. Conjugation with L-glutamine is most common in humans. Taurine, arginine, asparagine, histidine, lysine, glutamate, aspartate, alanine and serine conjugates also have been found. For example, benzoic acid (commonly used as a food preservative) is conjugated with glycine and then excreted (Fig. 16.13).

Phase III (Transportation/Efflux of xenobiotics)

- A family of ATP-dependent transport proteins found in the plasma membrane is involved. For example, P-glycoproteins MDR1 and MDR2 are responsible for Multiple Drug Resistance of some tumours.
- They act as ATP-dependent efflux pumps to remove a wide variety of toxic compounds.
- Their physiological role is in lipid transport across membranes.

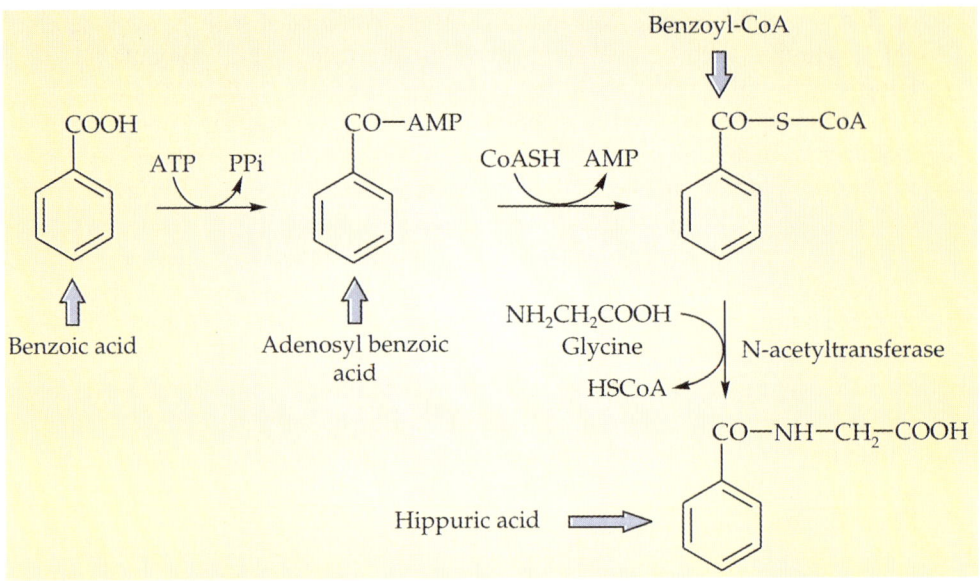

Fig. 16.13. Conjugation of benzoic acid with glycine.

Q. 4. Give examples of the reactions of xenobiotic metabolism participating in metabolism of endogenous compounds.

Ans. Conjugation and excretion of:
- Bilirubin – glucoronidation
- Bile salts – conjugation with taurine and glycine
- Catecholamines like dopamine, epinephrine and norepinephrine, serotonin and melatonin – oxidation, methylation, glucoronidation and sulphation
- Steroid hormones – glucoronidation and sulphation
- Thyroid hormones – 30% of T4 and T3 are conjugated in the liver to form sulfates and glucuronides
- Degradation of vitamin D and A.

Cytochrome P450 enzymes are involved in the synthesis of:

- Steroid hormones in adrenal, ovaries and testes
- Thromboxane A2, arachidonic acid and fatty acid metabolism
- Bile acid synthesis
- Cholesterol synthesis – lanosterol 14-alpha demethylase/CYP51A1.

Q. 5. Give examples of some xenobiotics activated during their metabolism.

Ans. *Activation vs Detoxification*

Activation and detoxification may occur as alternate pathways or as sequential reactions. The fate of any particular xenobiotic depends upon the competition between activation and detoxification reactions. Figs. 16.14, 16.15, 16.16 & 16.17 show the pathways of bioactivation and detoxification of some common xenobiotics and their harmful effects on body.

Xenobiotic Metabolism, Antioxidants and Biochemistry of Ageing

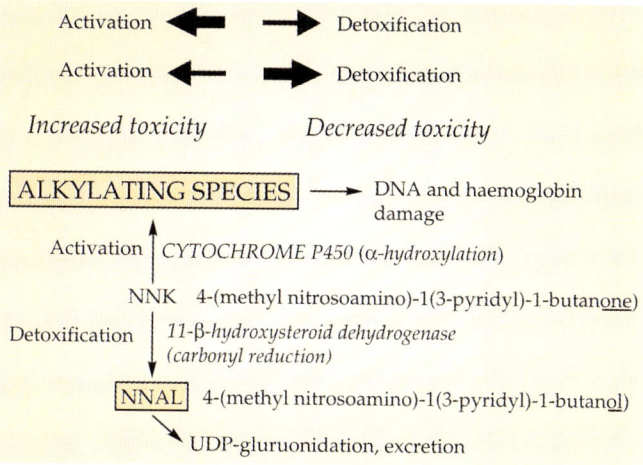

Fig. 16.14. Balance between activation and detoxification. For example, activation and detoxicification of NNK found in tobacco smoke.

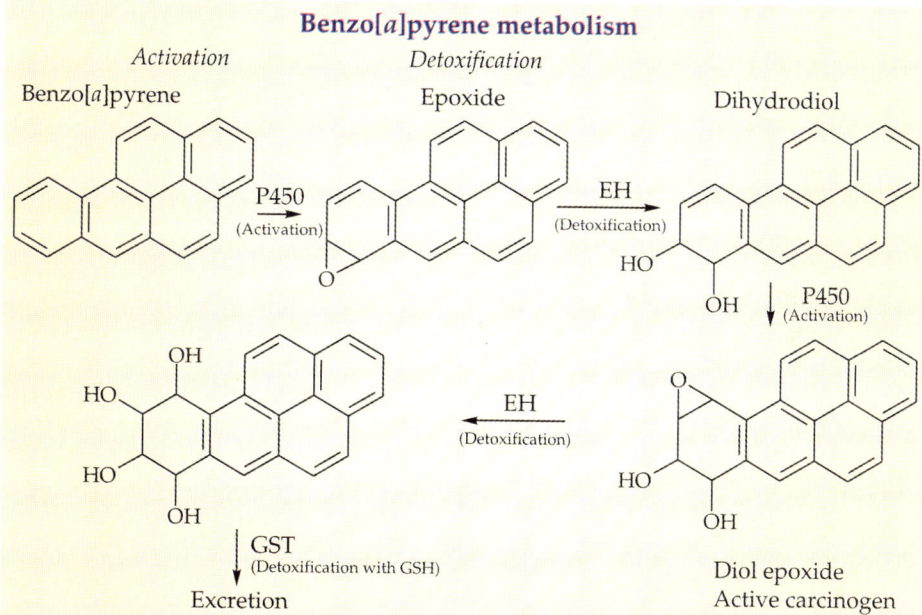

Fig. 16.15. Activation and detoxification of benzo(a)pyrene found in vehicle exhaust and tobacco smoke. EH = Epoxide hydroxylase.

Polymorphisms of different enzymes involved in these pathways can alter the genetic susceptibility to damage caused by these xenobiotics.

- NNK in tobacco smoke (nicotine-derived nitrosamine ketone) (Fig. 16.14).
- Benzo[a]pyrene (Fig. 16.15).
- Quinones (Fig. 16.16).
- Acetaminophen (crocin or paracetamol) (Fig. 16.17).

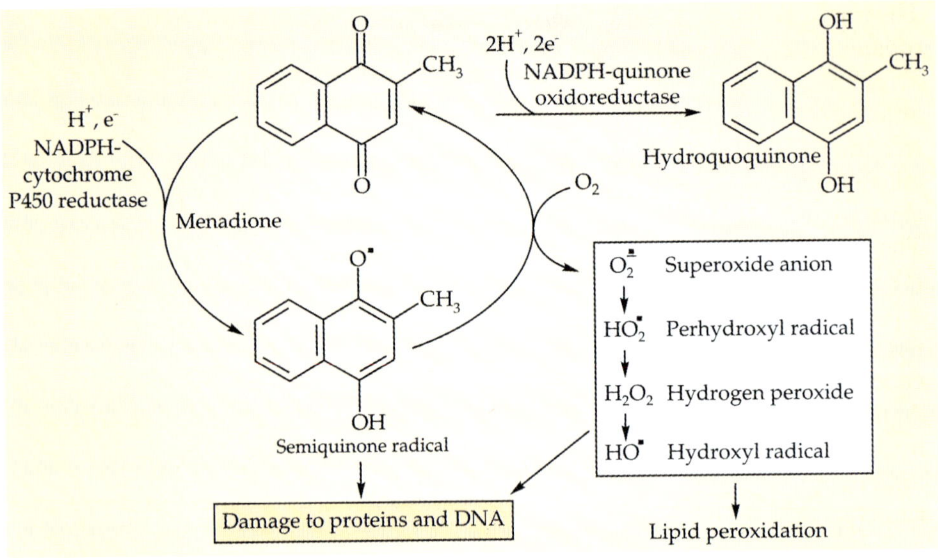

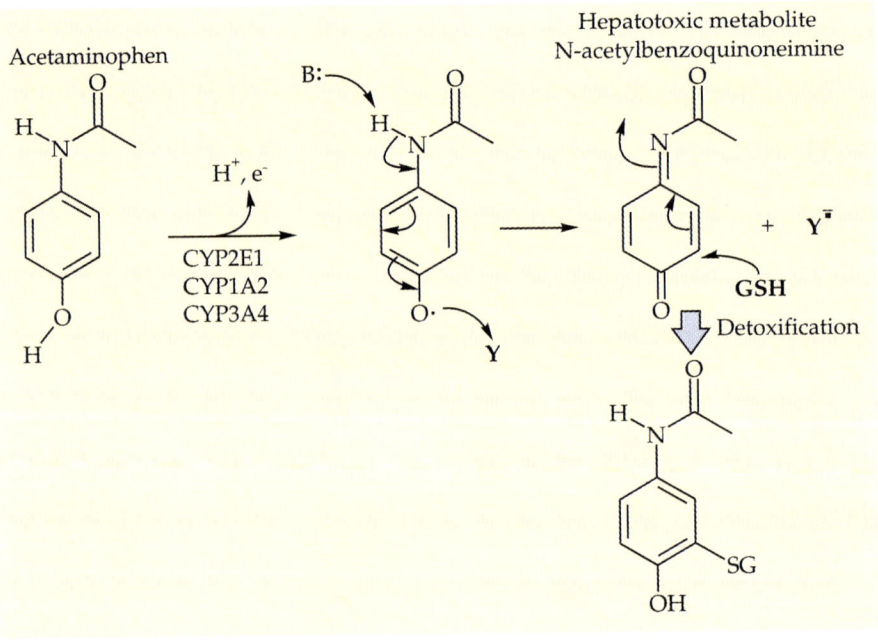

Fig. 16.16. Bioactivation of quinones and further detoxification to hydroquinones.

Fig. 16.17. Bioactivation and detoxification of paracetamol (acetaminophen).

Q. 6. What is the effect of caloric restriction on longevity?

Ans. *Caloric restriction and longevity*

- Early nutritional studies showed that rats fed a low-calorie, but balanced and nutritious diet lived nearly twice as long as rats with unlimited access to food (2.4 years versus 1.3 years).

- The relationship between diet and longevity was found to be a general one applicable for organisms from yeast to mammals.
- To achieve this effect of caloric restriction (CR), animals are given a level of food that amounts to 60% to 70% of what they would eat if they were allowed free access to food.
- In animals, CR results in lower blood glucose levels, declines in glycogen and fat stores, enhanced responsiveness to insulin, lower body temperature, and diminished reproductive capacity.
- The extended life span due to CR has evolutionary advantage: Any animal that could slow the aging process and postpone reproduction in times of food scarcity and then resume reproduction when food became available has better chances of survival.
- CR also diminishes the likelihood for development of many age-related diseases, such as cancer, diabetes, and atherosclerosis and reduces chronic inflammation.
- At metabolic level, caloric restriction with adequate nutrition has been shown to improve insulin sensitivity, reduce fasting glucose and insulin concentration, reverse the abnormal lipid deposited in large adipose cells, and prevent obesity, type 2 diabetes, hypertension and chronic inflammation.
- In humans also research has also shown that caloric restriction to 600 kcal/day can potentially cure patients with recent onset type 2 DM.

Biochemical mechanisms of the caloric restriction effect on metabolism: Action of SIRT1 protein – Sirtuin protein SIRT1 connects nutrient availability to the expression of genes controlling metabolism.

- Sirtuins are NAD-dependent protein deacetylases which remove acetyl groups from lysine residues of histones, the core proteins of nucleosomes. Acetyl groups inhibit interaction of histone with DNA and removal of acetyl groups allow the nucleosomes to interact more strongly with DNA, thus inhibiting transcription.
- Sirtuin activity is controlled by NAD/NADH ratio which is an indicator of cellular energy status. Nicotinamide and NADH are strong inhibitors of the deacetylase reaction. High NAD levels activate sirtuin action, while high NADH levels inhibit activity.
- Mitochondrial oxidative metabolism converts NADH to NAD and so enhances sirtuin activity.
- Caloric restriction leads to increased number of mitochondria in liver, fat and muscle, which act to raise the NAD/NADH ratio and thus increase sirtuin activity.
- SIRT1 interaction with PPARγ (peroxisome proliferator-activator receptor-γ) leads to inhibition of genes regulated by PPARγ. These genes promote adipogenesis and fat storage. SIRT1 binding to PPARγ represses transcription of these genes, leading to loss of fat stores, the main effect of caloric restriction.
- Because adipose tissue functions as an endocrine organ, loss of fat has significant hormonal consequences for energy metabolism, decreasing insulin resistance and chronic inflammation.
- In liver, SIRT1 interacts with and deacetylates PGC-1 (peroxisome proliferatoractivator receptor-γ coactivator-1), a transcriptional regulator of genes involved in glucose production. Thus, CR through increased sirtuin levels leads to increased transcription of the genes encoding the enzymes of gluconeogenesis and repression of genes encoding glycolytic enzymes. Thus gluconeogenesis is increased and glycolysis decreased.
- Caloric restriction leads to reduction in the production of damaging ROS.

Resveratrol, a phytoalexin compound found in red wine, is a potent activator of sirtuin activity. Phytoalexins are compounds produced by plants in response to stress, injury, or fungal infection. Resveratrol is abundant in wine grape skins as a result of common environmental stresses, such as infection by *Botrytis cinerea*, a fungus used in making wines. Resveratrol might be the basis of the French paradox—the fact that the French people enjoy longevity and relative freedom from heart disease despite a high-fat diet.

Q. 7. Describe the relative importance of various antioxidants. Why exogenous antioxidant supplements have little effect or may even be harmful?

Ans. *Antioxidants*

Multiple substances provide physiologic antioxidant action. Besides bilirubin and GSH, uric acid, ascorbate, vitamins A and E, ergothioneine, and possibly melatonin are physiologic antioxidants. It is difficult to assess the relative importance of these substances. Physiological antioxidants include:
- Endogenous: bilirubin, melatonin, GSH, and uric acid
- Exogenous: such as vitamins A and E, ascorbate, and ergothioneine
- Lipophilic: bilirubin, vitamins E and A
- Water soluble: GSH, ascorbate, uric acid, and ergothioneine

- **Melatonin:** It is a direct scavenger of radical oxygen and nitrogen species including OH, O_2^-, and NO. Melatonin works with other antioxidants to improve the overall effectiveness of each antioxidant. Melatonin has been proven to be twice as active as vitamin E. An important characteristic of melatonin that distinguishes it from other classic radical scavengers is that its metabolites are also scavengers in what is referred to as the cascade reaction. It has particular role in the protection of nuclear and mitochondrial DNA.
- **Vitamin E:** It reacts with lipid peroxides to reduce them to fatty acids, itself forming the relatively stable tocopheroxyl radical, which persists long enough to undergo reduction back to tocopherol by reaction with vitamin C at the surface of the cell or lipoprotein (Fig. 16.18).
- **Ascorbate, uric acid and a variety of polyphenols derived from plant foods** act as water-soluble radical trapping antioxidants. These form relatively stable radicals that persist long enough to undergo reaction to non-radical products or to be excreted in urine. Ubiquinone and carotenes similarly act as lipid-soluble radical-trapping antioxidants in membranes and plasma lipoproteins.
- **Vitamin C:** On reaction with free radicals it is converted to monodehydroascorbate radical which then undergoes enzymatic reduction back to ascorbate or a nonenzymic reaction of 2 mols of monodehydroascorbate to yield 1 mol each of ascorbate and dehydroascorbate (excreted in urine).

Other antioxidant mechanisms

- Metal ions that can generate oxygen radicals by non-enzymatic reactions (Fenton reaction, etc.) are bound to proteins as the prosthetic group, or to specific transport and storage proteins keeping them unreactive. Iron is bound to transferrin, ferritin, and hemosiderin, copper to ceruloplasmin, and other metal ions are bound to metallothionein.

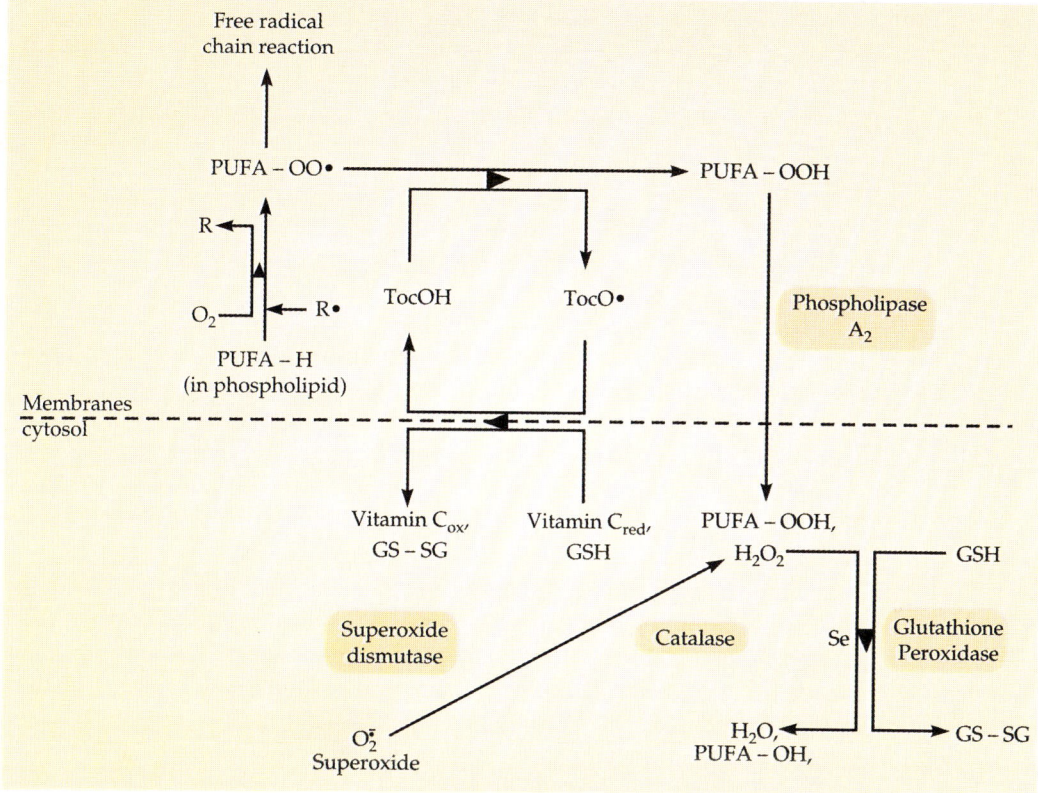

Fig. 16.18. Recycling of vitamin E with the help of vitamin C and GSH.

- Protective enzymes:
  - SOD and catalase: Superoxide is produced both accidentally and also as the reactive oxygen species required for a number of enzyme-catalyzed reactions. A family of superoxide dismutases catalyze the reaction between superoxide and protons to yield oxygen and hydrogen peroxide. The hydrogen peroxide is then removed by catalase and various peroxidases: $2H_2O_2 \rightarrow 2H_2O + O_2$.
  - Glutathione peroxidase: The peroxides that are formed by radical damage to lipids in membranes and plasma lipoproteins are reduced to hydroxy fatty acids by glutathione peroxidase, a selenium-dependent enzyme.

Exogenous antioxidant supplements are little helpful or may even be harmful under some conditions:

- Early epidemiological studies suggested that vitamin E is protective against atherosclerosis and cardiovascular disease. However, clinical trials showed increased mortality among those taking (high dose) supplements. Vitamin E acts as an antioxidant by forming a stable radical that persists long enough to undergo metabolism to non-radical products. However, it also means that the radical also persists long enough to penetrate deeper into the lipoprotein, causing further radical damage, rather than interacting with a water-soluble antioxidant at the surface of the lipoprotein!

- Antioxidants can also be pro-oxidants:
    (a) Vitamin C: Large concentration of vitamin C can also be a source of superoxide radicals by reaction with oxygen, and hydroxyl radicals by reaction with Cu^{2+} ions, but usually such concentrations cross renal threshold and vitamin C is lost in urine. Excess vitamin C can be metabolized to oxalate and excess vitamin C in urine can promote growth of bacteria acting as risk factor for urinary tract infections.

    $$Ascorbate + O_2 \rightarrow O_2^{\bullet} + Monodehydroascorbate$$
    $$Ascorbate + Cu^{2+} \rightarrow Cu^+ + Monodehydroasacorbate$$
    $$Cu^+ + H_2O_2 \rightarrow Cu^{2+} + OH^- + OH^{\bullet}$$

    (b) Though carotene was suggested to be protective against lung and other cancers, intervention trials showed an increase in death from lung (and other) cancer among people given supplements of β-carotene. Although β-carotene is a radical-trapping antioxidant under conditions of low partial pressure of oxygen, as in most tissues, at high partial pressures of oxygen (as in the lungs) and especially in high concentrations, β-carotene is an autocatalytic pro-oxidant, and hence can initiate radical damage to lipids and proteins.
- Exogenous antioxidants once oxidized need to be excreted or recycled to reduced form with the help of endogenous antioxidants like GSH and bilirubin. Further, the oxidized form of exogenous oxidants in large concentration may themselves act as oxidants. Endogenous antioxidants are present in low concentration and yet very effective due to rapid recycling in the body.
- One approach to consider the relative importance of antioxidant substances is to compare their endogenous concentrations. Circulating and tissue GSH levels range from 1 to 10 mM, probably the highest of the physiologic antioxidants. The approximate circulating concentrations of other substances are 30–100 μM ascorbate (vitamin C), 0.3–0.6 μM β-carotene, 2–28 μM α-tocopherol (vitamin E), 1 mM ergothioneine, 0.2–0.4 mM uric acid, 50 pmol/L melatonin, and 5–15 μM bilirubin, while tissue concentrations are significantly lower. The levels of oxidant species are in the mM range i.e. 1000 times higher than many of these antioxidants! In cytoplasm the –SH groups of GSH system are the most important antioxidants.
- The reducing power for endogenous antioxidant GSH and bilirubin/biliverdin is ultimately derived from NADPH which is available abundantly and freely from glucose metabolism (HMP pathway). It is evident by the clinical consequences of G-6-PD deficiency.

    Such comparisons can, however, at times be misleading. The antioxidant actions of bilirubin may be amplified 10,000 times or more by the BVR (Biliverdin reductase) cycle. GSH undergoes some cycling with GSH peroxidase oxidizing GSH to GS-SG, after which GSH reductase recycles it back to GSH. Lipid and protein oxidation increases manifold by BVR and GSH depletion respectively in knockout experiments. This implies that these 2 substances are the major physiologic antioxidants.

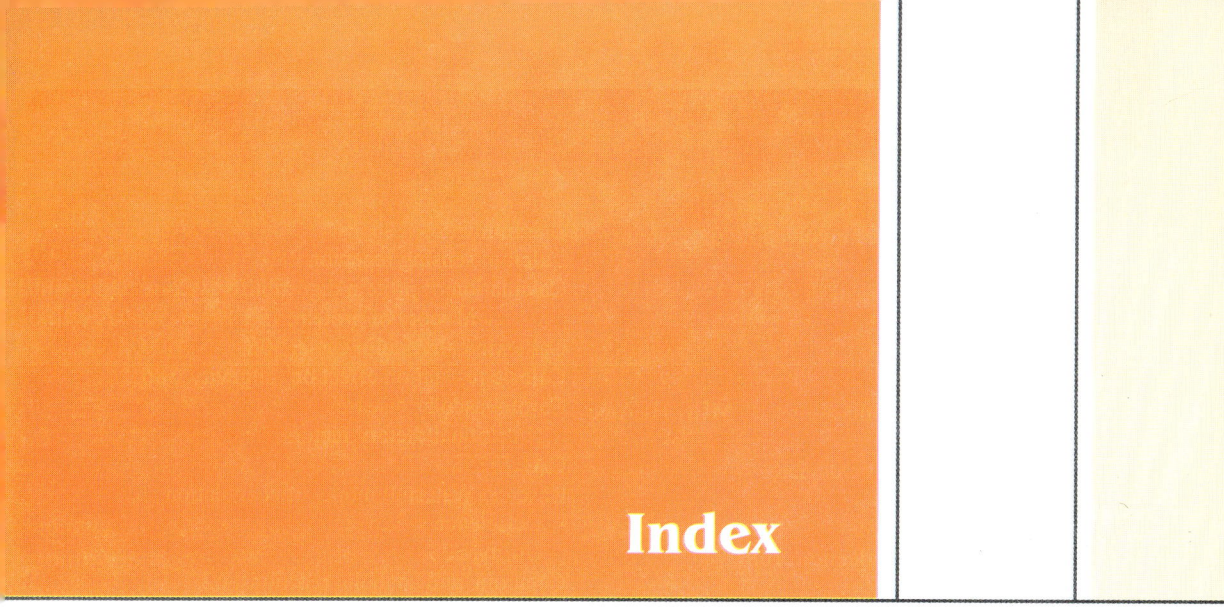

Index

A

ABC transporters, 252
   Clinical significance, 252
   Present in human tissues, 253
Action of ionophores, 252
Action of telomerase, 223
Activation and detoxification of benzo(a)pyrene found in vehicle exhaust and tobacco smoke, 385
Activation by selective proteolysis of pro-enzyme
   Advantages, 58
Activation of procarcinogen benzo(a)pyrene to active carcinogen, 214
Acyl CoA synthetase, 42, 66
   Converting ATP to AMP rather than ADP, 65
   Energetics, 67
Acute hyperammonemia,
   Treatment, 162
Adenylate kinase reaction and the relative changes in concentration of ATP, ADP and AMP with ATP use, 269
Adipose tissue
   Adipokines and other factors responsible for consequences of obesity, 273
Aerobic metabolism, 95
Agents interfering with oxidative phosphorylation, 69
Aggrecan structure, 299
AGRP, 256
β-Alanine
   Physiological significance, 180

Alanine cycle, 264
Aldehyde dehydrogenase, 68
Allosteric enzymes, 54
Allosteric modulator, 54
Allotypes, 367
Amino acid transporters and associated disorders, 158
Amino acids
   Nutritionally essential and non-essential, 143
   Transport across cell membranes, 157
22nd Amino acid, 12
β-Aminoisobutyric acid
   Physiological significance, 180
Ammonia toxicity, 161
Ammonium sulphate, $(NH_4)_2SO_4$
   Use for salting out, 26
AMP-activated protein kinase, 269
AMPK regulated enzymes in liver, 270
Amphipathic molecules, 2
Anaemias due to defect in enzymes involved in RBC metabolism
   Biochemical basis, 91
Anaerobic exercise training
   Effects on glycolysis in athletes, 80
Anaerobic metabolism, 96
Analogous proteins, 40
Anaplerotic, or "Filling Up", reactions, 103, 105, 106
Anorexia nervosa, 260
Antioxidants, 388
Antiviral defence of innate immune system, 338
apo B100 and apo B48 producion from same gene, 127

391

apo B-containing lipoproteins
   Inherited causes of low levels, 140
Apolipoproteins and enzymes involved in lipoprotein/lipid transport
   Function and consequences of defects, 135
Arginine synthesis, 154, 155
Arthritis, 304
Ascites in cirrhosis, 314
Association of autoimmune diseases with MHC/HLA alleles, 349
Asymmetric distribution of lipids, 240
Atherosclerosis, 304
   Role of LDL and HDL, 135
ATP depletion and urate production, 108
ATP energy transfer, 65
ATP synthesis on inner mitochondrial membrane, 76
ATP-producing processes
   Activation by AMPK, 270
ATP-requiring processes
   Inhibition by AMPK, 270
Autoimmune diseases, 348
Autoimmunity, 348

B

Base stacking in ssDNA on interaction with water, 3
BCAA catabolism in muscles
   Contribution to glucose alanine cycle, 151
BCKA dehydrogenase complex, 152
Benzoic acid, conjugation with glycine, 384
Benzo(a)pyrene 4,5 epoxide, 379
   DNA adducts, 214
Beta-oxidation, 116
   Inborn errors, 118
BH4
   De novo synthesis, 164
   Regeneration, 165
   Requiring enzymes, 163
Bioactivation and detoxification of paracetamol, 386
Bioactivation of quinones and detoxification to hydroquinones, 386
Biochemical basis for co-operativity, 55
Branched and unbranched chains of glycogen, 111
Branched-chain amino acid metabolism, 149, 150
Branched-chain keto acid dehydrogenase complex regulation, 151
Bulimia, 260
Bulky adduct formed by benzo(a)pyrene, 214
Butylated hydroxyanisole (BHA)/E320, 122

C

Calcimimetics, 280
Calcium sensing receptor, 280
Calculation of protein digestibility – Corrected amino acid score of protein, 195
Calnexin/calreticulin cycle, 306
Caloric restriction effect on longevity, 386
Cardiovascular diseases
   Nutritional/dietary factors, 196
CART, 256
Cascade/Waterfall model of coagulation
   Deficiencies, 328
   Utility, 328
Catabolic and anabolic reactions, 62
Catalysis mechanisms, 47
Caveolae, 241, 244
Caveolae and planar lipid rafts, 245
Caveolin, 246
CBP300, 287, 289
CCK, 256
Cell-based model of coagulation, 327-329
   Advantages, 336
   Phases/stages of coagulation, 332
Cellular transport of lactate, 97
Central and peripheral tolerance, 344
Central control of appetite, 255
Central role of thrombin, 336
Ceramide-containing compounds, 128
Child-Pugh classification of cirrhosis, 327
Cholecalciferol synthesis from 7-dehydrocholesterol in skin, 189
Cholesterol balance in cells, 132
Cholesterol in plasma membranes
   Role and functions, 234
Cholesterol metabolism
   Regulation role of liver X receptors, 127
Cholesterol synthesis pathway
   Useful compounds synthesized, 121
Chylomicrons, 127
Citric acid cycle
   Key role of vitamins, 90
Class, 36
Co-activators, 285
Co-factors, 47
Co-factor, co-enzyme and prosthetic group
   Differences, 47
Co-operative enzymes
   No hyperbolic dependence of the velocity on substrate concentration, 56

Coenzymes, 47
Cold agglutinin disease, 371
Cold agglutinins, 369
Compartmentation/separation of anabolic and catabolic pathways involving same metabolites, 57
Conditions limiting the rate of cellular respiration during exercise, 72
Configuration and conformation, 19
Conjugation of benzoic acid with glycine, 384
Consequences of covalent binding of xenobiotics to cellular macromolecules, 377
Consequences of DNA damage and mutation, 215
Conserved residues in enzymes, 48
CoQ, 121
Cori's cycle, 264
Coupling of catabolism (exergonic) and anabolism (endergonic), 63
Covalent modification by phosphorylation
    Advantages, 58
Covalent modifications to regulate enzyme activity, 58
Cryoglobulins, 369
'Curd' formation, 78
Cyanide toxicity
    Mechanism and features, 71
    Symptoms, 72
    Treatment, 72
Cystic fibrosis
    Coconut oil for malabsorption, 118
CYP450, 378

D

Death fold, 39
Decorin and TGFβ action, 297
Degradation of intracellular enzymes, 58
Dehydrogenases, 68
2-Deoxyfluoroglucose (FDG)
    Clinical significance, 87, 89
Depurination of DNA, 212
Development of autoimmunity, 351
Dextrose and dextrin
    Differentiation, 81
$\Delta G°$, $\Delta G°'$ and ΔG
    Difference, 61
Diabetes mellitus
    Type 1, metabolic defects, 279
    Type 2, metabolic defects, 277
Dietary bases and nucleosides from nucleic acids in food
    Fate of, 170

Dietary goitrogens, 198
Dietary therapy used for refractory seizures, 119
Dipole, 1
Distribution of Tyr and Trp in integral membrane proteins, 237
Disulfide bonds, 27
    Formation, 32
    Production in proteins, 31
    Role in hair curling and straightening, 30
    Significance, 28
D-Lactic acidosis, 99
DNA damage, 209, 210, 215
DNA mutation, 209, 215
DNA replication, 220
    Eukaryotes and prokaryotes in DNA replication
    Similarities and differences, 223
DNA tautomerization, 207
2,4-DNP or 2,4-dinitrophenol, 69
Dolichol, 121
Domain, 33
Domains or modules
    Examples, 37
Double-stranded DNA, 3
Drugs used to prevent graft rejection, 364

E

Eadie–Hofstee equation, 52
Early fasting state, 262
Eating behaviour
    Regulation in humans, 255
    Satiety control, 255
Effect of cholesterol on transition temperature of membrane, 235
Effect of pH on enzyme activity, 51
Effect of pH on protein solubility, 24
Effector mechanisms of graft damage, 358
Electrophiles, 3
Electrophoresis of lipoproteins, 127
End replication problem, 220, 221
Enhancers, 284-286
Enolase
    Clinical significance, 87
Enzyme activity effect of substrate concentration, 51
Enzyme classification, 46
Enzyme functioning by covalent catalysis, 48
Enzyme-dependent movement of lipids, 241
Eruptive xanthomas, 130
Essential fatty acid deficiency, 125
Essential and non-essential amino acids, 144
Essential fatty acids, 124
Evaluation of abnormal liver function tests, 326

F

Factors released by adipose tissues responsible for consequences of obesity, 273
Familial hypercholesterolemia, 130
   Treatment, 134
Family, 39
Farnesyl anchor, 238
Fatty acid synthesis
   Factors regulating, 124
Fatty acids
   Shapes, 247
FDG applications, 89
Fed state, 260
Feeding and satiety
   Disorders, 260
Feed and starve cycle, 260
Fibrous, globular and membrane proteins, 18
Fibrous proteins, 17
FIGLU test, 184
Fischer's 'lock and key model', 48
Fish oil – protection against myocardial infarction, 126
Folate deficiency, 184
   Biochemical and clinical consequences, 186
Folate functions in body, 184
Folate metabolism and folate trap, 188
Folate trap, 186
Fold, 37
Folding of a polypeptide due to interaction with water, 4
Folic acid deficiency tests, 186
Fredrickson classification of hyperlipoproteinemia, 135
Free carnitine decreased levels, 118
   Biochemical basis, 118
   Clinical manifestations, 118
   Diagnosis, 118
Free radicals, 73
Frohlich's syndrome, 260
Frostbite, 9
Fructose metabolism, 106, 107
   Harmful effects of excess consumption, 106
   In sweetened beverages, 106
Fuel metabolism in starvation, 262
Functional enzymes of blood, 49

G

G6PDH deficiency, 93
GAG types, 294
GAGs structure of different types, 296
Galactosaemia, 80
Galactose
   Compounds derived from, 80
Gaucher's disease, 128
Gene expression
   Effect of hormones, 284
General acid base catalysis, 47
Geranylgeranyl anchor, 238
Ghrelin, 258
Globin fold, 37
Globular proteins, 17
GLP-1 and related drugs
   Action, 90
Glucagon-like peptide (GLP)
   Clinical significance, 87, 89
Gluconeogenesis
   Role of beta oxidation of fatty acids, 114
Glucoronidation of a xenobiotic R and enterohepatic circulation, 380
Glucose homeostasis, 260, 266
Glucose tolerance test, 191
Glucose utilization by various processes, 77
Glutamate aspartate exchanger, 74
Glutamate aspartate transporter (GLAST), 74
Glutaminolysis in intestinal epithelium, lymphocytes and macrophages, 264
Glutathione, 32
   Conjugation, 382
Glycemic index, 191
   Classification, 192
Glycemic load, 191
Glycerophosphate and malate aspartate shuttle
   Differences, 73
Glycerophosphate shuttle, 73
Glycine cleavage system, 146
Glycine metabolism, 145
Glycine metabolism and associated clinical implications, 144
Glycogen metabolism in liver and muscle
   Differentiation, 83
Glycogen structure (Whelan's model), 110
   Advantages, 112
Glycogen storage diseases, 85-87
Glycolysis
   Feed forward activation, 102
   Inhibition by arsenite and arsenate, Differences, 82
   Inborn Errors of metabolism, 91
Glycoprotein
   Actual proportion of complex glycans, 292

Glycosaminoglycans, 294
    Different types, 294
    Structure, 296
Glycosylation, 291
Goitrogenic factors, 197
Gout, 179
    Role of alcohol, 178
Graphs to study the relation of Vi versus substrate concentration, 52

H

Haemoglobin
    Role in the action of nitric oxide, 44
Haemolytic anemias, 91
    Enzyme defects, 92
Haemophilia, 336
Hanes equation, 52
HDL metabolism – High levels of HDL-C
    Genetic disorders, 142
HDL metabolism – Low levels of HDL
    Genetic disorders, 140
HDL
    Role in atherosclerosis, 135
Heme A, 121
Heme degradation products, 166
Heparan sulphate, 304
Heparin, 304
Heparin and heparan sulfate
    Differences, 305
Heterotropic effect, 54
Hexokinase IV/glucokinase, 94
Hexokinases I, II, and III, 93
Hill equation and plot, 52, 53
Histidine metabolism, 185
HIV treatment combination therapy, 218
HIV virus
    Life cycle, 219
HMG CoA synthase
    Inborn error of metabolism 117
Hofmeister series, 26
Homogentisate oxidase, 68
Homologous proteins, 40, 41
Homotropic effect, 54
Hormones with cell surface receptors regulating transcription, 289
HRE, 284, 286
HRE, AFE, the hormone receptor complex, and the coactivators, 286
Human erythrocyte
    Actual glycocalyx, 292

Human proteins and their functions, 17
Hydrolases, 46
Hydroperoxidases, 68
Hydroxylase cycle, 68, 69
3-Hydroxylation of lignocaine by CYP450, 378
N-Hydroxylation of 2-acetylaminofluorene, 379
Hyperammonemia
    Effects on brain, 160
Hyperbilirubinemia
    Isolated, 318
Hyperlactatemia and lactic acidosis, 98
    Biochemical basis of causes, 98
Hyperlipoproteinemias
    Fredrickson classification, 135
        Type I, 136
        Type IIa, 136
        Type IIb, 138
        Type III, 138
        Type IV, 139
        Type V, 139
Hyperuricemia
    Causes, 176
Hyperuricemia in Von Gierke's disease
    Mechanism, 109
Hyperviscosity syndrome, 9
Hypothalamic satiety network, neurochemistry, 256
Hydroxylase cycle, 378

I

Idiotypes, 367
Inhibition of glycolysis by arsenate, 82
Inhibition of glycolysis by arsenite, 82
Inhibitors and uncouplers
    Difference, 71
Inhibitors and uncouplers of ETC, 71
Inhibitors of ETC, 69
Initial rate/velocity of reaction, 51
Insulin
    Glucose homeostasis, 261
    Promoter, 285
    Regulation of eating behaviour, 258
Integral and peripheral membrane proteins, 236
Interaction of amphiphatic phospholipid molecules, 2
Intolerance to milk, 79
Intramitochondrial NADPH, 73
    Sources, 73
Intravenous imiglucerase or recombinant glucocerebrosidase use, 128
Intrinsically unstructured proteins (IUPs), 20, 21
    Significance, 22

Iodine deficiency disorders, 198
Iodine excess, 204
Iodine intake
   Recommendations by age or population group, 198
Iodine nutrition based on median urinary iodine
   Concentrations in school-age children, 204
Ionophores, 249
Irreversible reactions, 50
Isoelectric pH, 13
Isoelectric pH of amino acids
   Calculation, 13
Isoelectric point, 13, 14
Isoenzymes, 59
Isoenzymes of hexokinase
   Differentiation, 93
   Metabolic significance, 94
Isoionic point, 13
Isomerases, 46
Isoprenoid anchors, 238
Isotypes, 367
Isotype, allotype, and idiotype determinants of an antibody, 368

K

Ketogenesis
   Regulation, 116
Ketogenic diet
   Uses, 119
Ketone and ketone bodies
   Differentiation, 114
Ketone bodies
   Organs consuming, 116
   Organs producing, 116
Ketone body synthesis
   Regulation, 116
Kinetics and Km of hexokinase and glucokinase, 95
Koshland's induced fit model of enzyme action, 48
Krabbe's disease, 129

L

Lactic acid production and utilization (Cori cycle), 97
Lactate plasma levels
   Clinical significance, 95
Lactate shuttle in cancer, 102
Lactic acidosis
   Biochemistry, 95
   Pathogenesis, 100
   Role of anaerobic metabolism, 95
   Types, 95, 98

Lactobacillus delbrueckii subsp. *bulgaricus*, 78
Lactulose and lactose
   Differentiation, 81
LDL
   Role in atherosclerosis, 135
Lectins, 308
Leptin, 256
Leucine glutamate cycle in neurons and astrocytes,s153
Ligases, 46
Limiting factor/states of respiratory control, 72
Lineweaver–Burk plot, 52
Lipid anchors, 238
   Types, 239
Lipid anchors for attachment of membrane proteins, 238
Lipid organisation in raft microdomains, 244
Lipid peroxidation, 123
Lipid raft, 241
Lipid storage disease causing severe demyelination, 129
Lipids asymmetric distribution in membranes, 239
Lipids
   Derived from ceramide, 129
   Types and significance, 230
Liposome, 2
   Use for drug delivery, 124
Liver diseases
   Grading and staging, 325
   Utility of biochemical tests, 316
Liver glycogenoses, 85
LPC and atherosclerosis, 122
Lyases, 46
Lysolecithin, 121
   Role in atherosclerosis, 121

M

Malate aspartate shuttle, 74
Maple syrup urine disease, 149
   Clinical phenotypes, 152
MCAD deficiency
   Most likely diagnosis, 118
   Treatment, 118
Measurement of Vi, 52
Mechanism of action of inhibitors and uncouplers of ETC, 70
Mechanism of proofreading, 220
Mechanisms for hyperuricemia in glucose-6-phosphatase deficiency, 110

Mechanisms linking excessive fructose intake to the development of metabolic disorders in the long run, 109
Membrane bilayer, 2
Membrane proteins, 18
Membrane-bound proteoglycans, 300
Membrane lipid distribution, 231
Metabolic abnormalities in type 1 DM, 279
Metabolic abnormalities in type 2 DM, 277
Metabolic budgeting by pyruvate kinase, 102
Metabolic syndrome nutritional/dietary factors, 196
Metabolism and excretion of xenobiotics, 377
Metabolism in various organs in different phases of feed-starve cycle, 270
Metabolism of xenobiotics, 375
Micelle, 2
Michaelis–Menten equation, 52
Mitochondria oxidants and free radicals produced, 73
Mixed lymphocyte reaction, 362
Motifs, 41
   Examples, 42
Movements of lipid molecules in membrane, 240
MSH, 256
Muscle glycogenoses, 86
Muscular cramps and pain associated with vigorous exercise, 78
Mutations 209, 213
Mutation due to tautomerization, 209
Myocardial infarction (MI) protection by fish oil, 126
Myoglobin, 43
   Physiological function, 43
Myokinase, 60
   Deficiency, 60

N

NAFLD, 277
Neuroglobin, 43
NH_3 toxicity
   Mechanism, 161
Niacin
   Pharmacological application, 195
Nitric oxide, NO, 44
Nitrogen balance or protein balance measurement, 143
Nitrogen transport from tissues for disposal, 155
Non-functional enzymes in blood and their diagnostic uses, 50
Non-ketotic hyperglycinemia, 145
NPY, 256
Nuclear receptor superfamily, 286

Nuclear receptors, 284
   Classification, 287
Nuclear receptors with special ligands, 288
Nucleophile, 3
Nucleotide excision repair, 227
Nucleotides
   Biological functions, 171
   Fate of dietary, 170
Number of enzymes required for the synthesis of amino acids from amphibolic intermediates, 144
Nutrients
   Quantities to be consumed daily, 183
Nutritionally essential and non-essential amino acids, 143

O

Obesity, 260
   Harmful effects, 272
Obesity, insulin resistance and diabetes, 274
Oligosaccharides role in protein folding, 305
One-way MLR, 362
Ontogenesis of thyroid function, 202
Organ-specific autoimmune diseases, 355
Organophosphate poisoning, 54
Orientation of cholesterol in membrane, 235
Ornithine synthesis in intestines, 154
Orthologous proteins, 40
Oxidase, 68
β-Oxidation of unsaturated fatty acids, 115
Oxidation-reduction reactions
   Classification of enzymes involved, 68
Oxalate synthesis, endogenous pathway, 148
Oxidoreductases, 46, 68
Oxygen dissociation curve of myoglobin, 43
Oxygenases, 68

P

P/O ratio, 76
'Paneer', 79
Paralogous proteins, 40
Passive regulation of enzyme activity, 56
Pasteur effect, 100
   Mechanism, 100
Pathogenesis of ascites due to cirrhosis, 315
Pathophysiology of gout, 179
Patterns of graft rejection, 359, 360
PCOS, 276

PDCAAS of some common food proteins, 195
Pentobarbitone
   Side chain oxidation, 378
Peptides and proteins
   Differences, 33
Peptides and their functions, 34
Peptides
   Important biological functions, 33
Peroxisomal biogenesis disorders (PBD)
   Common lab findings, 120
pH, 4
   Significance, 7
pH in living systems, 6
pH scale, 5
Phases of glucose homeostasis, 266
Phosphofructokinase positive co-operativity with fructose-6-phosphate as substrate, 56
Photoreactivation, 217
Physiological uncouplers, 70
pKa, 4
   Significance, 7
pKa values and the isoelectronic point, pI, for the 20 α-amino acids, 15
Plasma lactate levels in emergency patients
   Significance, 95
Polymorphisms in non-MHC genes associated with autoimmune diseases, 349
POMC, 256
Pore-forming toxins, 249
Prenyl, geranyl and farnesyl groups, 121
Primary hyperoxaluria
   Type I, 147
   Type II, 148
Prolonged fasting state, 265-267
Proofreading by DNA polymerase, 219
Prostaglandins
Phospholipase involved in production, 128
Prosthetic group or co-factors
   Role of metal ions, 47
Prosthetic groups, 47
Protein antigens
   Factors that determine the immunogenicity and tolerogenicity, 343
Protein catabolism
   Disposal of amino group, 156
Protein quality, 192
Protein quality assessment, 192
Proteins binding to sulfated glycosaminoglycans, 303
Proteins
   Biological functions, 16
   Domains, 38
   Folding, 4,306
   Membrane, 236
   Modular structure, 38
Proteoglycans, 293
Proteoglycans and diseases, 304
PTH activity, 282
PTH release via CaSR inhibition by calcium, 280
Purine and pyrimidine bases
   Maximum light absorption, 168
Purine synthesis
   Regulation and clinical implications, 174
Pyrimidine 52-nucleotidase (P5N) deficiency, 93
Pyrrolysine, 12
Pyruvate kinase, 102
   Feed forward activation, 102

R

Rate limiting enzyme of a pathway, 57
Rate of cellular respiration during exercise
   Conditions which limit the rate, 72
Rate of enzyme catalysed reaction
   Effect of changes in temperature, 51
   Effect of change in pH, 51
Reaction catalysed by myokinase, 60
Reaction of acyl CoA synthetase, 66
Reaction rate factors, 50
Reaction rate of a multi-substrate reaction effect, 52
Reactions used for measurement of glucose, 49
Recombinant DNA technology
   Production of eukaryotic proteins in bacteria, 33
Recombinant glucoceribrosidase, 128
Recommended Dietary allowance, 183
Recycling of vitamin E with the help of vitamin C, 389
Regulation of purine synthesis, 175
Relation between calcium and PTH release, 280
Relative changes in ATP, ADP and AMP concentration, 61
Release of energy from 'high energy phosphate bond', 64
Renal handling of uric acid, 178
Reversible reactions, 50
Rheumatic heart disease due to molecular mimicry, 353
Ribozymes, 49
RNA editing for production of apo B100 and B48, 128
Rossman fold, 37
Rotenone, 70
Rothera's test
   Ketone bodies detected, 117

S

SAAG and ascetic fluid protein levels, 314
Salting in and out, 23-26
Salvage pathway, 171
SCOP classification of protein domains, 39
Secondary hyperoxaluria, 149
Secretion and action of 3-aminoisobutyric acid, 181
Selenium, 11
    Deficiency, 12
    Toxicity, 12
Selenocysteine, 9
    Insertion in translation, 11
Selenosis, 12
Serum–ascites albumin gradient, 313
Shapes of different lipids in membrane, 232
Significance of isoenzymes in our body, 59
Simple proteoglycans
    General structure, 295
Single gene mutations leading to autoimmune diseases, 350
Skin ageing, 304
SNAP-25 bound to BoNT/A, 22
Specific acid base catalysis, 47
Specific dynamic action, 183
Spherical β particle of glycogen, 112
Spontaneous deamination, 211
Starve–feed cycle, 260
    Substrate and hormone levels in different phases, 267
States of respiratory control, 72
Steady-state amounts of DNA damages, 215
Streptococcus thermophilus, 78
Structural classification of proteins (SCOP), 36
Structure of glycogen, 111
Structure of telomeres, 222
Sugar code of life, 290
Suicide enzyme, 125
Suicide enzyme and suicide inhibition
    Differences, 125
Suicide inhibition, 126
Sulfation of paracetamol, 381
Superantigens, 365
Superantigens in human disease, 367
Superfamily, 39
Supersecondary structures, 41
Supersecondary structures or motifs, 42
Sweetened beverages, harmful effects of excess consumption, 106
Sympathetic ophthalmia, 354
Synthesis of glycine from choline, 146
Synthesis of unsaturated fatty acids, 125
Synucleinopathies, 23
Systemic autoimmune diseases, 353, 355

T

T cell anergy, 346
T loop at the end of a chromosome, 222
Tautomerization
    Effect on base pairing, 208
Tautomers of thymine and guanine, 207
Telomere shortening, 221
Teriparatide use for the treatment of osteoporosis, 282
Tetrahydrobiopterin deficiency, 163
TG synthesis
    How adipose tissue obtains glycerol-3-phosphate, 128
Thermic effect of food, 182
Thiamine deficiency and TPP stimulation, 88
Thioredoxin, 28
Titration curve for alanine, 13
Titration curve of aspartic acid, 14
Titration curve of histidine, 15
Tolerable upper intake level for iodine, 204
Tolerance biochemical basis, 342
Tolerance therapeutic applications, 342
Toll-like receptors, 339
    Structure and function, 340
Toxicity of galactose
    Signs, 80
    Symptoms, 80
Transcription
    Regulation and control, 284
Transferases, 46
Transketolase
    Clinical significance, 87, 88
Transplant graft rejection, 354
    Immune mechanisms, 354
    Methods to prevent graft rejection, 354
Transport of cholesterol and LDL metabolism, 133
Transport proteins
    Classification, 248
Transporters in inner mitochondrial membrane, 74
Transudate and exudate
    Differentiation by biochemical tests, 316
Treatment of chronic angina
    Use of drugs which inhibit fatty acid oxidation, 117
TT dimer generated due to UV light, 213
TTAGGG repeats in telomeres and the T loop, 222
Tumor cell migration, 304
Tumor lysis syndrome, 173

Type 1 interferons
  Actions, 341
Types of transfer potential, 62

U

Ubiquinone, 121
Uncouplers, 70
Uncouples and inhibitors of electron transport chain
  Differences, 69
Universal solvent, 1
Unsaturated fatty acids
  Effect on membrane fluidity, 247
Unsaturated fatty acids synthesized in human body, 124
Unstructured proteins, 20
Urea bicycle, 157
Urea cycle defects
  Clinical features, 159
  Management, 161
Uric acid
  Renal handling, 177
Use of NH_3 generated from Gln to excrete H^+, 8

V

Vi vs [S] relation, 57
Viscosity, 9
Vitamin D
  Actions, 190

W

ω3 and ω6 fatty acids, 126
  Beneficial actions, 126
Warburg effect, 100
  Mechanism and advantages, 100
Water
  Properties, 1
Whelan's model of glycogen structure, 110

X

X-linked adrenoleukodystrophy, 120
Xanthine oxidase and xanthine dehydrogenase
  Difference, 181
Xanthomas of the eyelid, 130
Xenobiotic metabolism, 374
Xenobiotics, 373
  Harmful effects, 376
  Metabolization, 376
D-Xylose
  Clinical significance, 87, 88

Y

"Yoghurt", 78

Z

Zellweger syndrome, 120